MW01200763

1001 Magical Plants

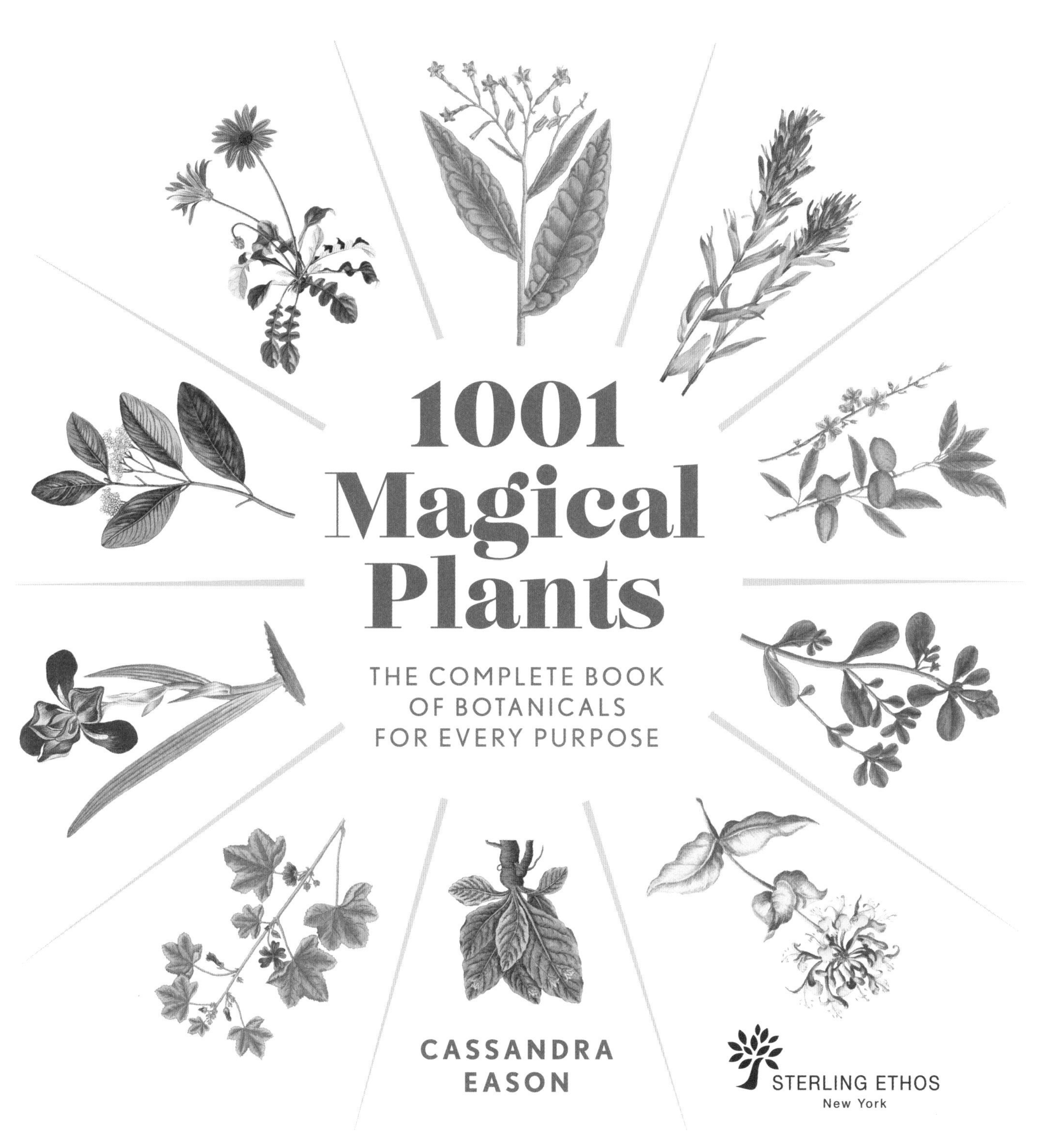

1001 Magical Plants

THE COMPLETE BOOK OF BOTANICALS FOR EVERY PURPOSE

CASSANDRA EASON

STERLING ETHOS
New York

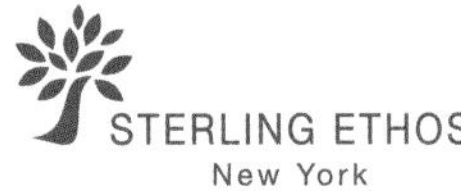

STERLING ETHOS and the distinctive Sterling Ethos logo
are registered trademarks of Sterling Publishing Co., Inc.

This publication is intended for informational purposes only. The publisher does not claim that this publication shall provide or guarantee any benefits, healing, cure, or any results in any respect. This publication is not intended to provide or replace medical advice, treatment, or diagnosis or be a substitute to consulting with a physician or other licensed medical or health-care providers. The publisher and author shall not be liable or responsible for any use or application of any content contained in this publication or any adverse effects, consequence, loss, or damage of any type resulting or arising from, directly or indirectly, the use or application of any content contained in this publication.

ISBN 978-1-4549-5209-1
ISBN 978-1-4549-5210-7 (e-book)

Library of Congress Control Number: 2025931433

For information about custom editions, special sales, and premium purchases, please contact specialsales@unionsquareandco.com.

Printed in China

2 4 6 8 10 9 7 5 3 1

unionsquareandco.com

Cover and interior design by Carlos Esparza
Picture credits appear on p. 541

Contents

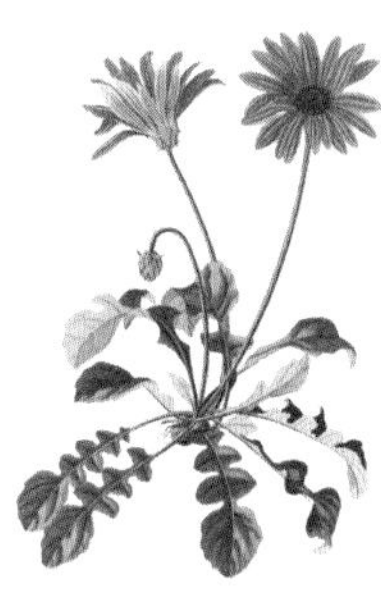

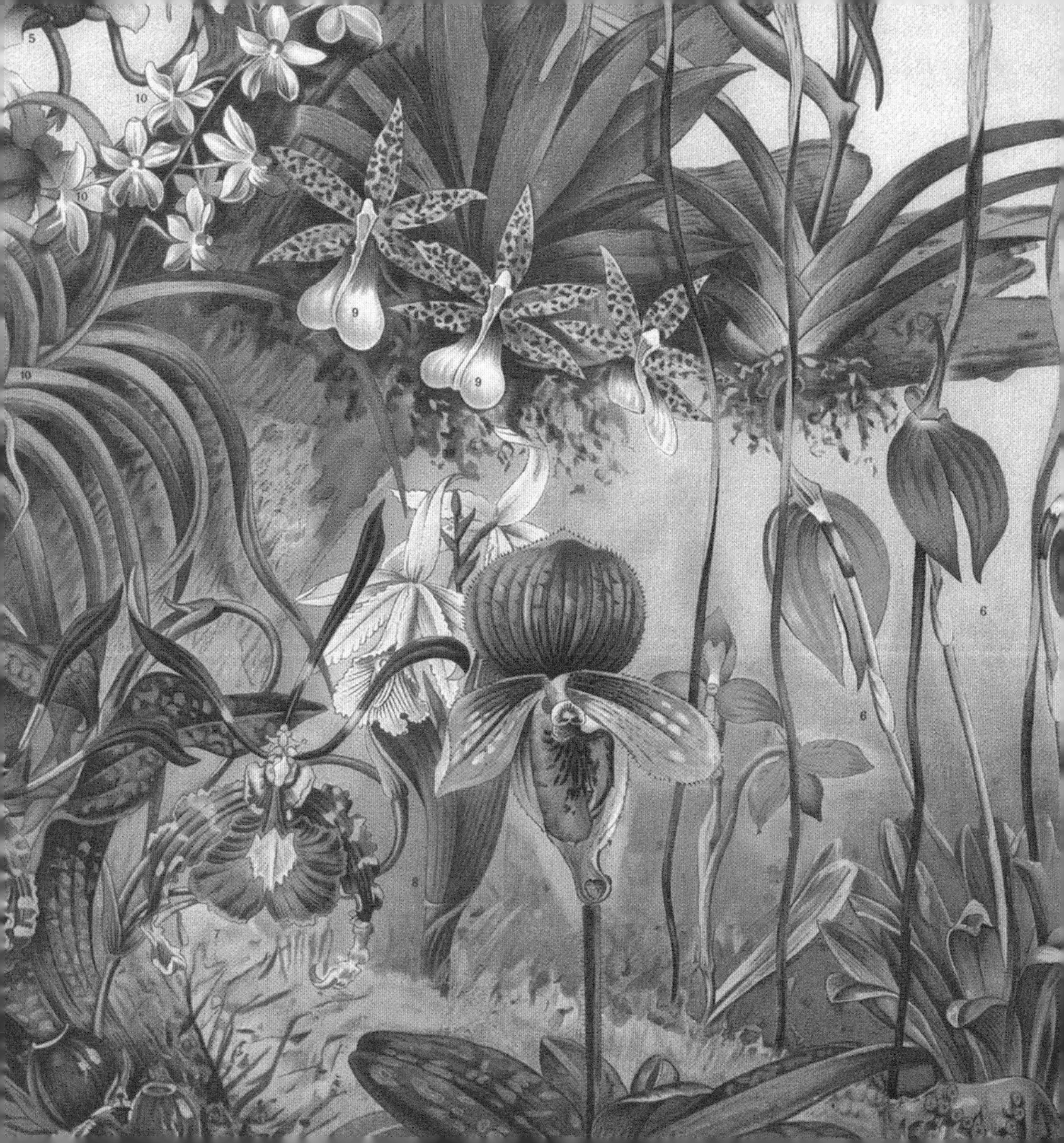
5
10
10
10
9
9
6
6
8
7

Introduction

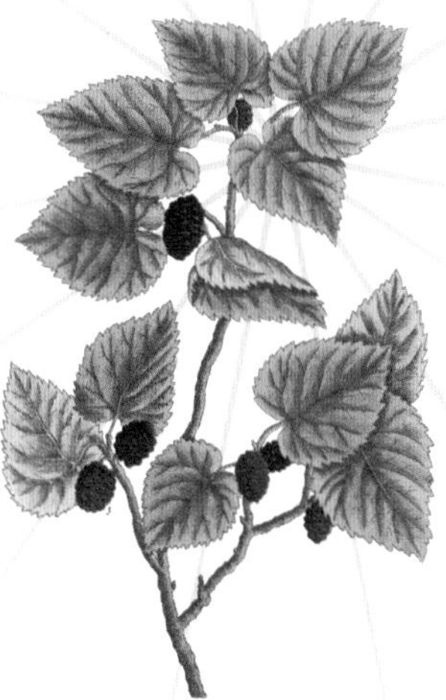

Every plant has its unique meaning: a story told, retold, and often reworked through the ages. Some plants, those found deep in the forests, may have encountered few humans through the millennia, while others have been cultivated for food, medicine, or ornament. Many offer healing, while others are beautiful but lethal to humans and animals. *1001 Magical Plants* describes how plants and the products derived from them have become a valuable part of our daily world, enriching our lives with their powerful spiritual gifts, which are often linked to their physical properties. Plants contain energies to transmit good fortune, love, happiness, and health. They can also help us protect ourselves and our friends and families (including pets!), as well as our homes and workplaces. There are myriad ways to add the powers of plants to our lives, whether we channel these properties through living, growing organisms or in any other form. This book teaches us how to observe the magical and energetic correspondences of botanicals, whether fresh or preserved, powdered, as resin, or made into herbal teas, oils, fragrance, or even as edible products like bread or syrup.

The information in this book comes from decades of research. Many healing remedies date from ancient Egyptian or Greek books of wisdom. Others have been passed down through families for many generations, with materials sometimes transported to other lands and across oceans as seeds or cuttings by explorers and settlers. Often, I have discovered the most fascinating magical strengths in plants as I have researched during my travels around the world. For more than forty years, I have talked with the Australian Aboriginal grandmothers and the Scandinavian wise men who keep the old traditions alive. I have also tried to respectfully acquire knowledge from living Native North American traditions and ancient lost peoples, such as the Mayans and the Aztecs, without claiming anything more than what is willingly offered. I hope that the information in these pages will prove useful to you.

Discovering the Plants

Even if you live in a cold climate, many of the exotic flowers and trees listed in this book can be found in botanical gardens, which often have greenhouses or dedicated specialty sections in which plants from different climates are grouped together. Arboretums, too, offer a wide range of trees you might not otherwise see around your home, grown and showcased far away from their native habitats. Cacti gardens are also a wonderful way to view succulents in temperate zones where they wouldn't normally be found. Vacations are ideal for discovering plants that do not grow in your region.

While it can be very therapeutic to plant, tend, harvest, and dry your own herbs, online sources are even easier ways to access them. You need not leave your home or even your room to find an array of herbs, dried flowers, and leaves, sometimes as powders, that may be used in spellwork or healing bags. Check your kitchen spice rack, the herbal teas in the local supermarket, and the ingredients in organic incenses and resins you burn or oils you diffuse or add to your bath after a quarrel or illness. Hold plants and listen to their wisdom. Just be sure to research the sourcing of these materials whenever possible to make sure they are derived from pure plants and are not synthetics. Local grocery stores, farmers' markets, and ethnic stores are a treasure house of magical ingredients all year round.

However, using locally sourced magical ingredients in season can make a strong connection with the location where you are magically connecting with the plants. Meditating close to a growing plant, sipping a pure herbal tea if work is stressful, scattering the blossoms of a flower in a bath to attract love, or sitting against a tree for strength all bring a powerful transference of healing and magical energies. If you do pick a flower for use in spellwork or healing, be sure to do so gently without harming the well-being of the plant from which it came. If picking endangered or rare flowers in the wild, check with the local conservation society or local regulations, and take only one or two flowers from each plant.

How to Use This Book

The A-to-Z Treasury of Magical Plants in this book offers detailed information and suggestions for using individual plants, both magically and physically, for healing and in everyday ways to attract what you most need in your life, whether it's personal harmony and quiet sleep, confidence, or to act as protection in the home or workplace. You'll gain an in-depth look into each and every herb, plant, flower, and other element named throughout the book, with a detailed history of the plants, where they grow, planets and elements for each plant, and how to magically use the plant, along with necessary cautions associated with each plant's use, for example, to not use certain plants internally with pregnancy or if suffering from certain chronic conditions.

This book describes the resources of 1001 plants as they can be used magically, energetically, and practically in the everyday world, rather than offering a scientific or biological list. Some of the plants in this book are grouped under a common name that may correspond to a number of species, or broken out into particular varieties or cultivars within an umbrella species because of their specific magical qualities. It is also, in spite of its breadth, hardly a guide to every plant in the world: some scientists believe that there are over 380,000 independent species of plants living on this planet. This is merely one resource to offer possibilities for making plants part of your life.

Are Plant Remedies Safe?

Beware of raw plants; however, cooking may destroy some toxicity. Plants growing wild may be polluted by chemicals or traffic fumes, so wash them thoroughly. Please consult a qualified herbalist or physician before taking remedies. Also consider using herbs as supplements rather than substitutes for conventional medicine if that is working for you. Many herbs have been central to folk medicine for hundreds of years but have not been tested as safe by modern research. That said, this book focuses mainly on safe ways that plants and their derivatives can enrich your home, working life, and personal equilibrium, making you more confident, tuned in, and resistant to spite and malice, and creating a calmer home and productive but harmonious workplace. Indeed, some plants do physically absorb pollutants from the atmosphere, and while some take nourishment from the soil, many more enrich it.

Each plant has meaning, and each adds to our lives, offering gifts revered by our ancestors. These plants can be treasured as a potted plant on a kitchen counter, in magical cooking, or simply as a beautiful feature of the natural landscape as we enjoy a day in the wilderness, taking in the healing and restorative powers of Mother Nature, which are free for us all.

Plant Energy

Each day plants that have flourished for centuries are found to aid modern ills, and despite deforestation and climate disasters, we still can access the riches of the natural world and gain strength and connection with our own roots. Plants may ultimately be the answer to many of the chronic and currently untreatable conditions created by modern life, but until then, their beauty and fragrance bring daily joy. May this book help you find ways to empower yourself with plants—from a sachet of luck-bringing herbs to a meditation in a grove of pines—by focusing on their living, growing energies and channeling them successfully to improve your life.

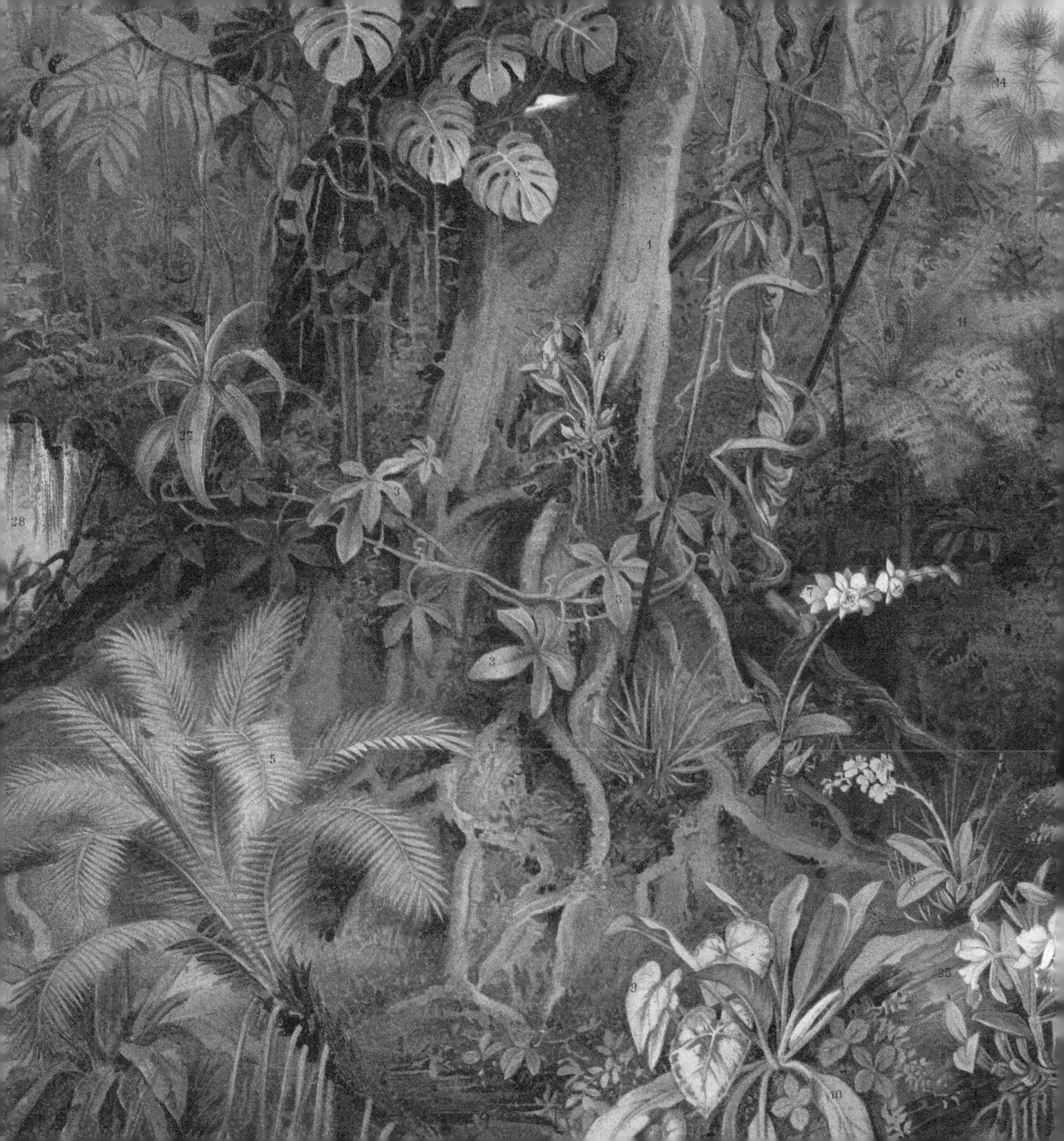
14
4
1
11
6
27
3
28
7
5
8
25
9
10

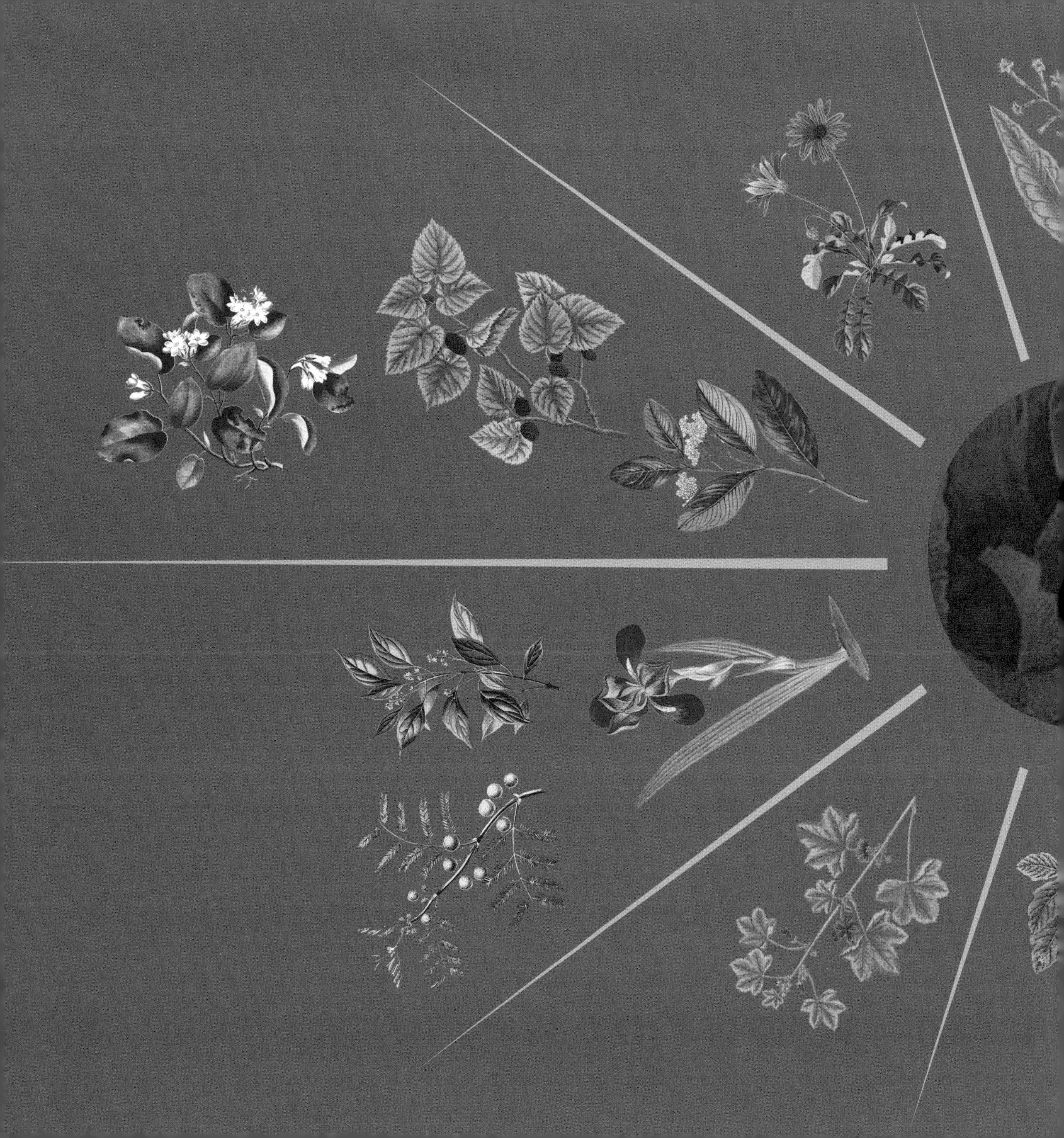

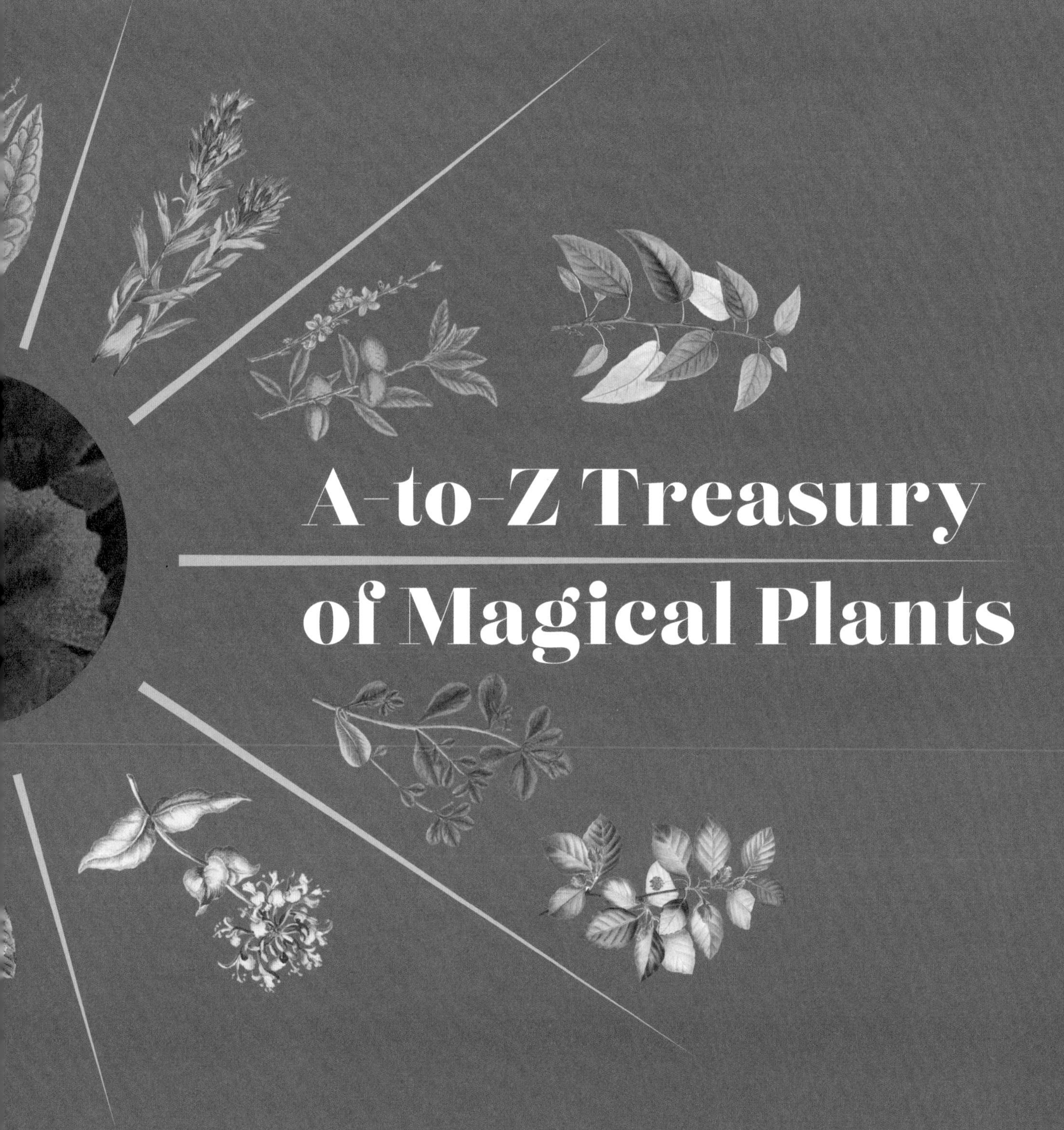
A-to-Z Treasury
of Magical Plants

Acacia

(*Acacia senegal*)

MAGICAL FORMS

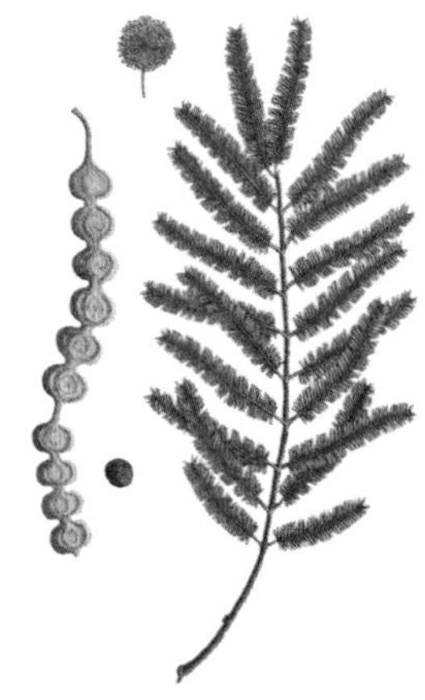

though it can grow as a tall tree, can be found in dwarf varieties or indoor plants (see "Gum Arabic Resin," p. 209, which is used in making incense and is from the *Acacia senegal* and *Acacia vera* trees) • magically use the growing plant, oil (made from the flowers), bark, flowers, and leaves

PLANET AND ELEMENTS

Sun • Fire/Air

MAGICAL USES

personal power • protection against paranormal evil • increasing psychic powers and mediumship • money • platonic love • secret love • friendship • if you have a big enough tree, the wood makes a protective wand to connect with the spirit world

HOW TO USE

Burn the leaves, bark, or the resin. • Acacia resin and sandalwood or frankincense together increase psychic powers. • When acacia oil is burned or diffused or the leaves are burned on charcoal, it aids meditation and brings visions of other worlds. • Mix with camellia oil and dilute well for personal anointing to connect with angels and guides. • Place a sprig of the blossom and leaves, a twig, or a sachet over the bed to drive away evil spirits, such as poltergeists, an incubus or a succubus, or sexual demons, and to prevent psychic attacks by night. • Contact spirits, especially deceased relatives, by anointing white candles with the oil. • Infuse the leaves to make sacred water to purify and bless an altar or tool.

CAUTION

Though regarded as nontoxic, it may react badly with some medications that are regularly taken for chronic conditions, so check with a pharmacist or herbalist. • A bad reaction may result if the fiber is directly inhaled or ingested.

Acacia, Sweet

(*Acacia farnesiana*)

MAGICAL FORMS

multi-trunked shrub or small tree • vaselike shape, ferny foliage with sharp thorns and highly fragrant, gold, puff-like flowers that bloom all year round with a peak in winter • grows naturally in central and southern Florida, Texas, and California and is cultivated in Europe for perfume • can be grown indoors in a pot in cooler climes • magically use the whole, growing tree; dried flowers; thorns; and perfume

PLANET AND ELEMENT

Sun • Fire

MAGICAL USES

combines both beauty and warning with its flowers and thorns, for protecting what is precious • in perfume, for setting boundaries where users are judged on superficial characteristics and not ability • protects the home if grown outdoors or in a container against those who appear welcoming but have hidden spite

HOW TO USE

Anoint your solar plexus in the center of and base of your ribcage and the middle of your hairline for your crown energy center in anticipation of situations during which you want and need to be valued on your merits if youth and beauty are taken as the criteria for success. • Use the dried flowers, dried leaves, and thorns in an amulet bag hidden in rooms where you keep precious items, or place a small bag with your computer, smartphone, or tablet when traveling in crowded places or if there have been a lot of thefts and muggings.

CAUTION

The seeds of sweet acacia are nontoxic for humans but toxic for dogs.

Acai Palm

(*Euterpe oleracea*)

MAGICAL FORMS

also known as the Assai palm • a tall, slender, tropical palm mainly found in the Brazilian rainforest and along the Amazon River estuary • grown for its fruit, which because of its perishable nature is exported to the USA, and increasingly worldwide, mainly as juice or frozen fruit pulp, and for the edible heart of the palm • the berries/drupes, with a single large seed, ripen as green bunches to deep purple from small brown-purple flowers • popularly considered a superfruit, tasting like a cross between an ordinary berry and chocolate • magically use the juice, acai products, and palm hearts (see "Hearts of Palm," p. 212)

PLANETS AND ELEMENTS

Jupiter/Sun • Air/Fire

MAGICAL USES

magical cookery, berries popularly used as puree in drinks, dried and powdered as a health supplement, smoothies, and health snack bars • products containing the acai berries can be empowered before ingesting or as part of your own, a teen's, or a partner's school or workplace lunch to give emotional strength, perseverance, vitality, and protection if there is a difficult day ahead • palm hearts are an aphrodisiac and attract love matches even with those who seem unattainable

HOW TO USE

Linked with the protection of Archangel Michael, ingesting acai in its many forms opens possibilities thought out of reach. • The berry juice can be used instead of wine as the Water element in archangel rituals, especially when offered to Michael with a spoken request or petition for an urgent or complex matter. • Drink the juice before divination to open your clairvoyant vision. • Share acai juice or a product made with the puree for the mutual growth and expression of love.

CAUTION

Acai is considered safe with pregnancy in moderate amounts. • Carefully source your acai products where possible as child labor is still sometimes used. • Buy it without impurities from a reputable source.

Acanthus

(*Acanthus mollis*)

MAGICAL FORMS

also known as Bear's Breeches • glossy leaves • black branched taproot • dusky-purple bracts/hoodlike modified leaves top the tall, spiky, white blossoms, which are tinged with pink • found mainly in gardens • other species of acanthus can grow up to five feet high and three feet wide • magically use the fresh and dried stems, flowers, leaves, and bracts

PLANET AND ELEMENT

Moon • Water

MAGICAL USES

from Greco-Roman times, the acanthus motif adorned classical and later neoclassical columns, friezes, official buildings, and fountains because of the perfect symmetry of its leaves • called the architect's flower, acanthus may be used as a gift for those graduating in the classics or design and for graphic designers • also a symbol for art or artistic endeavors • acanthus is used as an altar flower for ritual magick, where there are distinct steps to follow and accuracy is important • for finding your soulmate intellectually as well as romantically

HOW TO USE

Place the dried, spiky-edged bracts, the thorniest part of the plant found just under the flower, in an amulet bag if you suspect a visitor has ulterior motives. • Hide it in your workspace or near a home computer to avoid deceivers, scams, and those who shake your equilibrium. • The flower is linked with long life, immortality, and rebirth and so is often part of funeral wreaths or left on tombstones on anniversaries of a death. • Cast the leaves and flowers off a bridge in memory of a loved one you cannot openly mourn. • The leaves, stems, and bracts can be cut and dried for several months. Because of their symmetry, harvest them just before the flowers appear and use as Thanksgiving or Christmas decorations for a harmonious gathering.

CAUTION

Considered nontoxic, it has been used medicinally since ancient Greek times but should only be ingested in an accredited remedy.

Adam and Eve Root

(*Aplectrum hyemale*)

MAGICAL FORMS

small roots from the rare curtain orchid • native to North America, but obtainable from magick stores worldwide and online • usually sold in pairs • the long, pointed one is called the Adam root and the round one the Eve root • in nature, the Adam root grows around the Eve root • magically use the whole, growing plant; flowers, fresh and dried; and roots, fresh and dried

PLANETS AND ELEMENTS

Venus • Water (Eve), Mars • Fire (Adam)

MAGICAL USES

to mend broken relationships • for love and fidelity • to bring a hesitant lover closer • Adam and Eve roots work equally well for heterosexual and LGBTQ couples

HOW TO USE

Keep them in a charm bag, either red flannel or green, to attract love or a marriage proposal. • If the roots are for attracting love, they can be anointed with a drop or two of rose essential oil before being put in the bag, saying, if you know the lover you wish to attract, *Be for me (name), think of me, be with me, constantly and willingly.* • If the lover is unknown, substitute for the name *Wherever you may be.* • The roots can be kept in twin love bags, and after commitment, one partner carries the Eve root and the other partner the Adam root.

CAUTION

Handle with care as these roots are poisonous, particularly for cats, dogs, and horses. • Keep away from children and pets, and never ingest.

Adder's Tongue

(*Ophioglossum vulgatum*)

MAGICAL FORMS

found in the northeastern USA and, relatively rarely, in Europe • also called Christ's spear because it is linked with the spear that pierced Jesus's side at the crucifixion • small, single leaf, and stemlike stalk resembling a snake's tongue • can be grown in gardens but often found in the wild • magically use the whole plant, fresh or dried

PLANET AND ELEMENT

Moon • Water

MAGICAL USES

all forms of healing, dream, and Moon magic • protection from spite and gossip and human snakes • rituals for transformation similar to the snake shedding its skin • sacred to serpent goddesses and women's mysteries • only appears above the ground June through August, the rest of the time hidden in the earth, so used for uncovering fears • overcomes fears of reptiles

HOW TO USE

The dried plant is beloved by writers, placed in a vase near where they create to reveal hidden talents and original ideas. • Carry the dried, crumbled plant in an amulet bag or hide the bag in your home or workspace if you are subject to gossip or spite. • Hang it on your side of a jealous or overly curious neighbor's fence to create a protective boundary. • Meditate on the plant before bed to discover answers in your dreams to a question written and placed under your pillow, to overcome traumas in sleep, or to incubate creative ideas. You may see the plant or a wise serpent goddess in your dream.

CAUTION

Adder's tongue is used extensively in folk and magickal healing. • It is not known for toxicity, but care should be taken around children and with pregnancy as it is a fern, which can have toxic properties.

Agapanthus

(*Agapanthus africanus*)

MAGICAL FORMS

also called the African lily or Our Lady of the Nile • huge, bell-like exotic flowers • magically use the whole, growing plant; cut flowers; fresh and dried petals; and flower essence

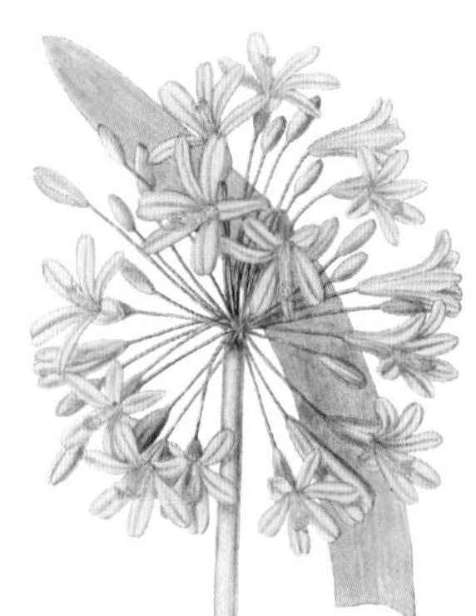

PLANET AND ELEMENT

Jupiter • Air

MAGICAL USES

hidden love • beauty in the later years • name means flower of love and the dried purple flowers especially are carried as a fertility charm and for healthy babies • as an aphrodisiac • by men to overcome impotence • brings authority and confidence, especially if self-esteem was diminished in childhood • gives a sense of the certainty of your own worth • its white Arctic Star form gives a tropical touch to a wedding • agapanthus protects against storms and fear of storms

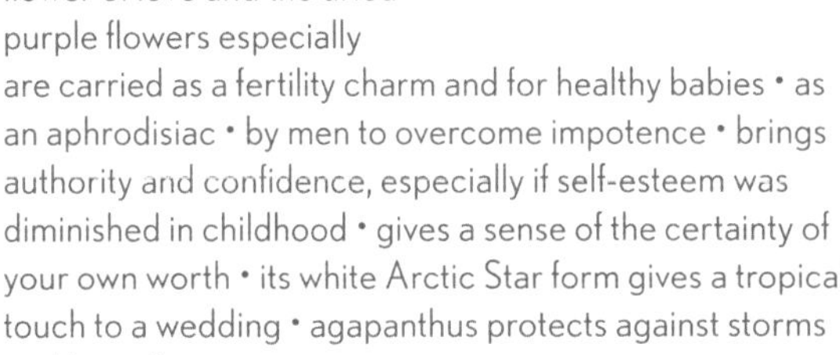

HOW TO USE

Sit close to the flower and pass your hands around it, palms flat, fingers together, tracing the shape of the flower a small distance away from it (not touching), to draw its psychological and psychic strength into your aura. • Keep it in your business or workspace as either cut flowers or a potted plant to impress others with your leadership qualities and to ignore detractors. • If you know others will try to override your wishes or take over your plans, spray the room or meeting place before anyone arrives or before taking a Zoom call with the flower essence diluted in water.

CAUTION

Agapanthus is toxic to pets, especially cats, and humans if the rhizome is ingested. • Beware also of the toxic sticky sap if the rhizome splits. • Be careful also of the leaves.

Agarwood

(*Aquilaria malaccensis* Lamk.)

MAGICAL FORMS

a resinous tree affected by overforesting that is now classified as critically endangered • wood chippings, called oudh, are burned as incense, releasing a heady musk fragrance • dark, fragrant resin appears when the tree is affected by mold • resin is made into a very expensive oil (said to be the costliest in the world) and known as "black gold" or "the fragrance of the deities" • the oil is distilled from the wood or by melting the resin • prized for centuries in India, Southeast Asia, the Middle East, China, ancient Egypt, and Assyria • first recorded in 1400 BCE, traveling down the Silk Road • used also in perfumes • magically use as wood chips, incense, resin, oil, and in fragrance

PLANET AND ELEMENT

Venus • Water

MAGICAL USES

oudh is used for sacred ceremonies and for inducing a deep sense of calm • for opulence and sensual experiences

HOW TO USE

Anoint the center of the brow or Third Eye energy chakra before meditation to experience powerful visions of spiritual realms and beings. • Gucci Intense Oud Cologne or Versace Pour Femme Oud Oriental perfume both contain genuine oudh oil that can be substituted for anointing as a less costly version. • Burn the chips, sticks, cones, or resin in incense in the bedroom before lovemaking or if you are going through a hard economic time to restore or bring luxury into your life.

CAUTION

Do not ingest. • Keep the room well-ventilated if burning incense; some people may suffer mild allergies.

Agave

(*Agave* spp.)

MAGICAL FORMS

more than a hundred species • large multispiked plant • *Agave americana* is an Arizona desert flower releasing great strength and survival instincts in harsh conditions • agave nectar/syrup from blue agave (*Agave azul*) contained in tequila • nectar often used instead of maple syrup • vegan, purely plant-based, and twice as sweet as sugar • native to Mexico and the Americas • also grows in the Caribbean and tropical areas of North America • *Agave salmiana* (also known as maguey pulquero) produces syrup and grows in gardens with a Mediterranean-type climate • magically use the flowers as an essence

PLANET AND ELEMENT

Sun • Fire

MAGICAL USES

to overcome fears of all kinds • known as the *late bloomer*, the essence is made from the pink, green, and yellow flowers for manifesting talents, especially later in life • for nervous pets who hide from strangers and are scared of loud noises and other animals

HOW TO USE

Since many agaves flower only once and then die, carry the dried fallen flowers as a reminder to enjoy every moment of a relationship or situation and not demand permanence. • Sip the essence in water or put it under your tongue before selling your artistic talents in the wider marketplace. • Spray your studio or creative workspace with agave added to water (ten-plus drops) to overcome inspirational blocks. • Add a little agave to desserts or serve instead of maple syrup with waffles and pancakes to put everyone in a good mood.

CAUTION

Agave can overstimulate the appetite. • It contains a much larger proportion of fructose (natural fruit sugar) than maple syrup. • Eat in moderation, especially during pregnancy. • These warnings do not apply to the flower essence, where you are absorbing the spirit of agave and not the chemical makeup. • Touching the plant can cause allergies.

Air Plant

(*Bryophyllum pinnatum*)

MAGICAL FORMS

also called life plant or miracle leaf • member of the bromeliad family and relative of the pineapple • more than six hundred varieties of air plants • though native to the West Indies, Mexico, Central and South America, they also flourish in California, Florida, Georgia, Louisiana, Texas, other southern states, and warm climates around the world • can grow indoors or outdoors • each variety differs in flowers, leaves, beauty, and structure, but all grow without soil and with visible roots, and are totally versatile whether at home or in the workplace • magically use the whole plant

PLANET AND ELEMENT

Mercury • Air

MAGICAL USES

though air plants attach themselves to different surfaces, they do not take nourishment from them and so are ideal for rituals of self-sufficiency whether setting up a business, growing and selling produce, or living and working cooperatively but not codependently • leaving home or encouraging a partner or adult child to move on peacefully if a situation is not working

HOW TO USE

After flowering, air plants produce offsets called pups that either become new air plants if removed from the mother plant or remain as clusters. • Use a cluster of new air plants next to the original air plant in fertility rituals where there is a need for medical or surgical intervention to conceive or if you hope for or expect a twin birth. • Surround the growing air plant with alternating gold and silver coins and, behind the coins, a circle of lighted yellow candles for swift growing or urgent money. • Surround the plant with light blue candles for slower but longer-lasting acquisitions. • Set your air plant in the Air/East segment of a magick circle along with a citrine or amethyst if you are using plants and crystals rather than ritual tools.

Ajwain

(*Trachyspermum ammi*)

MAGICAL FORMS

also known as carom • a fragrant herb, popular in Indian cookery • can be grown in the garden or in a pot in the kitchen • leaves taste like thyme when eaten raw in yogurts or salad • the bitter pungent seeds, actually small green to brown fruits, can be eaten raw but mainly are purchased roasted before adding to a recipe • the seeds resemble cumin seeds and may be ground as a spice or whole in a variety of dishes, tasting like a mixture of thyme, oregano, cumin, and anise • obtain the seeds online, in Asian grocery stores, or grow your own in temperate zones • magically use the seeds whole, ground, or powdered

PLANET AND ELEMENT

Sun • Fire

MAGICAL USES

reduces desire for excess alcohol • for overcoming image problems, especially connected with weight • promotes youthfulness

HOW TO USE

Decorate the top of bread with seed outlines of what you most desire and need. • Use the flower for love, a baby, or fertility. • Use the seed or fruit for money, a plane or boat for travel, scales for justice, a key for a new home, a book for learning, or a path up a mountain for career advancement. • You can create symbols for joint family or business aims and share the bread. • If you crave excess food, cigarettes, or alcohol or if you are addicted to online gambling, take a jar of the seeds outdoors. Bury a few where nothing grows with a symbol of what you want to give up, whether candies, a crumbled cigarette, or pouring out alcohol that you had been hiding. Repeat this, dispensing a few seeds each time, and by the time your jar is empty, you will be reminded of your new resolve.

CAUTION

Though used traditionally in Ayurveda and generally medicinally, not enough is known about the effects of carom during pregnancy and breastfeeding, so avoid. • Only a little is needed in cooking; excess can cause health problems.

Alder Tree

(*Alnus* spp.)

MAGICAL FORMS

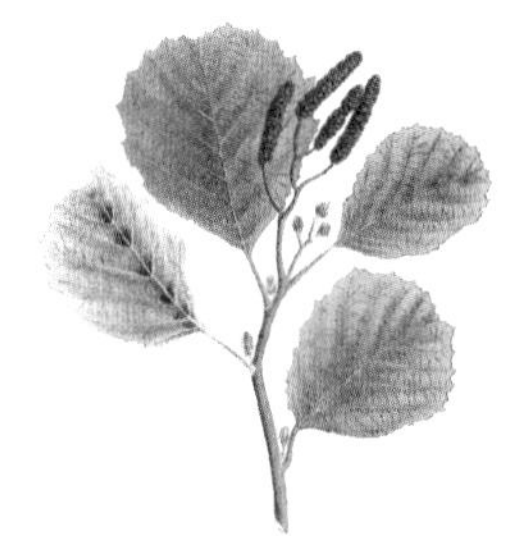

includes red/Oregon alder (*Alnus rubra*): native to western North America • common/black alder (*Alnus glutinosa*): native to most of continental Europe, the United Kingdom, Ireland, and introduced into the USA • white alder (*Alnus rhombifolia*): found in the Rockies from Idaho and Montana south to southern California • magically use the growing tree in situ, wood, fresh and dried leaves, catkins, and cones

PLANETS AND ELEMENTS

Moon/Jupiter • Water/Fire

MAGICAL USES

known as the tree of Bran the Blessed, a mighty Celtic hero giant whose head (regarded as the seat of power and the soul in Celtic times) is said to be buried under the White Mount or Tower Hill in London, as security that his beloved land will never be invaded • a tree for protective rituals and amulets from attack and natural disasters • a fae tree, offering a gateway to visions of the world of the alder tree spirits by sitting against the tree at twilight

HOW TO USE

One of the Celtic sacred trees, alder wands are used for empowerments and wishes for security, stability, and all property matters. • Dried leaves of alder and rowan trees are mixed in a cloth bag and buried beneath an alder tree on full-moon day for fertility or creativity. • Buy or make a whistle of alder wood, traditionally used to summon and control the four winds, for resistance to emotional blackmail and mind games. Attach it to a tree or bush in a high place. If you cannot obtain an alder whistle, tie an alder cone or catkins with red thread to any wooden whistle.

CAUTION

Alders generally are nontoxic, but beware of the buckthorn alder (*Frangula alnus*), which is not a true alder.

Alfalfa

(*Medicago sativa*)

MAGICAL FORMS

magically use the whole, growing plant; sprouting leaves, fresh and dried; dried flowers and seeds; and oil

PLANETS AND ELEMENT

Venus/Jupiter • Earth

MAGICAL USES

Roman author Pliny the Elder, 23–79 CE, records alfalfa was brought to ancient Greece by Darius, king of Persia, when he was trying to conquer Athens • one of the ultimate moneymaking and preserving-resources herbs, because alfalfa is a major food for cattle • cattle represented a major source of wealth in times past, and there is a Viking rune, *feoh*, that means both cattle and the portable wealth that was taken on the longships for colonization in the form of cattle • it is said a pinch of powdered alfalfa in your wallet, purse, or cash register will ensure you are never without money

HOW TO USE

Alfalfa is used magically either as the whole plant or dried, chopped, and ground into incense. • However, the dried plant is used more in ritual than the incense or oil. • A sealed jar packed tight with dried sprouting plants and kept in a kitchen cupboard is an amulet against there not being enough for the basic needs for the household. • Carry a charm bag containing chopped dried alfalfa, mint, and basil with you when applying for loans or grants, negotiating debt repayment, entering competitions, or expanding business. • When seeking money owed to you, sprinkle on an invoice printout and release the herb outdoors. • On Fridays, create a bundle of fresh alfalfa loosely tied with red thread to call an absent or unknown lover. Choose a windy day or a high open place, undo the thread, and let the alfalfa fly in all directions.

CAUTION

Do not take alfalfa alongside anticoagulant medications, such as warfarin. • Avoid the seeds. • Do not use large amounts with pregnancy or if suffering from autoimmune conditions.

Alkanet

(*Anchusa officinalis*)

MAGICAL FORMS

also called common bugloss • native to Europe and Asia, introduced to the New England states • purple-blue flowers and gray-green hairy leaves • magically use in root form, which contains a red dye that is an ingredient in the New Orleans Red Fast Luck Oil

PLANET AND ELEMENT

Venus • Water

MAGICAL USES

for money, business success, games of chance, and good fortune • deters unfair competition • the root keeps away hostile spirits in a red amulet bag

HOW TO USE

Use the chopped root in a money wish jar with shredded dollars, dried basil, and dried orange peel. • Bury the root at or near a crossroads if you believe you have been hexed, jinxed, or cursed. • The root is traditionally burned with patchouli as incense to attract wealth.

CAUTION

Alkanet can cause skin irritation and should not be used during pregnancy or while breastfeeding. • Though traditionally regarded as a medicinal plant, alkanet should only be used on medical advice and not in excess quantities.

Allium Ornamental Flower

(*Allium* spp.)

MAGICAL FORMS

called flowering onions; related to chives, onions, and garlic • shades of purple, blue, white, pink, and yellow flowers on tall stems, growing in late spring and early summer, some as late as the fall • *Allium aflatunense* 'Purple Sensation' have deep purple, rounded flowerheads • *Allium giganteum* can grow up to six feet tall with dense round purple flowerheads, made up of dozens of starlike flowers • the flowers do not smell of onions, only the foliage if crushed or bruised • leaves fade early • native to the Middle East, they grow worldwide except in the tropics and New Zealand • magically plant in the garden or use as cut or dried flowers in the home

PLANET AND ELEMENT

Mars • Fire

MAGICAL USES

traditionally flowers are regarded as protectors of those who grow them • considered sacred in ancient Greece as ritual offerings • banish curses and hexes • purple and pink alliums are an alternative seventy-fourth wedding anniversary flower, stripped of leaves • some are sweet smelling

HOW TO USE

Plant or have fresh or dried cut allium flowers in the home, especially hung over doors, or in a vase near the front door to act as protection against earthly and paranormal harm entering. • Provide shelter for the house guardians by removing the leaves and weaving the dried flowerheads on a circlet to display in the main room, bringing harmony, health, and good fortune.

CAUTION

The flower can cause an allergic reaction in those sensitive to onions. • Do not use if taking anticoagulants. • Though considered edible by many sources, the ornamental flowers are not generally eaten, as the flavor is too strong, and some consider them mildly toxic. • Avoid or seek advice before ingesting even medicinally any allium flowers if pregnant or breastfeeding.

Allspice

(*Pimenta dioica*) or (*Pimenta officinalis*)

MAGICAL FORMS

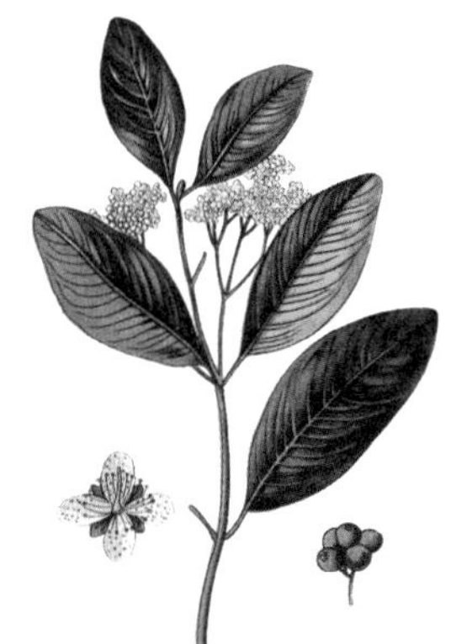

medium-sized evergreen tropical tree, a relative of cloves • tiny white flowers producing berries • indigenous to the West Indies, Central and South America, especially Mexico • available worldwide as incense, oil, and spice from leaves and berries • magically use the berries, dried and whole; as powdered spice; and as essential oil

PLANET AND ELEMENT

Mars • Fire

MAGICAL USES

in incense and magical cookery to attract money, good luck, and success • for past-life recall • as a charm to enhance love and passion if a guy has issues with virility • enhances the power of spells with the assurance that what is desired will be manifest and eradicate doubts

HOW TO USE

Burn or diffuse the oil to lift exhaustion and bring optimism, especially for empowering home businesses running out of impetus. • Add empowered spice to a meal, cakes, or cookies if those in a position to financially advance your career will eat them. • Add the powder to cornstarch, and sprinkle a little of the mix outside the workplace or hide in a plant pot for successful interviews. • Cleanse a room or yard with lemon, pine, and allspice oils in hot water to drive away malevolence and disperse lingering misfortune while attracting prosperity.

CAUTION

Allspice is only toxic if the spice is used in large quantities. • Dilute the oil well, and do not use the oil during pregnancy. • Take care around the eyes, mouth, and nose if using it as a massage oil.

Almond Nut and Paste

from (*Prunus dulcis*)

MAGICAL FORMS

grown primarily in lands with Mediterranean climates, with 80 percent of the world's almonds coming from California • the nuts are frequently used in baking and paste made as marzipan to cover cakes, in and as candies • the nuts are not true nuts but seeds enclosed in a hard covering • the nuts, both eaten and in paste, magically absorb the power of the almond tree in concentrated form

PLANET AND ELEMENT

Mercury • Air

MAGICAL USES

attracting and keeping prosperity through generating moneymaking endeavors • as a fertility charm, traditionally given or thrown at weddings • learning traditional wisdom

HOW TO USE

As you ice a cake with a layer of marzipan or add paste to the top of a cake or dessert, gently mark with a knife your magical intention and then smooth over it. • While outdoors, add to a bag an almond for each hundred or thousand dollars you urgently need. Shake the closed bag the same number of times as almonds in the bag, swirl your body around clockwise with the bag that number of times, and scatter the nuts in all directions. • Eat a sugared almond or almond candy before meeting a new partner's relatives if you suspect they may be hostile, and take a box of the candies along as a sweetener.

CAUTION

Avoid almonds totally if you or a recipient have any nut allergy. • Sweet almonds are safe to eat, but bitter almonds (*Prunus amygdalus* var. *amara*) are poisonous and banned in the US.

Almond Tree

(*Prunus dulcis*)

MAGICAL FORMS

nuts are mainly grown in California • magically use the growing tree; blossom, fresh and dried; as sweet almond nuts; and as sweet almond carrier oil

PLANET AND ELEMENT

Mercury • Air

MAGICAL USES

abundance, prosperity, fertility, and love without limits • the blossom in May Day celebrations • the wood as magical wand used in rituals for power and authority, a purpose dating back to the rod of Aaron in biblical times • also a wand shared by two magical practitioners who have a love connection for joint magical rites for passion and prosperity • to ease alcohol addiction

HOW TO USE

Anoint white candles with almond oil, filling the candle with your love intention as you burn it, if you want to propose marriage or seek a proposal or major commitment. • Add a drop of the oil to a prosperity bag with bay leaves, dried almond blossom or leaves, a gold-colored stone or piece of jewelry, saying nine times *May all I need come my way.* • Place five almonds in your pocket or purse when bargain hunting or visiting garage sales for unexpected treasure. • Like many nuts, almonds can be used as fertility charms, collecting one on a white cloth for each night from the crescent to full moon night (can vary by a day according to the lunar month), with the final being added on full moon night and shared by the couple before lovemaking.

CAUTION

Avoid all almonds totally if you have any nut allergy. • Sweet almonds are safe to eat, but avoid ingesting bitter almonds (*Prunus amygdalus* var. *amara*), which are poisonous and banned in the US, though the trees can be grown.

Aloe, Bitter

(*Aloe ferox*)

MAGICAL FORMS

also known as cape aloe • a relative of *Aloe vera* • woody flowering plant native to South Africa • can grow in tropical regions of the USA and in pots in other regions of the USA and the world • though the bitter medicine is found in the sap of this and some other aloes, magically use the small, dried, bright-orange or yellow flowers in liquid form or the dried powder, which can be bought from health or magick stores

PLANET AND ELEMENT

Mars • Fire

MAGICAL USES

deters gossip and false friends, hostile neighbors, and jealous colleagues • use only when in a calm mood and always with blessings for the purpose of defense and not attack, as it is magically very strong

HOW TO USE

Add a little of the liquid mixed with sour red wine to defensive bottles. • Alternatively to stop lies being told about you, add a few drops of liquid or powder to sour milk and vinegar and tip the contents of the bottle (having shaken the sealed bottle well) down a drain or under a running hot water tap. • Add the flowers/powder to an amulet bag and bury the bag against a boundary fence for defense from abusive neighbors. • Keep a defensive bag in your workspace if cliquey colleagues are causing trouble for you or you have a bullying boss.

CAUTION

Though traditionally used medicinally, ingest *Aloe ferox* medication only on expert advice and not with pregnancy, breastfeeding, or in excess. • While used in cosmetics, nevertheless, the plant/sap may cause skin irritation.

Aloe Vera

(*Aloe barbadensis miller*)

MAGICAL FORMS

can be grown outdoors in warm climates or in indoor prosperity gardens • magically use the whole, growing plant; firm, clear gel from leaves; flowers; juice; skin products and drinks; and as carrier oil

PLANET AND ELEMENT

Moon • Water

MAGICAL USES

draws luck and money into the home • health and healing • prevents accidents in kitchen and from fire • the flower in spells increases charisma and radiance • give extra care if aloe vera wilts as it has absorbed a lot of negativity from hostile visitors and neighbors • for fertility • female rites and mysteries

HOW TO USE

Use the dried leaves in incense blends, empowered on the full moon as part of Moon Goddess rites. • The juice is used in anointing rituals at full moon. • Aloe vera juice on the Third Eye opens clairvoyant powers. • Leave aloe vera hung over doorways or as part of wreaths with garlic and lucky charms to attract moneymaking opportunities to the home. Replace the fresh aloe on the wreath when it withers, and bury the old garlic to keep luck and money sources continually inflowing.

CAUTION

Do not ingest the yellow latex layer surrounding the gel under the tough green leaves of the plant as it can cause stomach cramps and diarrhea. Though it has low toxicity for humans, aloe vera can cause skin rashes on sensitive skin. • Aloe vera is toxic to cats, dogs, and horses. • If in doubt as to quality, use commercial gels and juice from a reliable herbalist store.

Alyssum

(*Alyssum* spp.)

MAGICAL FORMS

some species called sweet alyssum • magically use the cut or whole, growing plant; flowers; and leaves

PLANET AND ELEMENTS

Venus • Water/Earth

MAGICAL USES

overcoming illusion and deception • defusing self-destructive anger and permanently angry people • increasing what is of worth whether love, money, or fulfillment • drawing to you empathetic caring people • sweetening the words and actions of abrasive people • flower psychometry

HOW TO USE

Traditionally it has been hung in the home to prevent others seducing away partners and lovers. • Also a pot of alyssum for his/her workplace can deter flirtations. • Grow it in an indoor or outdoor garden to keep away ill-wishing and those who would deceive, especially through flattery. • Carry a fresh sprig in a purse if there are a lot of dramatics and histrionics at work, and replace it as it fades or crumbles by burying the spent sprig where nothing grows. • Keep the fresh plant in a vase or pot next to a family photograph to bring peace and deter overreactions at family gatherings. • Flowers frozen in ice cubes in drinks will, as they melt, thaw difficult relationships and interactions.

Amaranth

(*Amaranthus* spp.)

MAGICAL FORMS

Amaranthus caudatus, also known as love lies bleeding because of its crimson flowers, and *Amaranth hypochondriacus*, also known as *Prince's-feather* • both species are ornamental • nearly all parts and almost all amaranth are edible • magically use the roots, seeds, leaves, flowers, and seed oil

PLANET AND ELEMENTS

Saturn • Earth/Fire

MAGICAL USES

called the flower of immortality because of its fresh appearance and color even after it has died • a sacred offering in ritual • easing the passing of a life and soothing grief • often featuring in burials in natural settings and remembering the ancestors • mends a broken heart • its use was forbidden among the Aztecs after the Conquistadors came as it was associated with rituals for fertility of the land involving blood • among the Hopi people, amaranth brings good luck, health, eternal love, and abundance.

HOW TO USE

Regarded as more sacred than grain in the Aztec world, amaranth was dedicated to the sun god Huitzilopochtli, to whom the priesthood made a seed and honey statue each year. • In magical baking, it is believed to endow supernatural powers as a plant of the Otherworld to those who eat it and to bring strength, psychic powers, and fertility. • Prickly seed heads or those varieties of amaranth with prickly leaves can be used in both love-attraction jars and in protective bottles. • Add the prickle-free leaves and dried flowers to abundance bags with coins, thread (representing enough clothing), and a small piece of wood (symbolizing fuel) to bring sufficient resources to the home and family.

CAUTION

Use gloves if handling the prickly leaves, and remove stickles from leaves before cooking. • Consuming amaranth is generally considered safe in moderation. • Consult your doctor during pregnancy, and avoid for pancreatic diseases and gallstones.

Amaranth, Globe

(*Gomphrena globosa*)

MAGICAL FORMS
often white or yellow with bright magenta, red, or orange bracts • a long-lasting flower that can also be used when dried, as it retains its color • blooms June to winter and grows around the world • magically use the seeds and as tea

PLANETS AND ELEMENT
Saturn/Venus • Earth

MAGICAL USES
provides protection against malevolent spirits in the home • calls benign spirits and ancestors • traditionally is used as a ritual offering in Hinduism • can be set on household altars to ask for blessings of abundance, health, and long life • carries these energies if used in magical cookery

HOW TO USE
The fresh blossoms can be used to create blooming tea, where buds blossom in the making. • Cut dried or fresh flowers to release their life force, energize, revitalize, and cleanse yourself of stagnation. • At weddings, they can be employed as a symbol of love that can never be broken or lost, especially when the flowers are red. • They also symbolize that love is forever and can be used to decorate a partner's or beloved relative's grave or favorite spot after they have passed.

Amaryllis

(*Amaryllis* spp.)

MAGICAL FORMS
also as the *Hippeastrum* genus, which is botanically unrelated but often sold under the common name "amaryllis" and shares its magical properties • also known as belladonna lilies but with absolutely no connection to the poisonous belladonna or poison ivy, which is a totally different species • magically use the whole plant, growing indoors or out; flowers, in bouquets or pots; and fresh or dried petals

PLANET AND ELEMENT
Venus • Water

MAGICAL USES

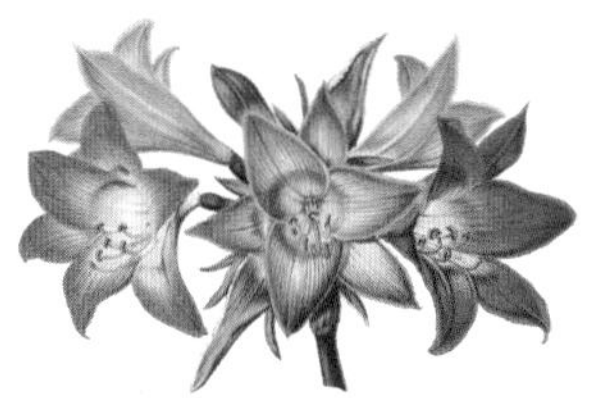

achievements especially in writing and all creative arts • encouraging the inner child and creativity for pleasure as well as for profit • connection with the Divine (purple) • a symbol of love that never gives up: The Greek maiden Amaryllis fell in love with the shepherd Alteo, but he rejected her. The Oracle of Delphi told Amaryllis to stand outside his home for thirty days and each day pierce her heart with a golden arrow. The drops of blood turned to a field of red amaryllis, and she won his love. • its name means in ancient Greek *horseman's star* because of its starlike shape and so is protective of travelers who follow their destiny

HOW TO USE
A bouquet or potted red amaryllis can be sent as a romantic gesture and the pink as a symbol of friendship. • In the language of flowers, amaryllis is the flower of those who create and is kept as inspiration in a writer's or artist's workplace. • Decorate the home around Yuletide with red amaryllis to welcome joy and, as in China, to attract good fortune and prosperity all year round. • Send white amaryllis to funerals or to comfort the bereaved. • Take also if undertaking a journey without certainty of outcome.

CAUTION
Amaryllis is toxic to humans and pets.

Amaryllis, Butterfly

(*Hippeastrum papilio*)

MAGICAL FORMS

a rare tropical evergreen amaryllis, with large flowers resembling butterflies • soft green and cream orchid-like flowers with burgundy stripes and touches of lime • green foliage, each stem producing two or three blooms • can be grown indoors • endangered in its native southern Brazil, but cultivated around the world, in many states of the USA, the UK, and the Netherlands • blooms twice a year in the spring and fall, year after year • magically use the growing plant in a pot, the cut plant, and the fresh or dried flowerheads

PLANET AND ELEMENT

Venus • Earth

MAGICAL USES

worth seeking for the seventy-seventh wedding anniversary with its health, travel, and renewed life-bringing powers, because of its connections with the Greek maiden Amaryllis who became goddess of spring and the rare transformative green butterflies, such as the emerald or peacock swallowtail and the tailed jay • use amaryllis evergreen (*Cybister amaryllis*) with large starry lime green petals associated with winter blooming or the smaller daintier Green Goddess Amaryllis (*Hippeastrum* 'Green Goddess') with apple green center fading to white for goddess rituals for new beginnings

HOW TO USE

Carry a fresh or dried butterfly amaryllis flowerhead as a reminder to seize opportunities, however risky, that may only come once. • Keep a green butterfly amaryllis in your business or workspace for seeking expansion beyond the safe zone. • If you see a green butterfly, take a photo, or download an image and set it in front of the potted or cut butterfly flowers. • Light a green candle, wishing for that seemingly impossible dream, especially involving travel, and blow out the candle, continuing nightly until the candle is completely burned.

CAUTION

Toxic to humans and pets if the bulb is ingested; to a lesser extent, even the leaves are toxic for pets. • Some people can experience allergic reactions with prolonged contact.

Amber

MAGICAL FORMS

organic gem that can be used as incense for very special mixes • from fossilized resin from coniferous trees existing more than thirty million years, many of which may be extinct • found especially on the Baltic shores • Mexican amber may be related to the *Hymenaea* tree • modern amber incense is usually created from beeswax, molasses, benzoin, vanilla, and labdanum, sometimes with frankincense added, the precise ingredients of which may be kept secret • the best sort will be plant derived and not contain chemicals

PLANET AND ELEMENT

Sun • Fire

MAGICAL USES

in fertility mixes • for contacting the ancestors • protects against physical danger and psychological and psychic attack and removes bad energies • a gateway to past-life recall and ancient wisdom • found in Palaeolithic graves, amber is said in China and the Far East to contain souls of many tigers and power of many suns • ancient Greeks believed amber was formed from rays of the setting sun upon the sea • found in many religions and different lands as sacred incense as well as the organic gem

HOW TO USE

Burn crushed amber resin (a small amount in a mix will do) before meditation, yoga, or other energy transference therapies such as Reiki and Tai Chi to shut out the daily world. • Empower amber jewelry with one of the amber incense stick substitutes. • If using the loose incense, it may be possible to find a small piece of amber to break up and add a little to mixes for higher spiritual work.

CAUTION

Do not burn during pregnancy or if you suffer from plant allergies.

Ambrette

(*Abelmoschus moschatus*)

MAGICAL FORMS

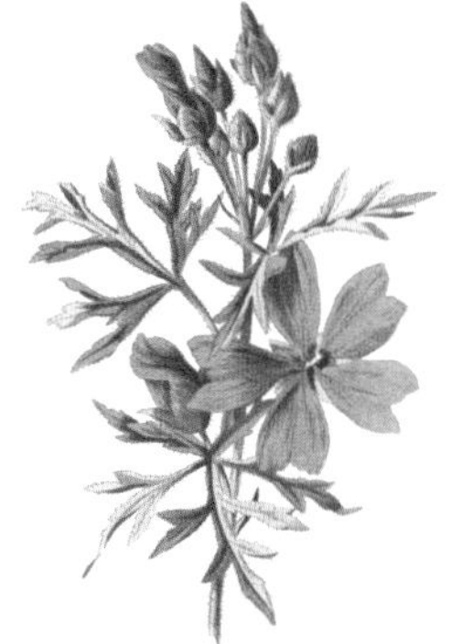

also known as muskdana or musk mallow • aromatic and medicinal evergreen plant, native to Australia and Asia • grows throughout tropical Asia and subtropical and tropical regions of the USA • can grow in cooler climes as an annual • yellow hibiscus-like flowers with purplish centers • flowers last only a day and give way to fruit capsules containing seeds with a sweet aromatic fragrance similar to musk • ambrette seeds are the best substitute for artificial musk • magically use the seeds, especially as essential oil or infused in oil for a month, and in incense

PLANET AND ELEMENT

Venus • Water

MAGICAL USES

linked with the Hindu goddess Parvati who brings not only sensuality but also lasting relationships • the flower is used in Indian weddings for good fortune • the diluted oil to anoint the brow (Third Eye) for enchantment in lovemaking • an ethical substitute for animal musk

HOW TO USE

Ambrette fragrance, a natural aphrodisiac, is said to steal away the heart. • Empower by anointing candles with a drop of the diluted oil and lighting them when you expect a lover or would-be lover to call. • Burn the ground seeds in incense in the bedroom in anticipation of a night of love. • Make a calming tea from the seeds.

CAUTION

Used in Ayurvedic and Indian folk medicine, ambrette is generally regarded as safe in food but not proven with pregnancy. • It should not be taken with antidiabetic medications.

Amyris

(*Amyris balsamifera*)

MAGICAL FORMS

also known as the West Indian sandalwood tree (not a true sandalwood) • flowering shrub/tree with white flowers • wild all over the island of Haiti, now grows from south Florida and Mexico through tropical USA and other parts of the tropical world • its resinous form is called torchwood because its branches easily ignite into torches • incredibly hard to find • magically use mainly as an essential oil made from the wood, or a perfume with Amyris fragrance

PLANET AND ELEMENT

Mars • Fire

MAGICAL USES

for astral projection in sleep if the oil is diffused or inhaled before bed • enhances, when diffused or inhaled, altered states during yoga, meditation, and energy therapies

HOW TO USE

Burn the oil for rites of passage in rituals, especially in wisewoman ceremonies, to combine youthfulness with experience. • Anoint your pulse points after empowering the oil as an aphrodisiac and to call back an absent love or your twin soul as yet unknown. • If you can find a fallen branch on vacation, cut and burn it in a safe place, as it is flammable, to connect with Fire spirits.

CAUTION

Avoid amyris when trying to become pregnant, during pregnancy, and while breastfeeding. • Do not use if suffering from epilepsy. • Never ingest the oil, and be aware that it may cause skin allergies in some people.

Anemone

(*Anemone* spp.)

MAGICAL FORMS

includes the meadow anemone or pasque flower (*Anemone pulsatilla*) • the blue, pink, or white Grecian windflower (*Anemone blanda*) • the florists' larger colorful anemones (*Anemone coronaria*) • the delicate wood anemone (*Anemone nemorosa*) • the ancient Greeks considered the wood anemone was a gift from Amenos, God of the Wind • magically use the whole, growing plant in an informal garden; florists' anemones as cut flowers or given in a pot; and fresh and dried petals in spells

PLANET AND ELEMENTS

Mars • Fire/Air

MAGICAL USES

calling back a lost love • keeping secrets, secret love • protects against illness, bringing health and healing • connects with the sylphs, the ruling spirits of the Air, and with all Wind magick

HOW TO USE

Traditionally, fresh anemone petals are carried in a red healing bag or a red cloth from when they first appear in the spring to keep away infections and illness and are replaced as they fade. • Red anemone flowers shield the home and family from negative energies, earthly and paranormal. • Burn the dried petals in incense to invoke the presence of Air spirits and call back a former love. • The petals are scattered to the four winds in Air magick spells to release a petition for manifestation and to telepathically connect with a secret lover. • Also burn at a natural burial service to call the soul to rebirth.

CAUTION

Do not ingest as it is toxic if the flower or bulb is eaten. • Though used worldwide medicinally for centuries, anemones should only be used medicinally under expert medical direction. • It must be avoided with pregnancy and breastfeeding, low blood pressure, bradycardia, and with some prescribed medicines. • Care may be needed in extensive handling as anemones can cause allergies with sensitive skin. • Nevertheless, it is an important magical flower and well worth the extra care.

Angel's Trumpet

(*Brugmansia* × *candida*)

MAGICAL FORMS

exotic small evergreen tropical tree with large leaves and big trumpet-shaped white, yellow, or pink flowers drooping downward • though from South America, especially the Andes, angel's trumpet will flourish in containers in frost-free environments and greenhouses • blooming mid-spring to fall and in a frost-free area, may flower all year • no longer grown in the wild • most fragrant at night attracting moths as pollinators • magically focus on the growing tree with care

PLANET AND ELEMENT

Mercury • Air

MAGICAL USES

for increasing clairaudience, psychic hearing, and receiving messages from angels, guides, and ancestors • practice sacred chanting in sight of the tree to initiate out-of-body experiences • smoked with tobacco by Indigenous shamans for astral travel, but it's toxic, highly hallucinogenic nature can make this dangerous

HOW TO USE

To contact the ancestors, write a message and bury it near your angel's trumpet tree to carry the words, especially if you cannot connect with a recently deceased relative. An answer will come in signs or dreams. • Powdered eggshells, known as cascarilla powder (compare with "Cascarilla or Sweetwood Bark," p. 104), can be scattered in a counterclockwise circle around the tree at full moon asking for justice where lies have been told or there is corruption. • Hang an empty sealed blue bottle safely on the tree where it cannot shatter to drive and keep away restless ghosts.

CAUTION

All parts of the plant are poisonous and can lead to death, especially the leaves and seeds if ingested. • Touch with gloves as a precaution and do not inhale when very close. • It may be that though this is considered a very powerful plant magically, and is beautiful when in flower, the risks of using it are too great if you have pets or children.

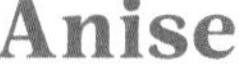

Angelica

(*Angelica archangelica*)

MAGICAL FORMS

magically use the leaves, stems, roots, seeds, candied, and oil from seeds and roots

PLANET AND ELEMENT

Sun • Fire

MAGICAL USES

calling love • seduction • increasing beauty and radiance • banishes hostility from others • protection, especially for children and against attacks on the home • brings energy • health • long life • associated with Michael, Archangel of the Sun and so a light bringer • angel, guardian angel, and archangel connections and making petitions

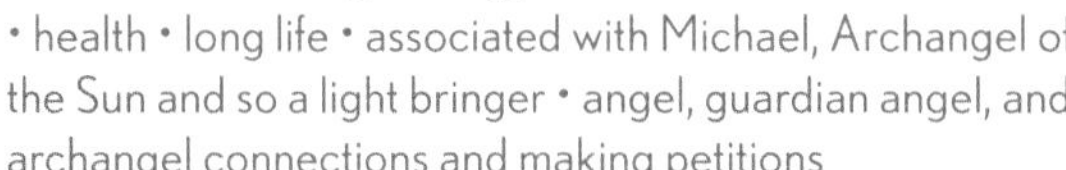

HOW TO USE

The stems are candied in magical cookery for romance and for enchanting a hesitant but willing lover. • The plant is worn or carried as an amulet in an herb sachet for good fortune. • Used as a defensive shield for domestic boundaries planted in the garden or in window boxes and in kitchen pots, it is reputed to be effective against evil spirits and infectious disease. • Use the seed and root, dried and chopped, in potpourri and/or with dried flowers to create a sleep pillow for prophetic dreams.

CAUTION

It may increase sensitivity to sunlight. • Avoid if pregnant. • Make sure the oil is diluted as it can cause irritation.

Anise

(*Pimpinella anisum*)

MAGICAL FORMS

also called aniseed • with a similar fragrance to licorice, is increasingly being grown in US gardens for its beautiful fragrance and magical properties • not the same as star anise (*Illicium verum*) • magically use the growing plant, seeds (despite the name aniseed, it is in fact a fruit), flowers, leaves, and essential oil

PLANET AND ELEMENT

Jupiter • Air

MAGICAL USES

reduces fears of attack and anxiety about aging and infirmity • drives off evil • assists overcoming and righting accidental harm • in magical cookery to keep a lover devoted and inspire passion • a potent cleanser of negativity, especially at home and a natural protector

HOW TO USE

The dried flowers can be burned in incense before psychic work, ritual, or meditation to call benign spirits. • Seeds or flowers in a sleep pillow guard against bad dreams. • The seed heads hung from the bed are a preserver of youth. • Cast the seeds or dried plant as a magical circle around you if carrying out antihex or curse-removing magick. • Draw an eye shape in the air over a sealed sachet of the seeds with a lighted incense stick in smoke, to guard against the evil eye. • Rub anise oil into a white candle to speed weight-loss spells. • Rub anise oil on twin red candles to keep a lover faithful. • Fresh leaves in potpourri or in sacred water banish evil spirits.

CAUTION

Avoid anise if suffering from hormone-sensitive conditions, endometriosis, during pregnancy, or while breastfeeding and if allergic to caraway, coriander, or similar plants. • For culinary purposes, sparingly use only food-grade anise oil safe for cooking.

Anthurium

(*Anthurium* spp.)

MAGICAL FORMS

especially *Anthurium andreanum* • also called the flamingo flower or painter's palette, originally a rainforest plant • magically use the whole, growing plant outdoors or indoors as a potted plant; cut flowers; and waxy bracts, fresh or dried

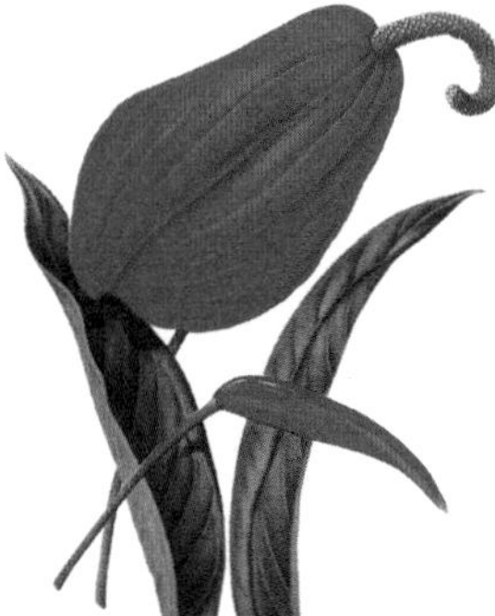

PLANET AND ELEMENT

Mars • Fire

MAGICAL USES

Anthurium clarinervium, the loving heart plant, is a perfect heart feng shui plant for ongoing health, love, and happiness for the seventieth wedding anniversary, platinum, or indeed for any couple who has shared deep love for years

HOW TO USE

Set a potted plant near the front door or in your workspace for a welcoming atmosphere and to attract inflowing resources, open communication, and cooperation. • Make a protection sachet against the evil eye of envy, using a turquoise crystal and the bracts/petals in a blue sachet. Draw over the sachet weekly in rose incense stick smoke the image of an eye. Set the empowered sachet between you and someone you know who envies you but whom you must see. The rest of the time keep the sachet in a jewelry box to endow the contents with protection. • Set coins in a circle on the surface of the soil around the stems of a potted plant to attract good fortune and money. • Keep the cut flowers on a table where you are sending out either written or email invitations to a celebration to ensure those who accept will enter into the spirit of the occasion. • Cast two bracts/petals into flowing water to free yourself from possessiveness in a relationship.

CAUTION

Anthurium is mildly toxic if ingested by pets and humans. • If you have sensitive skin, the sap may cause irritation.

Apple

(*Malus domestica*) or (*Malus sylvestris*)

MAGICAL FORMS

Malus domestica is known as the domestic or orchard apple, and *Malus sylvestris* is known as the crab apple • the Celtic Tree of Life and of the sacred Isle of Avalon, the Otherworld, whose fruit gave healing, rebirth, and immortality to deities and hero/ines • King Arthur was taken to Avalon after his death to await the return of the Golden Age • apples were brought to North America in the 1700s with the first settlers from the UK and Europe • the crab apple is native to the USA • the spread of the apple tree is credited to John Chapman (better known as Johnny Appleseed), a US missionary nurseryman who became a legend and planted apple seeds throughout the Midwest, giving thousands of apple seeds to nineteenth century pioneers, many of whom created their own orchards • magically use the tree, wood, and fruit

PLANET AND ELEMENTS

Venus • Water/Earth

MAGICAL USES

healing • brings fertility in every way, good fortune, and self-love • restores health and optimism • red apples for love, green for prosperity • for a good pregnancy, birth, and joy through babies, children, and families • the birth of boys (pears are for girls) • happy marriage

HOW TO USE

Share an apple with a lover or desired lover, afterward burying any discarded seeds or peel, so that commitment will grow. • Brush your hair a hundred times while gazing into a mirror and eating an apple by candlelight at midnight to see your future love reflected in the glass. • Bless golden apples in a fruit bowl with health, prosperity, and happiness and offer to friends, family, and visitors. • Use apple wands to connect with the fae and for fertility rituals.

CAUTION

Do not ingest apple seeds, as they are poisonous when crushed, containing amygdalin, a cyanogenic glycoside composed of cyanide and sugar.

Apple Blossom

(*Malus* spp.)

MAGICAL FORMS
often as *Malus pumila* and *Malus domestica* • state flower of Michigan and Arkansas • magically use the blossoms, growing on the tree or fresh and dried

PLANET AND ELEMENT
Venus • Water

MAGICAL USES
fertility, especially for a first child • good fortune • new beginnings • for all goddess rituals, especially beneath a blossoming apple tree or within a circle of dried apple blossoms • for enhancing beauty and creating enchantment in love

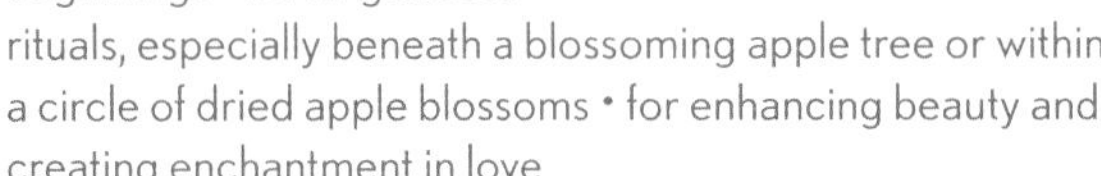

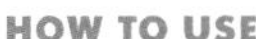

HOW TO USE
Roll in fallen apple blossom to conceive a child, increase your prosperity, or attract the right love. • Burn dried apple blossom as incense before divination or meditation to connect with other realms, especially if you have Celtic ancestry. • Add to bath sachets to attract new love or before lovemaking. • Share enchanted apple blossom tea with a hesitant lover or on full moon night if you are trying for a child and anxiety seems to be hindering conception. • Alternatively, set a tiny basket with a ceramic or clay babe resting on a bed of fresh or dried apple blossoms on a window ledge facing the moon, make love, and the next morning float the basket on gently flowing water, saying *From the rivers to the sea, return as a healthy babe within me* (or for my partner and me). • Sprinkle a trail of apple blossom tea drops from your boundary to your front door every Friday, the day of love, to call home an absent love.

CAUTION
Do not eat the seeds.

Apple Cider Vinegar

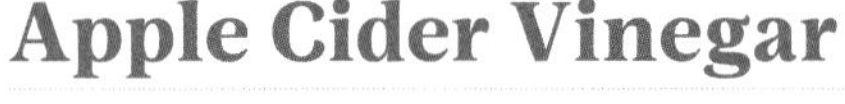

MAGICAL FORMS
bio-converted from cider made from fermented apples • traditionally and still used as an ingredient in the ancient Four Thieves' vinegar with such ingredients as garlic, peppercorn, thyme, lavender, rosemary, peppermint, and cloves, soaked for about a month in the vinegar and strained • it was said four thieves in southern France broke into plague houses to steal and did not catch the disease if they covered themselves with the mix • as a result it gained a reputation as a cure-all • apple cider can be empowered magically to increase its accepted earthly boost for health and energy or in a drink or added to recipes, in salad dressings and even for shiny hair and youthfulness

PLANETS AND ELEMENTS
Mars/Venus • Fire/Water

MAGICAL USES
mentioned with honey as a remedy for infections in the Old Testament and by Hippocrates the ancient Greek father of medicine to treat wounds • used by soldiers in the American Civil War as disinfectant • protects against psychic and psychological attack • empowered, it calms cravings, especially for food

HOW TO USE
It is used largely defensively either as the Four Thieves vinegar or ordinary apple cider vinegar as the liquid in spell bottles to break curses, hexes, jinxes, and ill wishing when it is placed in a dark high spot in the home and poured down a drain after a week, the jar washed in very hot water. • Apple cider vinegar can be sprinkled around boundaries or a small quantity added to floor and doorstep washes to repel all those with malicious intent, both unwanted earthly visitors and restless spirits who may still occupy the land.

CAUTION
Be careful with topical use as it can burn the skin. • Also avoid with pregnancy and breastfeeding as effects have not been fully researched.

Apricot

(*Prunus armeniaca*)

MAGICAL FORMS

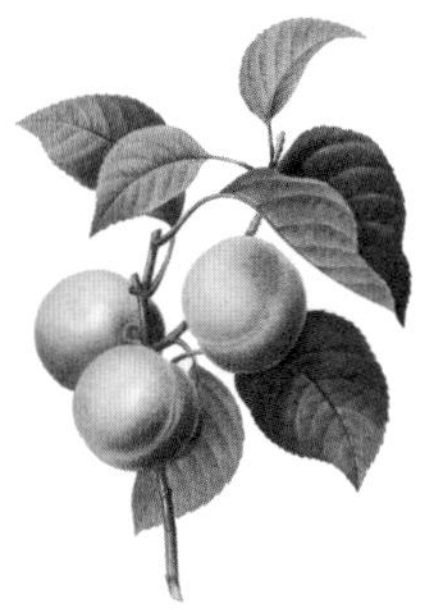

a small tree that loves the sun • blossoming in spring with fruit in the summer • native to Armenia and China, where it has been prized for thousands of years, apricots now grow in the central valley of California and Washington, Spain, southern Italy, and in sunny spots, especially in pots or containers, and in the UK • magically use the growing tree, blossoms, fresh and dried leaves, fruit, and carrier oil

PLANET AND ELEMENT

Venus • Water

MAGICAL USES

love, romance • health and healing • luxury, sensuality, and fertility • the Chinese goddess Xi Wangmu grew an orchard of magical apricots that promised immortality and the preservation of youthfulness and the apricot is still widely valued for its beauty and radiance-enhancing qualities • the kernel can be ground into healing incenses • in ancient Greece and Rome the blossoms and fruits were made as offerings to the love goddess Venus for fertility of people and land, planted near her temples

HOW TO USE

More delicate and smaller than the peach, eating or sharing apricots increases sweetness of response and turns away harsh words, especially spoken between lovers. • The carrier oil made from the kernel increases love and fertility, bringing properties of the essential oils with which it is mixed, and in massage enhances gentle spiritual lovemaking.

CAUTION

Do not use the oil or inhale the kernel incenses if you have a nut allergy. • Pregnant women should not eat unripe apricots. • Sulphites in dried apricots can trigger asthma in those susceptible.

Arabic Lump Resin

MAGICAL FORMS

true lump resin is a very pale pure resin from flowering small thorny acacia trees (see p. 14) that grow especially in Kordofan region of Sudan • a close cousin and variation, or some say the highest grade, of gum arabic resin • available from specialty magick stores and online • unusually free of human intrusion, as during drought the bark splits to allow the sap to flow out, releasing its treasure • dries into glassy tears used for special ceremonies

PLANET AND ELEMENT

Sun • Fire

MAGICAL USES

despite its less than exotic name, makes for a very spiritual incense that blends together different powers in an incense mix for positive results that are different from and greater than the individual properties

HOW TO USE

Crush and mix with oil or water for painting sacred, or divinely inspired, pictures. • Gives off an extra-rich smoke when burned on charcoal. Burn with frankincense and myrrh for visions of other realms and connection with ancient worlds, if you recall ancient wisdom without knowing how, or with dragon's blood for visions to astrally explore the world of distant ancestors and walk in their shoes. • Arabic lump resin is one stage higher than Gum Arabic resin if you crave to know more about higher realms, though they may be sold as the same thing.

CAUTION

Regarded as nontoxic generally, but use with care, as the dense smoke may cause allergies.

Arborvitae Tree

(*Thuja occidentalis*)

MAGICAL FORMS

also called the northern white cedar, eastern white cedar, or swamp cedar • a coniferous slow-growing evergreen, native to southeastern Canada, north central and northeastern USA • also found as dwarf and miniature forms • the first North American tree introduced to Europe • when crushed, its foliage smells of apples • magically use the essential oil, the leaves in tea (in moderation), and the wood

PLANET AND ELEMENT

Jupiter • Air

MAGICAL USES

arborvitae means "Tree of Life"; the oldest existing is a thousand years old • sacred to the Ojibwe people as one of the four major plants set in the north of the Medicine wheel • in Japan, the Japanese arborvitae (*Thuja standishii*) is one of the five sacred trees from which Shinto shrines are built • the oil in a burner or diffuser protects against psychologically and psychically toxic people and atmospheres and brings the power to overcome hardships

HOW TO USE

Since the wood is rot resistant and may lie fallen on the earth for a hundred years without decaying, use the wood for making wands for stability, security, long-term aims, and incorruptibility against injustice. • Make a tea from the dried leaves and sprinkled around a magical circle or around artifacts for purification and protection or to mark out sacred space for earth rituals. • Burn the wood or the oil to attract money. • Anoint, with a single drop of the oil, anything precious to you (underneath if it would stain) that you do not wish others to take or handle.

CAUTION

Avoid during pregnancy and while breastfeeding and if you suffer from low blood pressure or seizures.

Argan

(*Argania spinosa*)

MAGICAL FORMS

a short tree with a spreading canopy and thorny branches, dating back to the Tertiary Period 65 million to 2.6 million years ago • the oil of the tree comes from the fruit • genuine high-quality oil is still harvested by the women of the Amazigh people and is found only in the semideserts between the Atlantic Ocean of Magharibi and the Atlas Mountains in what is now a UNESCO-protected forest • introduced also into the Canary Islands • the oil has been used in Moroccan cookery and Berber medicines for many centuries • magically use the carrier oil, and argan oil in its many forms, added to shampoos, moisturizers, and bath products, all of which can be magically empowered

PLANET AND ELEMENT

Sun • Fire

MAGICAL USES

called liquid gold because of its value and rarity and the Tree of Life because its extraction gives the local people a major source of living and its deep roots enrich the soil so grass grows for the animals • the oil in its purer forms can be used to enhance its known physical benefits and ease moving to the next stage of life, embracing the right to claim happiness, enhancing beauty and radiance, and counteracting aging

HOW TO USE

Use the oil where its physical, psychological, and psychic properties overlap with anything with which it is mixed. • Empower any argan product used for massage and beauty treatments and absorbed through the skin or hair as its liquid gold qualities to bring health, wealth, and a sense of well-being to daily life. • Give empowered argan oil products to loved ones filled with blessings, especially if they are sick or sad. • Use the pure carrier oil for anointing your energy centers located at your pulse points for protection against loss or others who would threaten your livelihood or security.

CAUTION

Argan is safe with pregnancy if used topically. • Avoid it if you have a nut allergy.

Arnica

(*Arnica* spp.)

MAGICAL FORMS

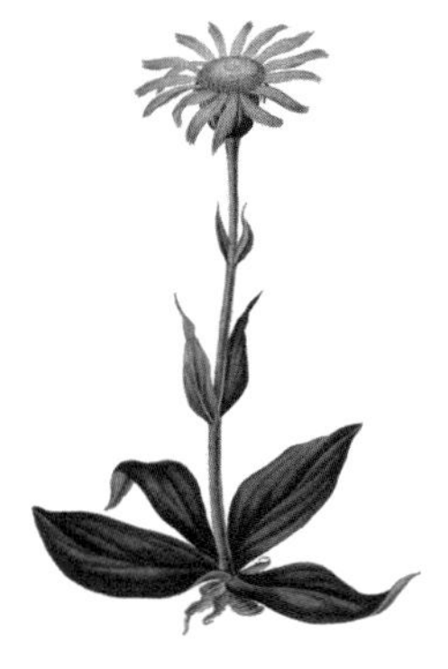

includes heartleaf arnica (*Arnica cordifolia*), mountain arnica (*Arnica montana*), and foothill arnica (*Arnica fulgens*) • heartleaf arnica is native to western North America in high places from Alaska to California and New Mexico and east to Michigan • grows also in Europe, Russia, India, the Far East, and Japan • all kinds of arnica have small bright yellow sunflower-like flowers with one to five daisy-like heads per plant, each with ten to fifteen rays • magically use the root/rhizome in a charm bag and the flowers, fresh (May to August) or dried (readily available online)

PLANET AND ELEMENT

Sun • Fire

MAGICAL USES

midsummer rituals, sun healing rites, especially of abuse and neglect • wish jars or charm bags to bring emotional and psychological strength as well as physical

HOW TO USE

For protection, arnica is traditionally buried in corners of fields at the summer solstice so that the harvest will be fruitful. • Burn the powdered plant in a protection incense if there have been arguments or external threats. • At the first grain harvest, mix the first seeds with dried arnica in a charm bag for fulfillment of wishes. • Carry the root for good luck in horse racing and competitions and as an amulet in a stable to keep the horse safe.

CAUTION

Do not take arnica internally or use it on broken skin, though excellent for clearing bruises on unbroken skin. • It may be restricted in some countries, though it has been used medicinally for many centuries.

Arrowroot

(*Maranta arundinacea*)

MAGICAL FORMS

can grow to six and a half feet high, with clusters of creamy flowers and numerous long-stemmed oval leaves • native to northern South America and the Caribbean, especially St. Vincent • cultivated worldwide in tropical regions • magically use the rhizome, which is easily obtainable in powder form from health shops and grocery stores, or the root, available online from magick stores

PLANET AND ELEMENT

Mercury • Air

MAGICAL USES

powdered as part of any wish powder mix • attracting good luck and money in its own right • named arrowroot because it was said to remove the poison from a wound inflicted by a poison arrow and so a natural protector from psychological and spirit attacks

HOW TO USE

Use in a charm bag to bring people together at home, in the workplace, community, or globally • Hang on a tree or over a door where air flows freely or in a room where the family will meet to celebrate or work colleagues will gather for meetings. • Add a root to a spell bag of crystals and herbs or add the powder to a wish jar to strengthen the power of the work by binding the different elements together.

Artichoke

(*Cynara cardunculus* var. *scolymus*)

MAGICAL FORMS

also called the globe artichoke and the French or green artichoke, with extra-large hearts • herbaceous thistle on a tall stem with young edible small buds and heart • if the buds are left to flower, they produce lavender-blue flowers from June to September but become more inedible past their budding season • native to the Mediterranean coast, artichokes grow in many lands, including Italy, the main producer; Peru; Argentina; the USA, especially in California and Monterey County; North Africa; China; and Egypt • magically use the seasonal buds and heart (March to May), the dried and fresh flowers, the flower essence, ready-prepared artichokes all year for magical cookery, and the whole plant at any time

PLANET AND ELEMENT

Mars • Fire

MAGICAL USES

a plant with many symbolic meanings, the flower signifying peace and prosperity in Libya, Egypt, and Somalia • once considered in ancient Egypt, Greece, and Rome as an aphrodisiac, bringing fertility • the whole growing prickly plant guards the home and family when grown in a garden or displayed in the kitchen before cooking • the dried or cut flowers act as a charm if an original opportunity has been lost or missed

HOW TO USE

Empower and cook fresh buds, the base of the buds, and the heart, or substitute canned hearts, if you have abrasive or sarcastic guests or family members. • Peel the layers of the whole plant at any stage of its development using a knife to remove problems or obstacles or break through resistance. • Ingest a few drops of flower essence or add it to a water-based spray at work before a meeting to overcome rigid beliefs and fears of change.

CAUTION

Though used medicinally for heart and liver health and weight control, keep to small amounts during pregnancy and breastfeeding. • Some people have an allergic reaction to it.

Arugula

(*Eruca sativa*)

MAGICAL FORMS

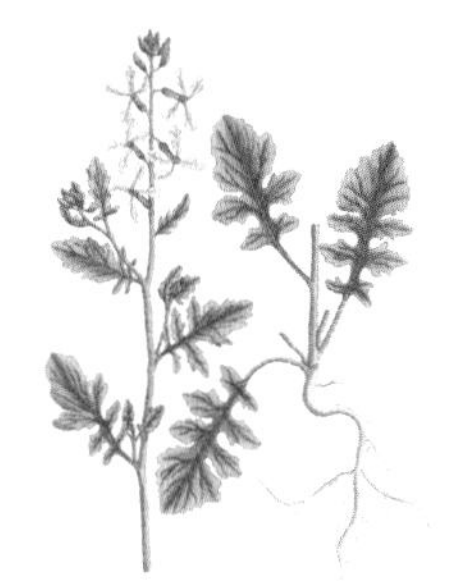

also known as rocket • rich green leafy vegetable/herb, belonging to the mustard family • hot and peppery, served raw in salad or cooked for a milder flavor • the white edible flowers that bloom from late spring or early summer, have four petals with green or purple veins through them, resembling a Celtic cross • often used purely as an ornamental flower • native to Italy, Morocco, Portugal, and Turkey, though not fully incorporated into US cuisine till the 1990s • magically use the flowerheads, fresh or dried; cut flowers; and the seeds, the empowered seed oil, and the ripe leaves in magical cookery

PLANET AND ELEMENT

Mars • Fire

MAGICAL USES

the ancient Egyptians, Greeks, and Romans regarded arugula, especially the seed oil, as an aphrodisiac and to increase male potency • in modern times eaten with tomatoes to enhance libido • grow in the garden to attract abundance

HOW TO USE

Use the cut, pressed, or dried Celtic cross flowers in your special place or growing in the garden as a focus of meditation to connect with past worlds, especially if you have Celtic roots. • Collect or buy the seeds for a charm bag to influence wise financial investments, especially if you are given conflicting advice. • Add the oil to an empowered beauty product such as shampoo, conditioner, or moisturizer or use as the oil if you like the pure fragrance, not only for hair and skin health and radiance but to attract the right people whether in love, friendship, or career.

CAUTION

Avoid in all forms if taking anticoagulants.

Asafoetida

(*Ferula assa-foetida*)

MAGICAL FORMS

also called devil's dung • a herb that can grow to six feet tall, from the carrot family, and has several varieties • native to Iran, Pakistan, and Afghanistan and a popular spice in ancient Rome • the dried gum from the fleshy tap root of *Ferula* plants is powdered as spice • the odor dissipates in cooking and tastes like onions or leeks • magically use mainly as empowered spice in cooking and in protection and banishing incenses outdoors or with open windows, as it has a very strong odor (as its folk name suggests)

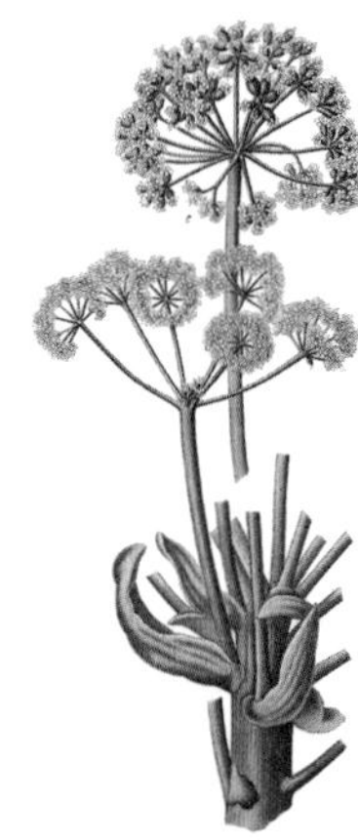

PLANET AND ELEMENT

Mars • Fire

MAGICAL USES

guards against having property stolen, damaged, or lost • in magical cookery as an even more powerful alternative to garlic (often added to East Indian recipes) • offers strong defensive powers against any malevolent forces

HOW TO USE

Sprinkle the spice around the outside of a home before going away to protect against intruders. • Use it in cooking to transform misfortune into fortune and replace ill-wishing against you with blessings. • Burn the powder in incense against unscrupulous debt collectors, bailiffs, and unjust legal or official accusations, with shredded paper naming the injustice or threatening organization. • Add fragrant herbs or resin to the incense.

CAUTION

Do not take with blood thinners or low blood pressure and not during pregnancy or while breastfeeding. • It may cause swelling of the lips. • Not enough research has proven its safety when applied topically.

Ash Tree

(*Fraxinus* spp.)

MAGICAL FORMS

including *Fraxinus americana*, the American white ash, and *Fraxinus excelsior*, the European common ash • most magical with a cleft • pieces of bark and leaves arranged in symmetrical pairs of two, six, or eight leaves, with one odd leaf at the bottom • winged fruits on female trees, called keys or helicopters because of their shape and the way the single wing clusters break off and come whirling down • magically use the growing tree, branches, bark, roots, and leaves

PLANETS AND ELEMENT

Mercury/Jupiter • Air

MAGICAL USES

the ash is a sacred tree to many of Celtic descent in the USA as well as Europe • after the Irish potato famine, emigrants carried shoots from the ancient ash of Creevna to the US to protect them in the new land • in Norse mythology, Ygydrassil, the world tree, was made of ash • protective against human spite (snakes) • pregnant women would embrace the tree for an easy and safe delivery

HOW TO USE

Make a broom for cleansing ritual spaces and the home with ash for the handle, and with birch twigs for the broom head, tied with willow. • Use ash for healing wands. • Place the keys in a sealed purple sachet beneath the pillow for prophetic dreaming and astral travel during sleep. • Carve poppets or dolls from ash roots for healing rituals. • If creating poetry or any inspired writing, keep the fresh leaves in a dish in your workspace. • For good fortune follow the traditional method of picking a sprig of the leaves and saying, *Even ash I do thee pluck, wishing you will bring good luck.* Carry or wear it, and each new day replace the old sprig, setting it free.

CAUTION

The tree as such is not poisonous, but leaves, bark, and fruit contain arsenic in concentrated quantities so do not ingest and handle with care. • Burn the wood outdoors or only in a well-ventilated space.

Ashwagandha

(Withania somnifera)

MAGICAL FORMS

also known as winter cherry or Indian ginseng • an evergreen shrub native to India, the Middle East, and parts of Africa, also cultivated in milder climate temperate regions around the world including the USA, especially in southern Oregon • the root and leaves have been used in Ayurvedic medicine for thousands of years • magically use the whole, growing tree; flowers; leaves; roots; and sometimes berries, to make restorative and calming teas

PLANET AND ELEMENT

Sun • Fire

MAGICAL USES

reduces stress and anxiety • brings strength and physical stamina at times when rest is not possible • enhances male potency • for tantric and sex magick • brings harmony to confrontational issues in relationships both workplace and domestic

HOW TO USE

Make tea as a decoction using the roots. The tea is regarded as an elixir of long life and health and when focus and concentration are needed for study, tests, examinations, or presentations. • Grow in the garden near the front door to ensure the free flow of the chi life force through the home or a home business whenever the door is opened. • Keep a dried chopped root with dried flowers and leaves in a dark-colored natural fabric protective amulet bag in your workspace if you are constantly drawn against your will into workplace disputes, are victimized by colleagues or seniors, or when dealing with complaining clients if you work in customer service, to keep your cool.

CAUTION

Do not ingest the plant in any form if you are pregnant or breastfeeding, have thyroid conditions, suffer with an autoimmune disease, or take central nervous system medications, such as sedatives.

Asian Watermeal

(Wolffia globosa)

MAGICAL FORMS

a kind of Duckweed • an aquatic plant that is the world's smallest flowering plant, native to tropical and subtropical Asia • availability is slowly increasing and can be found in California, Florida, and Hawaii • Asian watermeal is made up of tiny vibrant green beads covering the surface of still or slow-moving waters, each about a third of an inch in diameter spreading rapidly, doubling in two days, floating without needing stems, leaves, or roots • occasionally flowers and from the flowers emerges the smallest fruit in the world • harvested from ponds and the surface of aquariums though very rare in the Western world • for centuries used in Thai cuisine as *khai nam* or water eggs • magically, it is worth searching for to grow if you have a small body of warm calm water • magically use as *mankai*, the cultivated form, frozen in ice cubes or powdered (increasingly available in the USA and other parts of the world)

PLANET AND ELEMENT

Moon • Water

MAGICAL USES

add *mankai*, or if you can obtain the true Asian watermeal, to food or drink to bring rapid growth into your life • blend a disharmonious family together by eating a Thai meal containing the watermeal • search on vacation or find the watermeal growing naturally in aqua nature parks • stir the water very gently with a reed to bring the health and energy-giving powers of the plant into your life

HOW TO USE

If you find or produce Asian watermeal, the Library of Congress estimates it will take five thousand beads to fill a thimble. • Collect a thimble full to represent the growth of whatever is most needed, whether urgent money, health, or a sudden career boost, and tip them back in the water to rapidly grow.

CAUTION

It is not considered toxic, but avoid with pregnancy.

Asparagus

(*Asparagus officinalis*)

MAGICAL FORMS

also known as sparrow grass • green, white, and purple flowering plant with delicate spears or shoots that for a short time each spring are eaten as a delicacy, cooked or raw • the tips are especially prized • feathery foliage • native to western Asia, and northern Africa, introduced to many areas of the USA from France in the 1600s and 1700s • grows along the eastern coast of the USA and in thirty-six states, both wild and cultivated • also in the UK, especially in Kent, southeast of London • magically use fresh and canned asparagus in empowered cooking or eating

PLANETS AND ELEMENTS

Jupiter/Mars • Air/Fire

MAGICAL USES

the Romans brought asparagus from the Middle East and planted it on their conquests of Europe • traditionally an aphrodisiac, especially for increasing male libido and potency

HOW TO USE

To conceive a child, share single spears before lovemaking. • Cook into a prosperity herb sauce to enhance the main herb's qualities: for example, a basil-based sauce attracts money; rosemary or parsley-based increases love or passion. • To call back a lost love, eat without sauce. • Adding lemongrass or lemon juice in the sauce provides protection against lies and spite. • Increase psychic powers, especially for astral travel, by eating it before meditation, visualization, or chanting. • Tie a bundle of raw asparagus together with red ribbon in three knots, and use as a wand to draw a counterclockwise circle of protection around the photo of a partner you fear may be tempted to stray.

CAUTION

Its foliage is toxic. • Avoid if you have hypertension or are taking diuretic medicine.

Aspen

(*Populus tremuloides*) and (*Populus tremula*)

MAGICAL FORMS

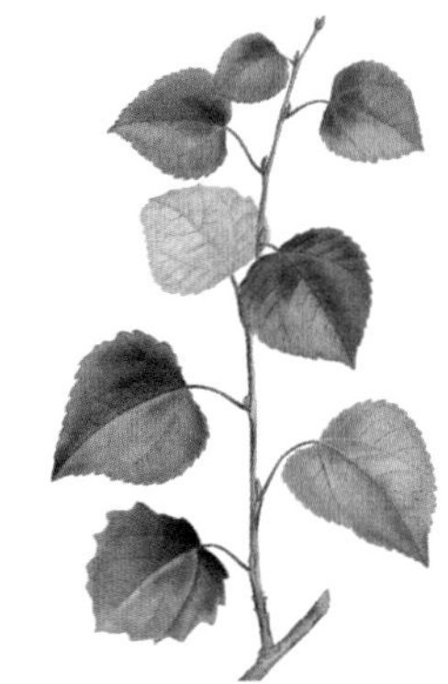

as *Populus tremuloides*, American aspen, growing across northern USA and Canada • glossy green leaves that turn golden in the fall • *Populus tremula*, the European aspen, is commonly found in cooler regions of Europe and Asia • both kinds are known as the shiver-tree because their leaves shake in the slightest breeze • magically use the whole, growing tree; fresh and dried leaves; and flower essence

PLANET AND ELEMENT

Mercury • Air

MAGICAL USES

European aspen was discovered fossilized in Turkey 64 million years ago • the root system of American trees can live for thousands of years • a colony of aspen in Utah is estimated to date back eighty thousand years • both European and American trees connect with past worlds and ancient lands

HOW TO USE

The golden leaves of the American tree in the fall are used in money spells and charm bags with a piece of gold. • Spray the home with a few drops of the Bach aspen remedy dissolved in water to remove free-floating fears of potential disaster and in the bedroom to drive away troubling dreams. • Put a little essence under the tongue for eloquence if you are speaking at a meeting or performing. • Burn the dried leaves in an incense mix to communicate with the ancestors at Halloween/Samhain.

CAUTION

Though the bark and leaves have been used medicinally for hundreds of years, the leaves may cause skin reactions. • Avoid with pregnancy and if you are allergic to aspirin.

Aster

(*Aster* spp.)

MAGICAL FORMS

genus of flowering plants named after the Greek word for star, because of their starlike blossoms • including the Michaelmas daisy, also known as the European aster (*Aster amellus*), the New England aster (*Aster symphyotrichum novae-angliae*), and the New York aster (*Aster symphyotrichum novi-belgii*) • magically use the whole plant, blossoms, and root

PLANETS AND ELEMENTS

Sun/Venus • Fire/Earth/Water

MAGICAL USES

star magic and contact with star beings • aligned with Astraea, a goddess turned into a star after Jupiter flooded the earth • when the flood receded, her tears for the sorrows of humanity fell and grew as asters • also called starwort • grown to attract and strengthen love • a Michael, archangel of the sun, flower associated with the fall equinox and Michael's special day, September 29 • associated with the banishment of all that is not from the light, especially malevolent spirits • for new beginnings in every area of life

HOW TO USE

Use a decoction of root or essence of the blossoms for cleansing an altar or sacred space. • Incorporate into goddess rituals. • Burn as incense to locate lost or stolen items. • Keep the growing or cut plant in a room to increase psychic powers. • Aster was first used in ancient Greece and Rome as a sacred offering woven into wreaths on altars. • Use the essence mixed with rose water to spray around your aura or a room to remove earthbound spirits or those seeking to enter the user.

Aster, China

(*Callistephus chinensis*)

MAGICAL FORMS

grows in a variety of colors, including a white 'Dwarf Milady' • close cousins/siblings of the Michaelmas daisy (the purple and yellow species) • in many colors, grown ornamentally in pots and containers, tubs, or in the garden • there are numerous species of asters native to the USA and worldwide and all share the same magical qualities • Chinese asters were cultivated in China two thousand years ago and were brought to Europe by Jesuit missionaries in the 1730s, thereafter they were taken to North America in the 1830s where their popularity rapidly grew • growing together they resemble one huge star • magically use the growing or cut starlike flower, and the petals

PLANET AND ELEMENT

Jupiter • Air

MAGICAL USES

delicate matters or negotiations • any astrological explorations and study, whatever the kind of aster, which is Greek for star • connection with stellar beings and much loved by people who consider themselves star souls • white asters are sent as a sign of sympathy after a bereavement • some say they will ease a passing and give sight of the afterworld when a person is ready to let go of earthly life

HOW TO USE

Victorians on both sides of the Atlantic regarded the Chinese aster as a symbol of love and higher feelings and so a bouquet of them or indeed any aster represents pure love. • When planted, cut, and placed in a vase on an altar, China asters offer a connection between the earth and heavens, following the magical principle *As above so below.* • Carry dried aster blossoms, especially pink, with a rose quartz crystal in a pink bag to call romance into your life or to rekindle it. • Also carry them to give you patience if love or better times are slow coming, and to speak with tact. • Plant a new aster in a pot to represent a new beginning, whether a new job, going to college, moving home, or living with a partner for the first time. Keep it as it grows in your workplace, new home, or college dorm.

Astilbe

(*Astilbe* spp.)

MAGICAL FORMS

usually grown in gardens • native to China • magically use the whole, growing plant; fernlike leaves; feathery flowers; and rhizome (an underground horizontal stem from which roots grow, producing new plants)

PLANET AND ELEMENT

Venus • Earth

MAGICAL USES

for passion • fidelity • for influencing people and meeting influential people • pink for maternal issues, white for first love or love after loss, and purple for enhancing spiritual gifts • flower psychometry

HOW TO USE

Grow in a pot to use as a gift for someone to express lasting devotion, promising to wait if you must be absent for a while. • Added to a wedding or anniversary bouquet as a pledge of lifelong loyalty. • Traditionally used for healing wounds and animal bites, in modern magick, a chopped and dried rhizome is carried in a brown bag as an amulet against physical, psychological, and psychic attack from humans. Bless this amulet on the last day of the waning moon before it disappears from the sky.

CAUTION

Take precautions if pregnant.

Astragalus

(*Astragalus mongholicus*)

MAGICAL FORMS

known in Chinese medicine for centuries as Huang Qi • has sweet roots, pendulous yellow flowers, and fernlike foliage that can be used magically, as well as the growing plant that can grow up to four feet • a member of the pea family • native to northeastern and eastern China and grown extensively throughout the USA, where it is considered endangered in the wild • magically use the tea made from the root for its health-giving properties

PLANET AND ELEMENT

Saturn • Earth

MAGICAL USES

antiaging rituals • protection against malevolence • resistance to and breaking hexes and curses • in magical cookery by adding the chopped roots to a dish being cooked

HOW TO USE

If you know who has wished you ill, etch their name on a root and take it far away from your home, burying it at or near a crossroads. • If the curser is unknown, etch *Whoever has wished me harm* on the root and again abandon it at a crossroads. • Grow astragalus along a hostile neighbor's wall, or put the potted plant between you and an unfriendly work colleague as a psychic shield. • Dry nine yellow flowers, and keep them in a yellow bag with nine gold-colored coins when you go shopping or to auctions and yard sales to attract unexpected bargains and treasure troves and prevent unwise impulse purchases.

CAUTION

Astragalus should not be used with medications to suppress the immune system, while pregnant or breastfeeding, or by anyone in excess.

Astrantia Maxima

(*Astrantia helleborifolia*)

MAGICAL FORMS

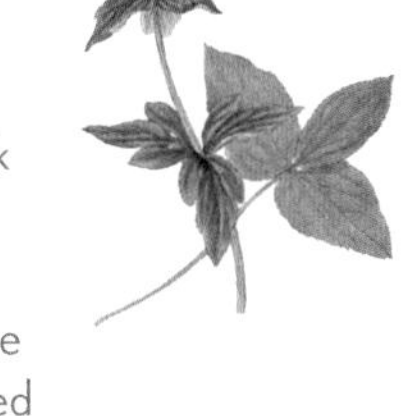

a very large flower, the largest form of the Astrantia/masterwort flowers • growing on both sides of the Atlantic, three feet tall and two feet broad • tiny soft pink flowers filling a dome-shaped flower head, sheltering within broad pink papery bracts • blooms from late spring to early summer • a flower representing the power of kindness • magically use the flowers, cut or growing; and fresh or dried flowerheads • if Astrantia maxima cannot be found, use any other large, pale-pink, multipetaled flower for similar effects

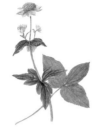

PLANET AND ELEMENT

Venus • Earth

MAGICAL USES

the softness of pink in such a large flower understates but never minimizes its power • a suggested alternative flower bouquet for the forty-seventh anniversary, an anniversary that in modern times has become associated with books as well as the balanced amethyst • a flower also for matriarchs and grandmothers who may hold a family together (the smaller pink Astrantia species is for younger women) • give the flowers also to a best friend you have known for years on their birthday • keep the flowers in a vase in rituals and bless them daily for restoring a family member to the right path with kindness but determination

HOW TO USE

Grow Astrantia maxima in the garden or keep one or two cut flowers in a vase of water inside the front door for creating an oasis of peace with boundaries so disruptive neighbors or family members are silenced or moderate their words and actions without knowing why. • Give the flowers to special friends you are leaving behind. • Before moving, pluck and dry petals for a sachet along with an amethyst or rose quartz for your new home when you invite neighbors to call. Carry it to your new workplace or leisure venue. • If you seek trustworthy online friends, keep the sachet near your computer when exploring friendship sites.

Astrantia, Ruby Wedding

(*Astrantia major* 'Ruby Wedding')

MAGICAL FORMS

Ruby Wedding astrantia is a form of astrantia • ruby pincushion flowers • blooms continuously throughout the summer and grows in eastern, northern, and midwestern parts of the USA, in the UK, and in other temperate lands (astrantia is not happy with continuous heat) • cultivar 'Burgundy Manor' also has ruby-red pincushion flowers • other ruby astrantia include the 'Claret' cultivar and *Astrantia carniolica*, called red masterwort (see "Masterwort," p. 285) and its red dwarf counterpart 'Rubra' • magically use the growing ruby plant; the cut, long-living flowers, dried or fresh; dried flowerheads; and petals

PLANETS AND ELEMENT

Mars/Sun • Fire

MAGICAL USES

any of the ruby varieties are a perfect fortieth anniversary gift, and in fact the 'Ruby Wedding' was created specifically for it • give a bouquet or cut flowers for reconciliation if infidelity has occurred but the couple wants to stay together • the flower of older women moving into a new phase • can be sent to an older woman by a younger man as a sign of serious love commitment

HOW TO USE

Like the ruby gem, whose possession is said to attract more gems, growing or buying oneself ruby astrantia flowers is a magical statement, particularly for a woman ready to welcome a new creative phase in her later years, as well as to revive or initiate a passion whether in love, career change, or travel. • Burn the ruby flowers in a hearth fire, a bonfire, or a deep, heatproof bowl and afterward scatter the ashes where nothing grows, naming whomever or whatever discourages you from the next phase of your life and development. • Whatever your age or gender, collect the dried petals daily in a glass jar, and when it is full, tip the jar from the highest place you can find to release money, good luck, and prosperity that have previously eluded you.

CAUTION

Astrantia is not considered toxic to humans or pets, but heed the warnings under the entry for masterwort (see p. 285).

Audumbar Tree

(*Ficus glomerata*)

MAGICAL FORMS

previously called *Ficus racemosa* • a sacred Indian fig tree, meaning in Sanskrit "the auspicious flower from heaven" • sacred to Lord Vishnu, created from the life force of the god Indra and planted wherever Dattaguru, the highest lord of yoga and a former monk who is venerated as a Hindu god, is worshipped • sold as pandit incense sticks, sometimes with added oils • if using incense magically, make sure you are buying incense that contains the fig tree or tree flower itself to give its unique sweet fragrance resembling sandalwood • magically use the incense and root

PLANET AND ELEMENTS

Venus • Water/Earth

MAGICAL USES

the tree is given water to bring the blessings of Venus for prosperity and good fortune and forms the center of many prayers and offering ceremonies within Hinduism • fights off rivals and foes • brings fortune, especially to those born under Taurus and Libra • known as the wish-fulfillment tree

HOW TO USE

The root can be carried as a charm in an adaptation of Hindu custom to bring about a successful marriage. • To call prosperity and property success, store in a bag with a silver charm placed inside, or carry it with you. • Burn the incense sticks to avert the evil eye. • Burn incense before and during yoga, meditation, or any transference of energy rites to connect with higher planes wherever in the world you live and whatever your belief system.

CAUTION

Use caution if suffering from allergic rhinitis or if pregnant; in these cases, seek medical advice before use.

Avens

(*Geum urbanum*)

MAGICAL FORMS

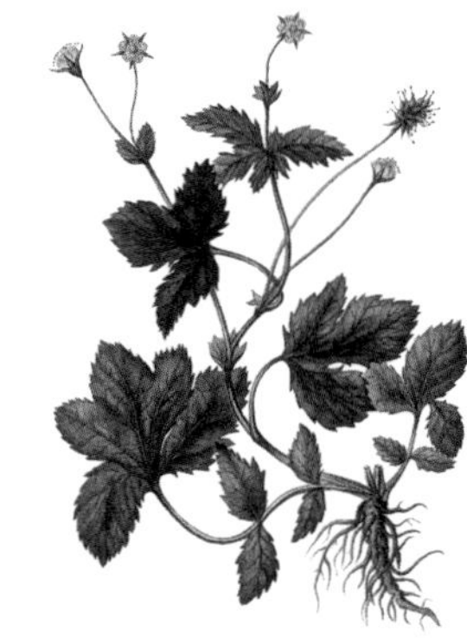

sometimes called the Blessed Herb or St. Benedict's herb • associated with the early saint, as some myths tell avens cured him of poison (see "Thistle, Blessed," p. 445) • the white five-petaled form *Geum canadense* is found more often in the USA and Canada but is often hybridized with *Geum urbanum* and has identical magical properties • magically use the whole plant, cut flowers, root, and five petaled starlike yellow, red, or orange flowers

PLANET AND ELEMENT

Jupiter • Air

MAGICAL USES

for exorcism and purification • overcoming all who are venomous, human and animal • the flower was traditionally worn by male North American Indians to attract the person they wanted to settle with, but worked for either sex • in medieval times the root was credited with magical powers to repel the Devil and was traditionally unearthed on March 25, considered the first day of the calendar year until 1752

HOW TO USE

The dried or fresh flowers are effective in love rituals either on an altar or outdoors. • A whole root is carried in a red cloth bag as an amulet of protection. • Burn a root outdoors on a bonfire or smaller pieces in an indoor hearth or in incense. The smoke from the root will guard the home and the family by creating a psychic fog around the home so evil will pass by unseeing.

CAUTION

Avens is not recommended to be taken internally. • Avoid during pregnancy, as avens may bring on menstruation. • Use medicinally with professional advice in small quantities and for a short period only.

Avocado

(*Persea americana*)

MAGICAL FORMS

tree indigenous to Central America • grows in tropical and subtropical areas of North America, California along the Pacific coast, Hawaii, Texas, and Florida • the West Indies, Israel, Spain, Australia, and South Africa • magically use the fresh and dried leaves, bark, fruit, seeds as oil, and as a potted plant

PLANET AND ELEMENT

Venus • Earth

MAGICAL USES

increasing the desire of someone for you • growth of beauty in self or environment, and/or moving to a beautiful place • manifesting intentions

HOW TO USE

Scoop out the flesh, and share the avocado with a lover to increase passion before lovemaking. • Bury a pit/stone in a pot of soil in sunlight, and keep in the home to increase family love, to attract love if you are alone, and when you move to a new home with a lover so that love will accompany you. • Dry the avocado skin, and grind it into a fine powder to add to an enchantment incense to make you irresistible. • Anoint a gold or yellow candle by rubbing in a drop of avocado seed oil to the unlit candle to bring luxury into your life or before bargain hunting for treasures or desired artifacts. • Oiling makes a candle more flammable for tangible rewards. • Keep a dish of avocado in the center of the living or family room if you have a volatile partner, outspoken relative, or confrontational teens.

CAUTION

Avoid if taking warfarin or allergic to birch pollen or latex.

Azalea

(*Rhododendron* spp.)

MAGICAL FORMS

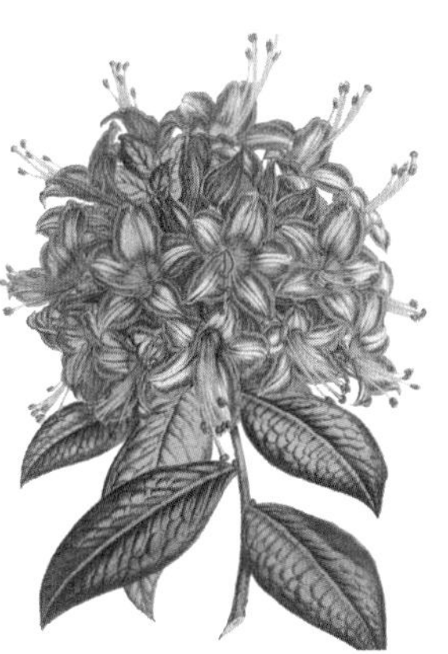

a flowering shrub in the Ericaceae family • a close cousin of the rhododendron • small colorful blooms, all the colors of the rainbow • unlike the rhododendron per se, with far fewer clusters and with tube or funnel-type flowers, where rhododendron has bell-shaped flowers • magically use the growing plant; cut flowers; petals, fresh or dried; and flower essence

PLANET AND ELEMENT

Saturn • Earth

MAGICAL USES

moderation • prudence • freedom from addiction • Alpine azaleas (*Kalmia procumbens*) are made into a flower essence with the same magical powers of American azaleas, increasing self-esteem and valuing the self

HOW TO USE

Assists binge eaters to be more moderate when a pot of the flowers is kept near the scale. • Since the Chinese have long associated the azalea with thoughtfulness, receiving a pot or bouquet of azaleas reassures you that the sender is reliable and will treat you respectfully. • Growing in a safe place in your garden or indoors, azaleas offer protection against hexes and those who threaten physical harm. • Keep on the altar for rituals for rites of passage into womanhood and into the wisewoman or wise man stage.

CAUTION

Any part of the raw plant is very unsafe for humans and pets to ingest, though it has been used in Native North American and Chinese traditional medicine and was popular among Victorians.

Azalea, Alpine

(*Kalmia procumbens*)

MAGICAL FORMS

also called trailing azalea • dwarf shrub that grows in high alpine regions of the northern hemisphere, with pink bell-like flowers in late spring, forming low mounds or spreading floral carpets • can be cultivated in the UK and European gardens as well as cool or alpine and subalpine regions of North America and Canada • magically use the dried flowers and as a flower essence

PLANET AND ELEMENT

Mercury • Air

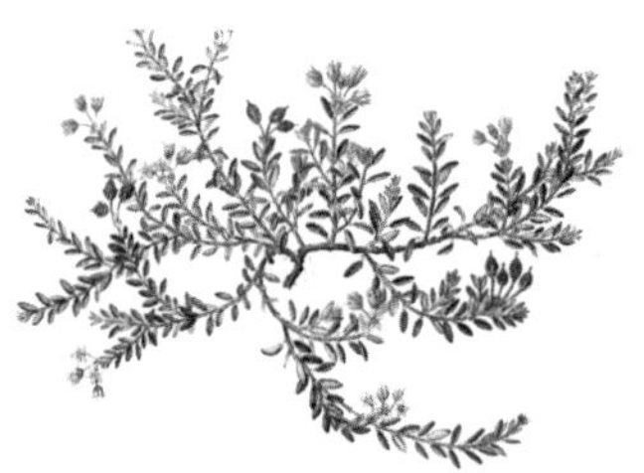

MAGICAL USES

overcomes fears, low self-esteem, dislike of body, especially if there are critical and discouraging people in your life • for pets who pull out their fur or feathers and shy from attention add a drop or two of the essence regularly to water or food

HOW TO USE

Put a few daily drops of the essence in an indoor water feature or spray spritzer bottle in water if the atmosphere at home or in the workplace is naturally pessimistic. • Use similarly if you are made to feel inferior or unattractive by jealous rivals, especially in highly competitive atmospheres. • Sip two drops of the essence four times a day in water to build up self-esteem and to overcome food issues or obsessions with cosmetic surgery. • Take the essence when you are hot and bothered emotionally as well as physically or when a temperamental family member or colleague is trying to provoke you. • Use the dried flowers in a charm bag for adventures, especially in mountains and to aim high in career or in spiritual exploration to connect with higher dimensions.

CAUTION

While the flower essence is quite safe, the plant is toxic if ingested and should be handled with care. • Avoid the plant during pregnancy as you may be extra sensitive to its effects.

Azalea, Golden Oriole

(*Rhododendron* 'Golden Oriole')

MAGICAL FORMS

flowering bush created by cross breeding of native USA and Asian varieties, with orange buds and yellow golden flowers in spring • in fall, leaves turn bronze • ideal in a natural garden • magically use the growing shrub, the cut flowers, the fresh or dried flowerheads, and the bronze leaves

PLANET AND ELEMENT

Sun • Fire

MAGICAL USES

oriole means "golden one" • this is the most dynamic of the usually cautious azaleas, filled with the energy of action and joy • a twenty-first anniversary flower • its name has magical associations with the Archangel Uriel/Oriel, who brought alchemy to humans (this is part of its association with the brass anniversary: a couple transforming their separate lives in a new and powerful way) • growing the flowering bush attracts prosperity and emotional abundance • linked also with the golden oriole bird that migrates between Europe and central and South Africa and sings to establish its territory • the flowering shrub or flowers are a talisman for any creative or performing ventures and for claiming your place in the sun

HOW TO USE

Spread the dried flowers and/or bronze leaves across a map of where you wish to travel, especially for fall or winter vacations (see where most land if you are undecided of your location). • Tip the petals and leaves outdoors (wait for a windy day) and ask the oriole bird to carry you on its wings to where you most want to be. • Surround yourself with golden flowerheads and light a circle of red or gold candles for Oriel/Uriel. • Blow on each candle, asking that specific restrictions in your life will be lifted and that you will be given the opportunities and resources to fulfill what may seem to be impossible dreams. • Blow out the candles one by one and put your flowerheads in a bowl of water in the center of your home until they fade as a reminder of the golden future you can make.

CAUTION

The golden oriole azalea is toxic to humans and pets.

Aztec Pearl Choisya

(*Choisya × dewitteana* 'Aztec Pearl')

MAGICAL FORMS

also called Mexican orange (*Choisya ternata* 'Sundance') • evergreen shrubs with glossy green leaves (the Sundance version having golden-yellow foliage) • Aztec Pearl buds are pearl-shaped and pale pink opening into star-shaped pure white, very fragrant flowers in late spring and again often in the fall • has golden-yellow leaves, while the leaves of Aztec Pearl are narrower, resulting in a less dense appearance • native to southern North America, Arizona, New Mexico, Texas, and Mexico • growing in other areas of the US, the UK, and southern Europe • though hardy, choisya does not tolerate frost • choisya shrubs have an orange-like fragrance in flowers and leaves, but do not produce oranges • magically use the growing plant in gardens or containers; as cut flowers; the blossoms, fresh and dried; and the leaves, especially the Sundance golden kind

PLANET AND ELEMENT

Sun • Fire

MAGICAL USES

a plant of the thirtieth wedding anniversary, pearl, as a garden gift or as part of a bouquet • associated with marriage, second or even third time around, especially for an older couple • instead of orange blossoms at weddings, especially at exotic weddings • the Aztec pearl flowerheads, buds, and/or Sundance leaves for prosperity and abundance charm bags

HOW TO USE

Bruise fresh leaves or hold the blossoms to inhale the orange fragrance (its scent and flowers resemble ordinary orange blossoms) to fill yourself with confidence and a sense of your own beauty/charisma if you have problems with body image or someone has denigrated your sexuality. • Meditate on the flowering plant to fill yourself with sun power when you need a burst of energy or enthusiasm or to generate it in others. • Add to a silver charm bag the dried star-shaped flowers (if fresh ones are not growing), dried silver buds from the Aztec Pearl choisya, and dried gold Sundance leaves with a small pearl, to carry to an audition, a presentation, an interview, or a social event where you want to make a major impression or need to take center stage.

Babassu

(*Attalea speciosa*)

MAGICAL FORMS

a palm tree with feathery leaves, growing wild in northeastern Brazil, with hard-shelled nuts in bunches of up to six hundred with one or two kernels in each • the nuts provide pale yellow babassu oil that is used for cooking and medicinally in South America • as a beauty product ingredient and in carrier oil to dilute essential oils in the Western world • resembling the heavier and stronger smelling and tasting coconut oil in its health-bringing properties • magically use the oil

PLANETS AND ELEMENT

Venus/Moon • Water

MAGICAL USES

as a carrier oil with essential oils or alone • mixes well with most oils and melts at body temperature from its creamy white more solid form at room temperature • for abundance and attracting success that may not seem possible • bringing harmony and sense of well-being to a mutual massage where one partner is uptight or cynical • in magical cookery with its soft nutty taste and mild smell for promoting a sense of well-being and kinship

HOW TO USE

As a Moon Goddess oil, anoint the womb or genitals with a single drop to call fertility at full moon. • Use the melting oil in a warm room, mixed with a drop or two of lemon essential oil or concentrated lemon juice, to bless wooden magical tools and wands and to polish wood in your home or workplace. • Make first counterclockwise and then clockwise circles to remove all negative influences and protect from future harm, spite, or potential loss of money and resources. • Massage yourself, especially your inner wrists for your heart energy center, with the oil to enhance radiance if you are feeling unattractive or past your sell-by date.

CAUTION

Avoid if pregnant, on blood thinner medication, or suffering from hyperthyroidism.

Baby Blue Eyes

(*Nemophila menziesii*)

MAGICAL FORMS

so called because two out of three species of the flowers are bright blue like a baby's eyes • sometimes called the Californian bluebell • a wild herb and garden plant, native to California, Oregon, and Baja California, that has spread to other states and will grow in the UK and Europe • six to twelve inches tall and with six petals, the number of Venus whose flower it is and so associated with romance • can bloom all summer • magically use the growing flower, wild if you need more spontaneity; the cut flower; the petals, fresh and dried; and as a flower essence

PLANET AND ELEMENT

Venus • Water

MAGICAL USES

a suggested flower for the forty-fifth wedding anniversary, sapphire, if you prefer an informal occasion • for a woodland wedding or informal commitment ceremony • in rituals for healing the inner child damaged by early relationship trauma with the father, especially for men who have become overly macho as a result • rituals connected with babies and children's health and happiness, particularly if a child is shy, withdrawn, or lacks contact with the father

HOW TO USE

On the crescent moon, if you have a body image problem, eating disorder, or are teased about your appearance, light a pale blue candle and encircle it with six dried baby blue eyes petals. Pass a pale blue angelite or blue lace agate crystal carefully around the candle clockwise six times. Extinguish the candle and with it your doubts and fears. Scoop up the petals with the angelite, and carry them in a blue charm bag as a reminder you are worthy of respect and admiration. • Spray the mist of the flower essence in water around your aura energy field to connect with your real self if you feel you are playing a role to please others.

Baby's Tears

(*Soleirolia soleirolii*)

MAGICAL FORMS

also known as angel's tears and mind your own business • as *Soleirolia soleirolii* 'Aurea' with gold foliage and *Soleirolia soleirolii* 'Variegata/Silver Queen' with silver-gray foliage • related to the nettle family but without its sting, this amazingly versatile plant forms a dense delicate green mat of round or bean-shaped leaves on short fleshy stems • blossoming late spring into delicate white flowers, forming the tears • grows outdoors in warm climates as ground cover, in rock gardens or hanging baskets, even in lawns and along ponds • indoors as a houseplant • baby's tears are much underrated magically, mainly used as a focus where it grows • magically use the growing plant and fresh or dried leaves and flowers

PLANET AND ELEMENTS

Saturn • Earth/Water

MAGICAL USES

first discovered in Corsica by French botanist Joseph-François Soleirol in the mid-nineteenth century • made popular in the USA in the mid-twentieth century • grown now around the world, indoors and out • mix golden *Soleirolia soleirolii* 'Aurea' with the silver leaves of *Soleirolia soleirolii* 'Variegata/Silver Queen' in an amulet bag for increasing wealth • considered good luck if planted in a vivarium or around a pond

HOW TO USE

Resembling hair hanging down in a basket or display, the plant lives up to its "mind your own business" name. • Kneel and whisper your secrets close to the plant, and it is said to hold them safe. • Grow the plant in your garden or indoors so that your family will never know sadness or loss (the plant has experienced the tears for you). • As angel's tears, meditate where baby's tears are growing in your lawn or rockery or with your houseplant, asking for connection with the angels to take away present worries and sorrows from your life, especially when the tiny flowers are blooming.

CAUTION

While nontoxic to humans or pets, it can occasionally cause skin irritation if touched.

Bakul Tree

(*Mimusops elengi*)

MAGICAL FORMS

also called the bakula tree, as well as the Spanish cherry tree • tree with tiny, highly fragrant yellow-white flowers, called perpetual flowers, as they bloom continuously from March to June • they are considered sacred in Buddhism and Jainism and are made as offerings to Lord Ganesha in Hinduism • the tree is native to southern and southeastern Asia and northern Australia and now grown in China • the dried flowers, which retain their fragrance, are worn as necklaces by women in India • the trees are found with their deep-green leafy branches in temple courtyards • magically use the fresh or dried flowers, or Hari Leela incense, which is made from the flowers

PLANET AND ELEMENT

Moon • Water

MAGICAL USES

use as daytime background incense • aids yoga, meditation, and energy transference work

HOW TO USE

Add the dried flowers or incense to a charm bag for self-love and self-confidence if you have been made to feel inadequate by spiteful peers or critical relatives. • Carry the flowers or incense charm bag on a date or if you are nervous about attending a special event, inhaling the fragrance to radiate charisma. • Burn the incense to create a sacred space for ritual and personal time out if you feel you are losing your identity beneath the demands of others.

Balloon Flower

(*Platycodon grandiflorus*)

MAGICAL FORMS

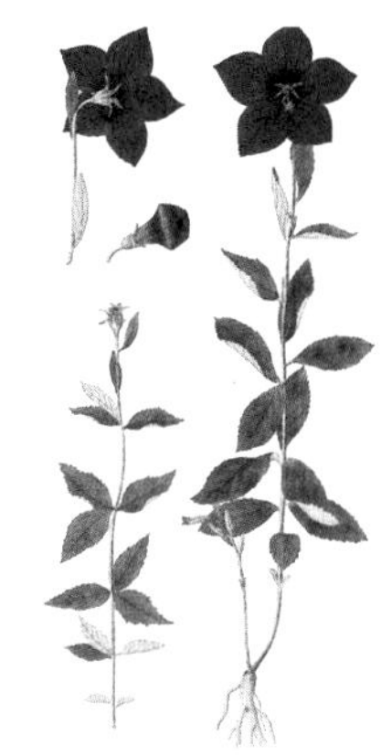

also called bellflower • the balloon-type flower opens to reveal the five-pointed flower • native to China, Japan, Korea, and Russia, it can grow as a houseplant in an indoor container garden • flourishes in the northeast, and in many other areas, of the USA • starting to become more obtainable in the UK • blooms all summer with intense violet color, also pink and white • the five-pointed flowers are magically highly significant • magically use the whole plant in situ and flowers, fresh or dried

PLANETS AND ELEMENT

Jupiter/Mercury • Air

MAGICAL USES

a sixth wedding anniversary flower for a very settled couple and a reminder that they can still have fun (candy as well as iron are the anniversary gifts) • the puffing up and popping open of the flower represent the release of magical power • the five points of the flower represent the five elements of Tao: wood, water, fire, earth, metal • in Wicca and other nature spiritualities, Earth, Air, Fire, Water, and in the center Spirit or Ether, the coming together of the elements

HOW TO USE

Place the cut flowers in your home or workplace where chi can circulate all around, bringing health, wealth, and harmony. • Send the flowers, before they open, to a loved one far away or to someone who is estranged, saying *I wish for your return, as these flowers unfold, I offer you my love.*

CAUTION

Valued medicinally and in cooking for centuries in China, Japan, and Korea, all parts of the raw plant are often considered toxic in the Western world. • However, the California Poison Control System says balloon flowers are not toxic, depending on the dosage and preparation. • Seek expert advice.

Balsam of Tolu

(*Myroxylon balsamum* var. *balsamum*)

MAGICAL FORMS

not to be confused with the related *Myroxylon balsamum* var. *pereirae*, the Peru balsam tree, which is also a species of the *Myroxylon balsamum* tree • a slow-growing, tall, white, flowering, rainforest tree • leaves and fruits are used by local populations • most commonly tapped for its resin from live trees • resin is initially brown, semifluid, and sticky • gradually becomes solid but brittle until melted as incense • native to South and Central America • has been introduced into southern Florida, Ceylon, India, and West Africa • magically use as resin incense made from its sap, which may be deep red; use also as essential oil made from the resin, with a warm vanilla-like fragrance

PLANET AND ELEMENT

Moon • Water

MAGICAL USES

for mediumship and calling benign spirits to manifest in the dense smoke • to reduce a sense of isolation and loneliness that can prevent social contact

HOW TO USE

Diffuse the oil or burn the incense before meditation to induce a trancelike state to connect with higher realms and past worlds of ancient civilizations. • Mix with other incenses, such as benzoin, cassia, black copal, juniper, patchouli, or sandalwood, to ease heartache and heartbreak. • Use only a little tolu balsam on charcoal as it will liquefy when heated. • Burn it to bring money through creative gifts.

CAUTION

The tolu balsam oil can, like the products of the Peru balsam variety, cause allergic reactions. • Dilute the oil well, and do a patch test if applying topically. • Tolu balsam has not been adequately researched, though it has been used as a folk medicine among the Indigenous people for thousands of years. • Seek expert advice if pregnant or regularly taking medication.

Balsam Tree, Arabian

(*Commiphora gileadensis*)

MAGICAL FORMS

also known as *Commiphora opobalsamum* • there are several forms in the modern world including the North American *Populus* × *jackii*, a tall hybrid between the eastern cottonwood and balsam poplar (*Populus deltoides* × *Populus balsamifera*) • *Commiphora gileadensis* is a medium-sized, fragrant evergreen tree growing in Yeman, Oman, Saudi Arabia, East Africa, Sudan, and southeastern Egypt • its aromatic sap hardens as sticky red resin used as incense or dissolved in oil • it has been identified, arguably, as the source of the biblical perfume Balm of Gilead • Balm of Gilead was used as a ceremonial incense twice a day in the Temple of Jerusalem, and is still a sacred incense in formal rituals and prized as an exotic, heady perfume • magically use the resin, incense, oil, and perfume

PLANETS AND ELEMENTS

Mercury/Venus • Earth/Water

MAGICAL USES

as incense, brings visions of other dimensions and spirits • protection • healing • purification of an area to be used for ritual magick • increases sensual pleasure

HOW TO USE

Carry the incense, resin, or the sticky buds in a red bag as a love amulet, to mend a broken heart, and attract new love. • Burn the incense or the oil or inhale the fragrance from a diffuser to connect with benign spirits and Ascended and Light Beings. • Burn or diffuse to add a spiritual dimension to lovemaking. • Rub the diluted oil into a white candle that is lit to bring wealth. • Pairs well with golden topaz in healing and prosperity ceremonies.

Balsam Tree, Gurjun

(*Dipterocarpus turbinatus*)

MAGICAL FORMS

grows in India and Asia • tall, with a canopy that stands above many other trees, reaching upward to the sky • introduced to Europe by medieval Middle Eastern traders • the oil is also produced in Europe and the USA, though the tree is in danger of extinction in its native lands • magically use as essential oil or empowered perfume

PLANET AND ELEMENT

Moon • Water

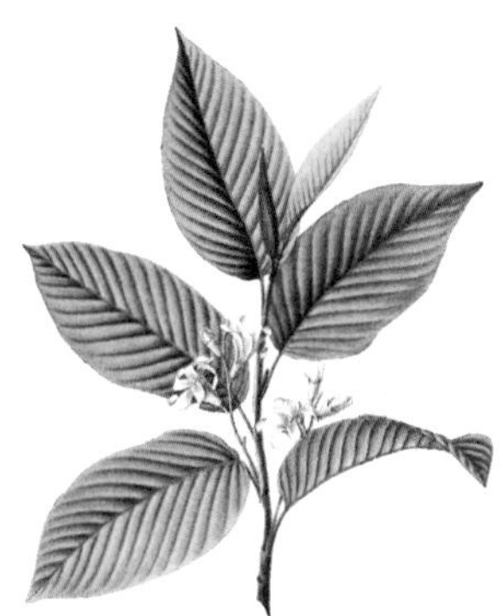

MAGICAL USES

brings youthfulness and calm to any environment • removes anxiety before challenging social situations and tests • inspires ambitions and positive solutions • for self-sufficiency and self-reliance

HOW TO USE

Add the oil to potpourri or diffuse to inspire all creative work and overcome artistic blockages. • Anoint the center of your hairline, your Crown energy center, with the diluted oil to reveal your talents at interviews and during assessments, examinations, auditions, and creative performances if you are aiming for the top. • Alternatively, to shine in any situation, wear a fragrance containing gurjun balsam. • At the end of the day, diffuse the oil to restore calm so you will not be buzzing all night.

CAUTION

Avoid if pregnant or breastfeeding.

Balsam Tree, Peru

(*Myroxylon balsamum* var. *pereirae*)

MAGICAL FORMS

related to Tolu balsam, a large tropical tree, native from Mexico to South America, especially San Salvador • prized by the Mayans, Incas, and Aztecs for medicinal and ceremonial purposes, Peru balsam was exported during the Spanish colonization to Europe and Asia and was once considered as precious as gold or silver • blooms with small, white, fragrant flowers • all parts of the tree contain the resin, which is dark brown or amber and semisolid • magically use the resin as incense on charcoal (remove seed from the fruit beforehand if included in the mix) or the essential oil

PLANET AND ELEMENT

Sun • Fire

MAGICAL USES

burn the incense or burn or diffuse the essential oil to catch glimpses of other dimensions and to dedicate yourself or reconnect with a spiritual cause or path if life or others have intruded

HOW TO USE

Prepare a room before private or guided communal meditation or visualization, yoga, or energy transference therapy sessions by adding the oil to small dishes of potpourri, then placing it near exercise mats or a massage couch. • Burn the resin with dry incenses to see guardian spirits, angels, and wise ancestors within the thick white smoke and to send prayers, or use the incense as an offering. • Burn or diffuse the oil or incense in formal rituals for the Air element as a substitute for other balsams (especially balsam of mecca, which is very hard to obtain), where healing is sought from higher sources. • If love has let you down or been denied, inhale oil dabbed or spritzed on a tissue or cotton ball, or apply a mini-roller or portable aroma tube diffuser whenever you sense or see the subject of your affections approaching to give you the necessary detachment and perhaps gently open or reopen channels between you.

CAUTION

Avoid the oil during pregnancy and breastfeeding. • Dilute the oil before using topically.

Bamboo

(*Bambusa vulgaris*)

MAGICAL FORMS

magically use the whole, growing plant; leaves; shoots; and as wooden stakes

PLANET AND ELEMENT

Moon • Water

MAGICAL USES

for immense good fortune • prosperity • protective from physical, psychological, and psychic harm, specifically for breaking hexes • granting wishes

HOW TO USE

Display nine potted lucky bamboo plants, each tied with nine red ribbon knots, and each holding a lucky Chinese divinatory coin, to mark the boundaries of a magical outdoor garden or as part of an indoor garden or workplace. • Attach wishes written on paper to growing plants with three red strings. • Break hexes by crushing the bamboo to powder and burning. • A potted or growing bamboo near the entrance, indoors or out, deters evil spirits. • A bamboo flute, however inexpertly played, attracts good spirits.

CAUTION

Do not ingest while pregnant.

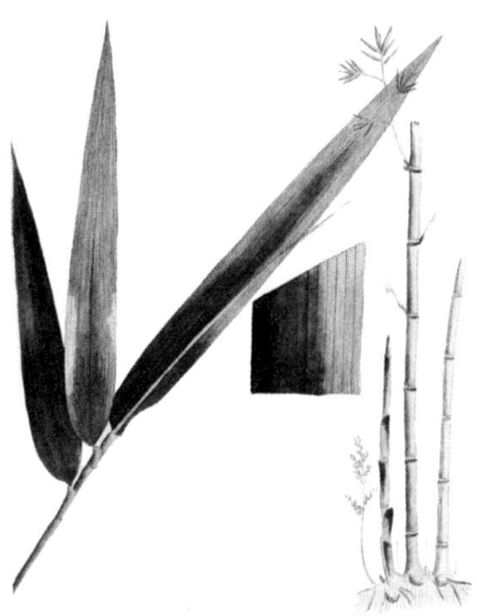

Banana

(*Musa* spp.)

MAGICAL FORMS

not a tree since it does not have a woody stem, but a large upright stalk from which bright green leaves grow • exotic flowers come in spring to be replaced by the ripening fruit • magically use mainly the whole, growing plant and fruit, but also the leaves and flowers

PLANETS AND ELEMENT

Moon/Venus • Water

MAGICAL USES

eating bananas absorbs the magick in empowerments and wishes for fertility, male potency, prosperity • especially favorable to those in the middle years • even as an indoor banana plant that does not bear fruit or a colder weather banana plant (most flourish in more tropical climates), the banana plant is a luck bringer to home or business • meditating on a banana plant or a bunch of the fruit, with its upward-reaching fingers, symbolizes and aids spiritual connections, shamanic travel, and reaching other worlds

HOW TO USE

To be married, hold a handfasting or commitment ceremony or make love beneath a large banana plant to bring prosperity, happiness, and fertility to the relationship. • Carry a banana in your travel bag to eat on or just before a journey to guard against accidents, loss of luggage or documents, and harm while traveling, especially by plane or road. • The skin, dried and crushed into powder, in a charm bag brings sexual stamina and protects against sexual cruelty. • On a nature altar, use a banana, as the God symbol along with a coconut or any round fruit with skin or shell for the Goddess, for fertility, sex magick, and increased libido rites. • Substitute large banana leaves and coconut shells on the altar instead of dishes in your nature rites.

CAUTION

If you are allergic to latex you may wish to avoid eating bananas.

Banana Flower Blossom Essence

derived from (*Musa × paradisiaca* L. *Nana*)

MAGICAL FORMS

from a range of exotic African Canarian essences • a crystal extracts the essence from the flower, which adds the living power of the crystal to the life force of the flower • distills the sheer power of the banana tree, including the way the white flowers grow within the trunk and ascend straight to the light, into pure yang energy • magically use the flower essence

PLANET AND ELEMENT

Moon • Water

MAGICAL USES

stimulates male sexuality, especially if work pressures get in the way and drain libido • can help couples when there is an inability by one partner to express feelings of affection and spiritual connection during and through lovemaking, as well as physical passion • assists to maintain opinions and viewpoints and clear cognitive focus in stressful situations or when being talked down to, when others are deliberately muddying the waters

HOW TO USE

If you are constantly pressured at work to meet unreasonable deadlines, complete a constant stream of urgent tasks, or make instant decisions, add a drop of the essence to spiky or carnivorous plants in your workspace to create a barrier of personal authority that will discourage others from approaching you unnecessarily. • If you swing between overassertiveness and backing off immediately when challenged, sip a drop or two of the essence mixed with water throughout the day to feel your balance restored. You can also drink the essence during a meeting where you need to speak or in your water bottle to remind yourself and others of your competence.

CAUTION

Banana blossom flower essence is safe, as it does not contain the physical qualities of the plant. However, if you are allergic to latex or have diabetes, check with an expert before using.

Banyan Tree

(*Ficus benghalensis*)

MAGICAL FORMS

also called Indian banyan and banyan fig • national tree of India • among the largest trees in the world because of its huge horizontal spread • some are more than 2,500 years old • aerial roots may form a tangle of secondary trunks • a banyan can have up to three thousand roots on a full-grown tree • native to southern Asia, Thailand, India, Burma, southern China • flourishes in the south of Florida and Hawaii, where it is also considered sacred • also grown as indoor potted plants and bonsais • magically use the leaves, fruit (not edible), figs, bark, and aerial roots

PLANET AND ELEMENT

Jupiter • Air

MAGICAL USES

sacred in Hinduism: Lord Vishnu in the bark, Lord Brahma, the roots, and Lord Shiva the branches • planted close to temples, Shiva is often portrayed sitting in the shade of banyan trees • a good tree to seek out on vacation and sit beneath to absorb its connection with the spirit world • brings good fortune, marital happiness • long life sought for a partner or beloved family member

HOW TO USE

If you can obtain a banyan leaf from a potted plant, bonsai, or an actual tree, etch on it invisibly with the index finger of your writing hand a special wish. Keep your leaf preserved between tissue or parchment paper between the pages of a heavy book until the wish materializes or the leaf is preserved. • Because it is called the strangler tree since it grows around a host tree (though the hollow inside is used beneficially by birds, small animals, and insects), cut a single root into pieces to break the stranglehold of a possessive relationship, restrictive practices, or takeover bids in business.

CAUTION

Although used medicinally for thousands of years in Ayurveda, should not be taken without expert advice, in excess, or while pregnant or breastfeeding, as effects are not yet well researched.

Baobab Tree

(*Adansonia digitata*)

MAGICAL FORMS

swollen trunk • one of the widest trees in the world, up to a hundred feet in diameter, holding up to 2,540 pints of water • indigenous to South Africa, Madagascar, and northwestern Australia • in the USA mainly grown in pots • magically use the dried and fresh leaves and dried fruit

PLANET AND ELEMENTS

Saturn • Earth/Water

MAGICAL USES

in Aboriginal myth the baobab tree, called gadawon or larrgadi, was punished for its arrogance by being pulled from the earth and replanted upside down • regarded as the Tree of Life because it has life-giving water in its trunk and branches • may live more than two thousand years • called also the miracle tree in Eritrea, eastern Africa, where there is a shrine to the Virgin Mary within a baobab tree • in World War II, two Italian soldiers were saved when a direct bomb on the tree under which they were sheltering failed to explode as they prayed for deliverance • use in rituals for antiaging, prophetic and happy dreams, to release money and opportunities, and as a gateway to the spiritual world

HOW TO USE

If you find a baobab tree (worth seeking on vacation or days out: there are five in the ArtsPark in Hollywood, Florida, and they can also be found in southern California and southern Florida), or using your potted baobab, put both hands on the trunk to free up trapped emotions within you, stagnant feelings, or situations. • Buy powdered dried baobab leaves or dried powdered fruit online, and place it in a charm bag to fill you with inspiration. • Hide it in your home if you have an undemonstrative or financially mean partner.

CAUTION

The fruit powder is generally considered safe, but avoid ingesting any part of the baobab if you are pregnant, breastfeeding, or trying to conceive, as it may interfere with fertility.

Barberry

(*Berberis* spp.)

MAGICAL FORMS

varies from dwarf varieties to quite tall so will fit in any garden or wildlife area • some species of Oregon grape are called barberry • magically use the leaves, berries, roots, and thorns

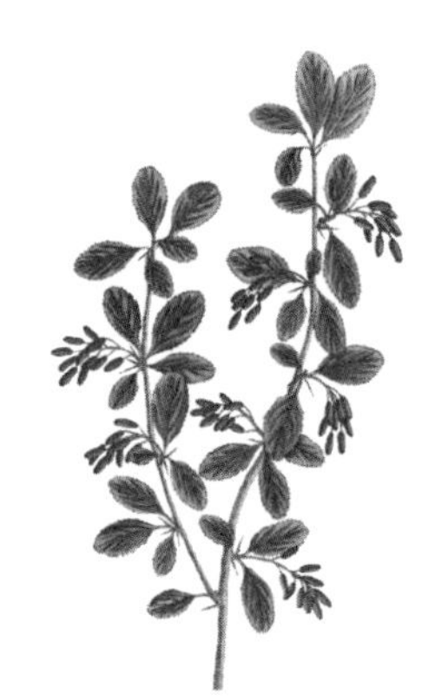

PLANET AND ELEMENT

Mars • Fire

MAGICAL USES

once called Holy thorn, because in Italy it was believed to be the crown of thorns Jesus wore • bars the home from all harm, when grown on a boundary • counteracts curses and hexes • takes away a sense of sorrow and evil in a new home that feels unlucky • magical cooking

HOW TO USE

Place the thorns and leaves in defensive spell jars and bottles. • If there are no thorns, substitute the dried berries and leaves for the thorns in spell jars and bottles. • Hide the root under a doorstep to bar the way from all who are ill-intentioned, earthly or paranormal. • Mixed with fennel, it makes a remedy from ancient Egyptian times to keep away illness (originally to prevent plague). • When defensive magick is to be practiced, place berries in a dish in the center of the altar to purify the ritual area and then pass the dish around the ritual circle before casting it.

CAUTION

Barberry is generally considered safe, but do not ingest excess quantities. • Avoid Japanese barberry, which is invasive, and choose a variety without thorns when very small children and pets are around, making sure they do not ingest it. • Do not use if pregnant or if you have a blood-clotting disease, diabetes, or low blood pressure.

Basil

(Ocimum basilicum)

MAGICAL FORMS

magically use the herb, dried or fresh leaves, well-diluted oil, and seeds from sweet basil

PLANET AND ELEMENT

Mars • Fire

MAGICAL USES

anti-bullying • guards against road rage • astral travel • conquers fear of flying • courage • divination with fire • fertility and male potency • good luck for new homes and house moves • increasing prosperity, especially to the home • love, fidelity • passion • purification and banishing harm, earthly and paranormal • protection of business premises, home, and vehicles against accidents, attack, and theft • water scrying

HOW TO USE

Use against intruders by hanging basil seeds in a net over the entrance. • For lovers, burn two leaves in a fire, one for each lover, to see if they come or stay together. • Burn leaves as options to questions, a leaf for each option. • Call fidelity in an absent partner by secretly surrounding baggage with dried basil circles before departure. • Add to charm bags. • Grow money by attaching Chinese coins to a strong growing basil plant. • Pour infusions down inside water drains to stop money from flowing out. • Use in magical cookery or work with its energy in magical gardening. • Plant along pathways to draw in money. • Use for magical saltwater scrying by sprinkling the herb on the surface of the water.

CAUTION

The oil is a skin irritant for children and babies unless well diluted.

Basil, Holy

(Ocimum tenuiflorum)

MAGICAL FORMS

also known as tulsi or tulasi • aromatic leaves, native to the mint family • found throughout southeast Asia • can be grown perennially in the hottest parts of North America and also annually in more temperate regions worldwide or as a houseplant • a part of the Ayurvedic healing tradition • magically use the whole plant, dried leaves in teas, and flowers, fresh and dried

PLANET AND ELEMENT

Sun • Fire

MAGICAL USES

a sacred plant in Hinduism, regarded as an embodiment of Lakshmi, goddess of abundance and light, and also associated with Lords Vishnu and Krishna • in this tradition, used in daily spiritual connections and the major commemoration of the cycle of life from weddings to funerals and rebirth • revered also within Christianity and used in making holy water in the Greek Orthodox church • can be used to cleanse sacred space, as well as in rituals to awaken the high spiritual self • increases life force

HOW TO USE

Drink the leaf tea or meditate on the fresh or dried purple blossoms to become aware of your spiritual guides and guardians. • Carry the dried, chopped herb in a charm bag for ongoing prosperity, health, and happiness. • Hang a sachet over the front door so that only good energies will enter and family and friends leave their troubles and any negative feelings outside. • Grow as potted plants or in the garden to create a protective boundary of harmony, as well as to keep away ill fortune and to welcome house guardians.

CAUTION

Avoid ingesting leaves or tea during pregnancy or while breastfeeding.

Basil, Lemon

(*Ocimum × africanum*)

MAGICAL FORMS

a hybrid between sweet basil (*Ocimum basilicum*) and American basil (*Ocimum americanum*), a member of the mint family • more commonly known as *Ocimum basilicum citriodorum* • also known as Thai lemon basil • lemon basil was and still is popular in Southeast Asia and northeastern Africa as a medicinal and culinary herb, reaching North America in the seventeenth century • mainly grown in gardens or specialty outlets rather than commercially in spite of its combination of lemon fragrance and anise-like taste • magically use the fresh and dried white flowers, which appear from late summer to mid-fall; the chopped or whole, growing plant, dried; and as tea

PLANETS AND ELEMENTS

Mars/Moon • Fire/Water

MAGICAL USES

fiercely defensive for creating barriers around the self in a hostile or overcompetitive environment • offer in a bouquet for a marriage proposal • brought back from their explorations and conquests by the ancient Greeks and used as a symbol of grief and an expression of mourning

HOW TO USE

Drink the tea for facing intimidation with words rather than actions. • Plant in a memorial place in the garden or in a pot indoors or where pets are buried to honor loved ones who have passed. • Carry as a love token if you lack the words or courage to approach a desired romantic interest.

CAUTION

Popular in Ayurveda, lemon basil leaves and flowers are edible for humans and not toxic to animals but should not be taken in excess. • Seek expert advice before using during pregnancy.

Basswood/Linden Tree

(*Tilia* spp.)

MAGICAL FORMS

common names for two trees in the *Tilia* genus, of which there are approximately thirty species • the common lime, or European linden (*Tilia × europaea*), grows throughout the USA, as well as the UK and Europe • linden trees, as they are usually called in the USA, are related closely to basswood trees • not the same species as the citrus lime tree (*Citrus aurantifolia*; see "Lime," p. 266) • the silver linden, *Tilia tomentosa*, is widely planted across the eastern USA • the silver linden has silver-green leaves in the summer and scented pale-lemon flowers emerging later from a bud than most of the species, which are very magical • magically use the growing tree, often with fragrant yellow flowers drooping down in bunches, heart-shaped leaves, and smooth, gray bark

PLANETS AND ELEMENTS

Venus/Jupiter • Water/Air

MAGICAL USES

the linden is considered sacred in eastern Europe, giving protection against evil spirits, curses, and storms • the tree was made into offerings in Lithuania in thanks for healing sorrows and sickness and to grant petitions • used in rituals for good fortune, long life, love, and marriage

HOW TO USE

The silver linden's heart-shaped leaves and fresh or dried yellow flowers can be made into a love charm, to be carried in a silk purse when you know you will meet the object of your desire socially. • If they do not notice you, scatter the contents of the bag on the path they have taken and say softly, *Silver tree, bring back to me [name], that we together soon shall be.* • Linden flowers and lavender mixed together in a sleep pillow aid insomnia and bring peaceful dreams. • Carve or write the name or number of your home on the bark of any of the *Tilia* genus trees. • Set the bark in a plant pot just inside your front door if you must go away and leave your house empty.

Basswood Tree, American

(*Tilia americana*), (*Tilia caroliniana*), or (*Tilia heterophylla*)

MAGICAL FORMS

Tilia americana is the only true basswood native to North America, from Maine to North Carolina and west to Missouri • introduced into the UK in 1752 • several cultivars/variations of the American basswood, including Carolina basswood (*Tilia caroliniana*) in southeastern USA and west to Texas, often found in temperate European botanical gardens and arboretums • the white basswood (*Tilia heterophylla*) grows in the Appalachian Mountains and, like other basswoods, is much beloved by bees • fragrant, yellowish-white flowers hang down in starry clusters • magically use the fibrous inner bark, or bast; the whole, growing tree; the fresh and dried leaves; and the fresh or dried flowers

PLANETS AND ELEMENTS

Venus/Jupiter • Water/Air

MAGICAL USES

creativity • Star magick and for Star souls • attracting love • enchantments to attract a desired lover or call one back • magical love teas

HOW TO USE

Use the fibrous inner bark as twine in knot magick, soaked and then boiled to separate fibers, to bind a lover to be true and to prevent love rivals from acting maliciously. • Make wands for rituals for uncovering truth, women's rites of passage, fair judgments, and justice. • Use the dried flowers, leaves, and bark as teas empowered to heal love. • Burn in incense on bonfires or hearth fires with wood chips for fidelity and to purify the home against malevolent land and earth spirits.

CAUTION

Do not use in excess medicinally, nor if you are pregnant, as not enough is known, if you have heart disease, or if you are taking diuretic medicine.

Bay Laurel Leaf

(*Laurus nobilis*)

MAGICAL FORMS

aromatic evergreen tree with smooth leaves • magically use the leaves, herb, tree, and oil

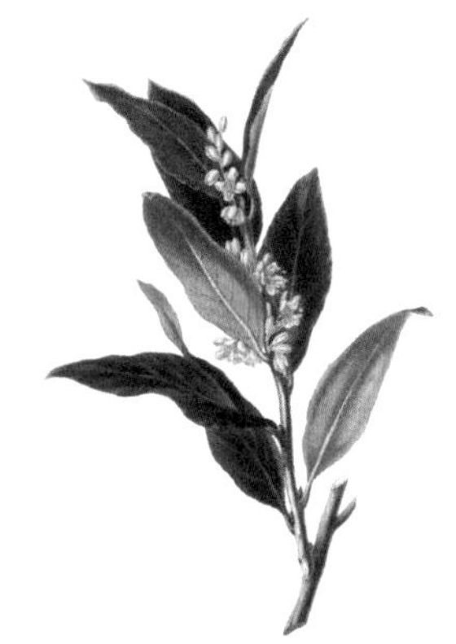

PLANET AND ELEMENT

Sun • Fire

MAGICAL USES

for fidelity in marriage • loyalty in all relationships • good fortune • health • attracting money • protects against lightning, poltergeists, curses, hexes, and misfortune • preserving happiness and security of property • brings victory

HOW TO USE

Burn as incense to increase psychic powers, especially clairsentience. • Place under pillows to bring dreams of the future. • Hang at windows or entrances to repel earthly and paranormal harm. • Mix with sandalwood and burn as incense to remove curses and hexes. • Plant near the front door to protect against sickness. • Scratch the same wish on a dried culinary bay leaf every day for seven days, and release each one to the winds. • As a symbol of lasting love, a bay twig is broken in half and one half kept by each lover when apart. • Attach coins to a bay tree for nine days and then cast into flowing water on the full moon to call money by the next full moon. • Create a fertility sachet, and then bury it on the full moon beneath a thriving bay tree or potted plant.

CAUTION

Bay leaves can be harmful to dogs, cats, and horses.

Bayberry

(*Myrica cerifera*) and (*Morella pensylvanica*)

MAGICAL FORMS

Myrica cerifera is also known as southern bayberry and *Morella pensylvanica* is also known as northern bayberry • small shrubs/trees native to North and Central America and the Caribbean with fragrant foliage, the *Morella pensylvanica* especially is found in eastern North America • the trees are grown for their silvery gray berries collected October through November or later • used in Yuletide aromatic bayberry candles and in making soaps • the berries are boiled and the wax extracted from the surface of the water • grown more widely around the world but not in Australia • magically use ready-made candles and dried berries any time of the year • alternatively grow your own shrub to make your own candles or buy the wax from a craft store

PLANET AND ELEMENT

Saturn • Earth

MAGICAL USES

fragrant candles from the *Morella pensylvanica* berries at Yule were first described by Robert Beverley in 1705 • the tree was said to give shelter to the Holy Family • lovers parted at Yule will be united through the delicate fragrance wherever they burn their bayberry candle • burning it all the way down on Christmas Eve brings luck throughout the year ahead

HOW TO USE

Add dried berries to a business prosperity charm bag. • Burn a bayberry candle completely, having scratched on the side with a pin the amount of money you need. • Sprinkle the powdered root in a jar of coins until it is full. Seal the jar and shake it every morning in the week before Christmas to draw money, family happiness, and business opportunities to you.

CAUTION

The berries are considered unsafe to ingest, especially by children, and while pregnant or breastfeeding. • Bayberry may cause an allergic reaction if applied to the skin. • Use bayberry medicinally only with advice and never in large quantities.

Beans, Green/Lima/Butter

(*Phaseolus vulgaris*)

MAGICAL FORMS

common bean, a flowering plant from the Fabaceae family • numerous varieties, growing either on an erect bush or climbing plant • bean plants produce beautiful flowers, especially green beans, whose pod is edible • flowers may be red, white, or the color of the bean • magically use the whole growing plant; beans, often in magical cookery

PLANET AND ELEMENTS

Mercury • Earth/Air

MAGICAL USES

magical cookery to absorb wishes, according to what is added in the empowerment • especially potent if grown in the garden • one of the oldest edible plants, their magical purpose is celebrated in the children's fairy tale Jack and the Beanstalk, where from Jack's five magick beans an enormous beanstalk took him to danger and rich reward in the giant's lair in the sky • beans in modern magick likewise are concerned with rituals of small beginnings to succeed in a major goal involving obstacles and initiative by the spellcaster • to increase sexual potency

HOW TO USE

In love magick, seven beans are placed in a circle and concealed under fallen leaves or small twigs on the path a desired or hesitant lover will take. • Use beans to make an impromptu rattle and shake around the home to remove negative earth energies and create a barrier of sound to guard against hostile earthly influences. • An old folk spell from my childhood to trap a poltergeist or unfriendly ghost suggested leaving beans and dried flowers from the springtime (optional) overnight in an open jar near the center of the house saying, *Here is food for you to eat, rest enter here, for you I greet.* In the morning, seal the jar, take the jar away from the home, shake out the beans (and hopefully ghost) saying, *Your dark forces be gone, begone, and done.* Wash the jar in hot water when you get home and leave outdoors. • To remove warts, spots, or skin lesions, rub a perfectly round bean over the blemish and bury the bean saying, *As you decay so may this—and only beauty regrow, it shall be so.*

Beansprouts

(*Vigna radiata*)

MAGICAL FORMS

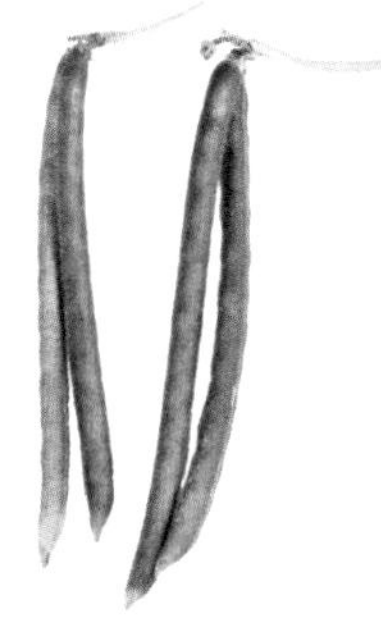

the most popular kind of these sprouting vegetables is from mung beans • the sprouts used in salad and Asian dishes such as stir-fries throughout the world • mung beans are upright plants or vines with clusters of yellow flowers at the top, pods becoming fuzzy and brown when mature • grown in Asia since ancient times • other popular forms of beansprouts come from soy beans • magically use beansprouts bought fresh from supermarkets or canned, or grow your own from mung beans or a chosen bean source

PLANET AND ELEMENT

Moon • Water

MAGICAL USES

eat the beansprouts, cooked or raw, for networking and bringing together new family members with existing ones • for acquiring money in numerous small amounts • grow beansprouts in a dark place for all new beginnings and business ventures in their early stages

HOW TO USE

Ask family or friends to join in cooking a stir-fry, adding beansprouts and making wishes for swift-moving ventures or relationships they seek. • As you grow your own beansprouts, which takes about a week (there are many online sites with precise instructions), endow the beans and the grown sprouts with whatever you want to manifest in your life (good for urgent matters), finally cutting the beansprouts free to mark freedom from all obstacles. • Shake beansprouts as you wash them in a colander to stir ongoing money coming your way fast.

CAUTION

Do not eat beansprouts raw if you are pregnant, older, or are medically vulnerable.

Bear Grass

(*Xerophyllum tenax*)

MAGICAL FORMS

also as *Xerophyllum asphodeloides*, turkey beard grass, and *Nolina matapensis*, Sonoran bear grass tree • the *Xerophyllum* forms have grasslike leaves • not true grasses, but from the corn lily family, native to North America • appearing in a huge variety of locations from subalpine forests, alpine meadows, high rocky elevations to desert regions • bear grass in all its forms becomes covered in small creamy flowers from late May to August depending on its location • magically use the cut ornamental grasses, fresh and dried, and the essence made from the flowers

PLANET AND ELEMENT

Saturn • Earth

MAGICAL USES

prevents outside influences, diverting or blocking intentions • overcomes fear of others' anger or disapproval • because bear grass is first to revive after fire, for all new beginnings • woven into baskets and used for adornment for centuries by Indigenous people • so named because young bears eat the tender stalks of grass and grizzlies use the leaves in their dens • the essence encourages a more creative, adaptable lifestyle

HOW TO USE

Add the foliage, sometimes sold with its creamy white, lilac-scented flowers (available online or from specialty florists) to wedding bouquets where the marriage is a second or subsequent one. • Use to mend a quarrel and to start afresh in a relationship, especially if ex-partners or stepchildren are causing trouble. • Sip the flower essence in water or add it to a water spritzer for your workspace to protect your aura energy field from intrusion or at home if overbearing relations are calling. • Use the essence regularly to discover or rediscover and reveal to the world your authentic self.

Bearberry

(*Arctostaphylos uva-ursi*)

MAGICAL FORMS

evergreen ground cover shrub with small leaves, shiny on the upper side • waxy bell-shaped pink flowers that give way to red shiny berries • native to Europe and found throughout the upper midwest of North America and Canada • berries are not generally eaten, though edible, but are loved by bears, hence the name • magically use any part of the plant dried, especially the leaves

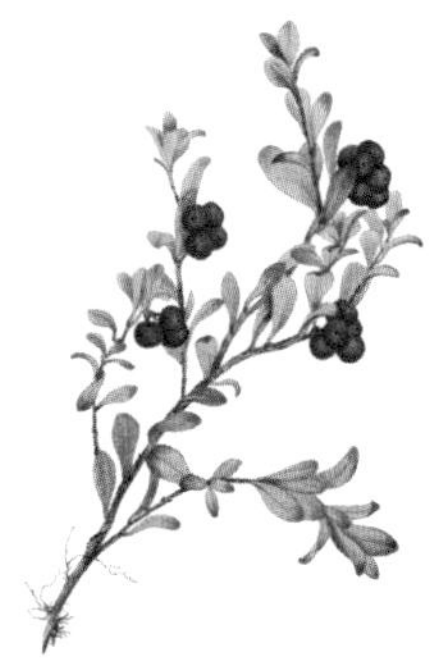

PLANET AND ELEMENT

Venus • Earth

MAGICAL USES

as incense or in a magical tea, made from fresh or dried leaves or from organic loose tea • increases psychic powers (traditionally used in sacred smoke mix by Native North American people) • for shape-shifting visions and shamanic rituals, especially involving bears • the tea shared for encouraging family traditions and the recalling of family legends

HOW TO USE

Sprinkle the dried leaves and flowers across the altar or a spell table to welcome the benign spirits. • Add dried berries to the dried leaves and flowers in a charm or medicine bag on vision quests or wilderness treks. • It is believed to protect children from all harm if they step over the dried leaves. • Tape a sachet of dried leaves to the underside of a doormat to extend the protection to family and visitors, and replace the sachet regularly, freeing the old leaves to the winds.

CAUTION

Avoid while pregnant or breastfeeding and if you have kidney disease.

Beech Tree

(*Fagus* spp.)

MAGICAL FORMS

in northern Europe, early manuscripts were written on thin tablets of beech wood and bound in beech boards, the name beech coming from the Anglo-Saxon and Germanic word for book • small edible nuts in fall, for animals, birds, and humans (with care) • magically use the branches; bark; leaves, especially the bronze leaves of the American beech (*Fagus grandifolia*) in the fall or the rare copper beech leaves from *Fagus sylvatica*; and nuts in their hard husks

PLANET AND ELEMENT

Saturn • Earth

MAGICAL USES

as wand for divining water and buried treasure • as a wand to call divine energy into a ritual circle • working with the husks and unripe nuts inside for preserving ancient wisdom and secret knowledge • the ability of a dying or apparently dead American beech to regenerate, assisted it is believed by living beeches around • for rituals to help those less fortunate personally, in community, and globally

HOW TO USE

A lucky talisman, the bark can be carried in a charm bag for success. • Alternatively, the bark can be powdered and a pinch put in the right shoe to guide the path to good fortune and advancement. • Burn in incense as chippings or powdered to increase creativity and formal learning. • Write wishes on beech leaves or small pieces of beech wood, and burn or bury them to allow the wishes to be fulfilled, not swiftly but in lasting ways. • For prosperity, display the dried or preserved copper leaves on a small branch from the American tree (in the fall) or the copper beech in your home or business.

CAUTION

Do not eat the nuts in excess as they do contain toxins, and, for security, roast them before eating. • Avoid eating them during pregnancy.

Beet

(*Beta vulgaris*)

MAGICAL FORMS

taproot of the beet plant, called beets in North America and beetroot in the UK • deep purple or dark red root vegetable, roasted, baked, boiled, or raw • the young green leaves are used in salad or boiled, tasting like spinach if they are older • beets can also be golden yellow, which is milder and sweeter, orange, or the Chioggia earthier sweet variety, pink-and-white striped inside • magically use the raw or cooked beets and leaves and the juice

PLANET AND ELEMENT

Saturn • Earth

MAGICAL USES

increases job opportunities • for all matters where practical action or input is needed • restores the reality principle in those prone to flights of fancy • use the juice instead of wine in a cleansing/purification ritual if a coven or psychic group has developed a toxic atmosphere

HOW TO USE

To attract love, trace invisibly on an uncut/uncooked/unpeeled golden or dark red/purple beet with your index finger, your name and that of your lover/desired love enclosed in a heart. Prepare the beet and eat or share it. • Use kvass, a fermented beetroot juice drink associated with the Norse god Kvasir, to invoke inspiration and poetry. • There is a low-alcohol version that is still popular in northeastern Europe and Russia that can also be used. • Generally pure beet juice or a meal including beets serves well as inspiration for creative writing, especially poetry. • Eat different shades of beets or different colored leaves to energize your rainbow aura energy field that surrounds you.

CAUTION

Eat beets in moderation. • Seek expert approval if pregnant, if you have low blood pressure, a tendency to low blood sugar, or gastrointestinal or liver problems, or if you suffer with gout.

Beet, White Sugar

(*Beta vulgaris* var. *saccharifera*)

MAGICAL FORMS

the white beetroot • white, conical, fleshy, root vegetable grown for its high sugar content • 20 percent of its contents are stored in the root • processed to extract sugar to make sucrose, molasses (see p. 293), and table sugar • while botanically linked, sugar beet is different from the purple vegetable beetroot (table beets in the USA) • sugar cannot be extracted from the purple table beet or beetroot • in contrast to sugarcane, sugar beet grows exclusively in temperate zones, especially in Russia, the USA, the UK, Turkey, France, and Germany • magically use the whole, unpeeled white beet or any of its products, such as organic beet sugar, molasses, or beet syrup (make your own syrup with water)

PLANET AND ELEMENT

Venus • Earth

MAGICAL USES

in spells, to sweeten people's attitudes or to make a gathering socially or at work more harmonious if there are going to be overly critical people present

HOW TO USE

If people take sugar in drinks, stir in the sugar clockwise before handing them the drink. When handing a drink to a would-be lover, touch their hand. If no one takes sugar, stir a teaspoon for every person present clockwise into a mug or jug of hot water, saying as you stir in each spoonful, *Sweet may our gathering be, filled with harmony*; leave until after the gathering, and, when cold, pour away under a running tap. • For fun and laughter, put sugar twists in baking paper and hide them in corners of a room before a celebration.

Begonia

(*Begonia* spp.)

MAGICAL FORMS

magically use the whole plant, especially a matching pair, and the flowers, fresh and dried

PLANET AND ELEMENT

Saturn • Earth

MAGICAL USES

warns of unreliable people • justice and court cases • anti-intrusive neighbors and gossip • love that faces opposition • bringing balance to a life that is all work • flower psychometry

HOW TO USE

To prevent workaholism or taking work worries home and conversely domestic anxieties into the office, set a begonia plant either side of your entrance. • Set a matching small potted begonia on either side of your workspace, and if one grows unduly, swap them over and beware of overload. • Add dried petals to a small brown bag with a brown agate or smoky quartz, empowered just after the full moon. Carry it to prevent gossip at work, or set next to a neighbor's adjoining wall or fence if they are rumor mongers. • Hide a tiny yellow bag of dried leaves and petals in your hand or pocket if you are meeting someone whose honesty you doubt. If possible, use your dominant hand (writing hand) to shake their hand or brush their hand or arm and you will feel either a positive or grating tingling in the bag. • Keep a small bowl of dried leaves and petals on top of any legal or official papers to strengthen your cause, and take a little of the mix with you to a hearing or investigation.

CAUTION

Begonia is toxic if ingested.

Bells of Ireland

(*Molucella laevis*)

MAGICAL FORMS

also known as the shellflower • called the Bells of Ireland because of the emerald green color of the large calyces holding the tiny fragrant white/purple flowers forming bells or shells, as Ireland is called the Emerald Isle • the shape and blooms of the Bells of Ireland have also been likened to the shape of an old Irish good-luck charm, another reason for its name and Celtic links, though it originated in western Asia • Bells of Ireland came to Europe in the sixteenth century and then traveled with the settlers to the USA and gained their present name and Irish associations in the twentieth century • magically use the whole, growing plant; cut flowers (half-open if fresh, fully opened if dried); and flower essence

PLANETS AND ELEMENTS

Venus/Saturn • Water/Earth

MAGICAL USES

in wedding bouquets, especially among those of Celtic origin • in many parts of the world used in St. Patrick's Day floral arrangements and parades • a symbol of good luck and said to give the ability to charm anyone with flattering words, sometimes called the gift of the blarney in Ireland

HOW TO USE

Use on the altar for Celtic rituals and while practicing Celtic tree stave divination. • Inhale the fragrance for awareness of past lives. • Meditate among the flowers to connect with nature spirits and the fae. • Crush and mix three dried calyces and flowers. Add three tiny green crystals and three silver-colored coins (they can be old ones not in circulation). Wrap them all in a green dollar tightly taped around the outside so the ends of the money bundle meet on top. Place this in a green bag so it all just fits, make a money wish, and bury the bag close to the plants saying, *I call on the luck of old Ireland to bring me wealth.* Do all this on St. Patrick's Day, March 17, and for luck put some coins in a collection box if possible during a parade. • For connecting with earth energies, use one of the long stems with attached calyces and flowers, having the whole plant facing downward. • Use it for dowsing for water or hidden treasure. • Place the cut flowers in the center of a nature or outdoor altar for earth rituals.

Benzoin Tree, Styrax

(*Styrax* spp.)

MAGICAL FORMS

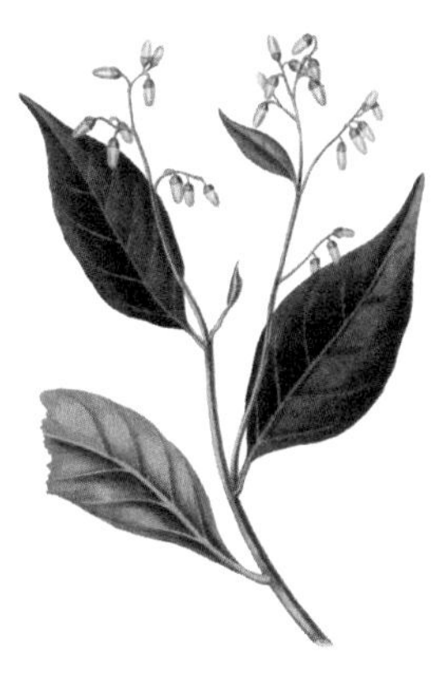

Styrax benzoin is also known as gum benjamin tree and Sumatra benzoin • *Styrax tonkinensis* is also known as Siam benzoin • two species of the tree commonly used to extract benzoin include *Styrax sumatra* and *Styrax siam* • has a vanilla-like fragrance • magically use the resin as incense, a magical fixative, and oil (dissolved in 30 percent ethylene glycol to make it the right consistency)

PLANET AND ELEMENTS

Sun • Fire/Air

MAGICAL USES

attracts riches and business success, promotion, or self-employment • as incense in ceremonial magick in any ritual or background to an empowerment • binding other nonresinous ingredients together in incense

HOW TO USE

In love magick, burn benzoin as incense with powdered cinnamon and basil to increase passion in a longstanding relationship or make a charm bag of the powdered ingredients, placing it beneath the mattress for spiritual as well as physical connection. • If you are a natural people pleaser or hold back socially, add a drop or two of sweet marjoram oil, a drop or two of benzoin, a drop or two of clary sage oil, and a drop of sweet orange to baths to create a sense of well-being.

CAUTION

Avoid benzoin if pregnant. • Do not ingest unless as part of an accepted remedy. • Though used medicinally as an ingredient in vaporizers and inhalers, some people have problems inhaling it. • Dilute the oil with carrier oil. • Siam benzoin is not used medicinally.

Bilberry

(*Vaccinium myrtillus*)

MAGICAL FORMS

the bilberry is a bush native to northern Europe, Scandinavia, Asia, the northern USA, and Canada and may grow wild in UK hedgerows • the berries are similar in appearance to blueberries, though smaller, and are called the new superfruit • small bell-like flowers become purple berries in the late summer and fall • magically use the berries, best when picked straight from the bush

PLANETS AND ELEMENT

Venus/Moon • Water

MAGICAL USES

called the *vision plant* in Japan • used in psychic work for increasing clairvoyant sight • also a remedy since the Middle Ages for eye complaints and eaten by the RAF during the Second World War to improve night vision • magical cookery • when the berries are eaten, raw or cooked, they offer protection against and removal of hexes and ill-wishing • associated with Lammas, the early August grain harvest celebrations • gathered at a festival held in Ireland on the last Sunday in July

HOW TO USE

Bake and serve empowered bilberry pies and cookies combined with flour for attracting abundance and financial fortune to the home. • Working with bilberries can offer awareness of unreliable people and situations before they manifest as a threat. • Powder the berries and sprinkle across thresholds and round boundaries, or burn in incense to create a safe space in the home if there is constant intrusion or external or internal hostility.

CAUTION

The leaves may be unsafe if eaten in excess or over a long period of time. • It is uncertain how safe bilberries are during pregnancy unless in normal food amounts. • They may react with certain cancer drugs, antidiabetes medicine, and blood thinners.

Birch Tree

(*Betula* spp.)

MAGICAL FORMS
silver birch (*Betula pendula*) is native to Europe, the UK, and Asia and grows across the USA in temperate zones • paper bark birch (*Betula papyrifera*) is native to Alaska, Canada, and the northern USA, often with orange or dark purple under-bark if grown in the UK • swamp birch or yellow or golden birch (*Betula alleghaniensis*) is native to northeastern North America • small to medium trees/shrubs found in temperate zones across the northern hemisphere • most birches have spectacular golden, fiery red, and orange leaves in the fall • magically use the growing tree, peeling bark of paper bark birch and silver birch, twigs, and branches

PLANET AND ELEMENT
Saturn • Earth

MAGICAL USES
one of the seven sacred Celtic trees, birch represents the first lunar month of the Celtic New Year calendar and is a feature of New Year celebrations throughout the northern hemisphere, to drive out the unwanted spirits of the old year • rituals for rebuilding ventures, projects, or traditions that have been destroyed • health • protection of animals and young children • used for cradles

HOW TO USE
Make or buy a birch staff or wand as a way opener, to become receptive to new influences and opportunities, especially in the natural world and for beginning the study of ancient wisdom. • Tie long birch twigs in a bundle with red ribbon to sweep out a home after illness, negativity, and stagnation. • Use fallen silver or paper bark, or during the fall the brilliantly colored leaves, to etch invisibly with your index finger, wishes for completion of tasks or rewards for efforts. • In old oracular style, leave them at the base of the tree to settle or blow free.

CAUTION
Although birch bark and other parts of the tree have been used in folk medicine for centuries, there are currently questions about its medicinal safety. • Do not ingest any part of the birch, especially the silver birch, except when approved by a medical practitioner. • Avoid during pregnancy.

Bird of Paradise

(*Strelitzia* spp.)

MAGICAL FORMS
also called the crane flower • includes *Strelitzia reginae*, with orange and blue flowers • native to South Africa, as landscape plants in warmer regions of the USA, including southern California, Florida, and Hawaii as well as other tropical lands • kept outside for part of the year in cooler climates • can be grown indoors • the official flower of Los Angeles • magically use the growing, flowering plant and cut flowers

PLANET AND ELEMENT
Jupiter • Air

MAGICAL USES
named after the colorful male birds of paradise, which display their exotic plumage to attract a mate • associated with the mythical golden phoenix of rebirth, the flowers and leaves resemble a bird in flight • a gift as a potted plant or in a bouquet for weddings, births, anniversaries (officially the ninth anniversary flower), relocation, or sympathy after loss • associated with empowerments for freedom from restrictions and breaking out of the comfort zone to use untapped potential

HOW TO USE
Cut a flowering outdoor plant, and display it indoors for removing stagnation and inertia. • Since the flowering plant has more than one color, choose the color to release the energies you most desire or need: neon orange flowers spread the energies of health, well-being, healing, and creativity; yellow for happiness, new opportunities, and when seeking a high profile; white for peace, contemplation, or courtship if a desired love does not notice you; red for major travel and for the performing arts; electric or deep blue for relocation; and purple for developing spiritual and psychic powers.

CAUTION
Bird of paradise is toxic to dogs, cats, and humans if ingested.

Bird Vetch

(*Vicia cracca*)

MAGICAL FORMS

also known as tufted vetch • a wild vine up to six feet in height with climbing tendrils and numerous bluish-violet, pealike flowers • a hermaphrodite, blooming from June to August with flower clusters on one side of the spike • native to northern Europe, Asia, and the UK, naturalized in North America from Canada to South Carolina and Minnesota • in some states it may be considered invasive, but it is still popular in temperate wildlife and informal gardens and ecologically valuable for fixing nitrogen in the soil and as a pollinator • magically use the whole, growing plant; tea; and flower essence

PLANET AND ELEMENT

Mercury • Air

MAGICAL USES

as the plant and flower essence, for overcoming sexual issues arising from childhood repression and confusion of sexual identity • resisting sex from being used as a weapon or power game • for helping people of all ages to be comfortable in their chosen sexuality

HOW TO USE

Use the essence either in water or under the tongue if you are suffering from impotence, vaginismus, or an inability to enjoy sex, or if you are concerned about gender issues, especially if you are being pressured or are suffering from prejudice. • Make vetch tea from the leaves (you can often buy it as part of other herbal tea mixes), sip a little, and then pour the rest on the ground or under running water to allow past sexual inhibitions to flow away. Alternatively, you can do this with the essence in water. You may need to do this many times.

CAUTION

Avoid in pregnancy and only use while breastfeeding under medical advice.

Bistort

(*Bistorta bistortoides*) or (*Polygonum bistorta*)

MAGICAL FORMS

also called snakeweed because of twisted roots or dragon's wort • magically use the growing plant, leaves, roots, rhizomes, and dried flowers

PLANET AND ELEMENT

Saturn • Earth

MAGICAL USES

for inflow of and attracting money for urgent and instant needs • for revealing hidden, disputed, or unexpected financial resources as in its folk name dragon's wort • protection against evil and poltergeists • fertility • increasing or restoring psychic powers if they are blocked

HOW TO USE

Burn or place in a prosperity herbal sachet to attract money. • Use in dragon rituals for retrieving what is owed or obtaining disputed inheritances. • A root of bistort shaped into an amulet is carried to bring conception. • An infusion of bistort sprinkled near the doorway of a house or business will deter ill-intentioned visitors, earthly and paranormal, and can be used in an exorcism mix. • Burned as an incense with frankincense, bistort increases psychic awareness and divinatory powers.

CAUTION

In excess, bistort can cause photosensitivity and prevent absorption of minerals. • Avoid with gout, kidney stones, or arthritis.

Bittersweet

(*Solanum dulcamara*) and (*Celastrus scandens*)

MAGICAL FORMS

also called European bittersweet or American bittersweet • dark purple flowers with yellow anthers and red berries • a climber vine that can grow to thirteen feet • native to Europe, North Africa, and northern Asia • naturalized in North America • common roadside plant • some practitioners prefer to buy bittersweet already powdered or to pick twigs in the spring and fall from a wild vine as bittersweet can suffocate nearby garden plants • magically use the wood or dried and crushed root

PLANET AND ELEMENTS

Saturn • Earth/Air

MAGICAL USES

use the dried pulverized root in a securely sealed amulet bag to bind or banish unfair competition or malicious opposition toward you physically, psychologically, or psychically • banish the negative actions but do not ill-wish the perpetrator, no matter how justifiable it seems • tie knots of biodegradable thread to a growing vine to let any stranglehold or regrets from your past life decay in its own time

HOW TO USE

Seal the dried chopped plant, crushed twigs, or powdered root in a small cloth bag, and hang it facing outward just inside and above your bedroom door lintel to forget a faithless or lost love who will not return. • Sprinkle the crushed herb or roots over the name, written in red ink on white paper with a diagonal red ink cross over it, of whomever is cheating or bullying you. Afterward, tip the herb away in an outside garbage can. • Secretly hide a twig bound in red thread somewhere inaccessible and dark to protect your home, business, or family from all harm, especially if a possessive relative or ex is interfering.

CAUTION

Though used medicinally, bittersweet, especially the American kind, is very toxic. • Take only under medical supervision and never raw or during pregnancy. • If grinding your own bittersweet, do not use your ordinary cooking utensils.

Black Caraway

(*Nigella sativa*)

MAGICAL FORMS

sometimes mistakenly given the name black cumin (*Bunium bulbocastanum*) (see "Cumin, Black," p. 146) • annual flowering plant native to southwestern Asia, the Middle East, and the Mediterranean region of North Africa, Iran, Syria, and parts of Iraq • oil is extracted from the seeds of this five-petaled blue or white flower that gives way to the ornamental seed pods • grows in the USA, the UK, and Europe • magically use the seeds, whole and ground in spice form, and the oil as carrier oil

PLANETS AND ELEMENTS

Venus/Mercury • Water/Air

MAGICAL USES

used in magical cooking and medicinally • like black cumin, regarded as a universal healer • favored by the ancient Egyptian queen Nefertiti to beautify herself • a vat of *Nigella sativa* was also found in the tomb of Tutankhamun • add empowered seeds when making bread to attract health, well-being, and protection to your home and those you love, making a blessing for all who will share the food

HOW TO USE

Add the carrier oil to or buy hair, skin, and beauty products containing the oil. • Empower them before use to relax if you bring work home or are constantly taking business calls all evening. • Trade massages with your partner using the oil mixed with rose, lavender, or jasmine oil, or enjoy a candlelit meal to which you have added the spice, before lovemaking to rediscover pleasure in each other if you have stopped communicating. • Use the spice to overcome addictions and cravings, especially for binge eating, bulimia, or anorexia. • Fill a small amulet bag with seeds you can hold when you feel you are losing control, and throw away a seed each time you succeed until it is empty.

CAUTION

Black caraway can be a skin allergen. • Avoid if you have kidney problems, are regularly taking diuretics, sedatives, serotonin, or other medications, or are pregnant.

Black Cohosh

(*Actaea racemosa*)

MAGICAL FORMS

also known as black snake root or squaw root • grows tall, belongs to the buttercup family • creamy white candle-like flowers • roots growing from the rhizome, the black horizontal underground shoot, root, and growth system • harvested after leaves die back in the fall • black cohosh originated among the Native North Americans, especially in the eastern USA and adopted by the settlers • magically use the whole, growing plant; root; and flowers

PLANET AND ELEMENTS

Saturn • Earth/Fire

MAGICAL USES

courage • protection • potency • all female mysteries, especially associated with the transition to wisewoman/crone and waning moon • famed for its benefits in menopause • restoring natural cycles and harmony to stressed modern lives, especially for older women • fertility

HOW TO USE

Use the root carved into a phallic symbol for fertility and potency. • A root carried in a white cloth gives courage to the fearful and gentle when facing intimidation. • Sprinkle a dried chopped root/rhizome infusion mixed with sacred water around the home to remove a sense of evil or malevolent spirits. • Use the candle-shaped flowers, often called silver primrose, as the God/Goddess candles on an altar and in the four quarters of the altar for sex and fertility magick. • Set three candle flowers in the center of a circle or altar in ascending size order to mark the transition from maiden to mother to wisewoman. • Sweep the dried chopped roots from doorstep to outside boundaries to undo hexes and curses. • If neighbors are terrorizing you, or an ex-partner or stalker will not leave you alone, bury the dried rhizome where your property ends to guard your boundaries (or in a plant pot outside your door if you have shared access).

CAUTION

Avoid during pregnancy or breastfeeding. • Excess doses can cause stomach upset and headache. • Do not use if taking HRT, birth control pills, or antidepressants or with heart problems.

Black Tupelo

(*Nyssa sylvatica*)

MAGICAL FORMS

also known as black gum tree • ornamental tree, native to North America, from New England to southern Ontario, central Florida, Texas, and Mexico • spectacular fall leaves turn purple, yellow, bright red, or orange • magically use the growing tree, dried or fresh leaves, bark, and fruit

PLANET AND ELEMENTS

Venus • Earth/Water

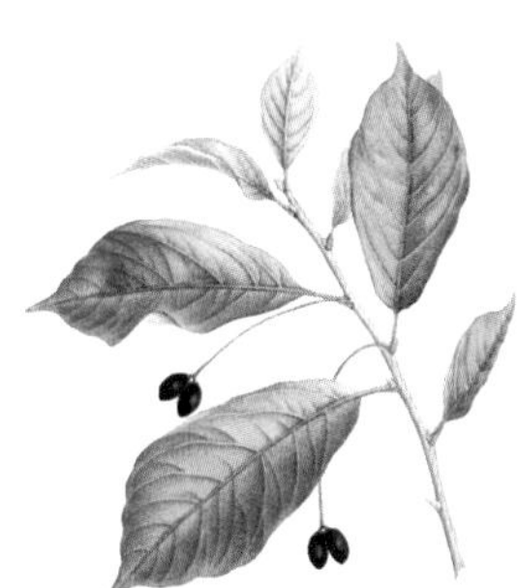

MAGICAL USES

since black tupelo loves living near water, it was named after the ancient Greek water nymphs the Nysiads (or Nysiades) • for increasing love • resolving old memories and overcoming karma from past lives • banishing parasitic relatives, friends, and neighbors • for water magick and celebrations since the nymphs reared the infant Dionysus, god of wine and ecstasy

HOW TO USE

Add tupelo honey to rose tea for romance and share with your loved one. • Drink it before bed alone to dream of past-life visions of your twin soul, whether known or unknown. • Hang dried fall leaves still on the branch, or if fallen tied with twine, over the front door to welcome the ancestors and benign house spirits. • Decorate your garden tupelo tree with solar lights to welcome visitors and especially call home relatives or friends who departed in anger or coldness. • Scrunch through the fall leaves as you did when you were a child to put behind your regrets for what went wrong.

Blackberry

(*Rubus fruticosus*)

MAGICAL FORMS

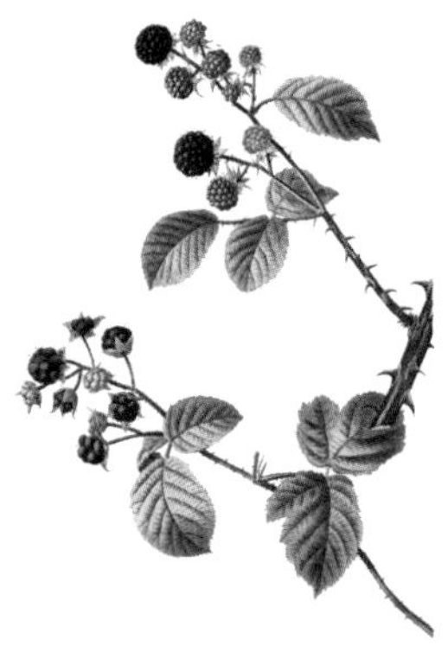

tall, prickly, brambly shrub with palm-shaped leaves, white to pale pink flowers, and clusters of black edible fruit • natural arches rooted at both ends are considered especially magical and, in folk traditions, were once used to cure those with various ills, especially affecting the skin or swellings • native to temperate Europe, naturalized in the Americas and Australia • magically use leaves; berries, whole or crushed; and as tea made from the leaves (remove prickles)

PLANETS AND ELEMENTS

Mars • Fire (the brambles and leaves), Venus • Earth (fruit and flowers)

MAGICAL USES

protective against earthbound spirits, emotional vampires, and mind manipulation • baked in pies at Lughnasadh, the first harvest at the end of July • leaves and dried berries in rituals and added to prosperity charm bags • a fae fruit and also associated with Lucifer landing in a bramble bush in his fall from Heaven, blackberries are said to be unlucky if picked after Michaelmas Day, September 29

HOW TO USE

Plant a blackberry patch in a wild area of a garden as a protective hedge against intrusive, gossiping, or hostile neighbors and against all harm, earthly and paranormal. • The fruit or leaves in tea, or the fruit eaten raw or cooked, creates an aura of protection around you. • The fresh berries shared before sex magick can heighten passion, but since it lowers inhibitions, set boundaries beforehand.

CAUTION

Beware of brambles when picking or if grown where there are small children or pets.

Black-Eyed Susan

(*Rudbeckia hirta*)

MAGICAL FORMS

from the family Asteraceae, as is the daisy and sunflower (see "Daisy," p. 151, and "Sunflower," p. 434) • a popular American garden flower, also found wild in all Canadian provinces and forty-eight American states • flowers bloom in the late summer and early fall • magically use the whole, growing plant; flowers, fresh or dried; and flower essence

PLANET AND ELEMENT

Mars/Sun • Fire

MAGICAL USES

assists in times of change or new challenging situations and environments • opens the veil between the dimensions in mediumship • justice after truth is revealed • said to be named after a poem by eighteenth-century English poet and dramatist John Gay about two lovers, Susan and her sailor love William (linked with the flower sweet William because they bloom simultaneously) • black-eyed Susan is the state flower of Maryland • protection • happiness through increased personal power

HOW TO USE

Meditate on the growing flowers, whether in the garden or a vase of cut flowers, to encourage transformation and making the most of a new situation even if not sought. • Release the flowerheads on flowing water to let go of grief or trauma, naming the sorrow or departed person and sending them blessings. • Use a drop or two of homeopathic black-eyed Susan flower essence in a spray mist or diffuser with geranium, lavender, and water to make a new home feel your own. • Press the dried petals between official documents causing problems.

CAUTION

Black-eyed Susan seeds are poisonous. • The hairs on the plant can cause a skin allergy in some people and bring on asthma in those who have lung conditions or are sensitive to the plant. • Do not ingest.

Blackhaw

(*Viburnum prunifolium*)

MAGICAL FORMS

close cousin of cramp bark (*Viburnum opulus*), also known as guelder rose, which is found more commonly in Europe and Asia • tall shrub with serrated leaves, clusters of white flowers, and blue-black berries • native to central and southern North America • magically and medicinally use the bark and root bark (the tough covering of the root stem)

PLANET AND ELEMENT

Moon • Water

MAGICAL USES

increases the power of other herbs, flowers, and crystals • use the tea made from the dried root bark or bought commercially as the Water element in goddess rituals, substituting the tea for wine in ceremonies for woman's rites of passage, especially wisewoman/croning rites • drink also during waning moon magick for women's mysteries/initiations

HOW TO USE

Keep the chopped bark or root bark in a charm bag for luck in gambling, gaming sessions, or lottery tickets, and replace after each major use. • Etch on a small piece of the fallen tree bark or cut root bark, the name of a company with whom you are seeking employment. • Seal the bark in an envelope with a paper naming your ideal salary and position and mail it to yourself. • To conceive a baby, on full moon night, place nine berries, which are edible, along with nine dried flowers in a natural fabric bag. If possible, tie it to the original blackhaw bush, otherwise attach it to any flourishing thick bush or tree where it cannot be seen.

CAUTION

Not generally recognized as safe by the US FDA, although blackhaw root bark has been used medicinally in folk healing for centuries. • Avoid if allergic to aspirin. • Seek advice if pregnant before ingesting blackhaw in any form.

Blackthorn

(*Prunus spinosa*)

MAGICAL FORMS

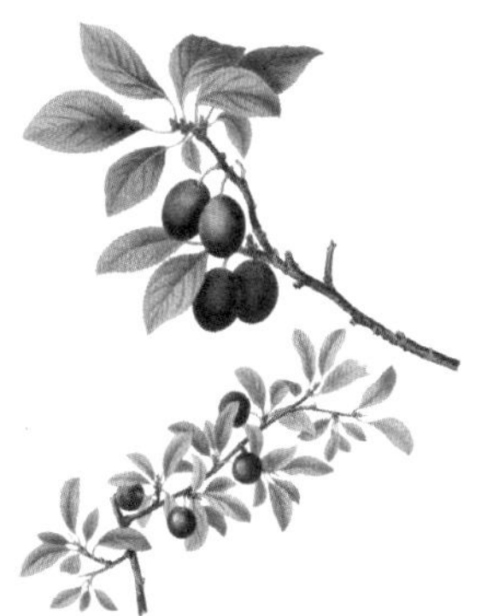

blackthorn usually grows as a bush, forming a hedge, but can become a tree up to twenty feet high with tangled branches • blackthorn is naturalized in the Pacific Northwest and New England and native throughout Europe • magically use the wood, thorns, fruits (as sloes they make gin), and fresh and dried blossoms

PLANET AND ELEMENT

Mars • Fire

MAGICAL USES

drives away evil and disasters • rituals for endurance and surviving hardship

HOW TO USE

The thorns can be added to dark glass witch bottles (those remaining on small segments of its almost black branches) along with watered sloe gin, as the ultimate protective guardian against all harm. • Unfairly considered an evil tree in the past, blackthorn represents the kindly Grandmother Goddess of winter and the waning moon. • The thorns can be carefully removed from a branch with secateurs, wrapped in thick dark cloth, and hidden at the back of a high, dark place or in a basement, and by naming for each a sorrow, loss, or misfortune, neutralize or banish the thoughts. • Blackthorn staffs, wands, and dowsing rods for recovering what has been lost or stolen, are protective and penetrate illusion to point to the way ahead. • When the flowers are in bloom, they can be used to decorate the wands, staffs, and dowsing rods as a symbol of rebirth (most bloom in spring).

CAUTION

Beware letting children near the bush because the thorns are fierce. • The fruit is edible, but not the flowers or leaves, and the seeds are poisonous.

Bladderwort

(*Utricularia vulgaris*) and (*Utricularia macrorhiza*)

MAGICAL FORMS

Utricularia vulgaris is native to Europe and Asia • *Utricularia macrorhiza* is the American species, also called common bladderwort • an aquatic carnivorous plant, with bright yellow flowers in the summer growing above the water • most of the plant is underwater • thrives in wetlands and shallow boggy waters with no roots • eats mosquitoes • in the fall, bladderwort forms winter buds that sink to the bottom • native to the northern hemisphere and present in all fifty of the US states, including Alaska • grows in habitats across the world, including damp peat bogs, along streams, and lakesides • bladderwort also flourishes in boggy garden ponds, greenhouses, and indoors in shallow water and keeps away mosquitoes • magically use the whole, growing plant; flowers, fresh or dried; and flower essence

PLANETS AND ELEMENT

Venus/Moon • Water

MAGICAL USES

to avoid being deceived • preventing self-illusion • a reality check rather than seeing what we want to happen

HOW TO USE

Take the essence for resistance to frauds and flatterers. • Sprinkle a few drops dissolved in water in counterclockwise circles around a paper on which you have written the names of those human mosquitoes in your life who cause you irritation and infect you with self-doubt, then shred and pulp the paper in cold water. • Meditate on the growing flowers and, afterward, snip off and dry a few of the heads to carry in a sachet as a shield when you are dealing with financial offers or brokers about whom you are uncertain and when on dating sites if a lover seems too good to be true.

CAUTION

However, there is not sufficient evidence about the plant to be sure it is safe to be used medicinally. For this reason, it is not recommended to be ingested during pregnancy. • The essence is generally considered safe, but check with your physician or an expert herbalist if you are pregnant or take medicine for chronic conditions.

Bladderwrack

(*Fucus vesicolosus*)

MAGICAL FORMS

olive-green to reddish-brown seaweed • can be up to three feet long, with bubble-like bladders • attached to rocks in the high intertidal zone, so spending much time out of the water • may cover rocky shores with its abundance • magically use the dried seaweed, whole or cut into small pieces, or pulverized into a powder

PLANETS AND ELEMENTS

Moon/Jupiter • Water/Air

MAGICAL USES

among the most ancient life forms on the planet, evidence of bladderwrack's use as a food and medicinal plant was discovered at Mount Verde, southern Chile, dating back twenty thousand years • for sea and full moon rituals by water • money spells • protection of those at sea or flying overseas (though you may need to leave your magical bladderwrack seaweed at home if traveling internationally by plane)

HOW TO USE

Cast it into the ocean, preferably where you found it, asking the sea spirits to bring good fortune and prosperity. • Leave it as an offering. • Make an infusion of the dried plant for a floor wash for your home to attract unexpected money or in a business for extra customers through the door. • Holding a long piece of bladderwrack, name all you wish to lose from your life, and then cast the seaweed into the ocean or a river, asking for and giving thanks for what you would wish to receive in its place. • Swirl bladderwrack over your head, and throw it high in the air from the shore into a rockpool to ask for the presence of the Air spirits for safe, happy, and, if appropriate, profitable travel or rising high careerwise. • As with all seaweed, keep a small piece of bladderwrack in a jar of whiskey for a year and a day, or until New Year's Eve, for ongoing financial security, then replace it.

CAUTION

The original source of iodine since 1811, only the tips are edible. • Seek expert advice before using bladderwrack medicinally. • Avoid while pregnant or taking insulin, or if suffering from thyroid problems.

Blazing Star

(*Liatris spicata*)

MAGICAL FORMS

a wild flowering plant, native to the meadows and prairies of eastern North America as *Liatris spicata*, with tiny bright purple, pink, and white blossoms and white leaves that turn bronze in the fall • *Mentzelia laevicaulis*, also called giant blazing star, has large yellow starlike blossoms and grows wild in western North America • the former is particularly popular as a cut flower • both grow in gardens in North America, Canada, Europe, and the UK • magically use the flowers, fresh or dried, and as flower essence

PLANETS AND ELEMENTS

Sun/Venus • Fire/Water

MAGICAL USES

to overcome drug and alcohol problems, destructive influences that peddle glamour, chasing after excitement and material riches • for expressing regrets in a bouquet and a desire to start over again • blazing star is not considered toxic to pets or humans and has been traditionally used medicinally in teas made from the ground root to cure sore throats, headaches, and arthritis

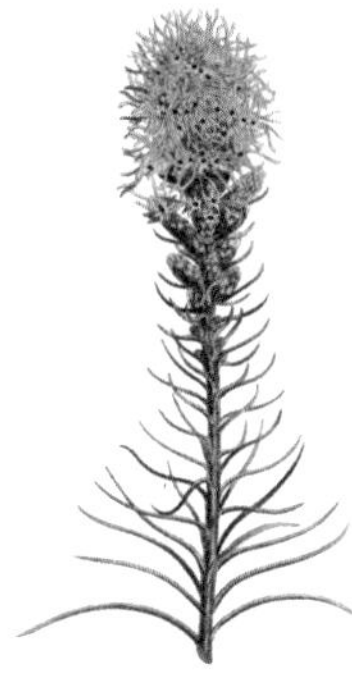

HOW TO USE

In meditation, hold the cut flowers under the stars to connect with stellar angels and higher starry realms and beings, such as Elaiah, angel of starlight surrounded by silver beams; Cochineal, starry angel of the planets, asteroids, and the Milky Way; Kokabiel, angel of the constellations; and Sandalphon, the tall archangel of transformation, in a shimmering robe of stars. • Give a drop or two of essence to teens to break the spell of friends leading them into trouble.

CAUTION

However, since blazing star is used to bring on scant menstruation, it is best avoided if trying to get pregnant or during pregnancy.

Bleeding Heart

(*Lamprocapnos spectabilis*)

MAGICAL FORMS

also called locks and keys • puffy heart-shaped pink flowers on large arching stems (rarely all white) so the flowers appear like a necklace or a key undoing a lock, with a protruding single white drop beneath the petals • blooms from April to June although in cultivation may be forced to bloom early around Valentine's Day • green fernlike foliage that turns yellow and drops after midsummer • native to Siberia, northern Japan, China, and Korea • includes the native eastern North American fringed bleeding heart (*Dicentra eximia*) and the western bleeding heart (*Dicentra formosa*), which is indigenous to northwestern USA • magically use the fresh or dried flowers, taking care to preserve the drop; fallen dried yellow leaves; and rhizome

PLANET AND ELEMENT

Venus • Water

MAGICAL USES

overcoming a betrayal or loss in love and moving on • forgiveness of self for letting a loved one down • unrequited love • on Valentine's Day, cut and send to an unresponsive or ex-lover for whom you still care

HOW TO USE

Plant in the garden to call love, for the return of a lover, or to protect the family from sorrow. • Give as a gift on Valentine's Day, or as a floral engagement or wedding gift, often accompanied by a necklace, as assurance love will always be true. • Carry the rhizome/root to further a love with whom you would like an affair but who may not yet be free.

CAUTION

Though used in folk medicine, raw bleeding heart can be mildly poisonous to humans and pets. • Avoid if you are pregnant, breastfeeding, have liver disease, or are taking prescribed sedatives. • It may cause contact dermatitis in some people.

Bloodleaf

(*Iresine herbstii*)

MAGICAL FORMS

colorful plant with variegated red to blood-red leaves • native to South America, especially Brazil, where it is used by shamans for trance flight • will grow in tropical and semitropical zones and as an annual plant in frost-free locations anywhere • indoors as a potted plant • magically use the fresh or dried leaves or the powder, obtainable online or in health and magick stores

PLANET AND ELEMENT

Mars • Fire

MAGICAL USES

for stopping gossip and keeping spiteful people from your life • to act as a shield if you are disturbed by paranormal dreams or spontaneous premonitions of disasters you cannot prevent

HOW TO USE

Mix the powdered herb with salt and sprinkle on doorsteps, sweeping outward to remove the presence of evil spirits and deter any earthly visitors approaching with malice in their hearts. • Use as an amulet, in a bag containing the powder or leaves, to take with you if you are ghost hunting or if moving to a property known for hauntings, to create a protective zone around you and your family. • Use the powder or leaves in a defensive bottle with sour red wine and rosemary sprigs to deter restless spirits if your home is built on an overactive energy line or close to where a massacre or disaster happened even centuries before.

CAUTION

Generally considered nontoxic, but evidence suggests it may have hallucinogenic properties, so seek advice before ingesting. • Traditionally used medicinally, but seek expert advice if pregnant or breastfeeding.

Bloodroot

(*Sanguinaria canadensis*)

MAGICAL FORMS

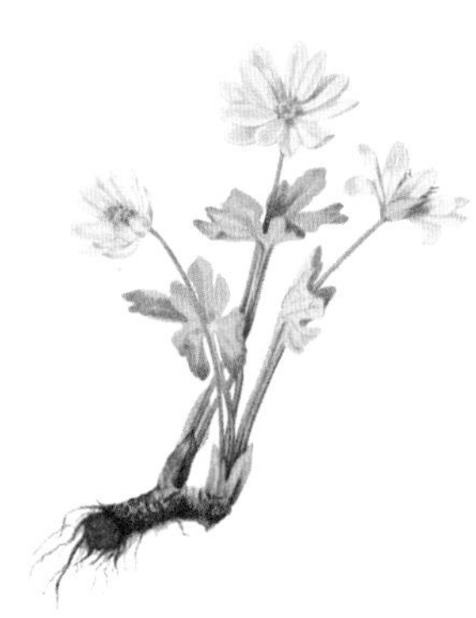

also known as red puccoon • related to the poppy family, with white delicate daisy-like flowers that bloom for a very short time • each flower stem is clasped by a leaf as it emerges just before the leaves open • native to eastern North America and Canada • can be cultivated in Europe and the UK • stems and roots contain orange-red sap when cut into • magically use the whole, reddish root (can be bought online), or the powdered root (can be bought online or from alternative health stores)

PLANET AND ELEMENT

Mars • Fire

MAGICAL USES

for reconciliation within the family • overcoming sibling and stepfamily or ex-partner rivalries • to prevent anyone tempting your partner to be unfaithful • to keep away hexes, curses, and jealousy by carrying the root as an amulet

HOW TO USE

Place the root over the front door lintel to deter evil spirits and malicious callers. • Hide the root in a room to prevent quarrels and jealousy. • If you sense the presence of restless spirits or ill-intentioned former residents within the home or children are afraid, hang a bag of powdered root over door frame lintels and above windows. • Burn the powdered root in incense to attract a lover. • Carry the root in a red bag to increase virility and courage.

CAUTION

It is poisonous to ingest, and the juices are also toxic and may cause skin irritation. • Avoid while pregnant or if you have low blood pressure or an irregular heart rhythm. • It interacts unfavorably with hypertension and blood coagulant medication.

Blue Cohosh

(*Caulophyllum thalictroides*)

MAGICAL FORMS

also called papoose root • magically use the whole plant, root, and berries

PLANET AND ELEMENT

Moon • Water

MAGICAL USES

primarily a woman's herb used in women's mysteries and goddess rituals • a powerful protection herb for making magical spaces and for children • though poisonous, a very sacred moon plant and as such worth planting in a safe place in your moon garden

HOW TO USE

Use for cleansing curses, hexed or jinxed clothing, artifacts, cars, and houses. • The tea can be added to a rinse or floor wash to remove a lingering sense of evil. • Blue cohosh root can be kept in charm bags or burned to bless a new home and clear energies from past residents and their ghosts. • Hang as bundles to guard children and babies, out of their reach so they cannot touch the plant.

CAUTION

Blue cohosh is no longer considered safe to induce labor or ease contractions. • Avoid blue cohosh while pregnant, breastfeeding, or trying to conceive, as not enough research has been done. • Berries, roots, and leaves can cause contact dermatitis so if sensitive wear gloves. • Berries are poisonous to children, and the whole plant is poisonous for pets, as is the plant for anyone to eat raw, so keep your blue cohosh in a secure place.

Bluebell

(*Hyacinthoides non-scripta*)

MAGICAL FORMS

also called the common bluebell • also including Spanish bluebell (*Hyacinthoides hispanica*), and mountain bluebell (*Mertensia ciliata*), found especially in western USA • protected in some countries, such as the UK, from being picked wild • magically use the whole, growing plant; fresh and dried bells; and flower essence

PLANETS AND ELEMENTS

Venus/Mercury • Water/Air

MAGICAL USES

shape-shifting • constancy and faithfulness, especially the true bluebell • brings understanding in relationships • good luck • flower of Beltane/May Day, the beginning of the Celtic summer • a fairy flower, called fairy thimbles and rung by fairies to call others to attend a gathering • a sign, especially if getting dark, that mortals should leave the place • if you trample on growing bluebells, the fairies will be angry and may make you lose your way • bluebells growing in a woodland indicate an ancient place of enchantment and you should not linger or pick the flowers (grow or buy your own)

HOW TO USE

As an incense blend, it dispels illness and aids healing. • A vase of bluebells in a room compels others to tell the truth and you to discover the facts in a situation, formerly shrouded in illusion. • Decorate an altar or a grave, especially with the rare white bluebell, on the anniversary of a death. • Alternatively, set a vase of the blue or purple flowers near photos of ancestors or beloved lost pets in the springtime for good memories. • Pink bluebells are given to indicate romance, to say thank you, and to welcome a baby girl (blue traditionally for a boy). • Send deep purple for regrets. • Bluebell essence overcomes low self-esteem, rooted in childhood.

CAUTION

The common bluebell and Spanish bluebell are toxic in all their parts if ingested. The mountain bluebell is safer and has been valued as medicine by the Cherokee and other Native North American nations. • Because of toxicity, it is not used in modern alternative Western medicine.

Blue Wild Indigo

(*Baptisia australis*)

MAGICAL FORMS

also called blue false indigo and *Baptisia* • a woodland and meadow large upright flowering wildflower • cultivated also in gardens because of its intense color in its native central and eastern North America • traditionally its seedpods were used by the Cherokee nation and traded by European colonists from the Indigenous people as a cheap source of blue dye, hence the name false indigo • indigo flowers from April through June, and the black seedlike pods appear after the flowers • magically use the growing and cut plant and the dried flowers and leaves

PLANET AND ELEMENT

Jupiter • Air

MAGICAL USES

planted in gardens to protect the home from danger of intruders and malevolent spirits and to surround the home with healing energies

HOW TO USE

In smudging, it is dried and tied as part of a smoke stick, frequently with sage, thyme, or rosemary, or chopped in incense with a resin, to clear a space for ritual or to remove sickness, misfortune, and unfriendly ghosts from the home or around the boundaries of the land. • The flowers, leaves, and stems, cut and placed indoors, welcome the ancestors and bring or restore good fortune. • Carry the dried chopped flowers and leaves in a purple amulet bag to ease emotional pain and protect against those you must still meet who make you unhappy or insecure.

CAUTION

Blue wild indigo should not be ingested by humans or pets as it is mildly toxic. • Its young shoots resemble asparagus and so are easily mistaken.

Blueberry

(*Vaccinium* spp.)

MAGICAL FORMS

native, growing both cultivated and as a wild bush, throughout the USA, reaching Europe in the 1930s, and also found in Asia • flowering and fruiting, close relative of the bilberry (see p. 61), huckleberry (see p. 226), and cranberry (see p. 140) • leathery leaves turn red in the fall • small bell-shaped flower clusters become the purple-blue fruit • magically use the berries, which can be bought from grocery stores all year; dried leaves, which can be bought from health stores; and in tea made from the leaves, berries, or both

PLANET AND ELEMENT

Moon • Water

MAGICAL USES

for enhancing memory • as an elixir for youthfulness • for bringing peace to the workplace, community, and the home • protecting the home and family against external psychic and psychological attack, especially when the fruit is shared at family celebrations such as Thanksgiving

HOW TO USE

Grow blueberry bushes or make the fresh or dried leaves, especially when red in the fall, part of homemade greenery circlet charms to hang around the home to prevent undesirable influences or restless ghosts from entering. • Eat blueberries or drink the tea on the full moon to strengthen your aura against psychic or psychological attack during the month ahead and on the crescent moon for the success of a new exercise or fitness program.

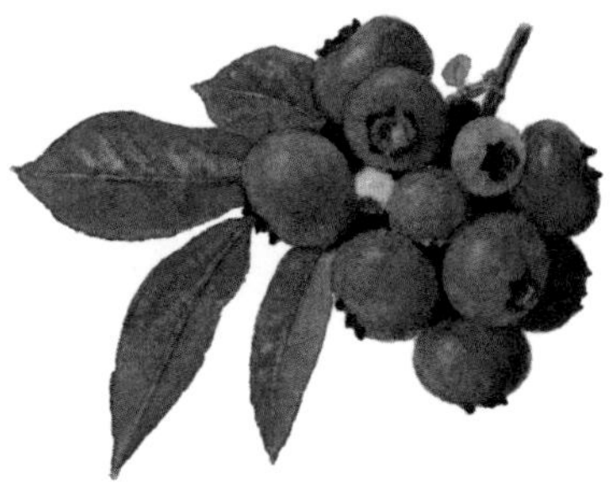

Bog Asphodel

(*Narthecium ossifragum*)

MAGICAL FORMS

sulfur-yellow spikes of six to twenty star-shaped flowers bloom June through August in damp environments such as peat bogs, heaths, and moorlands • native to northern and western Europe • as they fruit in the fall, the plants change color to amber/orange and color the peat bogs • magically use the flower essence, unless you start your own bog garden as a source of dried flowers or find the flower on vacation

PLANETS AND ELEMENT

Sun/Moon • Water

MAGICAL USES

bog asphodel essence, made with flowers and vodka, counteracts the willing-slave syndrome, the person whose life is centered around fulfilling the needs of others while neglecting his or her own well-being • especially those who take the role of nurturing mother/father into the workplace

HOW TO USE

In Scotland it is called the *lighthouse of the bog* for its yellow flowers that can be seen even in mist. In this tradition, put a drop or two of the flower essence under your tongue to absorb light into your aura so you no longer live in the shadows of others but shine like the flowers. • In Scotland the dried plant was hung over the front door to keep away evil spirits. • In parts of Europe, the flowers were cast, instead of rose petals, after a wedding as a fertility and happiness symbol.

CAUTION

Dried leaves were traditionally used to make tea to bring calm and to soothe digestion and respiratory problems, however, modern research does not yet confirm the safety of the plant for human consumption. • It can, however, be handled and taken in the small diluted quantities of the essence. • Bog asphodel is toxic to sheep and cattle.

Bok Choy

(*Brassica rapa* subsp. *Chinensis*)

MAGICAL FORMS

member of the mustard family, also called *pak choi* or Chinese cabbage • a leafy green and white vegetable eaten raw, cooked, or as juice • leafy green blades and a smaller bulbous base instead of a head • cultivated in eastern Asia, China, Vietnam, and the Philippines, Mexico, California, Hawaii, Arizona, and Texas • a cool weather vegetable, it can be grown in containers • imported seasonally, especially in spring or fall, sold in Asian specialty stores and supermarkets worldwide • magically use the whole vegetable, cooked or uncooked

PLANET AND ELEMENT

Moon • Water

MAGICAL USES

for clearing business difficulties • a Chinese New Year food representing long life • in family meals brings connection with the ancestors

HOW TO USE

Very nutritious physically when eaten, bok choy is filled with the life force. • Hold your hands an inch or two above a bundle of raw bok choy on the kitchen table, fingers and palms downward to absorb the flowing chi if you are tired or dispirited. Afterward, wash it well under cold water to replace the energies it has offered. • Name problems as you cut/clean/prepare bok choy, discarding worries as you work. • Allow it to cook, sautéing, and as you drain cooking water/steam, see urgent matters or any lingering misfortune or obstacles flowing away.

CAUTION

Take medical advice if you suffer from thyroid problems or take blood-thinning medication.

Boneset

(*Eupatorium perfoliatum*)

MAGICAL FORMS

a relative of the more attractive herb gravel root or Joe Pye weed • has numerous fluffy, white flowers and stiff stems that give the appearance that the leaf pairs on either side are single leaves, perforated through the stem • native to eastern North America and eastern Canada and now more widespread in Europe and the UK • magically use the dried leaves and dried flowering tops mixed together (you can buy them chopped or powdered and dried online from a magick store or an alternative health store) and the dried, cut flowers and leaves on the erect stem

PLANET AND ELEMENTS

Saturn • Earth/Water

MAGICAL USES

for endings, cutting cords, and letting go when a quarrel cannot be mended • attracts benign spirits • opinions differ over whether boneset is named after its reputation of the leaves being used for setting bones or its ability to assist recovery from a virulent influenza strain in the 1800s, akin to dengue fever where the pain was as bad as broken bones

HOW TO USE

Use as an infusion or powdered herbs, scattered on doorsteps, swept or mopped away to banish and deter paranormal specters, poltergeists, and restless ghosts. • Cut straight down a stem with a sharp knife to split the seeming single leaf perforation to mark an ending, especially in love, and cast the halves in opposite directions. • A parcel of dried leaves and an angelica root tied with devil's shoestring, burned on an outdoor fire, removes jinxes, curses, and hexes. • The fresh stem with flowers and leaves, secured with a honeysuckle vine and reattached to the honeysuckle vine, restores peace after harsh words.

CAUTION

Though used medicinally in folk traditions, it is generally considered unsafe to ingest boneset or to use it topically except under medical supervision.

Bonsai Tree

MAGICAL FORMS

many trees and shrubs worldwide are cultivated as miniature bonsai trees • originating in China and called *pun sai*, the bonsai, representing the perfection of nature written small, may have first been created around 600 CE; some believe a millennia earlier • bonsai reached Japan around the twelfth century, where they were adopted by Zen Buddhists, samurai warriors, and royalty • the smaller the tree, the more magical • magically use the whole, growing plant in situ

PLANETS AND ELEMENTS

Saturn/Jupiter • Earth/Air

MAGICAL USES

for contemplation, meditation, and in the home or workplace as a focus to raise spiritual awareness, bring harmony, peace, wealth, and radiance to any place, person, or situation • a reminder, too, with twisting branches that there must be effort and persistence

HOW TO USE

Some of the most popular bonsai include cedar (*Cedrus* spp.), offering long life and promises of better times. • Dwarf boxwood (*Buxus* spp.) keeps away malignant influences and spirits. • Chinese elm (*Ulmus parvifolia*) brings good fortune and protection and gives insight into the future. • Flowering cherry (*Prunus serrulata*), as the blossom is so fleeting, tells us that we must enjoy every moment of happiness. • Gingko (*Gingko biloba*) is called the fountain of youth, for people of any age to rediscover their inner child. • Ginseng ficus (*Ficus microcarpa*) and other bonsai figs are aligned with abundance and happiness. • Dwarf jade (*Portulacaria afra*) is good for wealth and fidelity. • Japanese red maple (*Acer palmatum*) brings balance and beauty to any situation or place. • Juniper (*Juniperus communis*) welcomes new beginnings and success in speculation. • Liquidambar (sweetgum) tree (*Liquidambar styraciflua*), with its fabulous fall leaves, helps you flow with the cycles of life. • Oak bonsai (*Quercus* spp.) represents wisdom and authority. • Pomegranate (*Punica granatum*) brings charisma and fertility. • Redwood (*Sequoioideae* spp.) is for family unity and loyalty.

Borage

(*Borago officinalis*)

MAGICAL FORMS

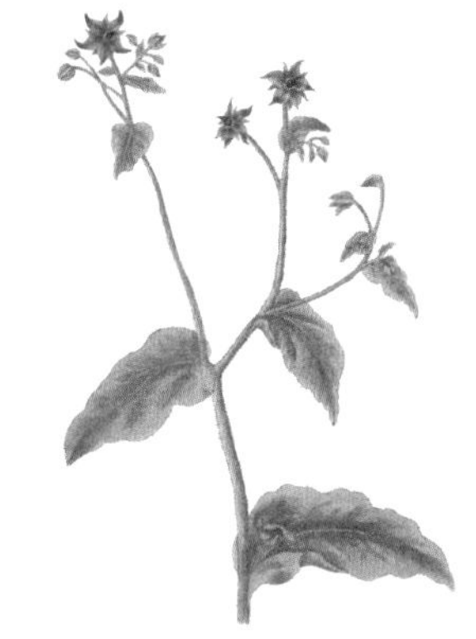

once popular in kitchen gardens, also called starflower because of the shape of its petals • magically use the growing plant, seeds, and flowers

PLANET AND ELEMENT

Mars • Fire

MAGICAL USES

courage • protection, both in and away from the home • increases the power of any spell or protective amulet • one of the magical herbs of the Celts, from a word meaning a brave person or warrior and given to medieval knights or embroidered on their doublets for courage in battle and jousts • star magick • the brilliant blue of the flowers was said to inspire Renaissance painters to create the robes of the Virgin Mary in celestial blue • color magick

HOW TO USE

Sprinkle the tea made from dried leaves or flowers around an area where you read tarot cards or other divinatory methods or keep borage flowers in a vase on the table to increase clairvoyance. • Carry the seeds in a sachet to overcome intimidation, bullying, or poltergeists and unfriendly spirits. • Use the star flowers, fresh or dried, for astral projection and communication with other dimensions. • Grow in the garden to bring peace and happiness in the home.

CAUTION

Although used for hundreds of years in remedies, in some countries borage is restricted medicinally except for the oil and oil products. • Keep safe from small children, cats, and dogs.

Boronia, Brown

(*Boronia megastigma*)

MAGICAL FORMS

a flowering shrub in most Australian states, native to bushland • can be successfully grown in the USA and Europe in warmer climates and in containers • also in the UK more rarely • member of the citrus family, the sweet lemony-scented brown boronia with cuplike yellow to dark brown blossoms with yellow inside, blooms throughout the spring and early summer • additionally as the fragrant bright-pink and red boronia (*Boronia heterophylla rubra*) • magically use the growing plant, cut flowers (though they can be short-lived), dried flowers, dried miniature flowerheads for making jewelry and crafts, as an essential oil, and as flower essence

PLANET AND ELEMENT

Saturn • Earth

MAGICAL USES

for breaking old patterns • moving on from a relationship that cannot be restored • as the oil or essence calming obsessive and circular thinking • to restore the life force after illness, misfortune, or loss

HOW TO USE

Cast the dried flowerheads into water to say goodbye to a love that cannot or can no longer be. • Use the flower essence daily to strengthen your resolve to not try to return to what was destructive or going nowhere, if necessary repeating the flower casting. • Anoint your Third Eye in the center of your brow with a drop of the diluted oil or the flower essence before trying new activities and experiences to reignite your inner life force.

CAUTION

Occasionally the oil causes an allergic reaction. • If pregnant or taking regular medication, consult a midwife or physician before using the oil as it is powerful. • Not to be used in the first trimester of pregnancy.

Bottlebrush, Crimson

(*Callistemon citrinus*)

MAGICAL FORMS

also as weeping bottlebrush (*Callistemon viminalis*) • native to Australia • multistemmed, shrub-like tree, widely grown in southern California and Florida • crimson bottlebrush spiky flowers continually bloom intermittently through the year in frost-free areas • grow in pots in more temperate zones, like the UK • weeping bottlebrush, native to eastern Australia, also grown in southern California, southern Florida, and other tropical and semitropical locations • weeping branches, red flowers resembling bottle brushes • magically use flowers and trees interchangeably, the essential oil, and the flower essence

PLANETS AND ELEMENT

Sun/Mars • Fire

MAGICAL USES

weeping bottlebrush for romance, especially restored or after betrayal • bottlebrush for abundance, banishing magick, fertility, celebrating birth, and new beginnings • bottlebrush essential oil in diffuser for harmony in the home, cheerfulness in face of adversity • although the seeds, leaves, and flowers of bottlebrush are traditionally empowered as an energy and medicinal drink

HOW TO USE

In Australia, bottlebrush is called the kookaburra plant. Wherever in the world, whether planted in the garden, potted at home, or in the workplace, like the kookaburra bird it welcomes each new day no matter how dismal the previous days. • Shred the many stamen flowers on the individual flower of the crimson bottlebrush or the weeping bottlebrush, and release them to the winds in a high place to clear misfortune and stagnation, inertia, and pessimism.

CAUTION

Bottlebrush has no toxic qualities but is not generally intended for consumption. • It has, however, been suggested by one or two sources that weeping bottlebrush has poisonous seed pods that hang down, and with the lack of contrary certainty, take care around children and pets.

Bougainvillea

(*Bougainvillea* spp.)

MAGICAL FORMS

magically use the growing plant, brightly colored leaves (often mistaken for the flower), flowers, and thorns

PLANETS AND ELEMENTS

Moon/Venus • Water/Earth

MAGICAL USES

self-esteem • socializing • self-image • new careers and businesses • bringing beauty into your life and home • flower psychometry

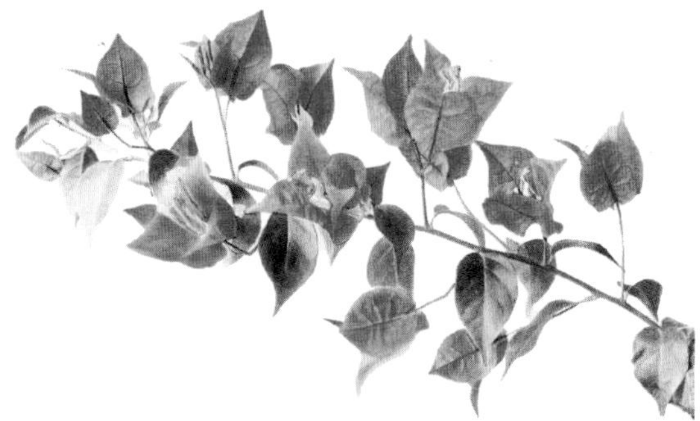

HOW TO USE

Use in meditation to restore self-belief and a strong self-image if others have made you feel inadequate or unattractive. • Place the papery leaves (sometimes called the *paper flower*) with notes or near a computer on which you are writing a novel or any creative projects. • Keep a pot or cut flowers near the computer if you are trading on the internet or overseas. • Place the fresh petals beneath the mattress to increase passion. • Scatter the petals instead of confetti for a joyous marriage. • Use the thorns, only with the greatest care and with clippers and tongs, in defensive bottles, buried under the doorstep to repel all harm.

CAUTION

Beware pricking yourself on a thorn, as this can cause skin irritation. • Remove thorns before using in flower psychometry. • Seek expert advice before ingesting the tea during pregnancy, and, if in doubt, avoid.

Bouvardia

(*Bouvardia* spp.)

MAGICAL FORMS

including *Bouvardia longiflora* and *Bouvardia ternifolia*, two of the most popular of the thirty species • these flowering evergreen shrubs with exotic flowers are native to Mexico, New Mexico, and Texas • they flourish outdoors in subtropical zones and extensively as hothouse flowers, especially in Holland • the firecracker bush with red-orange blooms is found in the southwestern USA • bouvardias are also grown as houseplants worldwide • bouvardias can be red, orange, pink, white, yellow, or combined colors • each stem resembles a bouquet • magically use the growing flower as a houseplant; the cut flowers, exported from greenhouses; the dried flowers bought online; and as a flower essence (available worldwide)

PLANETS AND ELEMENT

Sun/Mars • Fire

MAGICAL USES

courage • strength • determination • optimism • overcoming avoidance of challenging and emotional issues

HOW TO USE

Set your bouvardias or bouvardia potted plant in the center of your home where the air can circulate, and add a drop of the essence once a week to the plant or dried arrangement to generate enthusiasm and vitality if you have a sullen family member. • Add extra drops to the soil or vase whenever you have matters of the heart to discuss. • Take the essence regularly if you are creative but suffer from artistic or writer's block.

CAUTION

Though the flower essence and tea are traditionally used for digestive and skin problems, to dispel anxiety, and as a diuretic, modern research has not yet confirmed the safety of ingesting it or of the topical application, so care is needed particularly with pregnancy.

Box Plant

(*Buxus sempervirens* 'Latifolia Maculata')

MAGICAL FORMS

found as a clipped formal plant or hedge • can grow more naturally • varies in size from a small tub plant to a shrub that can grow twelve to fifteen feet if not clipped • small glossy tightly packed green leaves, with tiny yellowish-green flowers in spring • 'Latifolia Maculata' has yellow leaves when young, maturing to green with yellow blotches in summer, and yellowish flowers • box is native to western and southern Europe and especially to the Mediterranean, East Africa, and Asia • American boxwood and other variations have become naturalized across the USA, especially in formal gardens • magically use the growing plant (with care in handling), fresh and dried leaves, and flowers

PLANET AND ELEMENT

Saturn • Earth

MAGICAL USES

a fifty-sixth wedding anniversary plant, given in the growth-size appropriate to the couple • a box plant set either side outside the front door is a fiercely defensive guardian of the home or home business • made into topiary shapes, animals, or birds, box brings the powers of the creature in the way most needed into your life • the customary ball shapes signify unity, health, and well-being and box topiary cones offer increase in every way, especially love and money

HOW TO USE

The slender complex weblike root system gives the plant its powers to unite different people, ideas, and points of view. • Loosely so as not to damage the shrub, weave green ribbons or threads all over the box when you know you are networking, acting as mediator, or in the middle of confrontational factions. • Stand firmly with your hands around but not touching the plant, to absorb its Earth energies if you are feeling panicky or disconnected. • Pack leaves, especially yellow-tinged ones, as tightly as possible in a yellow purse, and hang it in a high place in your home or workspace to attract abundance and prosperity.

CAUTION

Box is harmful if ingested. • Handle with care, as it can be an irritant.

Bracken

(*Pteridium aquilinum*)

MAGICAL FORMS

also called eagle fern because of the shape of the leaves, which have tall fronds divided into three, resembling an eagle's claw • bracken is grown in gardens as well as wild in North America • grows in temperate and subtropical regions in both hemispheres, including Australia and Japan • the most profusely growing fern in the UK on heathland, moorlands, and in sandy areas • in fall, bracken turns reddish brown and dies back • magically use fresh and dried fronds, roots, and dried in incense

PLANET AND ELEMENT

Mercury • Air

MAGICAL USES

protective • in northern France shepherds made bracken crosses to guard themselves and their flocks from perils of the night while sleeping out on lonely hillsides • tied in the hair before swimming in Slavic lands against the rusalki, the freshwater sirens who hid in rivers • in Eastern Europe considered proof against werewolves • in Scotland the sliced stem was believed to reveal the Devil's footprint or the Greek initial of Christ's name • in Ireland called the fern of God • the marked stem was preserved as an amulet against harm in a charm bag • use the chopped or powdered plant with coins in a charm bag to turn an unprofitable business around

HOW TO USE

Since bracken is over 65 million years old, meditating near the growing plant or cut fronds or burning the incense brings visions of earlier times often containing an answer to or explanation of a present-day dilemma. • Because male and female cells for reproduction are within the same plant, use dried chopped bracken in fertility spells, especially if artificial insemination or IVF are being attempted. • Burning fresh or dried fronds are popularly believed to make rain fall.

CAUTION

Bracken is toxic if the fronds are eaten. • Avoid picking in the late summer to the fall, when toxic spores are released and could be inadvertently inhaled.

Brazil Nut Tree

(*Bertholletia excelsa*)

MAGICAL FORMS

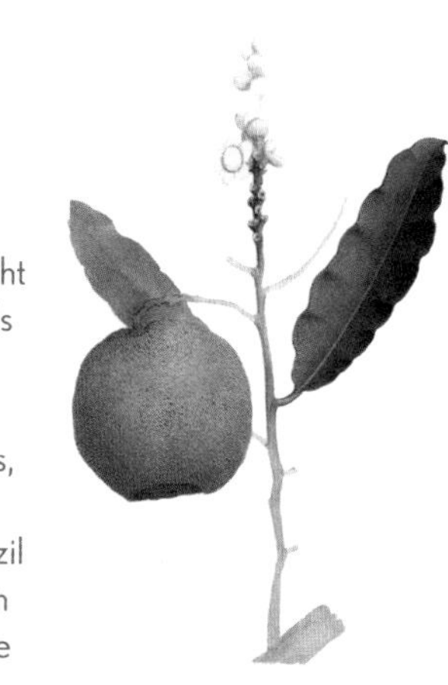

large South American tree, one of the tallest in the Amazonian rainforest, with a small crown and without branches for much of its height • hard coconut-like seed pods containing ten to fifteen dark brown triangular seeds with hard shells, known as the nuts, with a creamy white edible inner kernel • also called brazil nuts • native to Brazil, eastern Bolivia, the main exporter, the Guianas, eastern Colombia, eastern Peru, and Venezuela • mainly grows wild • the nuts are distributed worldwide • magically use the unshelled nuts and inner kernels

PLANETS AND ELEMENTS

Sun/Mercury • Fire/Air

MAGICAL USES

a good luck token particularly in love • consume a few daily if seeking to build up your authority and prestige for a major move forward or promotion • for concentration and recall in formal learning

HOW TO USE

Associated with fertility, empower brazil nuts and eat a handful the evening before IVF or any fertility treatment or tests. • If you are wishing to conceive naturally, eat one a day from crescent moon to full moon. On the night of the full moon, leave the unshelled nut on the window ledge so the full moon can shine on it. Shell and eat the nut on the following morning, having first pricked the shell with a sharp knife.

Bread

MAGICAL FORMS

though not a plant, it can be made with a variety of grains and as such has powerful botanical associations • an essential staple through the ages, called the "staff of life," bread has always been endowed with magical significance both in its making and eating • it can be magically empowered to bring sufficient resources, security of property, employment, prosperity, health, family love, happiness, and fertility, especially if the bread-making process is a family activity or shared with a partner

PLANET AND ELEMENT

Saturn • Earth

MAGICAL USES

at ancient celebrations for Lammas/Lughnasadh, the festival of the first grain harvest, the first grain to be cut was symbolically made into the first loaf of the new season, representing the spirit of the grain, who sacrificed his life so the people might be fed throughout the year • still commemorated as Lammas in churches at the beginning of August, where a freshly baked loaf is offered on the altar, sometimes in the shape of a sheaf of grain

HOW TO USE

Scatter crumbs from a freshly baked or bought loaf outside the four corners of your home or on the nearest plain as an offering to the spirit/goddess/god/guardian of the land, to give thanks even if life is not going well and to ask for blessings. It is especially effective when done the morning of Lughnasadh, August 1. • Decorate a loaf before baking with an image of what you most need as opposed to want. Or purchase an unsliced loaf and trace the image invisibly with a knife on top. • Take turns kneading and mixing bread dough to restore familial or marital harmony.

Breadfruit Tree

(*Artocarpus altilis*)

MAGICAL FORMS

thrives in the West Indies, Indonesia, Malaysia, and the Pacific Islands • grows in southern Florida and imported from Jamaica to the USA for most of the year and throughout the world, especially in Caribbean food stores and markets • magically use the fruit; leaves, sold dried for tea; and seeds, which some breadfruit have

PLANET AND ELEMENT

Saturn • Earth

MAGICAL USES

believed in Polynesia to be the first food created by the gods • famed for *Mutiny on the Bounty* connections when in 1789 Captain Bligh's crew mutinied off Tahiti and cast him adrift on the sea, in a bid for freedom, throwing the cargo of thousands of breadfruit saplings into the sea • for beauty and radiance, abundance • for spells to prevent cravings for unnecessary luxuries • breaking free of convention and seeking a better lifestyle as Bligh's men attempted (and most succeeded for a number of years, some permanently)

HOW TO USE

Set a breadfruit or its dried leaves (obtainable online or from health stores) on your altar on full moon night to call prosperity, success in career, home-based businesses, and self-sufficiency. The following evening, cook and eat the breadfruit with friends and family. • If you want to get pregnant, place forty breadfruit seeds on the night of the crescent moon, one for each of the forty weeks of pregnancy (you can buy seeds online), inside a breadfruit in which the inner part has been removed. Replace the top half and tie it together with nine knots of thread. Float it on flowing water or on the outgoing tide.

CAUTION

Avoid if taking blood thinners. • Seek expert advice if pregnant or breastfeeding, as in some traditions seeds were used as birth control. • Avoid with low blood pressure or kidney disease.

Broccoli

(*Brassica oleracea* var. *italica*)

MAGICAL FORMS

belongs to the cabbage family • as calabrese broccoli, native to Italy • grows widely, including the western USA (especially California), the UK, and Europe • deep, dark-green edible flowerheads and stalks • the carrier oil is made by cold pressing the tiny seeds and is pale golden green • magically use the vegetable, raw and cooked, and the carrier seed oil externally

PLANET AND ELEMENT

Venus • Water

MAGICAL USES

gaining and maintaining a steady source of income, when the vegetable is eaten on the full moon • protective if you are overgenerous or underappreciated • an aphrodisiac for men eaten or in massage • to the Romans the vegetable was considered a giver of physical strength and leadership qualities • the seed oil is increasingly used to moisturize skin, nails, and hair and in beauty products, bringing good fortune, youthfulness, and protecting against negative energies and entities • both the vegetable and seed oil reduce stress

HOW TO USE

Use as a fast-acting boost to your aura energy field when eaten or the oil when added to shampoo if your willpower to say no is wavering. • Keep broccoli in your vegetable rack or in your freezer to attract health and prosperity, replacing it with the fresh broccoli as needed. • Cook it before it discolors as an ongoing domestic charm.

CAUTION

Because of the slight smell of broccoli in the seed oil, add a little fragrant essential oil when using the oil, such as helichrysum or a fragrant herbaceous oil like rosemary. • Not enough is known about the longer-term effects of the seed oil with pregnancy or breastfeeding, so ask an expert. • Do not use broccoli in any form if you have thyroid problems.

Bromeliad

(*Cryptanthus* spp.)

MAGICAL FORMS

magically use the growing plant, spiky flowers, and protective encircling leaves

PLANET AND ELEMENT

Sun • Air

MAGICAL USES

for money, business affairs, and security • bringing abundance and sensual pleasures • protecting the aura and chakra inner energy centers from earthly and normal attack • regarded as a gift from the gods • flower psychometry

HOW TO USE

Near the entrance doors, inside or out depending on climate, the main spiky flower emerging from the colorful bracts (the part of the plant between leaf and flowers) repels spiteful or threatening visitors, relatives, or neighbors. • The bromeliad species, *Ananas comosus*, which grows a small pineapple on top of the flower spike, represents fertility and the unity of ovum and sperm. Split and open the fruit on the full moon, inserting a pointed clear crystal inside, then binding with twine and casting, in a small basket, into fast-flowing water on the morning after lovemaking. • Since bromeliads detoxify the air at night, they can be empowered as a guardian to keep away specters of the night and filter bad dreams, leaving the sleeper refreshed. • Some bromeliads, such as air plants, will grow attached to a block of wood instead of being planted, mimicking the way they can grow in South and Central America attached to trees. • Buying a ready-attached air bromeliad is excellent for attracting independence and freedom from the clinging possessiveness of others. • Attaching coins to the wood will draw money as the plant grows.

CAUTION

Avoid medicinally if you're pregnant, have liver problems, are taking blood thinners, or are allergic to pineapples.

Broom

(*Cytisus scoparius*) and (*Genista monspessulana*)

MAGICAL FORMS

the English twelfth-century Plantagenet dynasty, which included Geoffrey of Anjou and his son King Henry II, were named after *Planta genista*, the old name for broom, and they wore sprigs of broom in their hats • Scottish broom was brought to the USA in the 1800s • grow wild and in gardens in golden bloom • magically use the golden tops, fresh and dried

PLANET AND ELEMENTS

Mars • Fire/Air

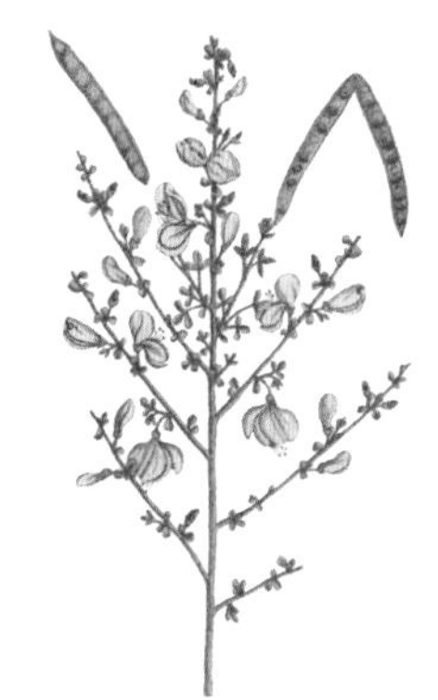

MAGICAL USES

long stalks of the cut broom plant are tied together with red ribbons for handfastings and woodland weddings, over which a couple leap hand-in-hand as a fertility symbol, and also so that the couple will always be prosperous • also as a broom to sweep negativity out of the home, or to sprinkle a ritual area, indoors or out, with sacred water • considered especially fortunate if the broom chosen grew nearby • hung in the home to bring good fortune and for protection • in a sleep pillow the dried flowers prevent nightmares

HOW TO USE

Burn broom on Halloween night for psychic visions and for connection with deceased relatives. • Cast fresh flowers into the air as tribute and for connection with the spirits of the Air, seeking their power to advance slow moving matters. • Calm a volatile situation by burning the flowers and burying the ashes where nothing grows, asking the Air spirits to cease their fierceness.

CAUTION

Broom is toxic to humans and pets, though it has been used medicinally in the past. • Broom is considered invasive in some states.

Brussels Sprout

(*Brassica oleracea* var. *gemmifera*)

MAGICAL FORMS

a cool-weather vegetable resembling tiny cabbages and probably the most underrated magical and culinary food, because too often they are served notoriously badly or overcooked • native to the Mediterranean, recorded in ancient Rome when the wild plant was first cultivated, spreading into northern Europe in the fifth century • so named in the thirteenth century for their cultivation around Brussels in Belgium • brussels sprouts reached Louisiana with French settlers about 1800 and are now grown around the American Pacific coast, the central California coast, and parts of New York, among other locations • magically use the cooked or raw vegetable

PLANET AND ELEMENT

Moon • Water

MAGICAL USES

one of the best vegetables (and quite delicious if cooked well) for attracting stability in earthly matters, such as property and daily living, antidebt, and persistence or perseverance • associated with Christmas in the UK because they arrived as a new vegetable to appeal to the wealthy at the same time as the Victorians began to celebrate Christmas • growing well in household gardens of ordinary folk in the winter who needed to bulk out the Yuletide fare

HOW TO USE

If steamed or lightly cooked on each of the three days before and/or the day of the full moon, money will flow in by the next full moon. • Growing on the stem in the garden or piled in a net in a vegetable rack, sprouts can be empowered to call security in times of change. • Cook and eat them to absorb the energies to overcome threats in the practical areas of life most needed. • Well-seasoned during cooking and served at a maybe unwillingly attended meal will unify the family over a contentious issue. • If sprouts are served to you overcooked, extra effort will be needed to break through fixed opinions.

CAUTION

Do not eat raw or not thoroughly cleaned if pregnant.

Buchu

(*Agathosma* spp.)

MAGICAL FORMS

Agathosma betulina, round leaf buchu, and *Agathosma crenulata*, oval leaf buchu, are two of the most popular forms • bushy shrub, stemless with leaves containing oil glands • native to dry mountainous regions of South Africa, a traditional remedy and sacred herb of the San and Khoisan people • adopted by Dutch settlers in the seventeenth century • buchu leaves came to the UK in 1790 and to the USA in 1860, where they were hailed a miracle cure-all and used for wounded soldiers in battle as an antiseptic • buchu is not widely grown in North America or the UK • magically use the dried leaves, loose tea, and tea bags (all of which can be bought online and from specialty health stores), as well as in spell bags

PLANET AND ELEMENT

Moon • Water

MAGICAL USES

connects with the ancestors and spirit guides • clears spirit and earthly negativity • increases psychic powers, especially clairsentience and prophetic dreams

HOW TO USE

Burned as incense or the dried leaves lit in a dish as smudge, it is used in ritual or home purification to banish malevolent spirits or unfriendly ancestors. • Burn with frankincense for prophetic dreams and visions of other worlds. • Drink the tea (from a reputable source as some forms of the plant can be toxic) before meditation and sleep for quieting the mind.

CAUTION

The oil is not used in aromatherapy, and the oil of the oval leaf should not be ingested in any form as it is toxic. • Buchu should not be used during pregnancy or while breastfeeding, if suffering from kidney or liver disease, or if taking blood-thinning medications. • Use medicinally on the advice of a physician or in officially approved remedies.

Buckeye Tree

(*Aesculus* spp.)

MAGICAL FORMS

includes California buckeye (*Aesculus californica*), yellow or sweet buckeye (*Aesculus flava*), red buckeye (*Aesculus pavia*), and Ohio buckeye (*Aesculus glabra*), which has the largest US distribution • found throughout the USA • the yellow buckeye was introduced into Europe in 1764 • all close relatives of the main genus horse chestnut (see "Red Horse-Chestnut," p. 373) • the yellow buckeye is best for lucky conkers, two brown nuts encased in a smooth, round husk • magically use the red buckeye's bright red flowers and the Ohio buckeye's yellow flowers and orange-yellow leaves in the fall

PLANETS AND ELEMENT

Mercury/Jupiter • Air

MAGICAL USES

as a gambling charm, for good luck in life, especially financial, also in sports • for male potency • keep the same nut/seeds in their casing from fall to fall • hide a spare from the same tree in case you lose the first to avoid losing your luck

HOW TO USE

Wrap a dollar bill, rolling it forward to enclose any buckeye seedpod, dried leaf, or conker casing containing the nuts, but especially from the yellow buckeye. Secure it with thin green twine, add a pinch of cinnamon powder, and keep sealed in a green bag when gaming, with lotto tickets, or when considering horse racing, sporting, or investment forms. • When playing cards, wear it on the right side of the body. • Some prefer to remove the seeds/nuts from the casing and use those as the charm. • To increase potency, a man should keep a red bag with a yellow buckeye casing that contains two nuts or the two nuts beneath the bed or mattress.

CAUTION

All parts of the buckeye tree are toxic and should not be ingested. • The Ohio buckeye fruit especially has a poisonous outer casing.

Buckthorn Tree

(*Rhamnus cathartica*)

MAGICAL FORMS

also called the common or European buckthorn tree • also as alder buckthorn (*Frangula alnus*) • not to be confused with a different plant, the Sea Buckthorn (see p. 406) • small trees with dense branches • small greenish-yellow flowers followed by red berries ripening to black that contain two or four seeds • the European buckthorn was introduced to the USA during the 1800s by colonists; now cultivated through northern central and northeastern USA and maritime provinces of Canada and growing wild • found in the UK and Europe • the *Rhamnus frangula*, or buckthorn alder, came across the Atlantic and is now regarded invasive • magically use the growing tree; fallen bark, alternatively sold as crushed bark (often from the alder buckthorn); small fallen branches; and fresh and dried leaves

PLANET AND ELEMENTS

Saturn • Earth/Water

MAGICAL USES

for justice in legal matters, banishing all harm, earthly and paranormal, to bring good luck • traditionally leaves or the crushed bark are cast in a circle at full moon to summon an elf who will, it is said, grant a single wish before escaping • leafy branches over a door will banish and keep away all malicious spells and attempts at mind control or possession

HOW TO USE

Burn the dried leaves or crushed bark in incense to create a sacred space for ritual and to drive away malevolent entities. • Scratch on the inside of bark the outcome you need in a court case, crumble, and bury it.

CAUTION

Buckthorn bark medicine is considered good for digestive problems, constipation, anal fissures, or hemorrhoids, but must be purchased from a reputable herbalist in capsule or lotion form, as the berries, seeds, and leaves from *Rhamnus cathartica*, *Rhamnus frangula*, and other kinds of buckthorn are toxic. • The berries are purgative if ingested. • Avoid while pregnant or breastfeeding, and if you have IBS or frequent diarrhea.

Buckwheat

(*Fagopyrum esculentum*)

MAGICAL FORMS

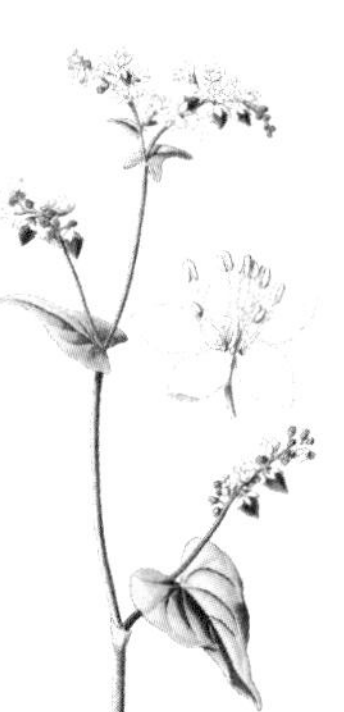

also known as Saracen corn • arrow-shaped leaves with white or pink flowers • native to central and northern Asia, but grown extensively in temperate zones, especially in the USA and the UK • magically use the cut and dried or whole, growing plant and dried seeds/grains

PLANETS AND ELEMENT

Saturn/Venus • Earth

MAGICAL USES

Called Saracen corn because it was probably introduced into Europe by the Crusaders in the eleventh and twelfth centuries • seeds in domestic amulet bags keep away poverty, debt, and malevolent influences, earthly and paranormal • ground as flour or flour purchased commercially for magical cookery to bring health and abundance, especially if the flour is kept in a jar in the kitchen and regularly held and asked for blessings

HOW TO USE

Eat buckwheat pancakes before a job interview or applying for a loan in person or online. • Create a display of dried cut buckwheat plus other grasses and grains in a vase in the center of your home to draw in money and keep it circulating. • Make your own buckwheat flour from hulled seeds in a grinder or blender, chanting all the time the intention you wish to manifest. • Add the flour to wishing powder (make sure it is finely ground by passing the ground flour through a fine mesh sieve) or wish jars for fertility and prosperity. • In an outdoor ritual, enclose yourself in three clockwise circles of the seeds, moving inward, to protect yourself and to welcome only benign nature spirits, and afterward let them blow away.

CAUTION

The plant is generally safe for humans when cooked, but not safe for pets or horses. • The leaves should not be ingested, as they are toxic.

Buffalo Gourd

(*Cucurbita foetidissima*)

MAGICAL FORMS

also called coyote gourd • edible, growing on a herbaceous spreading or climbing vine • indigenous to the semiarid and arid deserts of central and southwestern USA and northern Mexico • a member of the cucumber family, the fruit (gourds), which are globe-shaped, are relatively small, about four inches in diameter • magically use the hollowed-out, dried gourd; the whole gourd; the seeds; and the flower essence (most easily obtainable worldwide)

PLANET AND ELEMENT

Mars • Fire

MAGICAL USES

the gourd for fertility, protection, and as lucky charms • the essence for reducing anxiety, stress, physical and mental tension, creating a calm inner center, and emotional balance while dealing with outer world challenges • for counteracting mood swings in children and adolescents • for stress-free travel

HOW TO USE

Remove the inner flesh and seeds through cutting a lid at the top, and leave the gourd to dry (or buy a ready prepared hollow one from a crafting online outlet). Fill it with the dried seeds and other fertility seeds, such as poppy, pumpkin, or sunflower, replacing the lid. Use as a charm if trying to conceive a baby. • Eat the flesh and seeds, and hang dried gourds on a string on the ceiling over the entrance to protect the home and all within from earthly harm and malevolent spirits. • If traveling, take the essence for a few days before a trip, or give to nervous family members, for a stress-free journey, especially if afraid of flying. • Dilute a few drops of the essence in water to sprinkle around luggage and travel documents the night before a journey.

CAUTION

Seek advice during pregnancy before ingesting medicinally.

Bunchberry

(*Cornus canadensis*)

MAGICAL FORMS

a herbaceous wild flowering shrub from the dogwood family often used as ground cover, native to much of the northern USA through Canada and Alaska to northeastern Asia and Russia • resistant to cold • while it can grow up to eight inches, the bunchberry plant is often shorter • clusters of white bracts or enfolding leaves with tiny yellow-green or purplish flowers in the middle • leaves that turn red in the fall and edible scarlet berries that may have as many as ten in a cluster, ripening in late summer or early fall • can be grown in gardens in the US, the UK, and northern Europe • the berries can be bought in farmers' markets or specialty food stores • magically use the berries, the fall leaves, and as the flower essence

PLANETS AND ELEMENTS

Mars/Saturn • Fire/Earth

MAGICAL USES

the plant and flower essence bring clarity of thought for those easily distracted, caught up in the demands and lives of others, continually running out of time, and missing deadlines • the plant or essence if you need to conceal matters or keep a very low profile

HOW TO USE

In magical cookery, add the berries to jellies, jam, or pies and, as you stir them in, name and shed in the mix any unnecessary demands or requests you fulfill out of duty. • Make a wire circlet of berries and leaves attached with thread near the entrance of the home for maintaining a low profile against unfriendly officials and complaining neighbors. • Sip some essence water whenever asked for an unreasonable request whether face-to-face, by email, or phone.

Burdock

(*Arctium lappa*)

MAGICAL FORMS

magically use the whole, growing plant; roots; leaves; and flowers, fresh and dried

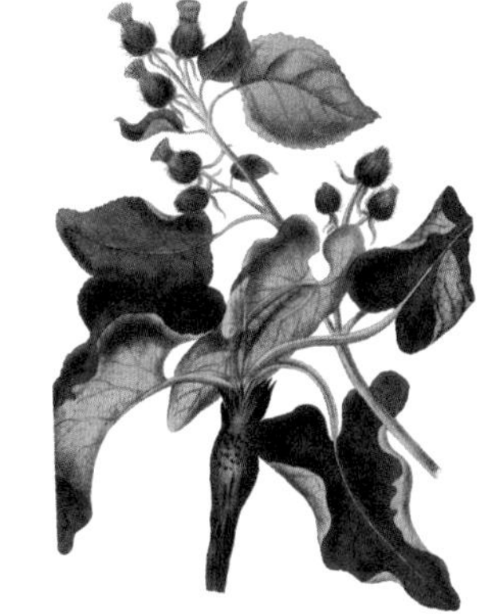

PLANETS AND ELEMENTS

Venus/Mars • Water/Fire

MAGICAL USES

protection against negativity • for healing • love and sex magick • good luck • carried for safety, especially in the USA, while traveling • used to prevent curses and hexes being sent • strong deep roots make it suitable in ancestor magick and when confidence is being shaken

HOW TO USE

Burn in protection incenses or powder and sprinkle around the home and land to create protective boundaries. • Burdock roots, most powerfully collected during the waning moon, are cut into even-sized pieces and worn on red thread as a necklace to guard against paranormal evil and ill-wishing. • Its rough sticky burrs are placed in sealed sachets to attract what is most desired, along with a coin or green dollar note for money, a silver heart or rose quartz crystal for love, an old travel ticket for a vacation or relocation, or a key for a new home. • Add it to potpourri to keep the life force flowing through the home. • Use it as a magical floor wash for removing lingering illnesses. • Use it in a tea, often with dandelion, or made into a pleasant cold drink to clear resentful, unduly competitive, and envious atmospheres in the workplace. • Use the chopped flowers, leaves, and/or root for the Earth element in healing rituals and as a tea made with the powdered root for the Water element. • Add to healing charm bags and bottles.

CAUTION

Remove burrs and make sure they do not stick to pets while the plant is growing.

Burnet

(*Sanguisorba officinalis*) and (*Sanguisorba minor*)

MAGICAL FORMS

includes *Sanguisorba officinalis*, greater burnet, and *Sanguisorba minor*, garden or salad burnet • often called the cucumber herb because of its taste • one of the few wild herbs providing edible greenery for most of the year • thrives in cooler regions of the northern hemisphere including northern Asia and the UK and can grow in pots in an indoor garden • arrived in the USA with the early European settlers • will bloom at any time spring to fall • dark red flowers on tall stalks looking like lollipops • the leaves for which it is mainly cultivated are eaten in salads, dressings, and marinades, especially with basil for lasting love and cilantro/coriander for protection from any loss, accident, or theft • magically use the herb in situ and the dried leaves

PLANET AND ELEMENT

Saturn • Earth

MAGICAL USES

dedicated in ancient Greece to Hecate who stood at the crossroads of past, present, and future • the herb is believed to increase clairvoyant powers if eaten • soldiers used the leaves in a tea during the American War of Independence to stop them bleeding to death if they were wounded and has retained its protective healing reputation • before magick rituals for courage to create boundaries with the daily world

HOW TO USE

Add the chopped dried leaves to incense with a tree resin to purify a space and to dedicate magical tools. • To reverse any ill-wishing, hexes, or spells cast against you, wash a hand mirror with burnet infusion counterclockwise, then rinse and dry the mirror. When you look in the mirror, the curse will be gone.

CAUTION

There are no known contraindications, but since burnet has not been fully researched, avoid while pregnant or breastfeeding, and do not take for prolonged periods.

Burning Bush

(*Euonymus alatus*)

MAGICAL FORMS

also known as winged spindle tree • flowering landscape shrub that can grow up to ten feet tall • though regarded as invasive where it grows wild in the USA in great profusion, it is prized and cultivated in gardens because of its brilliant scarlet fall leaf colors and red berries, with orange seeds inside a split purple husk that gives its name • first introduced from northeastern Asia to the USA and the UK in the mid-1800s • magically use its corky wings on twigs, fresh and dried fall leaves, and berries

PLANET AND ELEMENT

Mars • Fire

MAGICAL USES

named like other *Euonymus* species, such as the European spindle tree (*Euonymus europaeus*), after Euonyme, Mother of the Furies, the sisters who took revenge against those who broke oaths, betrayed their families, or harmed women and children, the burning bush is largely used in defensive magick • the dried leaves and berries carried in a sealed amulet bag or hung out of harm's way in the home to protect against hostile spirits and earthly visitors and also against fire damage • because of its kinship with the spindle tree, burning bush is popularly grown in the gardens of craftspeople and other creative people or the dried berries kept in a secure charm bag with creative tools to attract sales and positive publicity

HOW TO USE

Collect in a glass jar as a focus for astral travel the small corky, woody wings less than one-half inch wide that appear on the branchlets of younger trees. • Bury the wings in a small wooden box fastened with an old padlock without a key if you are suffering rumors or gossip, saying, *May [name of offender] be silenced against speaking ill of me or someone I love.*

CAUTION

The berries especially and the whole plant are highly toxic to animals and humans. • Use magically with great care, handling with gloves. • Avoid while pregnant or breastfeeding, or if you have a weakened immune system.

Butterbur

(*Petasites hybridus*) or (*Petasites japonicus*)

MAGICAL FORMS

also called Japanese giant butterbur • the giant butterbur emerges in spring as clumps of cauliflower-shaped white flower posies • by summer it grows three-foot rhubarb-like leaves • originates in Asia, introduced to the USA via British Columbia and to Europe by Japanese settlers • the *hybridus* form has small yellow flowers and large, heart-shaped leaves • native to central Europe from the UK as far as southern Scandinavia, now also growing in North America and Asia • magically use the roots, chopped dried leaves, and the seeds of either species

PLANETS AND ELEMENTS

Mercury/Saturn • Air/Earth

MAGICAL USES

the large leaves were used to wrap butter in the summer, hence the name • make a tea decoction from the root of the *hybridus*, not only to counteract seasonal allergies and prevent migraines, but to protect against the effects of those who intrude on personal space and disrupt well-being

HOW TO USE

According to the folklore of the Ainu Indigenous people of the northern Japanese islands, the *Korpokkur*, short fey fisherfolk, lived under Japonica butterbur leaves. • A root or chopped dried leaves can be hung above and inside the main doorway in an amulet bag to protect from bad weather and all danger and to attract abundance. • Traditionally the seeds are used in love sachets. • In a modern adaptation of an old European folk custom, plant in a deserted place if seeking a lover. It is said a vision of the lover may appear instantly (or later in a dream) and the two will find each other.

CAUTION

Use approved commercial brands, and avoid the unprocessed kind if suffering from liver or gastrointestinal complaints. • Not enough is known about its effects during pregnancy. • Do not use if allergic to ragweed, marigolds, daisies, or chrysanthemums.

Buttercup

(*Ranunculus* spp.)

MAGICAL FORMS

including bulbous buttercup (*Ranunculus bulbosus*), meadow buttercup (*Ranunculus acris*), and creeping buttercup (*Ranunculus repens*) • magically use flowers, fresh or dried

PLANET AND ELEMENT

Sun • Fire

MAGICAL USES

increasing wealth • energy • abundance • prosperity (bringing gold) • sharing resources • divination and psychic powers • happiness • protection • advancement in career • recalling ancient folk wisdom • for spells for children's well-being and releasing the inner child • slowing down the pace of life • called Shakespeare's cuckoo buds • called coyote's eyes in Native North American lore because they gave him acute vision if substituted for his eyes when he tossed his own eyes too high and lost them

HOW TO USE

Use as part of a wildflower planetary garden or lawn to attract butterflies for wishing and Air magick. • Place the flowers with a silver dollar or green dollar bill in a green purse for attracting wealth in daily life. • Grow to attract the fey to your garden, but put on the doorstep on May Eve to prevent mischievous spirits entering. • Shining a buttercup on someone's chin reveals if love is true and if you will be rich. • Place in potpourri for happiness and abundance.

CAUTION

Do not ingest buttercups or their roots. • Use the fresh plant with care, as it can cause reddening or even blistering.

Butterfly Pea Flower

(*Clitoria ternatea*)

MAGICAL FORMS

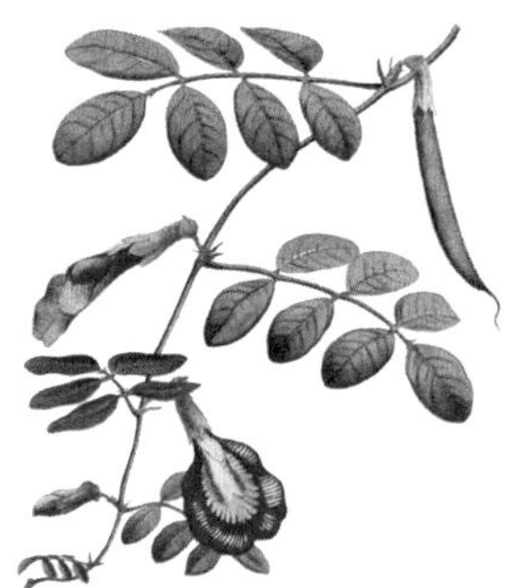

climbing tropical vine, used mainly for its vivid edible blue or purple flowers blooming in summer • though they only last a day or two, the flower can be picked fresh or wilting and left to dry • long flat pods producing six to ten peas each that are edible when the peas are young • the vine is native to Indonesia but grows well in warmer climates within the USA and other countries • the dried flowers can be purchased online or from tea outlets, the flowers used as a healing and magical tea • magically use the flowers, fresh, dried, or as powder; peas; and peapods

PLANET AND ELEMENT

Venus • Water

MAGICAL USES

protection, serenity, enhanced body image, self-esteem, antiaging • the flower is used in daily offerings in India and is a welcome gift on any altar, replaced once it wilts • in Thailand it is told a woman Isra was taken by the kinnary bird (half woman, half bird), shown the plant, and told to cultivate it for healing • in rituals for women's mysteries and rites of passage

HOW TO USE

Base rituals of transformation on any aspect of life as the blue flowers, resembling the butterfly with half-folded wings, turn tea blue and then if lemon is added changes the color to purple. • Split a pod when the peas are young and place the peas in a natural fabric purse or bag, for fertility or prosperity, each day splitting a new pod until the bag is full, then hide the bag in a tree with blue twine on a windy day to release in its own time the attracting powers. Do not go back to look at it.

CAUTION

Do not drink the tea or eat the peas or flowers while pregnant.

Cabbage

(*Brassica oleracea* var. *capitata*)

MAGICAL FORMS

edible green, white, red, purple, or pale-green leaves and heart • descended from the wild cabbage • the first cabbages originated in the Mediterranean more than 2,500 years ago, reaching England in the fourteenth century and the USA with the French explorer Jacques Cartier around 1541 • valued on ships to keep away scurvy • magically use the raw and cooked cabbage and cabbage blends, such as sauerkraut and coleslaw

PLANET AND ELEMENT

Moon • Water

MAGICAL USES

fertility, especially if eaten on the full moon • planted in the garden of a married or newly committed couple to bring good fortune and lasting happiness • in love divination, the Scottish poet Robert Burns described how at Halloween would-be lovers should be blindfolded and asked to pick from a selection of cabbages to determine the nature and wealth of a future lover and number of children • Lycurgus, the Spartan lawyer who was bound to a grapevine for life when he tried to stop the intoxication encouraged by Dionysus, god of ecstasy, was said to have wept with his tears forming tiny cabbages • eating cabbage is said to cure cravings and addictions • served in parts of the southern USA on New Year's Day with black-eyed peas for luck

HOW TO USE

Hold the whole cabbage, naming before cooking what most you seek for yourself and for any sharing the meal. • Use white cabbage for health and unexpected benefits, green for growth in any matter, red for a financial boost, and purple for power. • Create a spell by mixing and empowering sauerkraut (while pickling) and coleslaw, or empower a purchased product with a chant while mixing to build up energies for a major step forward, whether in love, fertility, or prosperity, to be shared with whomever eats the empowered mixture.

CAUTION

Be moderate if you suffer from low blood sugar or use blood thinners. • It may cause colic in breastfed babies.

Cacao

(*Theobroma cacao*)

MAGICAL FORMS

also called cocoa • evergreen tree that may be more than twenty-six feet high with large pear-shaped red-yellow seed pods • native to Mexico and South America but grown throughout the tropics • a pod can contain up to fifty beans and is harvested by hand several times a year • a source of chocolate flavor • as it contains endorphins, chocolate is a natural soother • magically use the beans, nibs (crushed beans roasted or just dried), powder, and numerous cacao/cocoa products

PLANET AND ELEMENT

Venus • Water

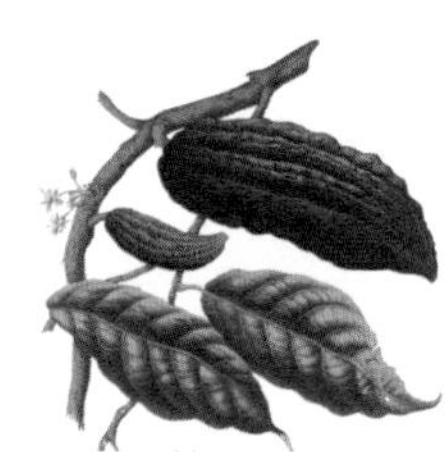

MAGICAL USES

celebrations • creativity • self-love • fun • sensuality • shared happiness • cacao, the pure form, is still a ceremonial drink from Vietnam to Central America • sacred to the Mayans and Aztecs, called by the Mayans the food of the gods, the meaning of the botanical name • cacao contains the "bliss molecule" anandamide, said to create euphoria and a sense of well-being

HOW TO USE

Make a drink from cacao powder or eat the nibs before meditation to open the heart energy center to universal love and compassion. • Cast cocoa beans into fast-flowing water naming for each a burden you wish to shed. • Make quiet time to share cocoa before bed if the family or your partner are super active or workaholics, or if you are alone, to wind down the day, sitting by fire or candlelight in companionable silence or sharing family legends. • Shake the beans in a dish passing them around a group, whether colleagues or family, for spontaneous brainstorming, each shaking the dish, speaking without formulating thoughts, and then passing the dish on.

CAUTION

Dark unsweetened chocolate contains caffeine. • Some people may have an allergic reaction after applying cocoa butter cream to skin.

Cactus

(*Echinocactus polycephalus*)

MAGICAL FORMS

magically use the living plant, spikes, flowers, and juice from the prickly pear (*Opuntia* spp.).

PLANET AND ELEMENT

Mars • Fire

MAGICAL USES

for fierce defense along boundaries or in the four corners, indoors or out, against intruders and unhelpful neighbors and colleagues • for survival if times are hard • absorbing negative vibes from the atmosphere • sprinkle a few drops cold water over your cactus monthly • repot the living cactus annually, and return the old soil to the earth to remove the negativity

HOW TO USE

Add the spines to a witch bottle, or protective bottle, along with rusty nails, rosemary, and rue and bury it near the front door to keep away all with ill-intent. • Carefully use a spine to scratch a banishing message with blessings on a candle or a cactus root and then burn or bury. • Set a cactus of the same species in windows facing the four directions to create a protective barrier against spite, jealousy, or resentment entering the home, especially caused by outsiders. • Yellow or orange flowering cacti are especially protective against troublemakers at work even when not in flower, but beware if offered one as a gift as intentions may not be pure.

CAUTION

Most cacti are poisonous if ingested. • Only the jelly-like liquid of the fishhook barrel cactus (*Ferocactus wislizeno*) can be consumed in an emergency and may have side effects. • To be safe, buy ready-made prickly pear juice.

Cactus, Christmas

(*Schlumbergera bridgesii*)

MAGICAL FORMS

Christmas cactus flowers in the northern hemisphere from late November to late January • a herald of the midwinter solstice, the return of light, and a symbol of Christmas • as an addition or substitute for poinsettia • from the mountains of southeastern Brazil, usually grown indoors in a pot • trumpet-shaped red, purple, pink, white, or yellow flowers, with flat segmented trailing stems • in the wild, Christmas cactus grows in rainforests not deserts • can last for many years and be handed on to the next generation • magically use the cut or whole, growing plant

PLANET AND ELEMENT

Sun • Fire

MAGICAL USES

as a centerpiece for Christmas celebrations • symbol of abundance, goodwill, and the coming together of family and close friends • give as a Christmas gift ahead of the holiday, along with an invitation to spend Christmas together • similar cacti appear around Thanksgiving (*Schlumbergera truncata*), their flowers peach, salmon, white, orange, or red with short bloom and spreading petals about a month earlier than the Christmas cactus bloom • the Easter cactus (*Rhipsalidopsis gaertneri*) with its starlike flowers blossoms in spring • grow all three as a reminder of the cycles of the year and personal transitions

HOW TO USE

Decorate your potted plant with red ribbons, greenery, and tiny baubles to set on the Christmas table as a reminder of the blessings of Christmas. • Each person can hold the pot in turn and make two wishes, one for themselves and one for others and the world. • If Christmas is not a happy time for you, light red candles around your cactus and, blowing softly into each candle, name the new beginning or return of light you most need.

Cactus, Compass Barrel

(*Ferocactus cylindraceus*)

MAGICAL FORMS

also called California barrel cactus • this tall, large barrel-shaped cactus is found extensively in southwestern USA and Mexico, especially around the Mojave and Sonoran deserts, on canyon walls, and rocky slopes • its flowers are red outside and yellow inside, blooming in the spring • the cactus is covered in sharp spines • can be grown in gardens in hot dry places as well as found in formal cactus gardens or in a pot indoors • most easily used as a flower essence, but magically use the whole plant in situ, dried, and powdered

PLANETS AND ELEMENT

Mars/Sun • Fire

MAGICAL USES

the plant and essence reduce anger and irritability, whether repressed or as irrational outbursts • for life makeovers and changes when they are feared, bringing clarity of the right way forward, preventing overthinking, and replacing living on autopilot with trust in inner wisdom • for moody adolescents and grumpy individuals who are constantly complaining but not solving their problems

HOW TO USE

So named because over time the compass barrel cactus in its natural habitat leans to the south, acting as a compass for Indigenous people for centuries and still by lost travelers. • Meditate on your potted plant, having added a few drops of essence to the soil. • Alternatively, or additionally, anoint your inner wrist points, solar plexus, and throat for the balance of heart, mind, and inspiration with the essence, and immediately afterward, pick up a pen, allowing your guides and the spirits of the plant (essence) to dictate, through the automatic movement of your hand on paper, messages indicating the correct path forward.

CAUTION

Use accredited supplements always on expert advice, and be extra cautious during pregnancy. • Beware of the sharp spines around pets and children.

Cactus, Jumping Cholla

(*Cylindropuntia fulgida*)

MAGICAL FORMS

called jumping cholla because the vicious spikes penetrate skin and remain there even if the plant is just brushed against • native to the Sonora Desert of central Arizona and Mexico, parts of the Colorado Desert, and the southwestern USA • can grow up to ten feet tall • there are about thirty species of cholla cactus • grows wild or in a cactus garden • resembles a tree, with thousands of hairy spikes covering its many branches • produces yellowish-green or deep-pink flowers, which are used to create a potent flower essence • magically work with the growing cactus indoors in a pot or not too close to the desert plant in situ, as well as with the flower essence

PLANETS AND ELEMENT

Mars/Sun • Fire

MAGICAL USES

take the flower essence for inner stillness if rushing frantically around • removes obsessive worries and helps in developing a controlled reaction to actual rather than feared crises • the plant is used for defense magic

HOW TO USE

Carefully remove nine spikes and transfer them to a small, dark, glass bottle, half lined with sand, then almost filled with sour red wine or vinegar. • Place it high in the home in a dark place to protect against sudden vicious attacks on your family and accidents with knives, saws, or other sharp implements. • Keep your potted cactus in a safe place near the front door to act as defense against intruders and those who come to your home with spite and malice in their hearts.

Cactus, Milky Nipple

(*Mammillaria mammillaris*)

MAGICAL FORMS

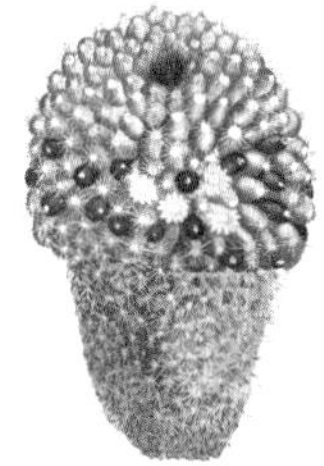

one of a number of flowering cacti with nipple-like protuberances over the body of the plant, that secrete white latex when the cactus is injured or broken • pink blooms emerge from the crown • native to Mexico and southwestern USA • also found under the same botanical name as the woolly nipple cactus in coastal regions of Venezuela, Antigua, and the West Indies, with woolly threads on the axils, creamy white flowers, and clusters of spines • another popular species is the smaller Texas nipple cactus (*Mammillaria prolifera*), with edible red berries that taste like strawberries • these cacti tend not to flower indoors • magically work with the growing plant, which can grow in pots in different regions of the world

PLANETS AND ELEMENTS

Mars/Moon • Fire/Water

MAGICAL USES

the flower essence counteracts the need for continual attention and approval of others • reduces codependency and replaces it with self-reliance • nurturing for children who cry when left at school or with another caregiver apart from the mother, and pets who yowl or bark incessantly if left alone

HOW TO USE

Make a collection of potted nipple cacti and meditate on them to strengthen your aura energy field if you are going through a period when you are under attack or vulnerable. • Add the flower essence to your food or drink if you have codependency issues with your partner or another relative. If possible, use in a spritzer when you are both present. • Add to drinking water of a pet who cannot easily be left and in children's water bottles to take to school.

CAUTION

The latex may be toxic, so handle the cacti with gloves. • Beware of the spines on nipple cacti, especially around children and pets, as these are very sharp.

Cactus, Organ Pipe

(*Stenocereus thurberi*)

MAGICAL FORMS

the second largest columnar cactus after the saguaro cactus in the USA • native and wild in the Sonoran Desert in Baja California, Sonora in Mexico, and southern Arizona, living for several hundred years • may be planted in a suitable clime in rows for hedges and fences • grows between sixteen and twenty-six feet high with tall column arms extending upward from close to or from the base, resembling a candelabra or organ pipes • stores water • gray or greenish-blue stems covered in spikes • in summer, white flowers tinged with pink or purple open at night • if you have the chance, visit the fabulous Organ Pipe Cactus National Monument in Arizona • the fleshy, sweet fruit is eaten by Indigenous Native Americans • magically use the whole plant if you see it, maybe at a cactus garden in situ • alternatively, grow one in your garden, asking an expert if this is possible where you live, or in a pot that can begin about a foot high but will grow to full height through the years • more easily used as essence

PLANETS AND ELEMENT

Mars/Sun • Fire

MAGICAL USES

as a flower essence, it is said to make the user feel nurtured and safe, calming worries, removing pressures, and healing both the physical and emotional self • the growing cactus absorbs and removes negativity from the atmosphere, whether a still relatively small growing potted version or one growing in situ

HOW TO USE

Sitting near a growing cactus, place your hands, palms upward, fingers outward, not touching the spiny exterior, but sufficiently close to allow all misfortune, anger, resentment, or jealousy (both your own and directed toward you) that has stuck in your aura energy field to flow into the plant. Move away when you feel clear and shake your fingers around your head and shoulders to absorb the refreshed energies. If potted, rinse the cactus with a little water or leave an offering.

CAUTION

Cactus spines are extremely sharp; even the growing potted plant should be kept away from children and pets.

Cactus, Prickly Pear

(*Opuntia ficus-indica*)

MAGICAL FORMS

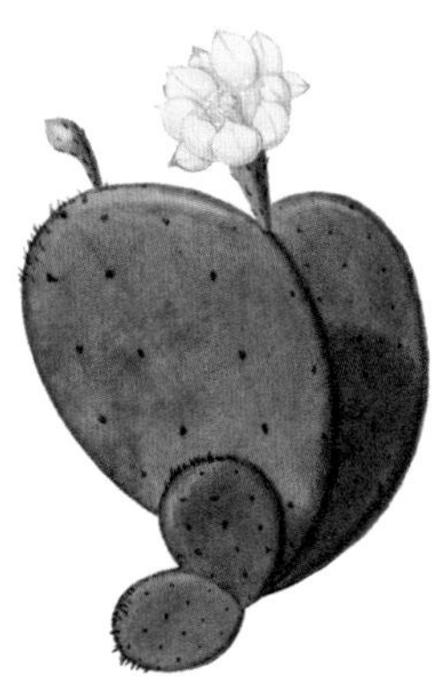

the cactus grows up to sixteen feet tall in the southern USA and Mexico • also in Australia, Africa, and the Mediterranean basin and exported widely • with flat, rounded, branching leaf pads and yellow to orange flowers, bright-red, egg-shaped fruit subsequently growing directly on leaf pads • two kinds of spikes, large fixed ones and small hairy spines that can pierce the skin • both leaf pads and fruit are edible but care must be taken removing the spines • magically use the fruit, potted indoor cactus (if you cannot see the large, growing one), and flower essence • for the use of the oil, see "Prickly Pear Oil" (p. 364)

PLANET AND ELEMENT

Mars • Fire

MAGICAL USES

as the cactus and the essence, for alleviating anxiety, stress, and tension by adapting to events and situations rather than trying to swim against the tide of life

HOW TO USE

A bowl of prickly pear fruits in the center of the home circulates prosperity, health, and wealth. Peel carefully and eat one every day, replacing it so your bowl is never empty. • Place the spines from the peeled skin or from your potted cactus in a thick protective brown bag to hang over the door for protection against earthly and paranormal malevolence. • Share the juice or the egg-shaped fruit with a lover to increase passion. • Anoint your breasts and womb or, for a man, just above the genitals with a drop of the flower essence well mixed in an almond carrier oil if you wish to conceive.

CAUTION

Beware of the spines on the plant and fruit.

Cactus, Queen of the Night

(*Epiphyllum oxypetalum*)

MAGICAL FORMS

flowering, climbing orchid cactus with sprawling waxy stems, exotic white flowers that open at night (but only on one night of the year and they wilt before the morning) • sweet-smelling • native to Mexico and South America • grows in tropical and semitropical climes • also as an indoor plant or in a hanging basket • magically use the indoor plant (if the growing one is not found or will not flourish in your area) and the flower essence

PLANETS AND ELEMENTS

Mars/Moon • Fire/Water

MAGICAL USES

for overcoming fears of all kinds, especially of open spaces • to get in touch with intuition and for men and women to connect with the cycles and energies of the moon • the rare bloom, while blossoming, is a token of short-lived but immense good fortune

HOW TO USE

In moon magick, set your potted plant (or hanging basket) in the moonlight or go outdoors in the full moon if the cactus is growing. Plant offerings in the soil around it: seven moonstones, making seven wishes to the queen of the night. • Take the essence for a lunar month, noting each night before bed how you have felt that day, whether energized, irritable, or weary. Check the moon phase with an online moon calendar each night and you may detect a moon pattern linked with your own energy and mood cycle. • Use the essence if you suffer from agoraphobia before going outdoors or spritz your aura with a few drops of essence in a water spray.

Cactus, Red Orchid

(*Disocactus ackermannii*)

MAGICAL FORMS

grows between two and ten feet high with long trailing leaves and, unusually for a cactus, non-spiny, broad, flat stems from which the flowers grow • large, exotic, usually-open, fragrant, red-orange flowers, though other varieties can be white, pink, or purple • flowers in spring or summer and, once open, blooms day and night, though some only at night • native to Central and South America • magically use as evergreen indoor plant, its main form (though it can grow outdoors in tropical or subtropical regions), and also as flower essence

PLANETS AND ELEMENT

Mars/Sun • Fire

MAGICAL USES

as the flower and flower essence, for women's emotional, physical, and psychological or psychic health, and the anima in both sexes • for diminishing being out of touch with real life instead of valuing every moment, as the flower is beautiful but short-lived

HOW TO USE

Send a night-blooming potted plant before it flowers to a love you must keep secret or when you cannot be together because of circumstances or distance (often called "nature's secret letter" because it blooms at night). • Carry out a goddess ritual with the potted plant in the center of the sacred space when sun and moon are both in the sky to manifest in real life what is dreamed of and desired but dismissed as seemingly impossible. • Use a few drops of the essence in the bath to reconnect with the natural cycles of life if a woman is in an overcompetitive environment or a man forced into a macho role by family or community demands.

Cactus, Woven Spine Pineapple

(*Echinomastus intertextus*)

MAGICAL FORMS

a cactus named because its spines weave around the cactus to resemble a woven basket or pineapple • native to the southwestern USA in New Mexico, western Texas, and Arizona in high, rocky outcrops • pinkish-white flowers, pale yellow around the base, with dark, pinkish-brown stripes underneath and red or pink stigma lobes • the flower lasts about three days • the cactus grows only six inches high • magically use the whole, growing cactus in the wild, in gardens, or in a pot (not easy to find, but worthwhile), and the flower essence

PLANETS AND ELEMENT

Sun/Mars • Fire

MAGICAL USES

for restoring energy and determination when you are overburdened by what you believe or have been told you should be doing • recovery from burnout, jet lag, exhaustion, or prolonged illness • releases what has been blocking your energies • the entwined spines make the cactus very protective against all forms of intrusion and threats

HOW TO USE

For long-haul flights, take the essence in water or under your tongue for a few days before the journey and a few hours before flying, on takeoff, landing, and on the way home (check beforehand with airline that it is permitted in cabin luggage). The cactus is empowering if you have a fear of flying. • Work in a cactus garden or, if you can, buy a cactus in a pot or visit one in its native habitat, perhaps while on vacation. Hold your hands above the plant with your fingers downward and together in a basket shape. Inhale the plant's fierce protection and exhale specific and general fears. • If you can't find the plant, download an image of one and use as a screen saver or lock screen for whenever you feel exhausted or overburdened.

Cajeput Tree

(*Melaleuca leucadendra*)

MAGICAL FORMS

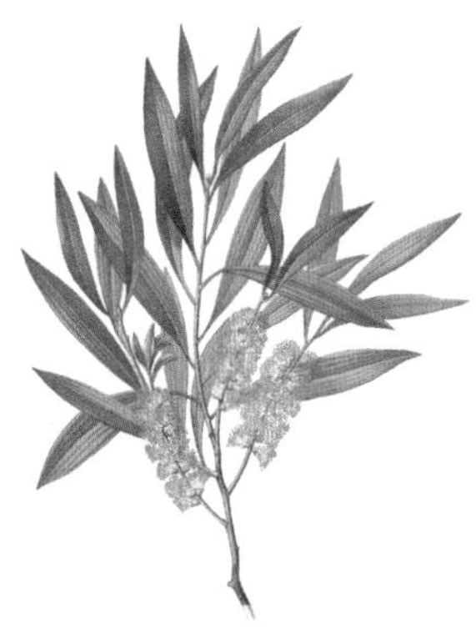

also called the weeping paperbark tree • milder than its cousin, tea tree, the cajeput tree has white spongy bark that flakes off the trunk • it can grow up to seventy feet • native to Western Australia, Northern Territory, and Queensland, the Solomon Islands, New Guinea, and Southeast Asia • its relative, the *Melaleuca quinquenervia* (see "Niaouli Tree," p. 307), the broad-leafed paperbark, has been introduced to the USA and is considered invasive in Florida, especially the Everglades • magically use the essential oil or, if on vacation, work with the fallen bark in situ

PLANET AND ELEMENT

Mercury • Air

MAGICAL USES

the oil will clear the mind if you are tired or have many demands on your time • increases concentration • inspires new options and solutions • kick-starts an ailing libido • for breaking bad habits and cravings

HOW TO USE

Burn or diffuse the oil to cleanse bad atmospheres and remove malevolent, spooky energies, and quarrels from the home. • Use before and during any creative work or a brainstorming session. • If you can obtain the fallen bark, write on it invisibly with the index finger of your writing hand what you most desire or wish to lose from your life and bury it beneath the tree.

CAUTION

Avoid while pregnant or breastfeeding. • Dilute the oil very well if you have sensitive skin. • If you have breathing allergies, be extremely cautious when inhaling.

Calla Lily

(*Zantedeschia aethiopica*)

MAGICAL FORMS

also called the arum lily • is not a true lily • a very popular flower that grows well in a pot in parts of North America, such as Florida and California, the latter where it is also found wild • magically use the whole, growing plant, outdoors or indoors as a potted plant; cut flowers; petals and spadix, fresh and dried; and flower essence

PLANETS AND ELEMENT

Venus/Moon • Water

MAGICAL USES

as wedding flowers, especially in white or pink for formal, traditional, and white weddings • vibrant reds and oranges and mixed colors for midsummer, Lammas, and the autumn equinox celebrations and as offerings in rituals • one myth says calla lilies were created from the Milky Way from drops of milk from the Greek Mother Goddess Hera's breast • where the milk touched the ground it formed calla lilies • for rebirth and new beginnings

HOW TO USE

As both a marriage and funeral flower, calla lilies may be planted in the garden as a private memorial to a secret love for someone whose death cannot be openly acknowledged. • The flower essence or a sachet of the white flower and the spadix, the yellow spike in the middle, can be placed under the mattress during sacred sex for intimacy on a spiritual as well as a physical level. • A sachet of just the dried flowers can be carried as a charm to enhance beauty, glamour, and sexual radiance. • Because of the shape of the flower and its spadix, calla lily is regarded as a symbol of male genitalia united with the female. • As a remedy for impotence, a fresh flower head with spadix intact is immersed in a sealed jar of olive oil, and the jar is secretly shaken nine times before lovemaking. • Use the traditional ritual by stroking the flower and spadix with olive oil before lovemaking.

CAUTION

Calla lily should not be ingested by humans or pets.

Camas, Blue

(*Camassia quamash*)

MAGICAL FORMS

with upright spires of star-shaped, clustered bright blue-violet flowers growing up to three and a half feet high, from spring to early summer • wild in meadows in the northwestern USA and southern Canada, with bulbs that were cultivated and cooked by the First Nations people • the large bulb was boiled down into sugar-like molasses, or baked as a vegetable tasting like sweet potato • increasingly appearing as an ornamental plant in gardens in the UK as well as in the USA and Europe • may be found wild growing with the creamy white poisonous death camas • magically use the bulbs in empowered cookery, as cut flowers, and as a flower essence

PLANET AND ELEMENT

Venus • Earth

MAGICAL USES

to find the balance between logic and feeling, head and heart, if moods alternate or one aspect of the personality is absent • for young people with learning difficulties, particularly dyslexia and dyspraxia • for remaining objective when being pressured to choose between people and decisions • grounding creativity in practical projects and seeing inspiration to change a mundane path

HOW TO USE

Grow in the garden or as cut flowers in the center of the home for tangible results for creative and artistic ventures and for encouraging overcautious family members to explore new possibilities and activities. • Regularly give a drop or two of the essence to children and teens or add to a nightly bath, explaining to older ones the benefits if they have learning difficulties, to give them the confidence to accept help, especially if they are teased about their challenges. • Massage a drop or two of the essence into your temples or that of a stressed-out partner, in a little lavender and coconut oil if you wish, when you feel tensions bubbling and overreaction or a quarrel looming.

Camas, Death

(*Toxicoscordion venenosum*)

MAGICAL FORMS

a toxic weedy plant flowering between April and July, growing across the western USA and the Plains states • two to three feet tall with long green narrow grassy leaves; creamy white, greenish, or pink clustered flowers • a poisonous plant, the mature leaves and bulbs being most toxic if ingested or held • sometimes found growing in a field of blue camas (*Camassia quamash*), which are nontoxic plants good for balancing logic and intuition • like blue camas, death camas is made into a flower essence • for safety, magically use death camas in its highly effective form as the flower essence containing the qualities, not the chemistry, of this attractive but lethal plant

PLANETS AND ELEMENT

Moon/Saturn • Water

MAGICAL USES

as the essence, death camas relieves anxiety, stress, and physical and emotional tension • fosters spiritual rebirth, easing rebirthing sessions with a practitioner • going with the flow instead of resisting unexpected or sudden change • for new beginnings and fostering new relationships

HOW TO USE

Mix the blue camas and death camas essences in a spritzer with water, and spray both on an old home before leaving and the new home on arriving if a move or relocation has been thrust unwillingly on you. • To assist with and accept new situations and work with the advantages rather than the drawbacks. • Sipping the death camas essence in water before going out socially, if you are dating for the first time or using an online dating site after a major relationship breakup, enables you to judge the new person or situation as unique and not through the eyes of past loss or betrayal. • Massage a little of the diluted essence into your limbs before taking up a new sports or leisure activity if you are physically tense as well as emotionally apprehensive.

CAUTION

Since all parts of the plant are poisonous, avoid it and focus on the essence.

Camellia

(*Camellia* spp.)

MAGICAL FORMS

the state flower of Alabama • pink, red, and white cuplike flowers • magically use the leaves, flowers, and as carrier oil made from seeds

PLANET AND ELEMENT

Moon • Water

MAGICAL USES

darker-colored flowers are more intense in spells • for wealth and beautiful acquisitions • the flowers attract precious gifts and luxury living or an indulgent vacation • pink in many shades signifying gentle love without limits or conditions or a beloved absent lover • white for young, first, or unconsummated love • red for romance and passion • all camellias for family loyalty at home or to a family business

HOW TO USE

Give flowers in an enchanted bouquet on love anniversaries and Valentine's Day to bring everlasting unity in love. • Use the leaves or dried flowers and leaf buds from *sinensis* for making black or green teas for tea leaf divination. • Grown in the garden, a camellia bush ensures the home will never run short of money. • Add the dried blossoms to a wealth potpourri in which three small gold objects such as earrings have been buried. • Place the dried flowers on a picture of a desired object or ideal home or failing business premises, then carry it outdoors and tip the flowers on to the ground to scatter with the winds, the picture then being pinned where the noonday sun will shine on it.

Camphor Tree

(*Cinnamomum camphora*)

MAGICAL FORMS

evergreen tree, native to Japan and China but found in parts of the southern USA • magically use the whole, growing tree; evergreen leaves with camphor fragrance; bark; resin, often sold in white squares; and oil, but only the white kind

PLANET AND ELEMENT

Moon • Water

MAGICAL USES

for health and healing • as incense or sitting beneath the tree during meditation to experience psychic visions • one of the seven sacred substances dedicated to Buddha, believed to offer enlightenment • the oil diluted in a diffuser mixed with sweet basil oil before sleep to bring prophetic dreams

HOW TO USE

Carry the bark and dried leaves as an amulet if sexual attraction is proving a problem in the workplace or the object of desire is committed elsewhere. • Use in rituals on the end of the wane/the dark of the moon to let go of a relationship that has ended or must end. Follow it with moon ceremonies on the crescent moon for new beginnings and the right love. • Add the gum resin in incense mixes to cleanse a ritual space or the home. • When you move to a new home, carry a heatproof portable incense holder (thurible) of camphor-based incense through the empty house to remove any lingering negative energies from the previous owner.

CAUTION

Camphor is toxic to humans and pets if ingested. • Avoid if you suffer from epilepsy or are pregnant or breastfeeding. • The oil can cause allergic reactions if applied to the skin. • Though used in modern aromatherapy, some experts believe it can be hazardous, so check.

Camphorweed Wildflower

(*Heterotheca subaxillaris*)

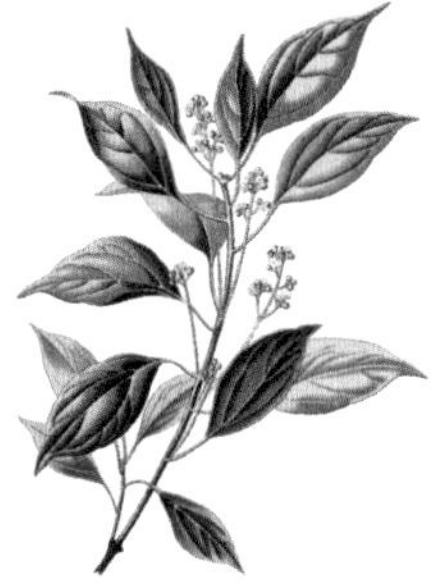

MAGICAL FORMS

wild flowering plant that can be seven feet tall, growing extensively in the USA from California to Massachusetts, west to Texas, and north to Kansas, and in Mexico and Belize • now can be found worldwide • a strong camphor scent when the leaves are crushed and bright yellow daisy-like flowers blooming July through November • magically use the growing and dried flowers and leaves, which are covered in white hairs, and the flower essence

PLANET AND ELEMENT

Mercury • Air

MAGICAL USES

for clarity of purpose • mental clarity • staying on track • letting go of old self-destructive patterns • bringing needs and desires to manifestation • slowing the adrenaline rush if you or family members, especially teenagers, are risk-takers and constantly push the boundaries

HOW TO USE

Crush the leaves and add to an incense mix for extra strength to any purpose and to cleanse a ritual space. • Take the essence daily to avoid burnout in a stressful job or accidents in a physically challenging activity. • Make a dried flowers amulet bag, adding a drop or two of the essence, to keep in the glove box of the car of a partner or teenager who takes risks or with athletic gear for extreme sports participants.

CAUTION

Camphorweed has not been fully researched, so use with care and in moderation.

Campion

(*Silene* spp.)

MAGICAL FORMS

consists of about nine hundred species throughout the world, as ornamental rock plants as well as wild or part of a wildlife garden • grows extensively throughout eastern and western North America and to the mountains in the north in its alpine form • includes red campion (*Silene dioica*), white campion (*Silene latifolia*), and bladder campion (*Silene vulgaris*) • magically use the growing plant, fresh or dried flowers, and flower essence

PLANET AND ELEMENT

Saturn • Earth

MAGICAL USES

hidden passion • forbidden love • secret meetings because some campions have their heads pointing permanently downward holding their secrets • red campion is associated with the mischievous fey who guard the plant at night • it is a Bach flower remedy for emotional balance if life is imbalanced • white campion is called the flower of mourning or the graveyard flower because it grows spontaneously on tombstones as a sign of eternal life

HOW TO USE

The bladder campion is used in decorative dried flower bouquets indicating love will last and win out. • It is also called the popping flower because of its balloon-like swelling behind its flowers. If you hold the flower and chalice in one palm and hit it with the other palm, you get a loud firecracker sound, an excellent conclusion to release the energy in a ritual if every member of a coven or group pops theirs at the same time, having empowered the flowers in the center of the altar during the ritual. • Make a spray mist with the flower remedy and water to bring the cloak of secrecy to a room if confidential matters are to be discussed. • Put a drop or two of the essence under your tongue so you will remain undetected if meeting a secret lover.

CAUTION

Campion is toxic to horses if ingested in huge quantities. • Avoid ingesting while pregnant or breastfeeding as a precaution.

Cananga Tree

(*Cananga odorata* var. *macrophylla*)

MAGICAL FORMS

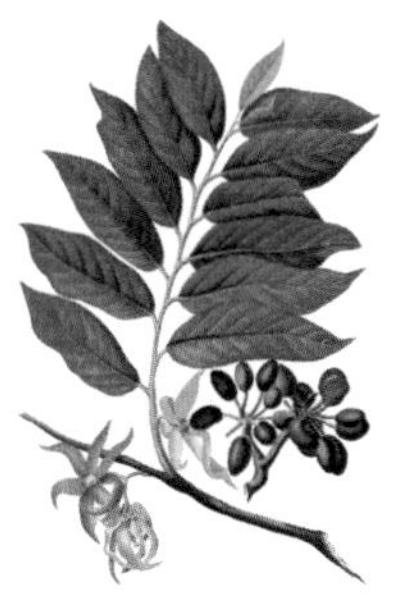

tree that can grow up to ninety-eight feet with large aromatic drooping yellowish-green petals • native to tropical regions of Southeast Asia and will grow in warm humid areas of the USA • similar to ylang-ylang, which also comes from the pure cananga tree species (*Cananga odorata* var. *genuina*) • often regarded as the economy version of ylang-ylang, but less intense, more floral, woodier, greener in fragrance, and chemically different • preferred by those who like more subtle fragrances • magically use the essential oil from this variety of the cananga tree and, if you can obtain them, the fresh or dried flowers

PLANET AND ELEMENT

Venus • Earth

MAGICAL USES

an aphrodisiac, encouraging gentle, spiritually focused lovemaking • connection with the ancestors, angels, and guides, for valuing self-time and overcoming loneliness and alienation from others who have different worldviews

HOW TO USE

Burn or diffuse the oil or use as well-diluted massage oil on your psychic Third Eye in the center of your brow before and during meditation, yoga, prayer, or chanting to connect with all those who have gone before you and receive messages from higher spiritual beings. • Listen to your favorite music with cananga as your background fragrance to connect with your authentic self and value your own company, filling your aura energies with the power to attract kindred spirits. • If you can get the flowers, cast them into flowing waters to call the one who will complete your life.

CAUTION

There is not enough research to determine its safety during pregnancy and breastfeeding. • Dilute very well if you have sensitive skin.

Candlewood Tree

(*Dacryodes excelsa*)

MAGICAL FORMS

large rainforest tree, also called tabonuco, whose indigenous name means "tree of incense" • grows to a hundred feet • the only tree of its kind, found in Puerto Rico and the Lesser Antilles from St. Kitts to Granada • once the dominant tree in the rainforest, now suffers from overharvesting and clearances • the endangered Puerto Rican parrot feeds on its seeds • its white, sticky, liquid resin hardens into a gum, smelling of a mix of menthol, camphor, and lemon • burned as resin, and the resinous wood has been used in torches since pre-Columbian times • Spanish settlers learned from the Indigenous peoples to tap the tree, especially at the full moon, for the flammable resin, which was used in ceremonies, prayers, and medicine, and to make sacred candles, hence the name candlewood tree • magically use the crushed resin or a powdered form in an incense mix

PLANETS AND ELEMENTS

Sun/Moon • Fire/Water

MAGICAL USES

use the resin for reviving what was given up as useless • for shamanic experiences • brings clarity and understanding to interactions

HOW TO USE

Burn the resin to overcome mind manipulation and power games if you or a loved one are being unwisely influenced, and to reduce cravings and addictions. • Light gold and silver candles for the sun and moon as you burn the incense for candle magick wishes and to connect with benign spirits and ancestors through the flame, framed by the smoke. • Although it is not always easy to find this resin online, if you can acquire it, use it for ceremonies connected with the full moons, the solstices in June and December, and the equinoxes in March and September to call the powers of fire and light into your life and to tap into the seasonal or lunar energies.

CAUTION

Use with caution if you have a chronic condition or are immunocompromised, or if you are pregnant.

Candystick

(*Allotropa virgata*)

MAGICAL FORMS

also called sugarstick • a plant resembling peppermint candy with red stripes twisting up the erect white stem • grows up to fifteen inches high • unusual since it is not a green plant and has no chlorophyll • gains nutrition through its roots via a fungus from the roots of neighboring host hardwood trees like the oak or western hemlock or conifers such as the Douglas fir • grows in the Pacific Northwest up to British Columbia and western states east to Montana and down to California • hard to cultivate • magically use the growing plant in situ to clear emotional blockages in meditation

PLANET AND ELEMENT

Saturn • Earth

MAGICAL USES

as an essence it can be used to tap into available resources to follow a unique lifepath • to take responsibility and consequences for choices (candystick neither helps nor harms its host) • to clear blocked energy around miscarriage, birth, and sexuality for women, especially linked with the pelvis and sacral energy center of emotions • for resolving anima issues among both sexes • accepting the free will of others to accept or reject our needs

HOW TO USE

Take the essence regularly if you are suffering loss or fears concerned with maternity (helpful for both sexes in dealing with a partner's miscarriage and for those who are afraid of the birth process or of becoming a coparent). • Also take the essence for resolving issues around relationship dependency, ideally sharing daily doses with a partner, particularly if you feel that you are not getting the support you need. • Scatter droplets around a printout if applying for resources or seeking funding or backing for a venture.

CAUTION

Candystick may be toxic if the plant is ingested medicinally in large amounts, but the essence is safe. • Seek advice from an expert if pregnant.

Candytuft

(*Iberis sempervirens*) and (*Iberis umbellata*)

MAGICAL FORMS

low-growing shrubs • *Iberis umbellata* is also called garden or globe candytuft • *Iberis sempervirens*, also known as snowflake candytuft, has clusters of fragrant snowy white flowers, blossoming in the spring, early summer, and again sometimes in the fall • deep evergreen foliage in warmer climates • native to the Iberian peninsula and southern Europe and naturalized in the USA, the UK, the Balkans, and northern Europe • some species have pink as well as white and purple cotton candy-like flowers, linking magically with candy (though named after its original location, Candia, now called Hiraklion in Crete) • magically use the whole, growing plant; taller varieties (twelve to eighteen inches high) such as snowflake or garden candytuft, as cut flowers, fresh and dried; and the fresh and dried flowerheads

PLANET AND ELEMENT

Venus • Earth

MAGICAL USES

a seventy-fourth anniversary flower for the young at heart, beloved in Elizabethan England as a garden plant • gift in a pot or as a mass of small flowers in a bouquet, accompanied by a box of favorite candies • ideal for children's first foray into gardening • associated with moon rituals for the white ones glow in moonlight

HOW TO USE

Associated with indifference and stoicism in the language of flowers, carry the dried flowers in a sachet to reduce obsessions, phobias, and crippling fears. Bury the contents where nothing grows, and replace each week. • To generate enthusiasm in yourself or a partner who is staid and will never have fun, surround a bunch of preferably fresh candytuft with your favorite candies. Light a white candle and say nine times fast, *Feel the joy, feel the sweetness, with unbridled happiness replace this neatness*, and then blow out the candle fast and put the candies in a bowl to be eaten or shared.

CAUTION

Candytuft is mildly toxic for dogs.

Canna Lily

(*Canna × generalis*)

MAGICAL FORMS

not to be confused with calla lily (see p. 94) • not a true lily, but related to ginger, bird of paradise, and bananas • also the hybrids (*Canna indica*) • exotic blooms in red, pink, orange, and yellow • dramatic foliage in maroon, green, or brown, with broad banana-like leaves • growing to a height of three to four feet in the dwarf varieties and up to eight feet or more in the giant kinds • magically use the whole flower in situ or cut for displays; flowerheads/petals, fresh and dried; foliage; and incredibly hard black or brown seeds, reputed to last centuries

PLANET AND ELEMENT

Jupiter • Air

MAGICAL USES

flower of the seventeenth wedding anniversary • favored in tropical/beach-based weddings, major birthdays, and spiritual/religious landmarks such as baptism/naming ceremonies or initiation into a spiritual/religious way of life • native to North, Central, and South America in tropical and semitropical zones • used by Native Americans for food and medicine for thousands of years, and centuries later naturalized in the northeastern USA, the UK (prized in Victorian England), Australia, Asia, and Europe • use the whole plant cut or growing for developing creative and artistic expression • for meditation and to clear doubts and distracting negative thoughts

HOW TO USE

A single cut or a small potted flower (dwarf variety) in the center of the altar or as a focus during spellcasting, lifts magical vibrations. • A natural symbol of perfection, beauty, prosperity, and good fortune, grow the lilies in the garden or keep one indoors in a container to cleanse all that is not positive (canna lily is a natural remover of toxins). • Use it to help older people to not regret the passing of youth.

Canterbury Bells

(*Campanula medium*)

MAGICAL FORMS

long-lasting blossoms with upright stems, two to three feet tall • cup and saucer/bell-shaped purple, pink, or white flowers and a clapper-like stamen in middle • native to the Pyrenees regions of France and Spain, Canterbury bells reached the British Isles at the end of the sixteenth century and have been naturalized in temperate regions of the USA • magically use the whole, growing flower; cut flowers; and bell-shaped petals and stamens, fresh and dried

PLANET AND ELEMENTS

Venus • Water/Earth

MAGICAL USES

a fae flower, the bells attract nature spirits, especially at twilight • as a symbol of support, fidelity, and constancy, Canterbury bells are a suggested choice for the twenty-fourth wedding anniversary as they make beautiful less formal bouquets as well as a potted or garden gift • they were known as Coventry bells, a cathedral city in the middle of England until the 1800s and then called Canterbury bells after the famous English cathedral • it may be they grew in profusion around these cathedrals, as one meaning given for *campanula* is tower of bells • whatever the connection, listen to church bells while meditating and holding the cut flowers for visions of past worlds when you heard other church or temple bells (a powerful if not totally explicable experience)

HOW TO USE

Pick the flowers, naming for each set of bells a happy memory. • In traditional fashion, press the flowers without the stems in pages of books between blotting or parchment paper to preserve joyous moments if life becomes hard. • Grow the flowers in your garden to keep away all harm from your home. • In matters of justice, make an amulet of the dried bells and stamens so that your cause will be heard and your words believed.

Caper

(*Capparis spinosa*)

MAGICAL FORMS

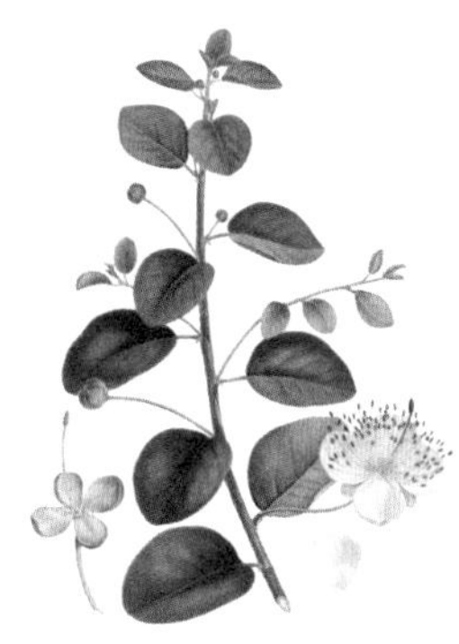

in summer the caper bush, with many spiny branches and round fleshy leaves, produces large pinkish-white flowers with four white petals surrounding a tuft of pink/white stamens • the unopened flower buds are the capers, and long-stalked olive-shaped caper berries (the fruit) are also edible • capers are generally salted or pickled before eating • often found growing wild in hot arid dry stony areas of the Mediterranean, on viny brambles in North America, and in lands including Pakistan, Egypt, Libya, Tunisia, the Asian Red Sea coast, Israel, and Australia • the bush can be cultivated in containers • magically use capers, ready pickled in brine or salt or raw in cooking to spice up any spell or empowerment

PLANET AND ELEMENT

Mars • Fire

MAGICAL USES

to have the courage to stand against bullying or being shouted down • to know who is lying or deceitful • drained from the brine as a nibble or garnish at a gathering to encourage sociability and lively communication • the flowers displayed to increase beauty in any place, person, or situation

HOW TO USE

Use in cookery to strengthen longer-term goals of the intention that the food represents, naming the purpose and time scale as you add the capers. • Add preserved, washed, and dried capers to an amulet bag on the outside of which you have invisibly drawn an eye to protect yourself and your home or workspace against the evil eye of jealousy and envy,and replace monthly. • Use to increase libido, especially for men. • Feed capers to yourself and a partner of either sex as a nibble or in a meal to raise the temperature in lovemaking and for sex magick.

Caraway

(*Carum carvi*)

MAGICAL FORMS

magically use the whole, growing plant; seeds; and essential oil

PLANET AND ELEMENT

Mercury • Air

MAGICAL USES

strengthens memory • guards against inconstant lovers • telepathically prompts communication with those whom you wish to reach • prevents social media attacks • alertness to potential scams • a charm to keep illnesses away from children • protection of property against theft or damage

HOW TO USE

Growing the plants in the garden or hanging the seeds in a net over entrances protects against evil spirits, thieves, and unwelcome visitors. • Seeds taped underneath precious artifacts guard against theft. • Use as part of an incense mix to drive away and keep away malicious fey who do not like caraway seeds. • Hold a sachet in your nondominant hand while activating a phone to prompt an absent friend or love to contact you or while turning on a computer when you are seeking information online. • The seeds in magical cookery in bread, cookies, or cakes act as an aphrodisiac, attract new lovers, and promote fidelity. • Sew one or two seeds in the lining of a child's garment to shield them from bullying or accidents when away from the home.

CAUTION

Avoid during pregnancy or if suffering from heavy menstruation. • Do not take the oil internally, and dilute it well, as it can irritate the skin.

Cardamom

(*Elettaria cardamomum*)

MAGICAL FORMS

also called cardamon or cardamum • sold as spice, made from whole ground dried fruits or seeds • tall herbaceous plant from southern India, Burma, and Sri Lanka, and produced extensively in Guatemala • can grow in tropical zones of North America • the spice dating back to the Bronze Age was introduced to the UK, Scandinavia, and Europe in the mid-sixteenth century • to make tea, use the crushed pods of green cardamom with honey or mix with green or black tea • black cardamom, Nepal cardamom (*Amomum subulatum*) is stronger in flavor and not as good for tea • magically use the pod, seeds, and the essential oil

PLANET AND ELEMENT

Venus • Water

MAGICAL USES

detoxification rituals • clear communication and public speaking or meetings • increases libido of reticent lovers when shared as tea or in magical cookery

HOW TO USE

Empower your spice (obtainable from any supermarket as powder or pods) with the purpose for which you intend it to be used. • For money or luck, burn the green pods or the powdered green seeds in incense. • Bleached white cardamom (from the green) is sometimes substituted in love, twin soul, or passion rituals. • Anoint a green and a white candle with a drop of cardamom oil diluted in a little olive oil, naming him or her, to call a desired love to your bed and to remain in your life.

CAUTION

Dilute the oil well as it can irritate or burn the skin.

Carnation

(*Dianthus caryophyllus*)

MAGICAL FORMS

flowering plant often used in wedding or anniversary bouquets • magically use the whole, growing plant; fresh petals in rituals; perfume; oil; and dried flowerheads

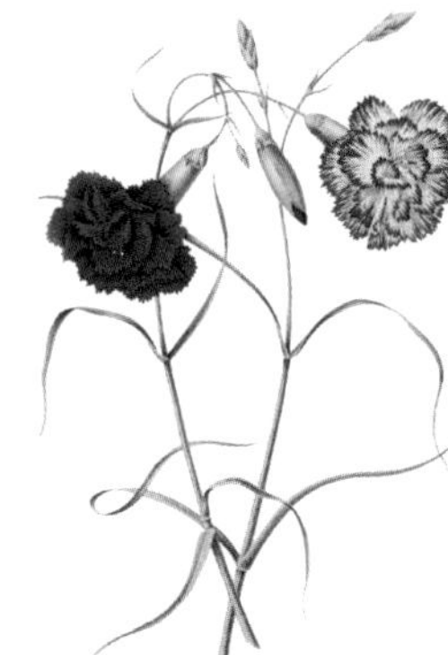

PLANET AND ELEMENT

Mars • Fire

MAGICAL USES

on Mother's Day: pink or red given in gratitude to living mothers; white to commemorate a mother who has died or is not in your life • pink also for romance and increasing friendship and team bonding • red for passion, long-lasting fidelity, courage, and, in sickrooms, for healing strength • yellow for calling back past love; also against spite, gossip, and overly critical neighbors, family, and colleagues • white for love in later years, truth in love, and overcoming grief because the tears of the Virgin Mary at the crucifixion were said to be transformed into white carnations • brown to overcome sibling rivalry, stepchildren issues, grief at the loss of a pet

HOW TO USE

Use the dried blossoms in incense and sachets for healing. • Use the living flower on an altar during healing and love rituals. • Hold a carnation in your nondominant hand and allow it to absorb all negativity before shredding the petals outdoors. • Use the dried carnation heads in tea or candied to decorate food in magical cooking for a lover. • Grow the plant in a garden to protect the home.

CAUTION

While carnations are generally very good-tempered, it is best to avoid during pregnancy. • Some people show skin and digestive oversensitivity if used to excess. • The oil should not be taken internally.

Carob

(*Ceratonia siliqua*)

MAGICAL FORMS

a rare evergreen tree that can reach fifty feet with large violet-brown seed pods, each containing between five and fifteen hard brown carob seeds/beans surrounded by sweet pulp • native to southeastern Europe, the Middle East, western Asia, and North Africa and grows in warm temperate regions including California • ripe, dried, and sometimes roasted, whole beans are often powdered for cooking and in drinks • considered a healthy substitute for chocolate • magically use the bean and powder as chocolate alternatives

PLANETS AND ELEMENT

Venus/Saturn • Earth

MAGICAL USES

once the seeds/beans were used in measuring gold, hence the word carat as a gold value • this has given carob beans their association with obtaining what is of worth whether at garage sales, treasure trove, or being given jewelry • protection of children • health • friendship • male potency • reduces cravings, particularly for candies

HOW TO USE

Carry a bag of beans to protect you as you travel or work. • Keep another bag in the home, replacing them every Friday, the day of Venus, and casting the old ones into water. • Drink carob or eat carob before bed for healing in dreams and to drive away fears of the night. • Share a meal or candies containing carob with a lover who has lost confidence in lovemaking to boost libido and reintroduce spontaneous pleasure if you are focusing on ovulation charts. • Offer carob cakes at a naming ceremony or christening to honor those who have passed over, especially when the name is to be recalled in the new child.

CAUTION

It is safe in moderate quantities but best to avoid during pregnancy and breastfeeding, as not enough sufficient research has been done.

Carrageenan

(*Chondrus crispus*)

MAGICAL FORMS

also known as Irish moss seaweed • highly branched, tree-shaped seaweed/algae, from dark or yellowish-brown to greenish-purple and purplish-red • grows in rockpools and on rocks attaching itself on a small stalk • the watery version of Irish Moss (see p. 297) • in practice you can use similar rituals for either form of Irish moss, especially when both are dried and crushed • grows throughout Atlantic coasts of Europe and Canada, on the shores of Japan and California, and the American North Atlantic coast • grows naturally in large quantities • magically use the whole plant, fresh or dried in the sun and pulverized, or purchased in herb or powdered form for ritual

PLANET AND ELEMENT

Moon • Water

MAGICAL USES

a plant sacred to the Celts, especially but not exclusively those of Irish descent, as a symbol of abundance and survival under difficulty • in Ireland, carrageenan provided food for the Irish living along the North Atlantic coastline during the potato famine of the nineteenth century • the algae was brought to the coasts of Massachusetts by the Irish settlers • for sea rituals connected with Celtic ancestry and connecting with their ancient wisdom and past lives (Scottish moss is similar)

HOW TO USE

Attach Chinese divinatory coins to a sturdy piece of dried seaweed for luck. • Add dried and pulverized carrageenan to a gambling sachet with a green dollar note and a lucky hand root. • Burn incense of dried carrageenan for protection against natural disasters. • Place it under a doormat to ensure only those with good intent will cross the threshold.

CAUTION

There is uncertainty whether processed carrageenan has side effects, though many consider the actual plant safe to consume. Talk with an expert you trust. • Magically there should be no problems as long as you do not ingest.

Carrot

(*Daucus carota* subsp. *sativus*)

MAGICAL FORMS

orange, herbaceous, cultivated root vegetable and cultivar descendant of the wild carrot (see "Queen Anne's Lace," p. 369) • a nutritious food with a distinctive sweeter flavor than the wild carrot • can be eaten raw, cooked, or made into carrot cake • the tap root growing beneath the ground is greatly enlarged from the wild version • magically use the vegetable, raw or cooked; the seeds, found under the umbel; and the many-rayed flower stems, which drop to the ground after flowering

PLANET AND ELEMENT

Mars • Fire

MAGICAL USES

may have been bred from the purple rooted wild carrots before a Dutch botanist developed the orange strain, reaching the USA with settlers in the seventeenth century independently of the wild kind • to increase fertility and act as an aphrodisiac, share a carrot cake, preferably homemade, on full moon eve, using a mix of full size and baby carrots, before lovemaking • traditionally believed to sharpen eyesight, eat a sweet raw carrot before divination to increase clairvoyance and intuition or if you need to see a person or situation clearly if motives are obscured

HOW TO USE

Seeds from the carrot can be ground and made into a tea with honey, stirred clockwise while naming the intention as a chant. • Add the ground seed to a flavorsome herbal tea to attract profitable ventures, especially through creative enterprises. • Share the tea for the success of joint or workplace ventures. • Dig up a carrot, or buy one with the greenery still attached, preparing and eating it for obtaining hidden resources or bringing to the notice of others previously unrecognized talents.

CAUTION

Avoid consuming large quantities if you are diabetic, and limit while breastfeeding, especially the juice.

Cascarilla

(*Croton eluteria*)

MAGICAL FORMS

known popularly as copalchi • large shrub/small tree with yellowish-brown bark and small white fragrant flowers • native to the West Indies, Bahamas, the tropical Americas, and the Amazon basin • magically use the essential oil, which is called sweetwood bark oil and is made from the bark, and the crushed bark, which is available (though not easily) online • note: cascarilla powder is made from crushed eggshells, popular in Santeria (an African diasporic religion) and Hoodoo, but is energetically and magically different from the oil and shrub

PLANET AND ELEMENT

Moon • Water

MAGICAL USES

the burned or diffused oil, or in a room spray, creates a barrier between seen and unseen worlds after divination, magick, or mediumship to restore you to everyday world consciousness

HOW TO USE

Carry the crushed bark in an amulet bag for protection against negative entities such as poltergeists, sexual demons, and lower life spirits called by mistake during a ouija board or amateur séance. • You can also add a drop or two of the undiluted oil to the bag. • Use the oil as a reassuring background fragrance, mixed with gentle oils. • Anoint your pulse points with diluted oil if you come home to a dark, empty house and feel spooked or anxious about intruders. • Add to lavender or rose potpourri to bless a gloomy home into which you have recently moved to clear the atmosphere and make it your own.

CAUTION

There is insufficient research on its safety during pregnancy or breastfeeding. • Though traditionally the leaves or bark are made into a tea, again there is insufficient modern research to guarantee the advisability of ingesting the plant. • Check with an expert for the latter, as the tea is sold online. • The oil should not be ingested.

Cashew Tree

(*Anacardium occidentale*)

MAGICAL FORMS

the cashew tree, native to South America, produces cashew nuts and cashew fruit (called apples) • the cashew nuts are edible only when peeled, roasted, or cooked, as the nut is surrounded by a double shell containing a caustic resin between the two shells • cashew trees can be cultivated in warm, humid locations worldwide • the cashew tree is grown from India to the tropical USA and the Caribbean and can flourish in cooler climes in a large container indoors (keep well pruned as they can grow up to thirty-five feet) • magically use the shelled nuts, butter, and oil, all available commercially and solving the risks of preparation and handling untreated nuts

PLANET AND ELEMENT

Sun • Fire

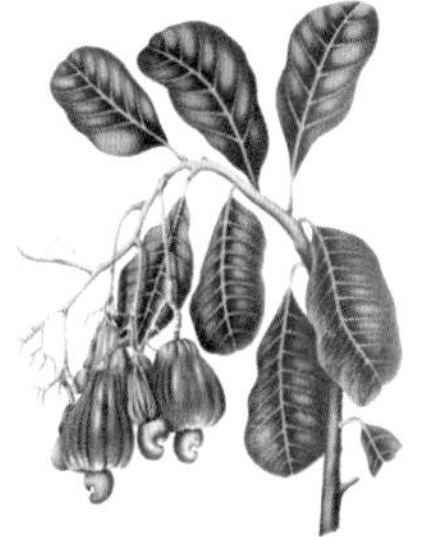

MAGICAL USES

a symbol of money, prosperity, and good employment if a few are eaten each morning with an empowerment of what you need in the day ahead • absorb focused energy for challenges by consuming morning cashew butter made with a little olive oil blended with ground nuts • add cold-pressed cashew oil to hair and skin products, in magical cooking, or as a food dressing for radiance, charisma, and making an impression • having dishes of peeled cashews at a party ensures guests will circulate, socialize, and offer networking opportunities

HOW TO USE

Eat the nuts before going for a job interview to fill your aura with high-flyer energies and radiate competence. • Because the raw nut is enclosed in toxic resin in nature, use only peeled and roasted nuts in an amulet bag against toxicity in people and situations.

CAUTION

Cashew nuts may cause allergies even if treated. • Avoid the oil if you have kidney problems. • Eat in moderation during pregnancy.

Cassava

(*Manihot esculenta*)

MAGICAL FORMS

also called manioc or yuca • a tuberous woody shrub that can grow to six and a half feet tall with large edible yellow-white fleshy roots, a tough papery bark, and large palm-type leaves • native to South and Central America, first grown in Peru four thousand years ago, the roots are the most widely grown food staple in the world • produced throughout the tropics, including warmer parts of the USA • both sweet and bitter varieties are poisonous if consumed raw • also found as tapioca or, popularly, deep fried as cassava chips • magically use the processed roots in their various forms in magical cooking

PLANET AND ELEMENT

Saturn • Earth

MAGICAL USES

cooked and eaten to keep away or reduce debt and ensure there will always be sufficient resources in the home • seen as a gift from the deities, or springing from the deities, in cultures as far apart as the ancient Mayans and the Yoruba people of Nigeria • seek blessings when using cassava flour or incorporating the vegetable in cooking as a substitute for potato (there are many recipes online for the sweet vegetable, whole and grated, or using the bitter kind safely processed as flour) • widely available in supermarkets and Asian or Latin grocery stores

HOW TO USE

Cassava is eaten as a way of honoring the land and connecting with the ancestors, not only one's own but the Earth guardians of your home, and as such, offer a little in a dish outdoors after a cassava-based meal as thanks for abundance to be received. • Make or buy a well-sweetened tapioca dessert to call fertility both to conceive a child and to launch a creative venture or business, stirring it clockwise before eating. • Share a meal containing cassava or cassava baked bread to restore unity to a family gathering.

CAUTION

Unless already prepared, always soak, peel, and cook cassava, even the sweet kind, as it is poisonous when consumed raw. • Only eat during pregnancy if well cooked.

Cassia

(*Cinnamomum cassia*)

MAGICAL FORMS

also known as Chinese cinnamon or cassia cinnamon • native to China, Japan, and Indonesia • grown also in the West Indies and Central America • formed as scrapings from the aromatic inner bark of the *Cinnamomum cassia* laurel tree • sometimes sold as the more expensive true cinnamon, Ceylon cinnamon (*Cinnamomum zeylanicum*) • cassia has a stronger flavor and coarser texture with the corky gray outer bark often left on the cassia scrolls, where cinnamon bark forms single quills • when ground into spice, cassia is reddish brown • cassia seeds are used to make tea • check which you are buying as properties differ • magically use the essential oil made from the leaves and twigs, the stems, and sometimes the bark

PLANET AND ELEMENT

Mars • Fire

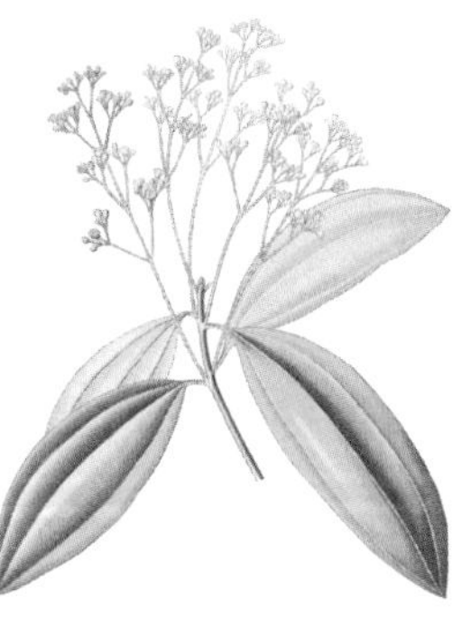

MAGICAL USES

used as a yang tonic in Chinese medicine • detoxifying • use in weight-loss rituals to support healthy eating programs • encourages money-making opportunities and initiative • strengthens psychic work especially using candles and crystals

HOW TO USE

Used in making teas, though stronger and more bitter than Ceylon cinnamon, it is good to kick-start the system emotionally and spiritually as well as physically if inertia or hopelessness sets in. • The oil is traditionally used in sacred anointing oils. • Apply extremely well-diluted oil on your Third Eye (keeping away from eyes and nose) to seal your spirit against everything not from the light to allow you to see true visions. • In a diffuser, the warm and spicy oil with a hint of cloves creates a sense of well-being in the home.

CAUTION

Avoid consuming the tea or spice in large quantities. • Do not ingest as an extract or use the oil during pregnancy.

Castor Oil Plant

(*Ricinus communis*)

MAGICAL FORMS

also known as castor bean • large herbaceous shrub/small tree • fast growing with star-shaped leaves, red flowers, seeds from the fruit, that resemble mottled beans, hence the name • native to southeastern Mediterranean, East Africa, India, and the USA and naturalized throughout Australia • only the bean is poisonous • magically use the bean, having removed the outer coat (with great caution; beware of the fine dust), and the safer oil from the beans/seeds

PLANET AND ELEMENT

Mars • Fire

MAGICAL USES

the beans/seeds are used for defensive purposes only as the husk contains a deadly poison called ricine • keep in sealed bags, away from children or pets, as an amulet against curses, hexes, and ill-wishing and to break these

HOW TO USE

To protect against the evil eye of envy, keep a single bean in a small purple bag and throw it away safely on the last day of the month. The bean will absorb the envious energies, so replace it if the jealousy is ongoing. • Alternatively, draw with a stick in a dish of the oil an eye on the surface (it does not matter if it instantly disappears). Afterward, dispose of both the oil and the stick. This method will not only remove envy but any other negative influence or addiction you name. • Seal beans in a dark glass bottle with sour red wine or vinegar and sprigs of rosemary to defend yourself or your home against danger, and keep it in a dark high place where children cannot reach it.

CAUTION

Wash your hands well after handling the bean or wear gloves. • Avoid both bean and oil during pregnancy or if you are in any way medically vulnerable.

Cat's Claw

(*Uncaria tomentosa*) and (*Uncaria guianensis*)

MAGICAL FORMS

bright green leaves on a woody vine with claw-shaped thorns, growing to great heights in the rainforests of Central and South America, especially around the Amazon • not to be confused with Chinese cat's claw (*Uncaria rhynchophylla*), which is a different plant with different properties and uses • magically use the rhizome, which is available online from magick or specialty herb stores, or as powdered rhizome or a bark decoction that can be bought as a tea from a health-food store or online

PLANET AND ELEMENT

Mars • Fire

MAGICAL USES

defense against spite and jealousy • protection of pets, especially cats • for rituals to awaken the hunting instincts of rainforest wild cats to attract resources and opportunities where there is competition • used ritually and medicinally for more than two thousand years by Indigenous peoples

HOW TO USE

Burn the powdered rhizome in incense or drink the tea before meditation or visualization to act as a bridge between the everyday and spiritual realms. • Add the powdered bark to a defensive bottle filled with apple cider vinegar along with any thorns, such as hawthorn or rose, since it may be hard to obtain the actual cat's claw thorns. Before adding the thorns say, *May these thorns act energetically as the claws of the fierce rainforest cats.* Make the bottle to protect your pets, especially cats, from being harmed by hostile neighbors or fierce dogs or to defend your own boundaries without malice. In either case, set the jar high in a garden shed or a low sheltered roof where it will not be disturbed.

CAUTION

Cat's claw should not be ingested except in officially approved medications. • Avoid ingesting even as tea if you're pregnant or breastfeeding, have an immunity problem or stomach ulcers, or are taking blood-clotting or blood pressure medicines.

Cat's Claw, Chinese

(*Uncaria rhynchophylla*)

MAGICAL FORMS

also known as gōu téng or fish hook vine • a flowering evergreen climbing shrub from southern China and Japan • a staple in traditional Chinese medicine for soothing agitation, for brain and cognitive health, and lowering blood pressure • Chinese cat's claw is different from cat's claw • magically use the dried and chopped stems, leaves, and twigs, which are available online • with diligence and luck you can grow the plant yourself in most soils and shade in the USA and the UK • use the flower essence made with alcohol and a small amount of apple cider vinegar and water

PLANET AND ELEMENT

Mercury • Air

MAGICAL USES

for increasing mental acuity, memory, especially if you are older or with information overload • for calm thinking in a crisis or if others are trying to pressure or panic you • for preventing subtle or financial bullying from adult children

HOW TO USE

Utilize its thorns not to attack but to climb up other plants to reach the light (you can obtain these packaged from a herbal apothecary store online). • Add them to a thick closed charm bag if you are going for promotion or where you need to shine. • Scatter the flower essence around the outside of your computer, books, or learning material to process the knowledge. • Drink a little of the essence in water before an interview, audition, or if you are acting as a witness or defendant in court or a tribunal to keep your mind focused and ahead of your questioner.

CAUTION

Do not ingest Chinese cat's claw while pregnant or breastfeeding. • If using medicinally, consult a traditional Chinese medicine practitioner or check with your physician on dosage, especially if you are taking other medication.

Cat's Ear

(*Hypochaeris radicata*)

MAGICAL FORMS

also known as false dandelion • resembles dandelions but smaller with only eight to twelve petals where the true dandelion has up to forty • has scales at the base and dense hairy lobe-shaped leaves resembling a cat's ear • true dandelion leaves are long and narrow • cat's ear is much shaggier than the true dandelion • its leaves are edible with a mustardy taste, as is the sweet root • usually bright yellow but can be white • blooms spring to fall • though native to Europe, cat's ear is found extensively in the USA, where it is regarded as invasive in some states • magically use the growing plant, the dried flowerheads, the dried leaves, and the seed heads

PLANET AND ELEMENT

Saturn • Earth

MAGICAL USES

much underrated magically, for increasing clairaudience • in amulet bags for healing spells for cats • for becoming aware of gossip, rumors, and concealed ill-will

HOW TO USE

Blow fluffy seed heads to disperse them on their silky parachutes to carry wishes and call protection, especially connected with your cats or other pets. • Since each morning cat's ear will not open until there has been an hour of light and will close in the late afternoon, it acts as a monitor of the changing energies around you. The dried leaves in an amulet bag act as a psychic radar, so as you touch it, you know the best time to speak, act, or remain silent. • Breathe in the gold of a meadow of the flowers to strengthen your power and persistence to come out on top if you have been overlooked or treated as second best.

CAUTION

Cat's ear is toxic to horses. • Seek advice during pregnancy, and beware of toxicity from chemicals used to control the plant.

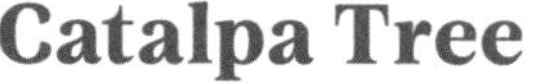

Catalpa Tree

(*Catalpa* spp.)

MAGICAL FORMS

genus of flowering deciduous tree • western catalpa (*Catalpa speciosa*) is a temperate tree, tougher than its southern counterparts, found along the Mississippi and Ohio Rivers and the western coasts in British Columbia, Washington, and Oregon • Farge's catalpa (*Catalpa fargesii*), from China, is grown extensively in Europe and North America • the Indian bean tree (*Catalpa bignonioides*), so named after the Native North Americans who wore its seeds as amulets, is distributed through southeastern USA • magically use the growing tree, seeds, dried and fresh leaves, dried and fresh flowers, and tree essence

PLANET AND ELEMENT

Moon • Water

MAGICAL USES

connects with nature spirits, guardians, guides, and angels • for developing unique gifts • against spite and jealousy • for meditation, sacred chanting, and for musicians

HOW TO USE

Sit beneath a tree, especially the more delicate Chinese form, on a windy day to hear messages in the rustling leaves from the otherworld, angels, and guardians of the trees. • Dry the trumpet-shaped flowers, and hold them in a closed white silk bag when you listen to sacred music, or join in sacred chants, to be carried on the sound to astral journeys. • Bind together seven fallen twigs that you find, and place them on your special place/altar, surrounded by white tea lights, to inspire your creativity whether for words, artistry, or creating/writing music.

CAUTION

Catalpa tree roots are poisonous, and some believe the leaves are, too. • The flower, if inhaled, and the wood, if excessively handled without gloves, can sometimes cause allergies. • Do not ingest any parts of the tree.

Catmint

(*Nepeta mussinii*)

MAGICAL FORMS

a gentler, more spiritual version of its sister, catnip, though they have similar properties and can magically be substituted if necessary • an ornamental plant often found in gardens, with aromatic gray-green foliage and vibrant blue-purple flowers, whose scent attracts cats • native to Europe, Asia, the Middle East, and Africa and naturalized in North America by the European settlers • magically use the growing and cut flowers and the flowers shredded and mixed with the dried fragrant leaves

PLANET AND ELEMENT

Venus • Air

MAGICAL USES

best known in cat toys, catmint flowers traditionally are a very spiritual flower, used in meditation for self-awareness of the deeper values of life • as a focus in rituals for treasuring what is beautiful, especially in nature • in goddess ceremonies as an offering

HOW TO USE

Like catnip, catmint is linked with the Egyptian cat-headed goddess Bastet, but in her aspect as goddess of music, dance, pleasure, and joy. • The herb is a perfect charm for releasing the inner child if life is overly serious and as a good luck charm for musicians who write, perform, or are attending auditions. • Also use as a charm for dancers, both professional and those who dance for pleasure. • Grown in the garden or hung over the front door, catmint attracts helpful spirits, well-intentioned visitors, and good fortune, keeping away all who come with ill intent.

CAUTION

Catmint is not safe during pregnancy. • It may cause allergies. • It should not be used with antihistamines or any medications with a sedative effect.

Catnip

(*Nepeta cataria*)

MAGICAL FORMS

not to be confused with catmint (*Nepeta mussinii*), its showier and more ornamental sister • heart-shaped ragged leaves and whorls of white flowers with purple spots • native to Europe but naturalized in North America • more aromatic than catmint • though there are many similarities in properties with catmint, catnip as its name suggests is more proactive, faster-acting • magically use all aerial parts, especially the leaves; flowers; and as oil

PLANET AND ELEMENTS

Venus • Water/Fire

MAGICAL USES

cat magick • working with animal familiars and spirit animals • telepathic links with pets, especially cats, some of which who love catnip, others preferring catmint • calling passion • sudden good luck

HOW TO USE

In fertility sachets with rose petals and a hint of ginger or cinnamon, it is said to bring fast results if ovulation charts have dimmed spontaneity. • Hide a sachet of dried catnip leaves or flowers in your bag or purse before meeting someone you would like to know better to have the confidence to make an impression. • Burn as incense for shape-shifting and astral travel to the temple of the ancient Egyptian cat-headed goddess Bastet, who offers protection against all harm. She bit the head off the Chaos serpent every dawn as he tried to prevent Ra the sun god rising, so this is the herb of tough love and fighting for what you want. • Sprinkle dried catnip under the mattress for more adventurous sex. • Before lighting a beeswax candle, roll it in honey and then catmint so that a little sticks to the candle to increase radiance in love and charisma to charm others to see life your way.

CAUTION

Do not use catnip in excess or if pregnant. • Avoid also if you have pelvic inflammatory disease or heavy menstruation.

Cattail

(*Typha* spp.)

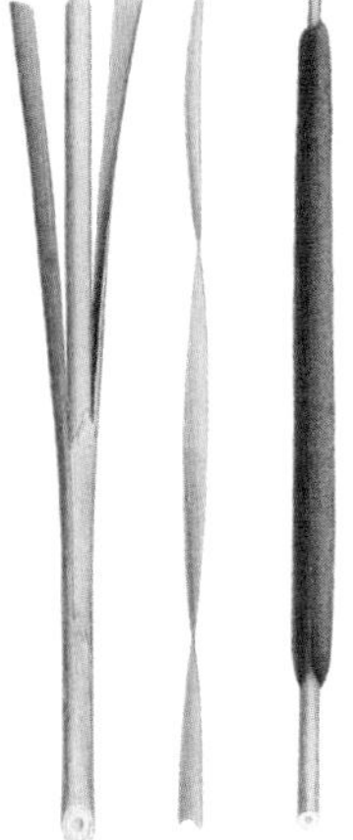

MAGICAL FORMS

including *Typha capensis*, also known as Cape bulrush, and *Typha angustifolia*, also known as lesser bulrush • tall reedy plants or rushes, semiaquatic, beige spikelike flowers, followed by decorative dark brown seed heads • valued by Native North American people as food, medicine, and clothing • magically use the cut or whole, growing plant; fresh or dried root; cattails; leaves; flowers; and pollen

PLANET AND ELEMENT

Mars • Fire

MAGICAL USES

for increasing female libido • prosperity • peace • natural ability over time to regenerate marshland into fertile earth and so a fertility symbol if conception is slow • rituals for the gradual growth of creative ventures and new businesses • for making the Celtic protective St. Bridget cross on February 1 in Ireland, her special day, and hung over doorways to keep away illness, misfortune, and all harm

HOW TO USE

Use the thick rhizome/root, ground into flour substitute (or bought commercially), in magical cookery to offer as cakes on abundance altars or as crumbs scattered on open land. • Bind dried cattails with red ribbon and keep in the bedroom to awaken passion, especially if trying to conceive has introduced anxiety into lovemaking. • Use the dried leaves in weaving magick to bind together (willingly) poppets (dolls representing lovers) or to bring different aspects of a spell together or to unite a number of people in a common cause. • Make a traditional witch's ladder. • Use the pollen fluff released from the flowers in Fire magick, but take care to use safely as they are flammable.

CAUTION

As a precaution, avoid ingesting during pregnancy.

Cauliflower

(*Brassica oleracea* var. *botrytis*)

MAGICAL FORMS

flowering plant with leaves that wrap round its stem • the florets on the head often called "flower of the earth" are edible • nutritious, cabbage-like, from which it is modified • an underrated magical plant in domestic magick • originally from Asia and still grown there • cultivated in European countries, also in North America • occasionally appears as orange or purple hybrids • magically use the whole vegetable, the raw and cooked florets, and as cauliflower rice

PLANET AND ELEMENT

Moon • Water

MAGICAL USES

eaten in Roman times as a luck bringer • carrying a small cauliflower floret as an amulet was, in the Middle Ages, considered proof against misfortune involving poverty or loss • in modern times kept in a vegetable rack to bring abundance and necessary resources to the home (not a symbol of huge wealth but ongoing sufficiency if replaced regularly and cooked to absorb the blessings)

HOW TO USE

A whole cauliflower should be blessed, before preparing and eating, on the full moon to bring protection to the home and family for the month ahead. • The cauliflower rice or vegetable should be served at a family meal where there are simmering disagreements and resentments or rivalry between siblings and different generations. • Purchase or grow a cauliflower with soil still attached, and, as you wash it, name any bad habits, worries, or negative influences you wish to shed.

CAUTION

Generally avoid it if suffering from kidney problems or gout.

Cedar Tree

(*Cedrus libani*)

MAGICAL FORMS

also called cedar of Lebanon, native to mountain forests of Lebanon, Israel, and southwestern Turkey • huge stately tree, with branches that sweep the ground • came to the USA in the late 1800s • one of the four true cedars, with dark gray-green needlelike leaves and oval cones • grows up to 130 feet • also is found in the UK • can live for a thousand years • dried leaves burned as smudge/smoke sticks from various species of cedar including the native California incense cedar (*Calocedrus decurrens*), a distant relative of the cypress, the western redcedar (*Thuja plicata*) in the Pacific Northwest coast and the UK, and the eastern redcedar (*Juniperus virginiana*) • magically use the whole, growing tree; wood; and leaves

PLANET AND ELEMENTS

Jupiter • Air/Fire

MAGICAL USES

the cedar of Lebanon was used in building the ceremonial barge dedicated to Amun Ra the Creator God in ancient Egypt, King Solomon's Temple, and Hanging Gardens of Babylon • cedar boxes are traditionally used for storing amethysts and sapphires • the cedar tree offers a magical space for meditation of other worlds and shelter in myth for unicorns • cedar as smudge or incense for removing negativity from situations, homes, and artifacts and so for cleansing magical tools

HOW TO USE

A bringer of abundance and financial good fortune, cedar relieves worries with debt by generating money-attracting energies. • Place dried leaves in wallets, purses, or cash boxes and with charge cards. • Also store it with special artifacts to preserve them from theft or damage.

CAUTION

Although used medicinally through the centuries and in modern times with expert advice, the raw fruit and bark can be toxic. • Avoid smudging and contact with berries and leaves during pregnancy.

Cedar Tree, Nootka

(*Callitropsis nootkatensis*)

MAGICAL FORMS

also known as the nootka cypress • indigenous to Canada and coastal regions of northwestern North America • can grow in the UK, Northern Europe, and other parts of the USA • reaches up to 130 feet tall, many branched with weeping tips • magically use the essential oil, which is not easy to find but worth searching for

PLANET AND ELEMENT

Moon • Water

MAGICAL USES

the oil for balancing and opening psychic channels • reaching new levels of awareness in meditation • the oil connects with nature even in a city, purifying the aura and home of inertia and misfortune • if you find the tree growing, astrally travel by sitting with your back against the trunk with eyes closed or looking directly upward within its shelter, and by either method following in your mind a branch ladder to the stars

HOW TO USE

Diffuse oil or add to potpourri in workspaces to constantly filter the atmosphere: a psychic air-conditioning system. This removes sluggish energies and speeds up a flow of clients, ideas, and opportunities. • Anoint your pulse points with diluted oil or inhale the oil through a personal inhaler with an inhaler pad inside, infused with nootka, before inducing breathwork, mindfulness, moving meditation, tai chi, or yoga. This keeps the life force circulating within you and takes away worries or self-consciousness about competence in performance. If you lose focus, re-inhale or use a tissue containing the oil tucked in your top pocket.

CAUTION

Consult a physician or midwife before use in pregnancy or breastfeeding. • Dilute very well for topical use.

Cedarwood Essential Oil

MAGICAL FORMS

created from the leaves, bark, needles, and berries from four main cedar trees: Himalayan cedar (*Cedrus deodara*) growing along the Gulf coast into Texas and along the Mississippi valley, around Vancouver and into California, the western Himalayas, the UK, and Europe • Atlas cedar (*Cedrus atlantica*) grows in the UK as well as in Algeria, Morocco, and the USA (though not naturalized) • Ashe juniper (*Juniperus ashei*), not a true cedar, is native to Texas, the southwestern USA, Mexico, and Central America • Virginian cedar (*Juniperus virginiana*) is native to eastern North America from southeastern Canada to the Gulf of Mexico • see "Cedar Tree" (p. 111) for magical uses of other parts of the cedar tree

PLANET AND ELEMENT

Jupiter • Air

MAGICAL USES

symbol of long life, increases sexual desire • protective, especially of property • speeds long-term plans or ambitions • brings justice by intervention of an unbiased authority figure • the oil has been used since biblical times and plays a part in formal rituals

HOW TO USE

Sparingly inhale from the bottle to suppress inappropriate anger even if justified. • Sprinkle a few drops on a cloth beneath your pillow (keep away from eyes and mouth) after a quarrel or injustice so you will not lie awake fuming all night. • Drop the oil into a bowl of water, swirl it nine times counterclockwise, and speak words of reconciliation, forgiveness, or letting go in peace. Stir again clockwise nine times, and pour the mixed oil and water under a fast-flowing tap followed by a rush of water.

CAUTION

Avoid the oil during pregnancy and lactation. • The oil should be very well diluted for topical use. • Do not ingest the oil.

Celery

(*Apium graveolens*)

MAGICAL FORMS

celery is grown for its long, thick, fibrous stalks, tapering into leaves, which are eaten raw or cooked • cultivated for at least three thousand years in Pharaonic Egypt and in China celery was recorded in the fifth century BCE • it came to North America in the 1800s from Europe and the UK and is cultivated especially in Michigan and California • magically use the seeds; spice, whole and ground in charm and amulet bags; and as the essential oil

PLANET AND ELEMENTS

Mercury • Air/Fire

MAGICAL USES

potency • money • protection • bringing travel • in magical cookery as celery salt • the oil burned or diffused with its sweet earthy smell, often with bergamot and lavender for a state of tranquility in the home and to overcome cravings

HOW TO USE

Add the seeds to a sleep pillow to discover what is hidden from you in dreams. • Add the ground seeds to an incense mix with orris root before meditation for sudden insight. • It can be used for astral travel when the seeds are chewed. • Secure in a poppet doll to increase libido. • Tie two poppets with enclosed seeds face to face if fertility attempts are hindering spontaneous lovemaking. • Alternatively, place the seeds in a charm bag hidden beneath the mattress. • Scatter the seeds over a map of where you wish to travel, scoop them up, noting where most land as an ideal destination, and then release them to the winds.

CAUTION

Celery can occasionally cause severe allergic reactions if ingested. • Do not ingest seeds during pregnancy or with kidney disease. • When using the oil medicinally, only apply it topically when it is well diluted.

Celosia

(*Celosia* spp.)

MAGICAL FORMS

known as woolflowers • includes *Celosia plumosa*, the plumed cockscomb, with feathery flowerheads • *Celosia cristata*, the crested variety, resembling a cock's comb, is often red, orange, or coral • *Celosia spicata*, the spiked variety, wheat-like at its point • grown in the USA since the eighteenth century • magically use the whole, growing plant; cut flowers; and flowerheads, fresh and dried

PLANET AND ELEMENT

Mars • Fire

MAGICAL USES

a symbol of undying love, because the flowers survive long after other flowers have faded in the fall and so are popular at weddings • the cockscomb represents good fortune in China and is associated with the proactive Chinese zodiacal rooster • the wheat-like *Celosia spicata* signifies fertility and abundance • celosia is associated also with mourning and with el Día del Muerte, the Day of the Dead, in Mexico, as the flame in the darkness leading the way to immortality

HOW TO USE

In some parts of Africa, it has been used as an aphrodisiac by women to inflame their husbands with passion. • Keep the cut flowers at home or a single large one in water in your workspace for courage and confidence if others try to intimidate or overshadow you. • Use them to inject fun into a celebration. • Display bicolor, purple, red, or orange celosias around a party or conference socializing room if organizing an event for people who do not know one another well or may be naturally restrained and not mingle.

Centaury

(*Centaurium erythraea*)

MAGICAL FORMS

also known as gentian • with care, centaury can grow in gardens as well as wild in Europe and the UK • naturalized in parts of North America, Australia, and New Zealand, in temperate climates • magically use the aerial parts, picked and dried, just before flowering; the pink-purple petals, fresh and dried; and as a flower remedy

PLANET AND ELEMENT

Sun • Fire

MAGICAL USES

for rituals to have the strength to say no • for valuing and caring for the self • counteracting curses and repelling malevolent spirits • traditionally keeps away snakes, reptilian and human spite

HOW TO USE

Because centaury opens in sunshine and closes as it gets dark or cloudy, use it for dual rituals of endings in the evening followed by new beginning as the flower opens again next morning or when the weather brightens. • Burn the chopped dried aerial herb in an incense mix to enhance psychic powers, especially clairvoyance, to connect with other dimensions. • Meditate on the whole plant with its leaves at the base and other leaves climbing the stem (hence, also known as "Christ's ladder") providing a gateway for visions of angels and protective spirits. • Mist around yourself with flower essence in water to help you to see clearly the truth of a situation or an elusive answer.

CAUTION

As a precaution, avoid during pregnancy or if suffering from stomach ulcers.

Cerato

(*Ceratostigma willmottianum*)

MAGICAL FORMS

small flowering shrub, between one and three feet tall • diamond-shaped green leaves with purple margins, becoming bright red in the fall • cobalt blue flowers from late summer to fall • native to western China, cerato is cultivated in gardens in the USA, the UK, and even southern Australia in all but the coldest areas • can be grown indoors in a pot • magically use mainly in its flower essence form, but the growing flowers and leaves possess the same powers

PLANET AND ELEMENT

Saturn • Earth

MAGICAL USES

relying too much on the advice and opinions of others • being easily misled, changing mind frequently, and trying one new solution after another according to the current seeming expertise offered by others • building confidence in personal decision-making

HOW TO USE

To prevent a pet straying or becoming lost, attach nine of your hairs and nine of the pet's to its collar, set the collar on cloth, and sprinkle four drops of the essence over the collar. • Take the remedy daily if you constantly follow the latest fad, fashion, or trend without considering the advantages and drawbacks for yourself. • If you grow or have access to the plant, as an indoor or garden plant, meditate on it, especially with the red fall leaves and blue flowers, to increase your self-esteem and confidence in your own expertise.

Chamomile

(*Matricaria recutita*) or (*Chamaemelum nobile*)

MAGICAL FORMS

Matricaria recutita is also known as German chamomile • *Chamaemelum nobile* is also called Roman chamomile • magically use the herb, leaves, flowers, and oil

PLANET AND ELEMENTS

Sun • Fire/Water

MAGICAL USES

anticurse and antihex • attracts money • babies and children • brings calm and peace to any situation • family happiness • fertility, especially first-time parents • gentle love • increases self-love after abuse • lessening obsessions and addictions • quiet sleep • removes restless ghosts • reconciliation • winning money or prizes • water scrying

HOW TO USE

Use charm bags with yellow dried flowers and gold earrings for wealth. • Use the oil, or use a porous bag of flowers, in the bath to attract love. • Enchanted teas deflect confrontation and bring financial gain or admiration from someone you want to attract. • Use as incense for meditation. • Use in an oil diffuser as background if your family is quarrelsome. • Water scry with the chopped flowers, chopped leaves, or dried chamomile, using Roman (English) chamomile for the best result, especially for family and fertility questions.

CAUTION

Avoid Roman chamomile during pregnancy. • Chamomile can also cause nausea or itchiness if the oil is applied directly to the skin.

Chaste Tree

(*Vitex agnus-castus*)

MAGICAL FORMS

also known as the vitex tree • an aromatic shrub or tree that can grow to twenty-three feet, with palm-shaped leaves and small, lilac flowers • native to Eurasia, but naturalized in the southern part of the USA • first cultivated in the USA in 1670 • the dark yellow-red berries, collected in the fall, can be dried in the sun and used to make tea • magically use the berries mainly, but also the leaves and flowers

PLANET AND ELEMENT

Moon • Water

MAGICAL USES

for positive mother/daughter interactions • Mother Earth ceremonies • in a charm bag, for the birth of new projects, ideas, and stages of life, as well as the birth of a child • for promoting fertility when trying for a baby if tests and charts have taken away the magic of lovemaking • originally used by virgins and those who had taken vows of chastity to reduce unwanted libido and sexual attention • as an amulet as far back as sixth century BCE to ward off evil, especially attacks by earthly and paranormal sexual predators, and unwise temptations

HOW TO USE

Add the dried leaves to incense for wisewoman rituals, and give the seeds sprouting from the fruit in a charm bag to a young person going through puberty. • The tea can be used ritually in goddess rites, especially on full moon, served in the chalice and offered to the moon first by raising it skyward, and then pouring some on the earth before sharing among participants.

CAUTION

Avoid if taking the contraceptive pill or undergoing medical fertility treatment. • Do not ingest vitex while pregnant. • While the berries are edible, they can occasionally cause a rash or stomach upset.

Cherry Plum Tree

(*Prunus cerasifera*)

MAGICAL FORMS

a plum tree, some of which produce sweet plums in shape of cherries • others are ornamental • the term sometimes applies to hybrids that are a cross between plums and cherries • an upright, rounded tree producing white or pale pink blossoms in early spring as the leaves appear and red, orange, or yellow fruit that ripens between early July and mid-September • native to southeastern Europe and western Asia, grows in the UK and is naturalized in the northeast and far west of the USA • magically use the fruit, the blossoming or fruiting tree, and the Bach flower remedy (also part of the all-purpose Bach Rescue Remedy)

PLANET AND ELEMENT

Venus • Earth

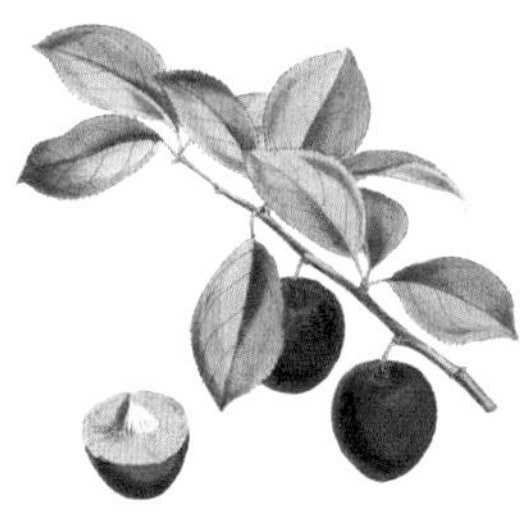

MAGICAL USES

the tree, like the flower essence, soothes shock, trauma, anxiety, and stress • as part of the Five Flower Formula, a fast-acting antidote to a sudden crisis, confrontation, or accident • support for an ongoing crisis such as divorce or major loss • minimizes tantrums in tots and teens and angry outbursts in inappropriate situations

HOW TO USE

Add the blossoms in a mesh net or a few drops of the cherry plum essence to a bath or to body lotion for a soothing massage. • Stand beneath a blossoming tree as flowers are falling, or pick and eat fruits, while wishing for inspiration and to bring inner peace. • Take the essence regularly if you are in a stressful situation where you cannot express your resentment or anger. • Where there are personality clashes or potential flashpoints, serve the fruit cooked, or have a dish of cherry plums in the kitchen for eating, to create a calm household.

CAUTION

The seeds (one within each fruit), leaves, and bark are toxic and should not be ingested.

Cherry Tree, Flowering

(*Prunus* 'Shimidsu Sakura')

MAGICAL FORMS

Japanese flowering ornamental cherry tree that does not bear fruit • one of numerous flowering cherry trees throughout the world • magically use the blossoms, fresh and dried or growing on the tree

PLANET AND ELEMENT

Venus • Water

MAGICAL USES

Japanese flowering cherries were first planted in Washington, DC, in the early decades of the 1900s as a gift from Japan, though not the first *Sakura* (cherry blossom) to be introduced to the USA • the first cherry blossom festival was held in Washington, DC, in 1935 and continues annually, recalling the planting of the early trees as a gesture of friendship between the USA and Japan • in Japan, the cherry blossom festival has been celebrated at the beginning of April for more than a thousand years as the springtime *hanami*, the viewing of the flowering trees that grow all over Japan • cherry blossom festivals are also celebrated in Korea, India, China, and Sweden to welcome spring • the fresh or dried blossom, or fragrances made from it, are magically symbols of new beginnings, good fortune, and of world peace as well as peace between families and individuals

HOW TO USE

According to the Japanese tradition, tie a single strand of hair (pulled out, not cut) to a blossoming cherry tree to attract love. • If in a relationship, you can tie a strand of hair for each child you want to conceive. • In traditional eastern European custom, a branch from a flowering cherry tree is taken indoors at Christmastime and nourished in a warm place in the hope it may blossom and bring blessings on Yuletide or Christmas Eve celebrations and yearlong abundance to the home.

CAUTION

All parts of the Japanese cherry tree, including the blossom, are toxic if ingested.

Cherry Tree, Sweet

(*Prunus avium*)

MAGICAL FORMS

also known as the wild cherry tree • magically use the growing tree, fresh and dried flowers, edible fruit, and cherry pits/stones

PLANET AND ELEMENT

Venus • Water

MAGICAL USES

new love • fertility • healing • increasing psychic powers • self-confidence • rituals for mending quarrels and calming anger in self and others • for those who have lost jobs to regain the right employment • *Prunus avium*, with its white blossoms and sweet fruit when ripe, came to New England with colonists in 1629, the seeds having originally been carried to Europe by birds from Asia Minor • cultivated in Asia as early as 8000 BCE and soon afterward in Greece

HOW TO USE

Carve or write the name of a person with whom you wish to be reconciled on the inside of a sharpened piece of the outer bark from an already fallen branch or solid twig. Point and throw it in the direction in which the person lives and when the wind comes from that direction so will peace. • Use the stones for love divination by counting cherry stones after eating a random number of cherries, asking "loves me/loves me not" as each stone is counted. This method can also be used with any other two-option question concerning love. • Eating a mix of black (yin) and red (yang) cherries calls your twin soul. • Cherry wood wands are used in love magick and to bring happiness after sorrow.

CAUTION

While the blossoms, leaves, seeds, and bark are toxic, especially if ingested in large quantities, they have been used medicinally in small quantities for centuries. • Buy commercial remedies or medicinal products from an expert herbalist.

Chervil

(Anthriscus cerefolium)

MAGICAL FORMS

sometimes called French parsley • magically use the whole plant growing outdoors or in a pot in a kitchen garden, fresh leaves, and infused oil

PLANETS AND ELEMENTS

Mars/Jupiter • Fire/Air

MAGICAL USES

chervil seeds were found in Tutankhamun's tomb, as a symbol of immortality • used in goddess rituals and initiations

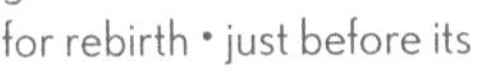

for rebirth • just before its flowering, add chopped chervil to olive oil and leave it to infuse for several days in a cool, dark place before straining • it smells like myrrh • can also be purchased commercially

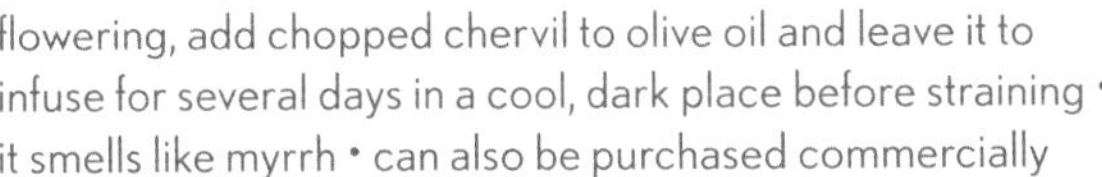

HOW TO USE

Anoint white candles with a little chervil oil in rituals to guide a soul peacefully who is ready to depart this life. • Burn in incense to enhance psychic awareness of other realms and for visions of the ancestors, past worlds, and the afterlife. • Inhale the smoke from the smoldering herb as you meditate on it to increase mediumship abilities and for more advanced meditation. • The fresh leaves, set in the center of a springtime altar, bring new beginnings, life, and health. • The fresh leaves can be chewed any time of the year, tasting like a mix of anise and parsley, for ongoing health and long life. • Dried flowers may be used in love sachets. • The chopped leaves, before flowering, may be used as a sweetener or in magical cooking (often a part of the culinary herb mix called "fines herbes"). • The flowers make a special garnish and can be endowed with wishes.

CAUTION

Beware of the poisonous hemlock, which can resemble rough wild chervil.

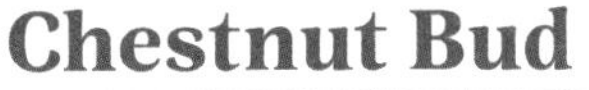

Chestnut Bud

(Aesculus hippocastanum)

MAGICAL FORMS

the buds from the European or common horse chestnut tree are dark red, brown, or black oval, shiny and sticky • native to the Balkans, the tree grows throughout Europe, the UK, and North America • the buds appear in spring, becoming clusters of white flowers in late spring to mid-May and, once pollinated, each flower develops into a conker or buckeye with a spiky shell • magically use the whole, growing tree and the essence

PLANET AND ELEMENT

Mercury • Air

MAGICAL USES

to avoid repeating the same mistakes in the hope it will be different this time • for assisting ADHD children to settle, absorb, and process information • for adults to focus on one activity or task without abandoning it for another immediately more attractive (see "Chestnut Tree," p. 118)

HOW TO USE

Sit beneath the budding tree and absorb its ability to progress through its natural cycle. • Give hyperactive children the Dr. Bach chestnut bud remedy, a drop or two daily, in food or water, to break old patterns, to assist them to concentrate, and to avoid impulsive behavior. • If you are aware that you are trapped in a cycle, for example picking the same kind of relationship or going back to a partner who has promised to change many times but never does, take the flower essence regularly until the cycle is broken. • If you feel you are slipping back into old patterns, repeat the essence cycle. • Massage the center of your throat and the middle of your hairline before study or examinations to concentrate and cut out irrelevancies by activating your focusing energy centers.

CAUTION

The horse chestnut tree is toxic, and the chestnuts should not be ingested.

Chestnut Tree

(*Castanea* spp.)

MAGICAL FORMS
genus including *Castanea sativa*, sweet chestnut, was brought into the UK and northern Europe by the Romans as food for themselves and their animals • introduced into North America in the early seventeenth century by colonists • *Castanea dentata*, American chestnut, is native to eastern North America, and has been devastated by blight, though efforts are being made for restoration • although not part of the *Castanea* genus, *Aesculus hippocastanum*, the European or common horse chestnut, grows throughout Europe and North America, and has similar magical effects • magically use the burred fruit of sweet chestnut with inner edible nuts; the creamy flowers of the horse chestnut and the inedible nuts (called conkers in the UK, and sometimes in the USA, but also known as buckeyes), covered in spiky green casing; and as sweet chestnut Dr. Bach flower remedy

PLANETS AND ELEMENTS
Venus/Jupiter • Earth/Air

MAGICAL USES
an offering for abundance both at the second harvest/autumn equinox and stored until Yule • sweet chestnut for abundance, expansion of opportunity, and employment • the horse chestnut for money, healing, courage, and justice • as a flower essence, the sweet chestnut represents replacing the dark night of the soul with light at the end of the tunnel

HOW TO USE
Carve the initials of you and your love or desired lover on a sweet chestnut before roasting it, and, as the shell splits, any barriers between you disappear. • Sit beneath the spreading branches of the tree to carry you back to past worlds, for chestnut trees have been planted for two thousand years and are a natural route to the past. • A horse chestnut carried as a fertility symbol in its green spiky case, should be opened at the precise moment of the full moon for conception after lovemaking. • Chestnut staves and wands keep away malevolent spirit and earthly influences.

CAUTION
Horse chestnuts are toxic and must not be ingested.

Chestnut Tree, White

(*Aesculus hippocastanum*)

MAGICAL FORMS
the white chestnut tree, with clusters of white flowers blooming in mid-spring • known also as the horse chestnut tree (see "Red Horse-Chestnut," p. 373), produces the Dr. Bach flower remedy known as white chestnut, prepared by the white blossoms being infused with sunlight • another Dr. Bach remedy called chestnut bud (see p. 117) is made from the same tree but is different because the white flowers are boiled to extract the essence, so produce another quality that prevents the repetition of old patterns of behavior • magically use the white chestnut essence, fallen blossoms, and flowerheads

PLANETS AND ELEMENT
Jupiter/Mercury • Air

MAGICAL USES
as an essence, the ultimate anti-insomnia remedy, both for difficulties going to sleep or waking in the night because of a mind whirling with old conversations from previous events and worries about the day ahead • as essence or blossoms, to calm an overactive mind • peace

HOW TO USE
Take the Dr. Bach nighttime remedy, which adds white chestnut to the Five-Flower Rescue Remedy mix (see p. 182); place under the tongue before bed to relieve insomnia caused by incessant reruns of old arguments, unfinished tasks, and the worries of the consequences of not sleeping and nightmares. • Give the nighttime remedy to teens in water at night if they are worrying about school or exams and cannot sleep, or in the morning if they are reluctant to attend classes. • Pick up fallen blossoms and hold them in the sunlight, allowing the warmth and light to flow through the flowers to calm the overthinking mind and to bring you peace and stillness; keep the flowerheads in water in your home office or workspace if you are worrying about unfinished tasks, deadlines, and anticipated criticism.

Chia Seed

(*Salvia hispanica*)

MAGICAL FORMS

tiny black or white seeds from the flowering plant, *Salvia hispanica*, a member of the mint family • native to Mexico and grown commercially there as well as in Guatemala, Bolivia, northwestern Argentina, the USA (especially Kentucky and Arizona), and parts of Australia

PLANET AND ELEMENT

Mercury • Air

MAGICAL USES

prevents gossip • detects false friends and deception • removes bad luck, especially from artifacts • a staple in the Mayan and Aztec diets, used also by them medicinally and ritually, the seeds were given as annual tribute to the Aztec rulers • seeds can be chewed, naming before each a wish or empowerment

HOW TO USE

Engrave on the side of an unlit soft wax or beeswax candle the name of an intimidating or overbearing person. Roll the candle in lightly oiled chia seeds, and light it (with care as it will be extra flammable). When it is completely burned, say, *May all malice be gone with the dimming of its light.* • Burn the seeds, whole or ground into powder, on charcoal in an incense mix with myrrh resin to remove bad influences on a family member or dragon's blood resin if there are serious threats to your safety, vicious slander, or intimidation of you or a family member (you are banishing the effects not harming the person).

CAUTION

Avoid if you suffer from high blood pressure, diabetes, plant allergies, or digestive problems.

Chickpea

(*Cicer arietinum*)

MAGICAL FORMS

also called garbanzo bean • flowering plant that can grow up to two feet tall • cultivated for its edible pealike seeds • two varieties, *desi*, small, yellow or green to dark brown with a thick coat, and *kabuli*, larger, creamy white with a thinner coating • part of dishes such as hummus, falafel, and couscous • a food legume from more than seven thousand years ago, chickpeas are grown both in subtropical and warm temperate zones • probably first cultivated in Turkey and the eastern Mediterranean, traveling via trade routes to southern Asia • now distributed worldwide, including California, Washington, North Dakota, and Idaho • magically use the cooked and raw chickpeas, chickpea flour, and dyed chickpeas for money spells (sold online)

PLANET AND ELEMENT

Venus • Earth

MAGICAL USES

to overcome competition, rivals, and opposition, especially by those who use unfair means • for mothering in all its aspects • preventing possessiveness in relationships • plant sprouting chickpeas in a pot indoors for slow but stable increasing money

HOW TO USE

Cast chickpeas along a path where an unscrupulous rival will walk. • Tape chickpeas beneath a doormat over which a love threat will tread. • If you are a mother or father with difficult children of any age, put one of the small desi beans in a bag for each child and a larger kabuli chickpea for each adult contributing to the problems, whether grandparents or a new stepparent. Shake the sealed bag morning and night, one shake for each of the chickpeas inside, chanting, *Mingle and mix, conflict we'll fix.* Add the chickpeas to a meal you are cooking for the family. • Serve hummus at a buffet when you know there may be a tense undercurrent.

CAUTION

Do not eat raw.

Chickweed

(*Stellaria media*)

MAGICAL FORMS

grows and spreads close to the ground, with white flowers resembling stars • native to Europe and Asia but is naturalized in many parts of North America and worldwide, taking over waste ground and meadows • often grown as chicken feed and sometimes regarded as a pest because of its persistent spreading under all conditions • magically use the aerial parts or the whole growing plant in situ

PLANET AND ELEMENT

Moon • Water

MAGICAL USES

charm bags or talismans for travel to far-off lands • telepathic communication with wild animals and birds • fidelity • extending influence and reaching the top by subtle, often unnoticed, efforts

HOW TO USE

Make a decoction from the leaves, and scatter it in all directions in circles in an open space if you need to succeed at networking, attract votes in your favor, or are planning a cooperative venture. State continuously as you turn what/whom most you seek to draw to support you. • On the full moon, set the seeds in a dish where wild birds gather or, with permission, where chickens feed to draw fertility to you, whether for a baby, to attain fame and fortune, or launch a creative venture. When the dish is empty, float the fresh or dried star flowers in water in the dish, and when they fade, cast them and the water from the dish into a fast-flowing source that they may return as your manifested wish.

CAUTION

Do not eat in excess, and beware of picking wild chickweed from polluted land. • Check with an expert before ingesting if you are pregnant or breastfeeding, suffer from a chronic condition, or have plant allergies.

Chicory

(*Cichorium intybus*)

MAGICAL FORMS

also called common chicory, a member of the daisy family • magically use the dried and fresh leaves and flowers, roots, and in flower remedy

PLANET AND ELEMENT

Sun • Fire/Air

MAGICAL USES

grown in ancient Egypt along the banks of the Nile and used magically as well as medicinally for power, success, and to remove curses • brought to Europe by people from the Netherlands in the eighteenth century and from there to the New World • used in the USA during the Civil War roasted as a coffee substitute • in rituals for removing obstacles • encourages saving • attracts favors • melts frigidity, both physical and mental • using the flower remedy reduces overconcern for the well-being of others • in magical potions

HOW TO USE

Use as incense to cleanse divinatory and magical tools. • Burn the powdered root in a mix with cinquefoil and cloves for psychic visions. • Cutting the fresh plant with a gold (or gold-colored) knife at noon or midnight on Midsummer Eve or Day is reputed to open locked boxes without a key and grant invisibility. • Dry and chop or powder the same chicory after Midsummer, and carry it as an amulet to lower your profile in times of confrontation and to uncover secrets. • Sit close to the fresh flowering plants or the cut flowers before they lose their freshness for astral travel where time frames are altered.

CAUTION

There are no known toxicities, but it may have a slight sedative effect. • Some experts advise to avoid ingesting it during pregnancy and with IBS or gallstones.

Chili Powder

MAGICAL FORMS

chili powder is the red dried pulverized fruit of one or more varieties of chili peppers, whose heat depends on the pepper chosen • the powder is usually sold or made with the addition of specific powdered herbs and spices that transform the powder magically as well as in taste • hotter forms often contain some cayenne pepper, adding fire to a spell if a need is urgent • cumin for good fortune • garlic powder for protection • oregano for justice • paprika for money • these form a mix often used in chili con carne or Tex-Mex • chili powder may also be made with cayenne pepper and unripe mild dried ancho pepper, or the ripened version, called dried poblano pepper • both are popular in Mexico and the southwestern USA and ancho may be substituted for paprika in the chili powder • magically use the powder, either pure or mixed with other powdered herbs

PLANET AND ELEMENT

Mars • Fire

MAGICAL USES

in amulet bags, especially as pure ground chili in hotter varieties, to silence gossip and banish ill-intent • should be used to attack behavior not the perpetrator as it is very powerful • believed to encourage troublemakers to keep far away

HOW TO USE

Stir spoken intentions into a pot during magical cooking, particularly chili powder with added herbs, to speed up stagnant or blocked matters or bring courage to end an overpossessive situation or relationship going nowhere fast. • Use to deter a stalker or unwelcome callers. • To deter a sexual predator at work, make up your own chili powder mix, adding extra cayenne pepper and oregano, or stir these into a commercial jar of the powdered spice. Name the intruder, writing their name on white paper in red ink, crossing through it, shredding it, and placing the pieces with the powder in a red bag. Tie three red thread knots round the bag to bind the person, and bury in the bag in a deep plant pot with either a Venus flytrap or a spiky cactus.

Chive

(*Allium schoenoprasum*)

MAGICAL FORMS

magically use the edible herb; budding purple and pink flowers, fresh and dried; and tubular grasslike stalks or scapes

PLANET AND ELEMENT

Mars • Fire

MAGICAL USES

abundance • aphrodisiac • breaks bad habits and addictions • brings unwelcome but necessary change • drives away evil spirits • magical cooking and eating empowered chives to absorb magick • protective garden • water scrying, the best herb as the separate stalks give distinct pictures • weight-loss rituals

HOW TO USE

Absorb the magick by eating or stirring scapes into cooking while visualizing who or what is most desired or which bad habits are to be broken. • Bouquets of the flowers in the home call to love. • Use it to banish addictions and draw money. • Prepare the herb by boiling and straining, or by pounding the stems with a little water and extracting the juice, and use for sprinkling outside home entrances, or, alternatively, hang bunches of the fresh herb over entrances, to drive away illness and evil. • Incorporate chive into your readings of Celtic tree or ogham staves to aid you in connecting with their meanings and energies. • Include it in all hawthorn tree protective rituals.

CAUTION

If allergic to onions, chives may cause problems.

Chrysanthemum

(*Chrysanthemum* spp.)

MAGICAL FORMS

includes *Chrysanthemum × morifolium*, known as florist's daisy, also called Ju hua in Chinese medicine • one of the four noble plants of China • *Chrysanthemum coronarium*, the most popular edible chrysanthemum for garden growing, is cooked as a green • magically use the growing plant, in flower arrangements, fresh flower petals, and dried flowers

PLANET AND ELEMENT

Sun • Fire

MAGICAL USES

flower and incense of Samhain/Halloween, the time of the ancestors to protect against restless ghosts and malicious spirits who wander free during the three days around October 31 • red for passion and power, marriage, and motherhood • yellow for ending relationships with kindness, but also the power of the sun to find new happiness • white for truth and love forever • orange for long life, stability, happiness in the fall, and leaving behind what did not work

HOW TO USE

Use it in rituals to celebrate the passing of the seasons and life changes. • Used especially in the Far East as a protective wreath on the front door or a front-facing window. • Grow it outdoors on a tree facing a difficult neighbor. • Suspend a mini one on the rearview mirror of a vehicle to avoid accidents and hostility from other motorists. • Place it in the workplace as a flower arrangement to draw business and financial success.

CAUTION

Avoid if you are allergic to sunflowers, daisies, or ragweed. • Wear gardening gloves if the plants irritate your skin or cause asthma-like symptoms. • Do not use while pregnant or breastfeeding. • Ensure that the chrysanthemums you grow are the less toxic kind; avoid *Chrysanthemum cineriaefolium* and *Chrysanthemum coccineum*, which are inedible and contain a lot of permethrin, which is used as insecticide. • If in doubt, buy chrysanthemum tea and commercial remedies from a reliable herbalist, and check with a pharmacist if taking other medication.

Chrysanthemum, Coppersmith

(*Chrysanthemum × morifolium*)

MAGICAL FORMS

native to Asia and South Africa, coppersmith flowers grow in many regions of the USA and Europe and can often be obtained from a specialty flower nursery or florist out of season • called a *cushion pom* because there are small petals in the middle that become larger moving outward (other copper chrysanthemums, such as the copper bronze spider mum can be substituted) • plants are covered in flowers from early to late fall • magically use the growing plant, the bright copper bronze petals, and the flowerheads, fresh or dried

PLANETS AND ELEMENTS

Venus/Sun • Earth/Fire

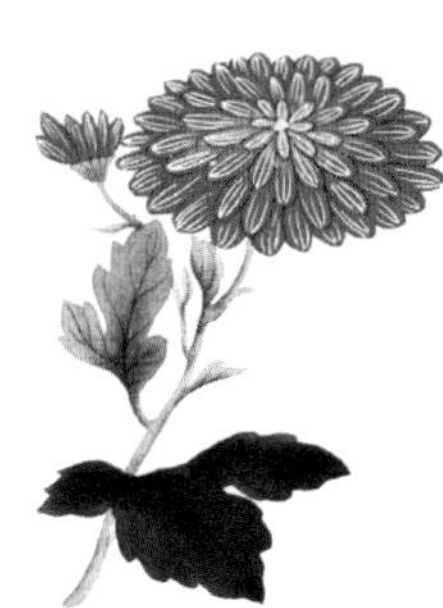

MAGICAL USES

as a bouquet or basket arrangement or as a garden gift for the twenty-second wedding anniversary (copper), often with metal copper roses or a piece of copper jewelry • send coppersmith chrysanthemums to older relatives for birthdays or for a second or subsequent marriage later in life

HOW TO USE

Use the fresh or dried petals collected during the fall in a charm bag with a copper nugget for attracting prosperity. • Substitute a copper ring and keep the bag under your pillow to dream of a lover known or yet unknown. • Surround a copper bracelet with the cut fresh or dried flowerheads and orange candles to transmit healing to an older friend or family member who is chronically ill or in pain, and afterward, send the bracelet as a gift.

CAUTION

It can cause allergies if ingested; if you are allergic to sunflowers, daisies, or ragweed; or if you are pregnant.

Chrysanthemum, Super Magnum

(*Chrysanthemum indicum* var. 'Super Magnum')

MAGICAL FORMS

from the Asteraceae family • characterized by very big single flowerheads • Super Magnum refers specifically to the large white flower, but there are other magnum chrysanthemums in red, yellow, pink, lavender, and even the lime green Magnum Spider Mum • magically use the magnum flowers, which can last up to fifteen days when cut; the whole plant, grown in a garden; and the dried petals

PLANET AND ELEMENT

Sun • Fire

MAGICAL USES

the filler or main feature of a bouquet, magnum chrysanthemums are a striking substitute for smaller chrysanthemums in brighter colors • given on the thirteenth wedding anniversary and also the nineteenth anniversary, where the white Super Magnum or red magnum promise the continuation of eternal love • burn magnum chrysanthemum petals, dried and shredded in incense, to greet the fall and the equinox around September 23 to let go of what is lost

HOW TO USE

Magnum chrysanthemums assist rituals, empowerments, and spells to go up a notch over the use of ordinary chrysanthemums. Use especially when there is an urgent or major wish or need. • For love questions if a relationship has broken up, pose the *Will she or he return, not return* by plucking every single petal and casting it on the ground for each response. • Leave a single white Super Magnum flowerhead on a grave, or cast into water, on the anniversary of the death of a love that ran deep but that you cannot openly mourn.

CAUTION

Super Magnum is not generally considered toxic, but avoid if you are allergic to sunflowers, daisies, or ragweed. • Beware of skin allergies or asthma-like symptoms. • Do not ingest while pregnant or breastfeeding.

Cinnamon

(*Cinnamomum verum*)

MAGICAL FORMS

also called true cinnamon or Ceylon cinnamon • bushy evergreen tree of the laurel family • magically use its spice from the dried inner bark of young shoots, either as sticks or powdered; the growing tree; essential oil; and as prepared powdered spice in a glass culinary jar from the supermarket

PLANETS AND ELEMENT

Mars/Sun • Fire

MAGICAL USES

success • healing powers • increasing psychic gifts • luck • attracting money • passionate love • courage • confidence • to increase concentration and focus • spice of New Year • for spiritual quests • in India, the Vedic books, written about 2000 BCE, list more than seven hundred substances, including cinnamon, ginger, myrrh, coriander, and sandalwood, that were used not only in ritual and perfume but also for healing • modern Ayurvedic medicine carries on this tradition • the ancient Egyptians used cinnamon oil for mummification

HOW TO USE

Add the spice to love and sex magick pouches, hidden beneath the mattress. • Traditionally it is part of a magical sachet for prosperity, with equal parts of cinquefoil, cinnamon, cloves, lemon balm, and a whole vanilla or tonka bean made on Thursday after sunset during a waxing moon and carried in a purple bag. • Purify a house or ritual space using cinnamon incense with sandalwood. • Add cinnamon powder to a defensive, psychic awakener, or passion-inducing jar, shaking all the ingredients together and then inhaling, keeping the jar sealed the rest of the time. • Carry the powder in a red purse, with a gambling chip or silver dollar, for gambling or for taking a chance on seemingly risky speculation with potentially great possibilities. • Mix in a wishing powder with peppermint, tarragon, and corn starch to sprinkle on the threshold of the workplace for promotion and recognition.

CAUTION

Use with caution during pregnancy and breastfeeding, and if taking regular medication or antibiotics. • Dilute the oil well, and do not use if you have sensitive skin.

Cinquefoil

(*Potentilla canadensis*)

MAGICAL FORMS

magically use the herb, leaves, and roots

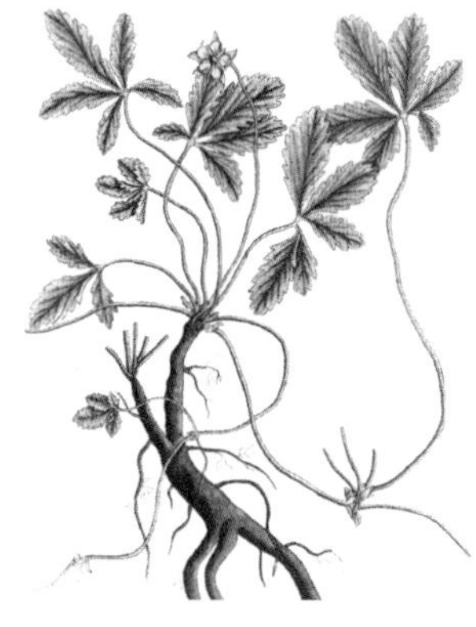

PLANET AND ELEMENTS

Jupiter • Earth/Air

MAGICAL USES

its five leaflet formations in a star shape offer five magical gifts: love, money, health, power, and wisdom (intelligence) • healing • peaceful sleep and prophetic dreams • increases successful fishing • drives away all evil, earthly and paranormal • for asking favors • successful court cases • herb of the spring equinox.

HOW TO USE

Because it has five leaves, it is magically associated with the pentagram and is generally used in magick involving fives, such as chanting five times or making five circles with the herbs. • Place dried yellow flowers in a love-charm bag. • For love divination, pluck the yellow petals. • Use in an infusion, rubbed into the forehead and hands, to remove curses and hexes. • A bundle of bound herbs hung over the entrance to the home keeps the property, and all within, safe. • In the workplace, hide a washed eggshell filled with the dried leaves or flowers to keep malice away. • Use in a sachet beneath the pillow to drive away night terrors, paranormal harm, and intruders. • Use especially the seven-leafed cinquefoil to bring dreams of an unknown lover. • Recite five times its five powers, while naming five times the favor or official matter to be resolved, all while dropping the leaflets of five cinquefoil from a bridge into running water.

CAUTION

Do not use cinquefoil in excess.

Citronella Plant

(*Pelargonium cucullatum* subsp. *cucullatum*)

MAGICAL FORMS

also called *Pelargonium citrosum* and known commonly as mosquito plant • an herb, member of the geranium family, whose green wrinkled lacy leaves when touched release a strong citrus scent that repels bugs, especially mosquitoes • small clusters of five lavender-pink petals, which are not scented • native to South Africa, Sri Lanka, and Java • grows in areas of the USA from Michigan to Texas and California and other parts of the world where it is warm, wet, and sunny • also in cooler regions as an annual plant • can be grown indoors in a pot • magically use the whole, growing plant; leaves, fresh and dried; scented candles; and as incense coils, cones, or sticks (rather than loose granular incense, made from the leaves and stems, on charcoal) • obtainable from camping stores as well as online • citronella oil is made from Asian citronella grass, often mistaken for the related lemongrass

PLANET AND ELEMENT

Mercury • Air

MAGICAL USES

deters overly curious neighbors, visitors who outstay their welcome, and emotional vampires • removes malicious thought forms and entities summoned in ouija board sessions or amateur seances

HOW TO USE

Burning citronella incense draws clients and new sales to a business and aids networking, brainstorming, and innovative solutions. • Grow the plant in a pot in your kitchen or office space, and crush a leaf or two to stop gossip, spite, and backbiting. • If it is mosquito season and you can wear a citronella-infused wristband on your dominant hand without attracting comment, move your hand subtly toward anyone who spreads negative energies when you are trying to raise enthusiasm or introduce new ideas. • Diffuse the oil or burn incense sticks in a new home, or in your personal space in a shared apartment, to imprint your own energies and personality.

CAUTION

The citronella plant is toxic to cats and dogs.

Cleavers

(*Galium aparine*)

MAGICAL FORMS

also known as goosegrass, because parts of the plant resemble geese's feet or may have been used for feeding geese (see "Lady's Bedstraw," p. 249, its close relative) • frequently cleavers are regarded as a garden pest as they spread rapidly and can choke out other plants • also good for butterflies, moths, and sun magick • valued by some for its medicinal properties • magically use the whole plant, stems, leaves, seed balls, and seeds, which all have the sticky hooks that characterize this plant

PLANET AND ELEMENTS

Saturn • Earth/Fire

MAGICAL USES

commitment • drawing closer in love after estrangement or seeming indifference • breaking possessive bonds with family or in love • persistence when you feel like giving up in any area of your life • butterfly and moth magick for sun and moon night magick

HOW TO USE

The chopped and dried leaves and/or sticky seeds are used in mojo bags to bring a couple or family together, especially if there have been quarrels or if one lover, or both, has been tempted to stray. • Stick coins into seed balls, one ball for each venture or financial need, carefully wrapped in a knotted blue cloth, and keep in a money safe or near a business computer so money will accumulate. • Cleavers near a boundary with a hostile neighbor, if you live in a dangerous area or have an intrusive ex-partner or stalker, provide natural protection. • Alternatively, fill a bag with the sticky seeds, adding on white paper in blue ink, the names of those who trouble you, and hang the bag on a tree away from the house saying, *The attraction of destruction is now bound, near me or my family home, shall you no more be found.* • Roll an old garment with sad memories in the sticky plant or seeds, and bury it away from where flowers grow free.

CAUTION

Some people suffer contact dermatitis from handling cleavers, so wear gloves while preparing spells.

Clematis

(*Clematis* spp.)

MAGICAL FORMS

part of Ranunculaceae (buttercup) family • over three hundred species suitable for gardens in many shapes and colors, a large number native to North America, such as the cultivar 'Bee's Jubilee' (*Clematis × jackmanii*), and in the UK, Old man's beard (*Clematis vitalba*) • some flowers bloom until the fall • clematis may be found wild and cultivated in Manitoba and Quebec, as far south as Alabama and Louisiana, and west all the way to Kansas • magically use mainly in its climbing plant form, as flower essences, and cut fresh or dried flowers

PLANET AND ELEMENT

Jupiter • Air

MAGICAL USES

linked with the clematis's ability to climb as high as it can, upward toward the light, twisting and turning to avoid obstacles • for problem-solving, travel, versatility, unstoppable ambitions, and aspirations • *Clematis* 'Huldine', with pearly translucent petals, and *Clematis* 'White Pearl', also with pearly white flowers and a pearl-shaped center, are flowers often associated with the sixty-ninth wedding anniversary

HOW TO USE

Use in rituals, meditations, and empowerments, the growing plant and fresh and dried flowers on the woody stem, to find new ways of achieving any aim if one route is blocked. • Tie paper luggage labels to your climbing clematis in ascending order of priority, naming for each the steps to success or a seemingly impossible travel venture until you can reach no higher. • Place two drops of the flower essence under your tongue to clearly speak your intentions in the workplace, in a relationship, or with neighbors, and refuse to accept half-truths or excuses in return.

CAUTION

Clematis leaves and flowers, though used extensively in Chinese medicine, can be toxic to people and pets if ingested raw and may cause an allergic reaction if you have sensitive skin.

Clematis, Wedding Day Variety

(*Clematis* 'Wedding Day')

MAGICAL FORMS

a clematis cultivar • magically use the whole, growing plant, often as a climber; cut flowers in bloom, in May/June and again in September; and fresh and dried petals of the creamy white and green banded flowers

PLANET AND ELEMENT

Venus • Earth

MAGICAL USES

blooming in May, June, and again in September but can be found at other times through florists or specialty growers • ideal in bouquets, as flower arches, or decorations at any wedding, large or small, formal or informal • substitute the fresh petals for confetti • representing a union blessed by the angels • for a couple who intends to travel, are planning major relocation after the wedding, or an extended honeymoon • also as cut flowers by those seeking marriage if a potential partner is slow to commit.

HOW TO USE

Make the wedding bouquet into an incense or potpourri mix to transfer the memories of the happy day into daily life. • If you want to find lasting love, pick the blooming petals or ask the bride for a single flower from her bouquet or take home a table decoration from the wedding venue to share her happiness. • Press a dried flower minus the anthers (the pollen-filled stamen) between tissue paper to make a bookmark, and keep it at the page for the wedding service or handfasting ceremony in any prayer book of your chosen religion. • Offer the flowers as a proposal of marriage with a ring concealed among the blooms. • If you are not allergic, collect the pollen and cast it to the winds to call an absent lover or an online love on the other side of the world.

CAUTION

Clematis can be a skin irritant and is harmful if ingested by pets.

Clove

(*Syzygium aromaticum*)

MAGICAL FORMS

an evergreen tree growing up to fifty feet with aromatic leaves • cloves are the dried flower buds of the clove tree, native to the Molucca islands of Indonesia • magically use the dried, small, brown, nail-like cloves, obtainable from grocery stores; as incense with whole cloves in the mix, whether on charcoal or powdered; or as diluted essential oil

PLANETS AND ELEMENT

Jupiter/Sun • Fire

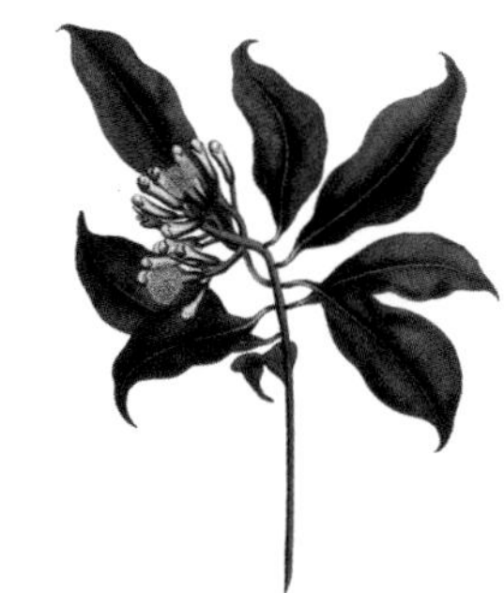

MAGICAL USES

burn cloves as incense, or release the oil in a diffuser, in your home for replacing what or whom is no longer wanted with new energies, opportunities, health, happiness, and success • a natural aphrodisiac, cloves both attract love and awaken sexual feelings • for those who have suffered loss, clove oil, well diluted for anointing the inner wrist points, offers solace

HOW TO USE

Rattle twenty-seven cloves (3 × 3 × 3) in a sealed tin every morning and night to prevent ongoing gossip, malice, and envy against you, saying continuously as you rattle it, *Three by three by three, no more your spiteful tongue/s shall trouble me.* Reduce the cloves by eating one each day until the cloves and problem are gone. • Hang a whole orange fruit over your altar or in your living space at Thanksgiving or Christmas, having pierced only the skin of the orange with whole cloves while making wishes for yourself and others or to restore good fortune. • If you suspect there may be falsehood or trickery around you, add cloves to magical cookery or make a tea with cloves, cinnamon, honey, and vanilla extract, stirring before offering it to those present whom you distrust, to discover the truth about a situation or person within a day or two.

CAUTION

Avoid if pregnant.

Clover

(*Trifolium repens*)

MAGICAL FORMS

also called trefoil • also many other species of the *Trifolium* genus • purple, red, and white flowers • magically use the whole plant, dried flowers, and small leaves (the number of leaves being especially important)

PLANET AND ELEMENT

Mercury • Air

MAGICAL USES

a four-leaf clover brings luck in every way, especially financial affairs and wins in speculation, gaming, or lottery • five-leaved clover attracts hoped-for financial rewards and unexpected sources of extra income • red clover encourages successful financial negotiations and passion • white clover breaks hexes and curses • purple brings love and fidelity • two leaves for love, three for protection, and four for good luck in every way • the herb of Lughnasadh, Lammas, the beginning of August

HOW TO USE

Place in a charm bag with dried St. John's Wort, vervain, and dill to see earthly and paranormal evil approaching and to drive it away. • Carry a four-leaf clover in a sachet with four wheat heads to attract sufficient resources. • Make as a wish tea, with rosemary, thyme, and honey to sweeten, stirring while making the wish and then drinking. • A two-leaf clover worn in the right shoe attracts a rich lover. • A three-leaf clover mixed with May morning dew preserves youthful appearance. • Seven grains of wheat set on a four-leaf clover brings the sight of nature spirits.

Clover, Red

(*Trifolium pratense*)

MAGICAL FORMS

one of the world's oldest crops • considered sacred and a symbol of wealth and immortality by the Celts and Anglo-Saxons • gathered two days after the full moon and kept out of sight of the sun once cut • magically use the whole, growing plant; leaves in triple-leaf formation; fresh or dried pink to purple egg-shaped flowers; flower essence; and oil

PLANET AND ELEMENT

Mars • Fire

MAGICAL USES

the three leaves growing on the plant signify the maiden, mother, and crone—birth, death, and rebirth cycles and the three main phases of the moon • use for consecrating copper ritual artifacts and tools

HOW TO USE

Grow in gardens or sprinkle the dried flowers and leaves on doorsteps (thereafter to be swept away) to banish restless ghosts, malevolent nature spirits, and too-powerful earth energies flowing unchecked from the home and land. In addition, this protects self, family, and pets and increases good fortune (doubled if a rare four-leaf red clover is found). • Red clover attracts benign fey to the garden. • Burn as incense to aid astral projection and connection with other dimensions and guides. • Bind together a whole, dried, white clover and a red clover, both with three leaves, and tape to the back of a photo of you and your twin soul to strengthen twin-soul love and fidelity. • Red clover is good, too, for reconciliation. • Regularly spray the essence in water around a pet bed to keep the animal(s) healthy. • Add a few drops of essence to water, or float the flowerhead in water, as the Water element in a ritual to heal a pet. • When you move house, sprinkle red clover infusion around the boundaries and just inside the front and back doors to remove any unhappy energies lingering and to make the home yours.

CAUTION

Red clover is edible, but do not use if pregnant, breastfeeding, taking blood thinners, or undergoing hormone treatment.

Club Moss

(*Lycopodium clavatum*)

MAGICAL FORMS

also known as foxtail, wolf's claw, and ground moss • not actually a moss, but a spore-producing fern • whole plant growing • dried stalk and mosslike growth crumbled together • not as incense as the spore dust is flammable (used by Victorian stage magicians when cast on flames) • magically use the cut or whole, growing plant and the spores

PLANET AND ELEMENT

Moon • Water

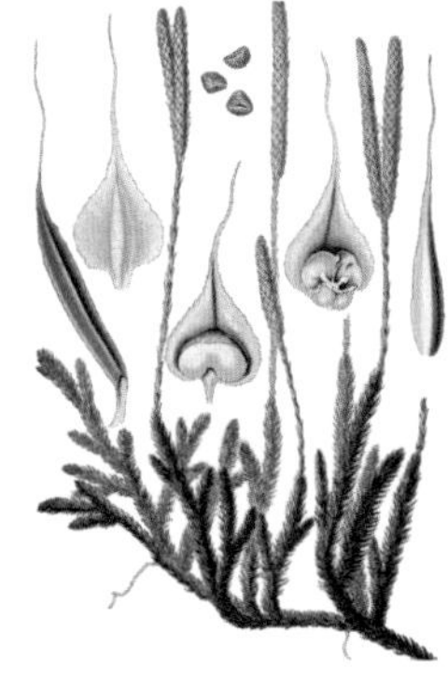

MAGICAL USES

the tips of the plant, extending from the end of a long stalk from the mosslike growth, resemble a wolf's claw and can be used in rituals and amulets for power and protection of the family and community • club moss is traditionally gathered ritually after a magical salt bath with the little finger of the dominant hand or the blade of a silver-colored knife • the plant is offered bread and wine on the ground around it before uprooting • this brings the blessings of the deities and guides and makes its use even more magical

HOW TO USE

The plant enables you to call on a power animal for courage and ingenuity in survival situations and for hunting for whatever is most needed or desired. • The oily spore dust was cast by Druids onto fires for visions of otherworlds. • For an urgent wish, cast just a little of the spores onto a well-guarded bonfire or fire pit (doing this with the utmost care).

CAUTION

Though used in homeopathy and medicinally by generations, including the Native North Americans, club moss should not be ingested during pregnancy, with a low heart rate, or if suffering from emphysema, asthma, or stomach ulcers. • It is recommended to take medical advice before self-medication with club moss.

Coconut Palm Essence

MAGICAL FORMS

made from the yellow flowers of the coconut palm (*Cocos nucifera*), growing in the tropics near water almost worldwide, including Florida and Hawaii • the essence is filled with the sunshine of its source and the life force of the crystal involved in its creation • magically use a coconut palm houseplant as a focus in combination with the flower essence

PLANET AND ELEMENT

Moon • Water

MAGICAL USES

helps sensitive people develop a protective outer shell, accept their own weaknesses, and learn self-love • protects the aura from negative influences and attacks while expanding psychic powers and safely receiving messages from the spirit world • shields single-sex couples who may be encountering prejudice or hostility and helps them overcome their difficulties conceiving a child

HOW TO USE

For those whose skin reflects stress as allergies or rashes, take the essence regularly. • Add a few drops to a coconut skin product to heal the underlying cause of the skin eruptions. • Meditate on a coconut palm houseplant, having added a drop or two of the coconut palm essence to the soil. Regularly add the essence to the plant soil, and set the plant in the center of a room or house so the life force, warmth, and laughter of its world will spread throughout the home on the coldest and darkest of days. • Anoint the center of your brow and your crown with the essence before meditation, breath work, or chanting to align and balance your inner self with the demands of the outer world so that you remain serene in the face of pettiness or undermining.

Coconut Tree

(Cocos nucifera)

MAGICAL FORMS

not a nut but a drupe, a fruit with a single seed • grows as an indoor plant • grows outdoors in Florida and Hawaii • magically use the growing tree, coconut fruit, oil, coconut water, natural fluid, and the milk extracted from the white meat

PLANET AND ELEMENT

Moon • Water

MAGICAL USES

the goddess symbol to the god icon, the banana • use empty shells as offering dishes, especially in full moon rites, along with banana leaves for a nature or outdoor ritual • for fertility, motherhood, the flow of new life and energies • gives protection against psychic attack

HOW TO USE

To conceive a child, on full moon break open a coconut, drink a little of the water, and eat a little of the fruit, saying, *The fruit is sweet with fecundity, the shell the womb, the water new life, Mother Moon by your bright light, I take this symbol of fertility*, then bury the remaining coconut, having tipped the rest of the water into the hole. • For protection of your home, halve your coconut, scatter any juice around the outside of the premises, fill half of the shell with protective herbs, such as basil, sage, and rosemary, then close the coconut and bury it outside your property or in a large plant pot near the front door. • To break a curse, hex, or malicious love spell, hammer a coconut until it splits into pieces and bury the pieces in different places away from your home so they can't rejoin. • Eat the white of the coconut for magical wishes. • Add the water or milk to bathwater for radiance.

CAUTION

Where possible, use the virgin unprocessed oil.

Coffee

(Coffea arabica)

MAGICAL FORMS

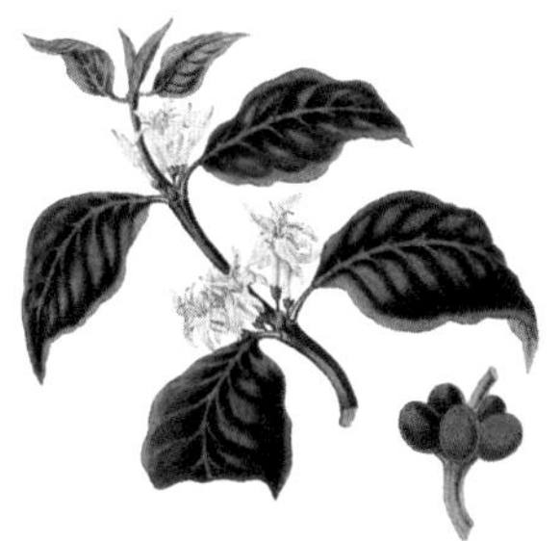

evergreen shrub or small tree that can reach thirty feet • star-shaped flowers becoming small red fruit, each producing two seeds/beans • native to tropical East Africa, reaching Yemen around the sixth century CE and then the Arabian peninsula • Sufi mystics drank it to stay awake in protracted rituals • coffee first reached the USA in the middle of the seventeenth century via British settlers • it now grows worldwide in tropical zones • magically use the beans, whole or ground; as instant coffee; and as brewed coffee

PLANETS AND ELEMENTS

Saturn/Mercury • Earth/Air

MAGICAL USES

sociability • networking • informal gatherings • speeds any slow-moving matters, especially using espresso beans and coffee • divining with coffee grounds

HOW TO USE

Swirl and read coffee dregs after drinking the coffee, or interpret images in the froth patterns on top of cappuccino coffee, to answer questions. • Shake coffee beans in a bowl, chanting slowly and rhythmically what or whom you most need, then grind the beans the old-fashioned way continuing the chant. Place the ground coffee into a French press, percolator, or drip coffee pot and add water (brewing it on the stove is even more magical than an electric device). Let it brew, and end the chant by clapping, stamping, or calling out the last words when the coffee is ready. You have just created the fifth magical element of ether where magical transformation is possible.

CAUTION

If pregnant, talk with your midwife or physician about what constitutes a safe daily amount.

Collard Greens

(*Brassica oleracea* var. *viridis*)

MAGICAL FORMS

also known as colewart • part of the cabbage and kale family, cultivated from the wild cabbage • edible leafy green vegetables with a thick stem • tough and bitter leaves unless well cooked, but with their own distinctive flavor • popular in the southern USA and increasingly worldwide because of their nutritional value • originating in ancient Greece and Rome, there are differing theories how they reached the USA in the 1600s • some say from Africa and that they became a staple food on the southern slave plantations • others believe they were introduced by Scottish and English settlers to the southern USA • the two ideas are not necessarily incompatible • magically use the growing plant, the uncooked whole plant, and the cooked leaves

PLANET AND ELEMENT

Mars • Fire

MAGICAL USES

protection for those who eat the greens from malevolent people and ill-intentioned spirits • on New Year's Day for the increase of money and good fortune when eaten with black-eyed peas • a dollar note representing currency can be tied around a few raw black-eyed peas with the same number of coins as peas and buried in offering to the earth at first light to greet the new year

HOW TO USE

A fiercely defensive plant, place the uncooked plant in a kitchen vegetable rack to shield the home and family from harm. • Cook and eat the leaves while still fresh to allow the protective guard to be absorbed. • Grow collard greens in the garden near the back door or door nearest the kitchen to allow only benign, luck-bringing energies to enter and attract prosperity. • Include collard greens in family recipes (numerous can be found online, many based on southern USA and soul food traditions) for celebrations, especially the return of absent members. • Take along cooked collard greens to share at community events to strengthen unity and kinship among relative strangers.

CAUTION

Take expert advice if used medicinally when pregnant.

Coltsfoot

(*Tussilago farfara*)

MAGICAL FORMS

native to Europe and parts of eastern and central Asia • naturalized in the USA and Canada • bright yellow dandelion-like flowers, distinguished by their scaly red stems • bloom in early spring before the leaves, which as they grow resemble a colt's foot and appear as the flowers fade • magically use the flowers, fresh and dried, but mainly the dried leaves

PLANETS AND ELEMENTS

Mercury/Venus • Air/Earth

MAGICAL USES

once used by apothecaries in Paris as a symbol of their trade in love rituals and sachets to attract a soul mate • induce peace of mind and tranquility • offers protection as amulets, especially to horses and all who travel • magically use the fresh flowers for seasonal springtime festivals

HOW TO USE

Coltsfoot aids in receiving visions when the dried leaves are burned as incense. • Use it as an incense to make connection with the spirit world before divination. • If using coltsfoot in incense or the leaves in a smudge dish, begin a ritual by acknowledging the six directions—east, south, west, north, upward to the sky, and downward to the earth—to welcome the elementals of Earth, Air, Fire, Water, Father Sky, and Mother Earth. • Use it in a floor wash to remove sickness and misfortune. • Place the dried flowers and chopped or powdered leaves into a wish jar to call back a lover, putting his or her photo in the bottom of the jar and covering in layers.

CAUTION

Though used medicinally for centuries and still commercially sold in teas (recommended to be limited in use) and remedies, coltsfoot flowers and leaves are regarded by some experts as toxic to the liver of humans if taken raw, and the root is generally off limits. • It is also toxic for pets and if ingested by horses (put protective coltsfoot amulets high in or outside a stable). • Do not use coltsfoot with blood pressure medication or liver problems, if pregnant, trying to conceive, or breastfeeding.

Columbine

(*Aquilegia* spp.)

MAGICAL FORMS

member of the buttercup family • includes *Aquilegia vulgaris*, or granny's bonnet, the flower looking like nodding bonnets in the breeze • *Aquilegia caerulea*, blue columbine • *Aquilegia canadensis*, eastern red columbine • magically use the plant, growing wild or in gardens, and the flowers, fresh and dried

PLANETS AND ELEMENTS

Venus/Mercury • Water/Air

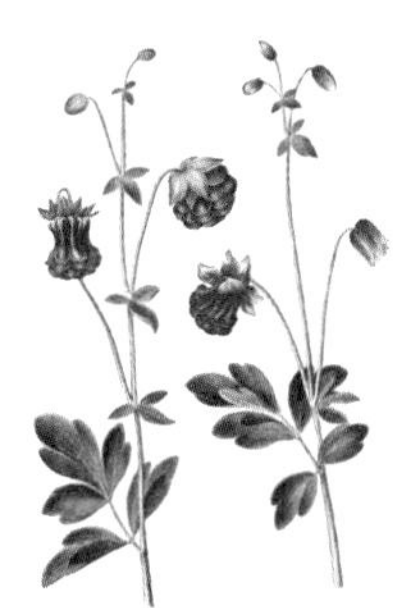

MAGICAL USES

for love magick • planted to attract the fey who are said to sleep in the flowers • blue columbine is state flower of Colorado • Air magick and connection with higher realms, as some columbine thrive high in the Rockies under inhospitable conditions

HOW TO USE

Meditate on the growing flowers for connecting with power birds and astral flight. • The Celts believed the flowers gave access to otherworlds. • Use for shape-shifting, as this has become a flower associated with the Norse goddess Freya who, in her cloak of swan feathers, led the Valkyries (the swan maidens) through the skies to choose the worthy from the battlefield to enter her halls. • Columbine has also come to represent, through modern goddess power rituals honoring this feisty magical goddess, a symbol of women's independence if there is prejudice or inequality in the workplace. • Keep the brighter colored petals dried in a scarlet charm bag in the workspace or a work vehicle. • Use for the reconciliation of opposites or seeming opposing views. • The botanical flower name *Aquilegia* has a dual meaning: Latin for *eagle*, because the shape of the flower petals resembles eagle's talons, and the common name, columbine, meaning *dove*, as the flower looks like five doves settled together. • Columbine can be used for dispelling jealousy powerfully but nonaggressively.

CAUTION

Columbine is toxic if ingested, especially the seeds and roots.

Common Agrimony

(*Agrimonia eupatoria*)

MAGICAL FORMS

also known as sticklewort • burrs on the fruit formed after the flowers die • named after Mithridates Eupatoria, king of Pontus in northern Turkey who died around 63 BCE and was an expert in plant medicine and antidotes to poison • magically use the fresh and dried flowers and leaves

PLANET AND ELEMENT

Jupiter • Air

MAGICAL USES

reverses ill-wishing and jinxes • acts as a psychic shield and returns curses to the sender • empowers any magical workings with authority • brings good fortune and blesses the home with health, wealth, and happiness • guards against goblins, orcs, and trolls

HOW TO USE

The flowers and leaves are used in herbal protection sachets until they lose fragrance. • Wrap dried agrimony inside a paper containing the name of a person who is hexing you and burn it, then scatter the ashes to the winds. • When added to a sleep pillow, it prevents nightmares and insomnia, especially when you are overtired. • The sticky burrs can be placed with care in a lucky witch bottle or wish jar to attract what is most wanted and in defensive bottles or jars to act as a barrier to harm. • Dried agrimony added to incense cleanses the aura and clears the air after quarrels or anxiety. • Mixed into a floor wash, it has the dual result of both cleansing and bringing love, success, and money to the home.

CAUTION

Agrimony is recommended medicinally only for short periods and in small quantities and only after consulting a medical professional. • Do not use if you are allergic to roses, pregnant, or breastfeeding.

Common Comfrey

(*Symphytum officinale*)

MAGICAL FORMS

in wild and informal gardens • native to Europe and Asia • grows naturally in forests from Nova Scotia to British Columbia, and from Yukon in Canada and south to New Jersey and Indiana in North America • magically use the growing plant, in situ or dried as decoration; the plentiful green foliage; the bell-shaped flowers; and the roots, chopped and dried

PLANET AND ELEMENT

Saturn • Earth

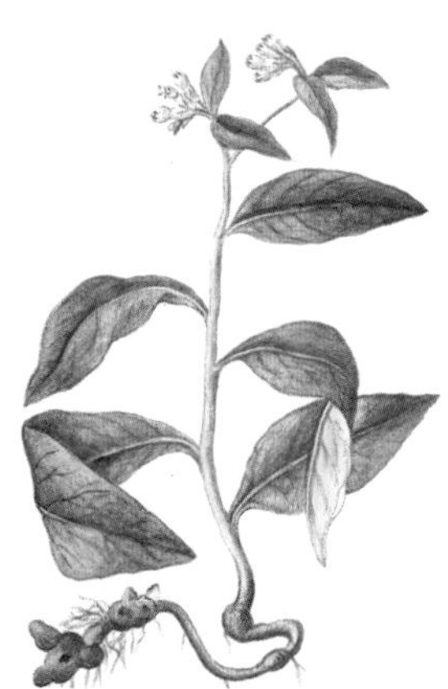

MAGICAL USES

as a talisman in a dried flower arrangement, including honesty and dried lavender in a room to encourage people to mingle socially or to regain assent if there have been disagreements at a previous meeting • hence one of its folk names is boneset or knitbone • a tiny piece of chopped root in a savings jar for spare coins attracts wealth

HOW TO USE

Make a sachet of the chopped dried plant, leaves, and flowers, and keep in a blue sachet in the glove compartment of a vehicle, in a pannier on a motorcycle, or on the handlebars of a bicycle or scooter for safety on long journeys and while commuting. • Scatter a mix of comfrey, elder, basil, and bay leaves on the doorstep to remove a curse from your home or business, and after sweeping it outward, stand the broom, with bristles upward, outdoors.

CAUTION

Though popularly used in folk medicine through the ages and still in parts of Europe, especially topically for bone injuries, comfrey is no longer allowed to be sold in oral medicinal products or in comfrey tea in the USA, the UK, Australia, Canada, or Germany. • Comfrey is toxic if the raw plant is ingested by pets or children.

Common Laburnum Tree

(*Laburnum anagyroides*)

MAGICAL FORMS

Laburnum anagyroides and *Laburnum alpinum* (Alpine or Scotch laburnum) are both native to southern and central Europe • Laburnum (*Laburnum* × *watereri* 'Vossii'), a hybrid between the other two, is called the golden chain tree in the USA, where it grows in temperate climates • beautiful yellow fragrant blossoms appear in late spring • not to be mistaken for the similar-in-appearance Golden Rain Tree (see p. 201), which is not poisonous • a powerful tree that must be handled physically with care • magically use the golden blossoms and the pods containing the seeds

PLANETS AND ELEMENT

Mars/Sun • Fire

MAGICAL USES

blossoms are used for bringing profit when blooming yellow • seed pods are excellent for use in defensive magic • anti-theft • breaks hexes, curses, jinxes, binding spells, and ill wishes • attracts money involving risks • good for spells associated with networking to bring financial profit • can help to overcome betrayal in love

HOW TO USE

Wearing gloves, collect the fallen yellow blossoms. Keep them in a sealed charm bag on top of investment papers or offers to make money that may be hazardous but would bring great returns. Before sealing, add eight golden-colored coins or disks and a piece of real gold, such as an earring, to the bag. Shake the closed bag nine times over the paper and say nine times, *Not without danger, risk is no stranger, yet shall I speculate, I shall not hesitate, winner takes all, I shall not fall.* • Take three pods with utmost care and bury them in or near the center of a three-way crossroads to break a hex or curse. • On top of that place, leave three crossed sticks, breaking them before leaving.

CAUTION

Do not ingest any part of the tree, and handle blossoms and pods carefully. • All laburnums are poisonous, especially the pods and seeds.

Common Toadflax

(*Linaria vulgaris*)

MAGICAL FORMS

also called yellow toadflax • often grows wild, with yellow and orange flowers tightly packed on tall spikes • appears in June until November • resembles the snapdragon • native to Europe, the UK, Ireland, Asia, and Siberia, and now common in North America • magically use the aerial parts, especially the flowers

PLANET AND ELEMENT

Moon • Water

MAGICAL USES

brings the power to see and connect with nature spirits • for breaking hexes and curses • reveals secrets because large bees settle and force open the mouth of the closed flower to reach the nectar • in China, the toad was believed to swallow the moon, causing an eclipse • use toadflax for eclipse rituals and on any full moon

HOW TO USE

Grow as part of a magical herb garden, placing a stone or metal frog with a coin in its mouth in their midst to attract good fortune. • Burn in an incense mix before meditation or divination for enhanced clairvoyance, adding more fragrant herbs. • Set amulet bags of the dried flowers at the four corners of the home or attach to a bamboo cane or tall bamboo plants tied with red twine at the four corners of your land to act as psychic boundaries against all living or spirit-unfriendly intentions. • During a lunar eclipse, toadflax will take away all curses, hexes, and jinxes if you pick petals or leaves when there is darkness or a ring around the moon, burying them before the light returns.

CAUTION

Some experts consider toadflax mildly toxic, but its odor and bitter taste generally deter pets and children.

Copaiba Balsam

(*Copaifera officinalis*)

MAGICAL FORMS

not a true balsam • native to Brazil, northeast and central South America • the oil is produced from the gum/resin of the many-branched densely foliaged tropical tree • magically use the essential oil and the resin as incense (usually sold as part of a mix, such as with frankincense, but hard to find)

PLANETS AND ELEMENTS

Sun/Moon • Fire/Water

MAGICAL USES

called the miracle tree in Bolivia by the Indigenous people because of its many healing and magical properties • protective against ill-wishing, hexes, curses, and mind manipulation • to bring a calm end to the day

HOW TO USE

To act as a destressor and to lower anxiety and fear, burn as an incense or oil mix or diffuse with lavender and sandalwood. • Massage the center of the brow and pulse points with the oil diluted in almond or jojoba carrier oil, if you are suffering panic attacks or psychosomatic illnesses before or after certain situations or with particular people. • Spritz your home and workspace with a water spray containing ten to fifteen drops of essential oil to half a liter of water in a pump action spray bottle if you sense you are being ill-wished, maligned, or jinxed.

CAUTION

It is uncertain whether the oil is safe with pregnancy and breastfeeding, so check with your midwife or physician.

Copal

from (*Bursera fagaroides*)

MAGICAL FORMS

Bursera fagaroides is also known as fragrant Bursera or fragrant elephant tree • sap from Bursera trees, especially in South America, Central America, and Asia, hardens as resin into small rocks or tears • resembles amber but is younger and softer • magically use as incense, resin, and jewelry

PLANET AND ELEMENT

Sun • Fire

MAGICAL USES

a sacred incense to both Mayans and among the Aztecs, in the early 1500s, copal was burned on Aztec braziers carved with the image of Chalchiuhtlicue, goddess of water and fertility, and was also sacred to her rain god husband, Tlaloc • copal is used to contact the spirits of the dead and is still burned in Mexican churches at the beginning of November on the Day of the Dead • solidified copal is a crystal of protection and brings abundance and fertility; it is found buried beneath the resin trees between the fresh and fossilized stages • copal has three forms: white, sweeter than black for connections with Divinity and sacred ceremonies, with a pine fragrance; gold, the sweetest copal for meditation and creating sacred spaces; and black, the least sweet for grounding and manifestation • it should be noted that when extracting the sap for both the gold and black copal, it is necessary to completely remove the bark, therefore it is ecologically ill-advised

HOW TO USE

Wear the beads as a necklace or burn it as incense to carry you in meditation or visualization for past-life recollections and visions of ancient lands, temples, and sacred ceremonies. • Gaze into the swirling smoke of crossed lighted incense sticks in front of the flame of a gold candle in darkness to connect with the angels and guides of healing and direct healing to a person, place, or animal. • Alternatively, send healing while gazing into a large resin rock or handful of the tears in a raised dish and naming the recipient of the healing.

CAUTION

Nontoxic, but do not use *Bursera fagaroides* resin with blood thinners.

Copal Tree, Protium

(*Protium paniculatum*)

MAGICAL FORMS

from the Burseraceae family, which contains many resin-producing trees, such as frankincense and myrrh • the Protium copal tree is endemic to Mexico and central Mexico • can reach almost a hundred feet and has long leathery leaves • magically use the resin and also as an oil made from the resin, quite rare but obtainable online and in specialty magick stores

PLANET AND ELEMENT

Mars • Fire

MAGICAL USES

used by Mayans and Aztecs in ceremonial magick as offerings to the deities for manifesting wishes and needs and providing stability in magick • for all night magick • contacting the ancestors and wise guardians • burned to remove and keep away hostile spirit energies and restless ghosts

HOW TO USE

Use the patterns of the thick smoke produced by the resin for divination or, in Mexican shamanic style, cast corn grains beneath the smoke onto the ground and through the smoke read their patterns to answer questions. • Black copal resin is burned in Mexico on *Día de Los Muertos* (the Day of the Dead), November 1, to guide the ancestors to the home. • Copal resin can be burned as incense to send blessings to beloved departed relatives. • Oil can be used in a diffuser/burner to induce a meditative state.

CAUTION

The oil should be well diluted but not ingested, as it can cause an allergy in some people. • Perform a patch test before use.

Coral Tree

(*Erythrina* spp.)

MAGICAL FORMS

includes *Erythrina variegata*, the Indian coral tree or tiger's claw, and *Erythrina × sykesii*, the Australian coral tree • Indian coral tree blossoms with scarlet flowers resembling coral and tiger-claw-like spines on branches • native to tropical and subtropical parts of eastern Africa, Indian subcontinent, northern Australia, and western Pacific east to Fiji • introduced into Arizona, California, and Florida • the Australian coral tree is native to South Africa • grows from California to Florida, with prickles on the trunk and scarlet flowers • magically use the growing tree, fresh and dried flowers, and thorns

PLANET AND ELEMENT

Moon • Water

MAGICAL USES

increase powers of attraction, good luck, fame, and fortune • new beginnings • shape-shifting • shamanic rituals • astral travel linked with fierce predators

HOW TO USE

Half fill a dark glass defensive bottle with the thorns from either variety of tree, adding sour milk and ginger powder if you are being threatened by a neighbor, bully at work, debt collector, or unscrupulous official. Seal the bottle and bury it deep in the garden, calling on your defensive spirit animal to drive off danger with their fierce claws. • Fill a small, red charm bag with dried, crimson flowers as a magnet to attract love, recognition, or success.

CAUTION

Do not consume raw parts of coral trees.

Coriander/Cilantro

(*Coriandrum sativum*)

MAGICAL FORMS

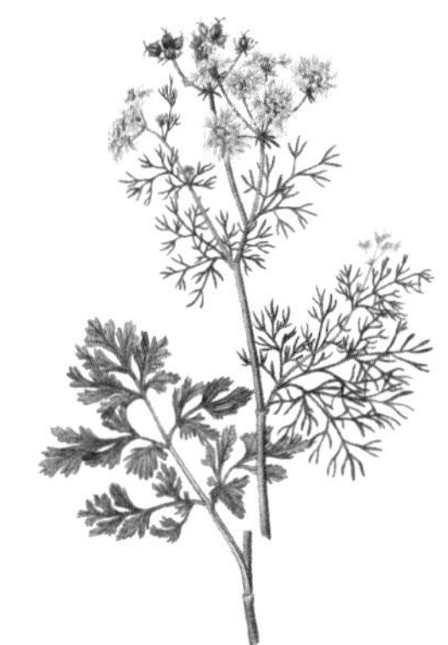

a popular culinary herb • cilantro is the name given to the leaves, also called Chinese parsley, often fresh or dried in tea • magically use the whole, growing plant; flowers; leaves; and especially dried fruit (often called seeds)

PLANET AND ELEMENT

Mars • Fire

MAGICAL USES

protects property if planted in gardens • removes negative energies • guards during astral travel • passion • love • health • encourages creativity • brings optimism • used by the ancient Egyptians to take them safely through the afterlife • as cilantro, connection with the earth, balance, peace to the home, detoxification, attracts clients to business

HOW TO USE

The growing plant, whether in an indoor herb kitchen, garden, planted near the house, or the seeds taped to the doormat, protects the property from harm, intruders, sickness, and sorrow. • To guard luggage while traveling, put the seeds in a sachet and place it in the luggage or scatter the seeds inside the luggage and around vital documents. • If you put nine seeds in a sachet, glued or sewed inside your bag or computer case, this aids memory and enables you to make a good impression with your knowledge. • The dried flowers are put in love sachets to attract love.

CAUTION

While generally safe, do not use if allergic to caraway, mugwort, aniseed, fennel, or dill. • Traditionally, pregnant women ate coriander to ensure their unborn children were quick-witted and creative in life, but check with a physician and herbalist as this may not be sound, especially in the first trimester.

Corn Silk

from (*Zea mays*)

MAGICAL FORMS

protective layer and nourishment for sweet corn kernels growing on the cob • shiny threadlike silky fibers that grow as a tassel protruding from the tip of the corn (can be purchased online, fresh or dried) • magically use in teas and as the silky fibers picked from corn before cooking

PLANET AND ELEMENT

Moon • Water

MAGICAL USES

corn silk is added to love spells to attract a desired mate, subject to free will • in Native North America, the silky hair of the Corn Mothers, for example, Selu, among the Cherokee nation, who allowed herself to be dragged by her hair in order to plant the corn that the people would be fed • for mothering and nurturing issues and helping adult children to let go of being overly dependent maternally, especially when the silk goes brown indicating the corn needs harvesting

HOW TO USE

Since every silk must receive pollen in order for the kernels to develop, to conceive a child corn silk is woven or tied around a clear crystal point or a small silver knife and left from crescent to full moon. The silk is then cut after lovemaking on full moon. • Brew tea using the golden threads, strain, and sip it to bring abundance into your life in the way most needed. • Sprinkle it around precious jewelry, especially that set in gold and silver, to protect against loss or theft and to settle disputes over inheritances of family gems.

CAUTION

It is generally used in indigenous, Chinese, and folk traditions of Europe. • Corn silk is safe when taken in food amounts but should not be taken during pregnancy, as it stimulates the uterus. • If taken medicinally, talk to a professional about safe doses and time frames for different conditions.

Corn, Sweet

(*Zea mays* L. subsp. *mays*)

MAGICAL FORMS

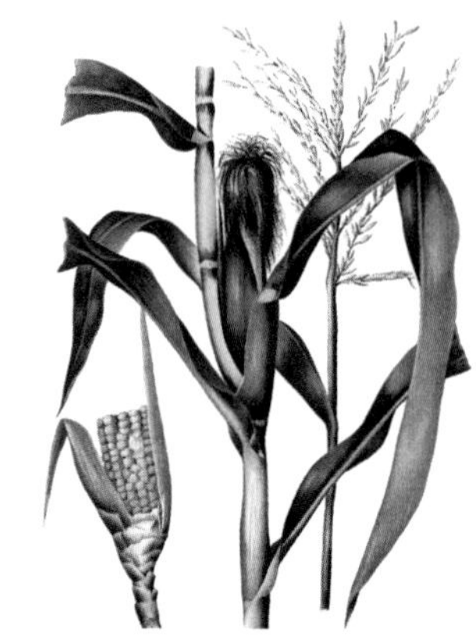

a cultivated form of sturdy maize grass that grows four to eight feet tall • high natural sugar content within the kernels • native to the Americas for thousands of years and now produced in many sunny lands, including the UK • pollinated by the wind and so representing independent thought and action • produces ears of yellow, white, or bicolored kernels on the central core within a leafy husk, with cornsilk protecting the packed kernels

PLANET AND ELEMENTS

Sun • Fire/Earth

MAGICAL USES

traditionally walk to pick (or indeed buy) ripe sweet corn and run at least part of the way home to speed ventures and bring a stagnant relationship or situation to fulfillment • the provision of what is most needed • abundance • good luck • fertility • beginning enterprises that will generate new energy and financial resources

HOW TO USE

On the summer solstice, around June 21, yellow sweet corn is eaten to further prosperity, marriage, or commitment and the confidence to achieve almost anything. • White corn, consumed before psychic activity, increases spiritual insights. • Roast whole cobs for manifesting creativity in the way most desired. • Corn mazes are often made in later summer, a throwback to ancient fertility rites. Walk one if you want a child or to connect with the Earth Mother for nurturing and mothering issues.

CAUTION

Sweet corn is safe during pregnancy and can be beneficial as it contains folate.

Cornflower

(*Centaurea cyanus*)

MAGICAL FORMS

also known as bachelor's buttons, often found growing with poppies • bachelor's buttons were so named because in Victorian times young beaus would wear a cornflower in their buttonhole when seeking or wooing a partner; if it rapidly faded, they knew their love was not returned • magically use the whole plant in a garden or in a vase and flowers, dried and fresh

PLANET AND ELEMENTS

Jupiter • Air/Earth

MAGICAL USES

the flowers were found preserved in the tomb of Tutankhamun and so became a symbol of rebirth and what is lasting • worn in France on Armistice Day and a symbol of enduring peace in a situation or relationship • in a fertility and abundance potpourri mix, enchanted at full moon • attracts the fey and their blessings • as incense burned so a storm will pass over without damage • color magick and flower psychometry in its bright blue shades

HOW TO USE

Make into magical inks for writing petitions, especially to Jupiter or his ruling archangel Sachiel, concerning justice, prosperity, commitment, or marriage. • A few dried petals in a tiny sachet sewn into the lining of a garment worn by an indigo child provides equanimity when they face the world. • Magical tea from the flowers increases clairvoyance if drunk before reading cards or used as the Water element in spellcasting. • Place the dried flowers in a fertility bag with a gold-colored bee charm, one of the oldest symbols of fertility, and empower it every full moon until conception. • At Lammas, the first harvest, walk through a field of cornflowers with a lover or alone to bring lasting love, youthfulness, and sufficient resources until the next Lammas.

CAUTION

Do not use cornflower if allergic to daisies, ragweed, marigolds, or chrysanthemums. • Avoid during pregnancy and breastfeeding.

Cornstarch

from (*Zea mays*)

MAGICAL FORMS

pure white powder, made by extracting the starch from corn kernels • gluten- and fiber-free and one of the most underrated ingredients in magick • obtainable worldwide (called corn flour in the UK) • discovered in 1844 when American Thomas Kingsford isolated cornstarch from corn originally for laundry • by 1850 it had become a food thickener • magically use the powder

PLANET AND ELEMENT

Saturn • Earth

MAGICAL USES

binds together magical ingredients in wish powders • in its own right absorbs negativity • when stored correctly, it lasts indefinitely and so can be added to longer-term magick bags • stir into magical cookery to emotionally bind together those who will eat the dish

HOW TO USE

Keep a small amount uncovered in the kitchen to absorb all negative energies entering the home, disposing of it weekly and replacing. • Add to charms, spell bags, and magical powders, in proportion of four teaspoons of herbs to one tablespoon of cornstarch, to combine different aspects of the mix according to the meaning of the individual herbs, thereby creating a power greater than the separate parts. • Use cornstarch separately in a unity amulet bag, hidden in a conference room or place where relatives will gather for a celebration, if there are underlying tensions, and throw it away after the event.

Cosmos

(*Cosmos bipinnatus*)

MAGICAL FORMS

also known as Mexican aster • magically use the whole, growing plant and cut flowers

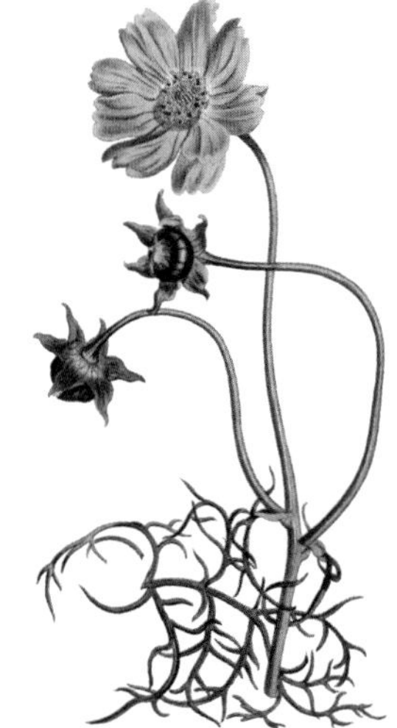

PLANET AND ELEMENT

Jupiter • Air

MAGICAL USES

for order where there is chaos or indecision • restoring harmony to life, family, or colleagues • originally named after the Greek word *kosmos*, meaning "order" because of its symmetrical appearance when grown as a garden flower in the Spanish missions in Mexico in the sixteenth century • in modern magick, because the flower cup when in full bloom resembles an upturned satellite dish, it is linked with star magick and extraterrestrial communication • also connects with the fey, both indigenous spirits and those that came with the flower to the USA in the 1800s • flower psychometry

HOW TO USE

The emblem of World Kindness Day in Tokyo in 1999, held annually on November 13, cosmos is a great appreciation and friendship bouquet. • It also is given after a quarrel when unkind words were spoken. • Give it to initiate romance. • The petals can be carried in a sachet if you have a speech to make or meeting or lecture to deliver. • If you have a lot of drama kings and queens in your life, grow it in the garden at home or use it as cut flowers for domestic or workplace peace.

CAUTION

While cosmos is not edible, it is regarded as nontoxic, though some experts warn that the flower should not be ingested.

Costmary

(*Tanacetum balsamita*)

MAGICAL FORMS

came from Asia to the UK and then traveled with the settlers to become popular in New England gardens and other parts of the USA such as northeastern Ohio • named after the Virgin Mary as Herbe Sainte-Marie because costmary was said to ease childbirth and also after Mary Magdalene, as the balsam with which she washed Jesus's feet • though much less popular today, those who practice herbal lore and love traditional plants are reintroducing it to gardens, for example in a reconstructed 1815 herb garden at Hale Farm and Village in Ohio • magically use mainly the leaves, traditionally used medicinally and in cooking

PLANET AND ELEMENT

Jupiter • Air

MAGICAL USES

called the Bible leaf because its leaf was used as a scented bookmark for the Bible and sacred books in church services • traditionally used magically for domestic cleansing and fragrancing to cleanse the home of sickness, sorrow, and misfortune • protective of babies and children in more hazardous times

HOW TO USE

Grow near the home to act as a magical barrier or to keep luck within and danger out. • Press a leaf and dry it between two sheets of paper, then use in bibliomancy or stichomancy by placing it anywhere between the pages of a sacred or common book, opening randomly to that page to give an answer to a question. • Add the dried lemony leaves to magical potpourri with rosemary, cloves, bay, and cinnamon to keep all harm from the home and attract abundance, health, and harmony. • Apply an infusion of the leaves created with hot water to the borders of yards to create magical boundaries against wandering spirits. • If there have been paranormal disturbances, add long dried leaves to a bundle of dried lavender and place on a white cloth on the bed to bless those who will later sleep in it and to bring them peaceful nights and protection while they sleep. Then, at sunset take the bundle outdoors and hang it outside the house to act as guardian until it crumbles.

Cotton

(*Gossypium hirsutum*) and (*Gossypium barbadense*)

MAGICAL FORMS

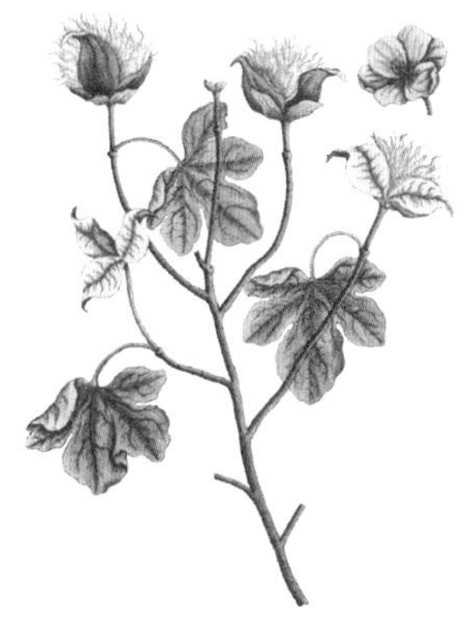

natural fiber, grown on a leafy green shrub related to hibiscus • native to the Americas, Africa, and Asia • grown in warm or tropical climates, such as parts of Australia • *Gossypium hirsutum*, American cotton, was cultivated by the Mayans and Aztecs for fiber and medicine • Columbus carried samples from his first voyage back to Europe • magically use cotton flowers, fresh or dried; cotton balls, the fluffy white tufts surrounding seed capsules; and woven into fabric or as undyed sewing thread

PLANET AND ELEMENTS

Moon • Water/Earth

MAGICAL USES

a cotton cloth on your altar adds spiritual dimensions, even to basic spells • carry dried cotton flowers or cotton balls in a cotton bag for prosperity, good fortune, or love, adding a favorite piece of jewelry to personalize the bag, and marking or sewing in cotton thread on the inside of the bag your initials and/or name of the person you want to attract

HOW TO USE

Make a featureless poppet out of pure white cotton, filled with cotton balls, adding lavender for healing, and dedicate it to yourself or an unwell person, sending or giving it if you know they would like it. • Tie a strong cotton thread with silver disks with holes on a tree near your home or a potted plant indoors near the front door to drive away ghosts as the wind blows.

CAUTION

Avoid raw cotton if pregnant. • The seed oil and root bark, formerly used extensively in magick and medicinally, are known to be potentially toxic, and seed oil may be implicated in infertility in men.

Cottonwood Tree

(*Populus* spp.)

MAGICAL FORMS

includes eastern cottonwood (*Populus deltoids*) • Frémont's cottonwood (*Populus fremontii*) • narrowleaf cottonwood (*Populus angustifolia*) • lanceleaf cottonwood (*Populus × acuminata*), a hybrid cross between the eastern and narrowleaf cottonwood without cotton fluff in the summer • swamp cottonwood (*Populus heterophylla*) • Chinese necklace cottonwood (*Populus lasiocarpa*) • American poplar/black cottonwood also belongs to the same genus as Poplar (see p. 358) • huge trees with fluffy cotton-like strands that appear in early summer growing in Europe, parts of Asia, in eastern, central, and southwestern states of the USA, and southern Canada • magically use the dried cottonwood tree buds or the fresh or dried cotton strands

PLANETS AND ELEMENTS

Sun/Saturn • Fire/Earth

MAGICAL USES

a cottonwood pole was traditionally used as the center axis of the annual Native North American sun dance, honoring the sun, the Great Spirit, and ancestors, now being carried out again after having been banned in the mid-1900s • use cottonwood magically for transformation, healing rituals using light, star magick, and star souls

HOW TO USE

Meditate or chant and dance around a cottonwood tree alone, with someone special, or with your magical group at midsummer to honor the sun and the natural world and to seek to connect with the Divine. • Use it when seeking to give up bad habits or destructive ways and relationships. • Collect the cotton strands in a sealed white bag as they fall from the tree and set them on your altar or special place, surrounded by a circle of white candles naming people, animals, and places that need light, healing, and hope.

CAUTION

The cotton-like strands can cause allergies, as can the pollen. • If you are affected by cotton, wear a mask and gloves when handling.

Cowslip

(*Primula veris*)

MAGICAL FORMS

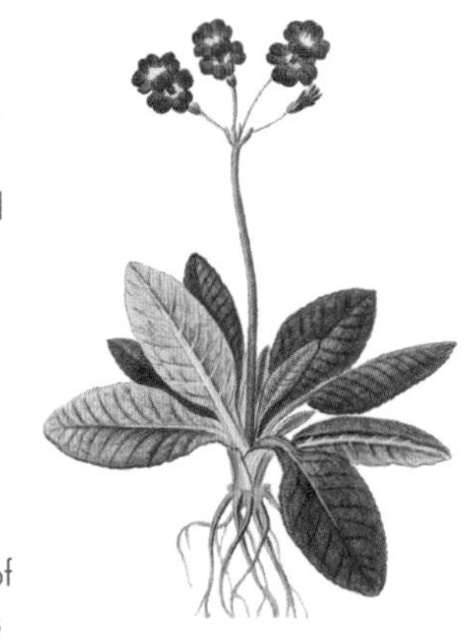

flowering plant related to the primrose • magically use whole, growing plant found in the wild or in a garden and the flowers, fresh and dried

PLANET AND ELEMENTS

Venus • Water/Earth

MAGICAL USES

learning and examinations • wise advice • flower of Beltane, May Day, the start of the Celtic summer, when it is made into garlands • finding treasure or lost objects • protects houses against intruders • for healing and preserving or restoring youthfulness • called fairy cups, a plant of the fey who are said to sleep within the bells and guard their fairy gold buried nearby that will turn to dust if mortals try to steal it • originally linked with Freya, the Norse goddess of beauty and magick, and in Christian times with the Virgin Mary

HOW TO USE

Place dried cowslips beneath the front step or a bunch over the front door to deter unwelcome or unfriendly callers. • Because they grow in clusters, cowslips are good in unifying rituals whether for the home or workplace, binding the plants together and naming those to be joined in harmony. • Hold a bunch in your hand, flowers downward to locate what is missing. • Restore youthfulness by adding dried cowslip flowers to your bath. • Cast cowslips on flowing water to call back a lost love. • A potted plant where you study will increase memory and focus. • Carry nine flowers, if possible in a cluster, in a yellow bag to an examination. • Keep a potted plant indoors or the cut flowers in a vase to restore calm and goodwill after quarrels.

Cranberry

(*Vaccinium macrocarpon*)

MAGICAL FORMS

small slender evergreen shrub with oval dark green leaves, pink flowers • round red berries, the main part used magically and medicinally • native to eastern North America, cultivated extensively throughout the northern USA, notably in Wisconsin and Massachusetts • introduced to the UK in 1808 • also found in northern Asia • magically use the berries

PLANET AND ELEMENT

Saturn • Earth

MAGICAL USES

for increased initiative • to resist bullies in the workplace and those in your life • passion • like its cousin the blueberry, a celebratory fruit at Thanksgiving and Christmas and other traditional formal and informal family occasions • in magical cookery as sauce, desserts, a juice, or tea made from the fresh berries, cinnamon, apple juice, and lemon (many easy recipes online) for allowing family affection to be expressed • as a substitute for wine in formal magical rituals

HOW TO USE

Share the juice or tea with your partner or lover at the end of the moon cycle, when the moon is no longer in the sky, to ensure none will come between you and that there will be no secrets. • Surround a purple candle with a circle of the berries and, while removing them one by one, ask Grandmother Moon to assist you in quitting a bad habit or assist a loved one to be free of an addiction or bad influence. Afterward, cast the discarded cranberries into running water or bury them and place a stone on top. • Use dried cranberries to decorate Christmas wreaths, and as you attach them, naming absent or estranged family members you wish to return to the family hearth and table.

CAUTION

While famed for its positive effects in curing bladder complaints, such as cystitis, do not ingest if you have kidney problems, unless under medical supervision. • Use in moderation during pregnancy.

Cranesbill

(*Geranium maculatum*)

MAGICAL FORMS

various species of wild geranium, growing up to three feet tall • many native to or naturalized in central and eastern USA and Canada • blooming pink, purple, or white from March until July • growing in forests, also in Europe • used by Native North American nations, especially as a tea for medicinal purposes, including mouth sores and stomach upsets • bright blue shining cranesbill (*Geranium lucidum*) is native to Europe, western Asia, and Africa and has been naturalized in gardens in the USA, sometimes becoming invasive • cranesbill is so called because the column of the fruit capsule, from the old flower, resembles a crane's beak and head • the column consists of five cells, each of which contains a seed, that spring open when ripe, casting the seeds over a considerable distance • magically use the roots/rhizome, the dried aerial parts, the beak still containing the seeds, and the seeds (see "Geranium," p. 192, and "Herb-Robert," p. 216)

PLANETS AND ELEMENTS

Moon/Venus • Water/Earth

MAGICAL USES

the root in an amulet bag, carried for all money transactions and speculation • the dried flowers made into a charm bag for success in artistic endeavors, especially the performing arts and dance

HOW TO USE

Release the seeds from the pods onto a white cloth, knot the cloth, and scatter the seeds in a high place to increase your influence and have your expertise recognized (the crane symbolically is a wise teacher). • Use for male potency if anxiety to conceive is causing impotence. • The tea, made as a decoction from the crushed root or purchased in herbal stores and online, should be sipped before major travel or sprinkled around travel documents and luggage to keep them with you until you reach your destination.

CAUTION

Generally considered safe, but do not use during pregnancy. • The root in excess can be harmful to the liver.

Craspedia

(*Craspedia globosa*)

MAGICAL FORMS

also known as billy buttons or sun ball • native to New Zealand and Australia but grows well in warmer parts of the USA • yellow pompom flower balls on long stalks • magically use the growing plant, fresh cut flowers, and, especially beautiful, dried flower balls

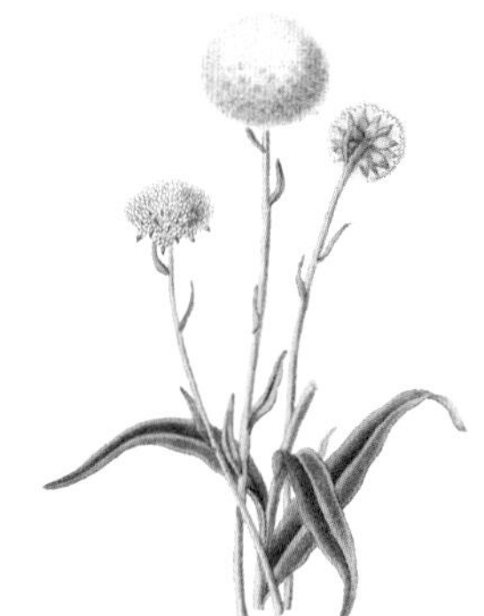

PLANET AND ELEMENT

Sun • Fire

MAGICAL USES

for informal and wildflower bouquets, boutonnieres, and table decorations for family weddings and handfastings • for good health and fertility • for a marriage based on laughter, fun, and goodwill • harmonizing different family members or rivals on the big day and in future married life • a sign of everlasting happiness

HOW TO USE

Use in sun rituals and astrology readings where sun signs are the main feature. • Keep three dried sun balls in a gold bag with three small pieces of gold, such as earrings, to attract money. • You can empower and re-empower the bag by leaving it in a sheltered place from dawn to noon on May Day morning, the summer solstice, or Lammas. • Place dried craspedia, along with dried wheat, corn, or any grain, in an arrangement in the home or a business to make the sun of well-being shine all year, bringing good love and abundance. • On family birthdays, Easter, Thanksgiving, or Christmas, set a basket of golden fruits and tiny wrapped gifts for all who visit, placed around craspedia flowers and grain to spread prosperity.

CAUTION

Craspedia is fatal for cattle to ingest and can be harmful to horses.

Creosote Bush

(*Larrea tridentata*)

MAGICAL FORMS

also known as chaparral • broad-leafed evergreen shrub • yellow flowers appearing after rain release their volatile oils • grows in desert regions in California, southern Oregon, the northern part of the Baja California peninsula in Mexico, the Sonoran Desert in Arizona, southern Utah, Texas, New Mexico, and other parts of the world that have a desert or Mediterranean-type climate • a long-living plant, the oldest being 11,700 years old near Victorville, California • so named because of the creosote smell of the bush and herb • magically use the flower essence, the dried and chopped herb (can be bought online), and as infused oil, usually in grape-seed or olive oil with honey (though its topical use is questioned)

PLANETS AND ELEMENT

Mars/Sun • Fire

MAGICAL USES

add a few drops of the chaparral essence to the chaparral crushed dried stem, leaves, and flowers as an amulet against disturbed sleep, nightmares, and specters of the night • the flower essence detoxifies all malevolent psychic energies and emotions without taking any chemicals from the bush

HOW TO USE

Add just a few drops of the oil or flower essence to a water spray with sweetening lavender to spray a room where there has been an angry exchange or there is a spooky atmosphere. As the oldest plant on earth (it clones new plants as one dies), meditate on the growing flowers or while holding the dried flowers in a charm bag to act as a natural past-life channel, especially lives associated with the industrial past. • If physical flowers are not available, use a downloaded picture.

CAUTION

However, the US Food and Drug Administration and Health Canada advise people against using chaparral medicinally. • It is agreed, even by herbal practitioners, that it should not be used if suffering from liver and kidney disease, if trying to get pregnant, during pregnancy, or while breastfeeding.

Crocus

(*Crocus vernus*)

MAGICAL FORMS

also known as spring crocus • more than fifty different kinds of crocus, all growing in the spring, including purple *Crocus vernus* ('Purpureus Grandiflorus') and snow crocus, *Crocus chrysanthus* • magically use growing flowers in a garden or pot, dried flowers, and flower essence

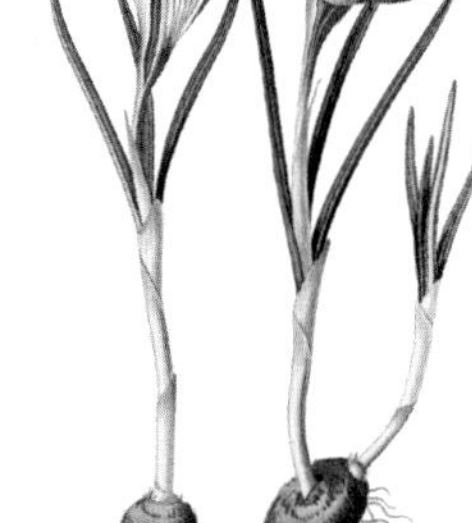

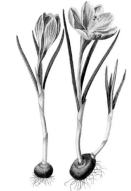

PLANET AND ELEMENT

Venus • Water

MAGICAL USES

for children and young people • joy • new beginnings • yellow crocus is a Valentine's Day flower traditionally worn on February 14 to attract a true love • flower essence resolves grief and loss • use as incense • an early flower appearing soon after the Imbolc festival in early February, growing crocus are placed on altars right through to the spring equinox to welcome ritually a new phase (once March 25 heralded the new year) • a good time for initiations and dedications and reaffirmation of New Year's resolutions

HOW TO USE

Keep a pot of crocus by your front door or grow in the garden to attract love, happiness, and new beginnings and to deter infidelity. • Meditating on an array of crocus in the garden or wild will take you to higher levels of consciousness. • Burn as incense to give a vision of a thief or deceiver. Can also help make connections with the spirit world, especially during divination. • Blow softly three times toward a bowl of crocus to make a love wish. • Mist the bedroom with rose or lavender water with a few drops of purple crocus essence added to prevent nightmares and around the home to reduce anger. • When peppermint is added to this spray, it is good to use as a mist around your aura to resist abuse or being disrespected.

CAUTION

Spring crocus can be toxic if ingested by pets.

Crocus, Saffron

(*Crocus sativus*)

MAGICAL FORMS

an aromatic plant with stunning purple flowers, grasslike leaves, and yellow stamens • each flower has three red, bright-orange, or nearly-purple stigmas • saffron spice is made from the stigmas, cut and dried to produce the thread-like saffron • grown in southern Europe; also its original home, India; in Russia; China; Japan; in the warm, dry parts of the USA; and especially in Kashmir and Iran • magically use the spice in empowered cookery and as incense made by grinding the powder and mixing it with wood shavings, beeswax, and essential oils, then forming it into cones, sticks, powdered incense, and coils (widely available online) • the more expensive kind of incense will contain a larger amount of the costly saffron

PLANET AND ELEMENT

Sun • Fire

MAGICAL USES

for increasing happiness and passion, and to enhance any love or money spell • reverses the outflow of money • offers second sight when consumed as a tea or as flavoring for rice

HOW TO USE

Burn saffron crocus as incense before and during prayers and meditation. • In India, a paste of saffron and sandalwood is applied as a *tilak*, a sacred mark of various kinds on the forehead over the Third Eye to enhance psychic powers and visions. • On Tuesdays, the saffron tilak is applied to the forehead to bring prosperity. • On Wednesdays, the day for new ventures, dedicated to Lord Vitthal, an incarnation of Vishnu, it is mixed with turmeric. • On Fridays, saffron paste is applied to honor the goddesses, and on Saturdays, it's worn while reciting prayers to Lord Hanuman, the deity of wisdom and self-awareness. • Marking the forehead with a saffron paste dot over the Third Eye taps into the tradition without showing disrespect—this is called applying a tilak, a symbol of the authority of God.

CAUTION

Use saffron crocus in moderation and avoid if pregnant.

Crown of Thorns

(*Euphorbia milii*)

MAGICAL FORMS

shrubby thorny plant whose stems can reach seven feet, with small white or red flowers, surrounded by red or yellow bracts, leaflike structures just below the flowers • the plant blooms all year but especially in winter months • native to Madagascar, it is often found as a potted houseplant growing to about three feet or outdoors in warmer regions of the USA, such as California, Florida, Hawaii, parts of Texas, and the Gulf Coast, and in other lands with Mediterranean-like or tropical climates • magically use the thorny stems, with care, and the flower essence

PLANET AND ELEMENT

Mars • Fire

MAGICAL USES

the plant and essence resolve unnecessary or past guilt that should be left behind • an antidote to the martyr syndrome where life is regarded as a constant struggle and happiness, love, or success only come at a price • avoiding setting impossibly high standards for self and not feeling worthy of love • named after the crown of thorns worn by Jesus on the cross because the red bracts represent the blood of Christ on the original crown of thorns

HOW TO USE

With care, seal the thorny stem in a dark glass bottle with a few of the petals/bracts, plus the essence dissolved in water, to represent the shedding of guilt or fear of not deserving happiness, and preserve the bottle in a high dark place where it will not be touched or opened. • Take the essence regularly to open yourself to unconditional love, happiness, and abundance.

CAUTION

Crown of thorns is poisonous to humans, pets, and livestock if any part is ingested, and handling it can cause skin and eye irritation.

Cubeb

(*Piper cubeba*)

MAGICAL FORMS

also called the tailed pepper or Java pepper • once grown only in Java and Sumatra, the cubeb tree now is more widespread • the berries are picked before ripe and left to dry in the sunshine till they become black and wrinkled • available in gourmet stores and some herbalists • magically use either as the berries, each about the size of a peppercorn, or crushed and powdered in incense

PLANET AND ELEMENT

Mars • Fire

MAGICAL USES

prized by the ancient Greeks, the spice traveled via the trade routes to the Middle East • recommended medicinally by the early German medieval mystic and herbalist Hildegard von Bingen • restricted by Java farmers to prevent it being grown elsewhere • the berries or powder increases the speed and intensity of any purpose in incense burning • cubeb increases potency as an aphrodisiac in incense or when added to food before lovemaking

HOW TO USE

Traditionally in Europe and China, cubeb pepper was burned in incense to drive away demons. • Its aromatic spicy fragrance similar to allspice is still used in incense mixes to keep away harm, earthly and paranormal, from the home. • The powder or berries can be sprinkled on doorsteps and swept outward to remove misfortune or anger. • Scatter the spice around a photograph of a lover you fear is straying or planning to stray to deter unwise passion. • Add cubeb to a love attraction bag along with any other spice, such as ginger, if the subject of your affection is not noticing you, spreading a little where she or he will walk.

CAUTION

Avoid excessive use, especially if you have gastric problems. • As with any spice, take care during pregnancy.

Cuckoo Flower

(*Cardamine pratensis*)

MAGICAL FORMS

commonly called lady's smock or mayflower, its numerous names reflecting its rich folk traditions • a wildflower in England and Europe and naturalized through cultivation in those parts of the USA where summers are cooler • growing plant, with pink, purple, or white flowers tinged with lilac color, closing during heavy rain and at night • magically use flowers and leaves, fresh and dried

PLANET AND ELEMENTS

Venus • Water/Earth

MAGICAL USES

called cuckoo flower because it appears in April at the same time as the cuckoo bird, both as first heralds of spring • for rituals and charms for new beginnings • mayflower and other popular names are linked with the old Maytime fertility festivals, romance, and lovemaking • in Christian times it is told the Virgin Mary left a smock behind in a cave near Bethlehem, found by St. Helena, that became a holy relic • April 25, being Lady Day, when Gabriel told Mary she would expect a child, is again a time when the flower first blooms and so strengthens the fertility link • a fairy flower, said to be unlucky to bring into the home without asking for permission, causing storms if disregarded

HOW TO USE

Carry nine fresh, if possible, or dried flowers in a charm bag with the same number of golden coins for prosperity. • Because of its association with Maytime fertility revels and Mother Mary, the flowers are considered a fertility symbol if collected at dawn on a May morning, or when the moon is passing through Scorpio, Cancer, or Pisces, each about two and a half days a month. • Place the petals in an empty eggshell, and bury it beneath growing cuckoo flowers or any other thriving plant. Because the cuckoo is heard but not seen and lays its eggs in other birds' nests, pick a closed flower and hide it in greenery if you have been unfairly blamed for another person's mistakes or to keep a low profile if excess burdens are being put upon you.

Cucumber

(*Cucumis sativus*)

MAGICAL FORMS
a creeping vine, belonging to the gourd family, grown for its edible fruit, usually in open fields in Arizona, California, Florida, Georgia, Michigan, and New Mexico • also throughout Europe, especially Spain, the UK, Russia, and Turkey • popular in ancient Greek and Roman times, its origins may date back to India more than four thousand years ago • magically use the fruit

PLANETS AND ELEMENT
Moon/Venus • Water

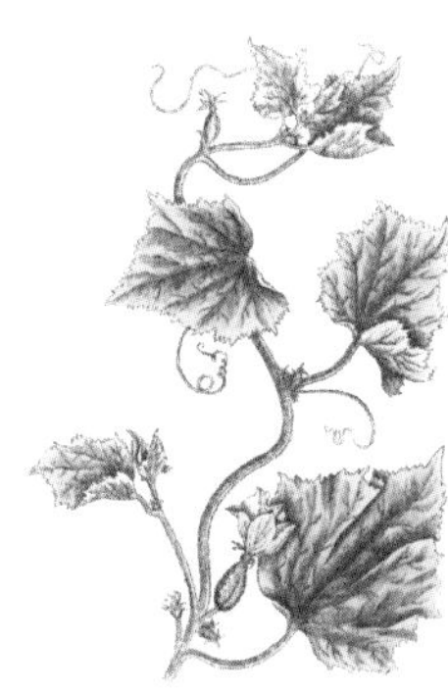

MAGICAL USES
deterring overly passionate lovers or workplace sexual predators • the dried seeds eaten for fertility if there is a lot of anxiety or conception has been slow • slices or the peel are used to ease eye strain, head pain, and stress • as a beauty treatment empowered as a mask or in lotions, especially with aloe vera, to preserve/restore youthfulness

HOW TO USE
A phallic symbol, the cucumber is offered whole to the full moon as part of a fertility ritual, bound with twine to a small melon with both attached to a flat piece of wood, then floated out with the ebbing tide or a tidal river. • Best used when the moon shines on the water to kindle male potency if the need to conceive a child has dimmed passion and to restore natural fertility cycles. • In contrast, peel and slice a cucumber and offer in a sandwich or salad to dampen lust in situations where sexual innuendos or approaches are a distraction or inappropriate. • Pickle small whole cucumbers and eat them to increase the power and lasting effects of any magical intention or spell.

CAUTION
While generally considered safe, they can occasionally cause allergic reactions. During pregnancy, cucumbers may be eaten peeled in small quantities.

Cumaru Tree

(*Dipteryx odorata*) or (*Coumarouna odorata*)

MAGICAL FORMS
a species of flowering tree that can reach over eighty feet high and three feet in diameter • producing almond-shaped seeds called tonka beans, which have a rough, black skin and are smooth and brown inside • native to central and northern South America • popular in perfumes for the tonka bean's beautiful fragrance, described variously as a mix of woodruff, caramel, vanilla, almond, and cacao • magically use the tonka bean in fragrances and the whole beans with care

PLANETS AND ELEMENTS
Venus/Jupiter • Water/Air

MAGICAL USES
for centuries, as part of magical practice, the whole tonka bean has been treasured and locked away (for safety) in a practitioner's ingredient store • in charm and mojo bags, in wish and protective jars, or carried wrapped in silk as a talisman to attract love; increase passion, money, and good fortune; keep illness away; and give courage to overcome any obstacles

HOW TO USE
Carry an odd number of whole beans—three, seven, or nine—in a red bag for love and enhancing sexual pleasure, green for money, brown for property, yellow for travel, and blue for employment. Anoint with a drop of whiskey before sealing. • Keep nine beans in a small bowl in the north or Earth realm of an altar or special space, making a wish for each bean. When the beans wither, dispose of them safely and replace, unless the wishes have been fulfilled or have changed.

CAUTION
If consumed in excess, beans can cause liver damage and can affect the heart. • Tonka beans have been banned for culinary and medicinal use by the FDA in the USA and restricted in parts of the European Union; some practitioners and cooks dispute this, but whatever the view, tonka beans should be avoided in pregnancy and around children and pets.

Cumin

(*Cuminum cyminum*)

MAGICAL FORMS

medicinally, almost always used as seeds • magically use spice in empowered cooking

PLANETS AND ELEMENTS

Mars/Mercury • Fire/Air

MAGICAL USES

anti-theft • loss of what is precious in every way • peace of mind • protection of homes, property, cars, and all within • fidelity

HOW TO USE

Scatter the seeds with salt on doorsteps and sweep outward to take away bad atmospheres and misfortune in the home. • Planting around the edges of a property, in a protective window box, or as pots of the growing herb at the four corners of a house or workspace prevents accidents, ill-intentioned visitors, and misfortune. • Drinking cumin seed, or the powdered seeds made into tea, increases psychic abilities, especially clairvoyance and telepathy over physical distance. • Sprinkle the infusion on unlucky objects or places to purify them. • Used as a spice in cooking, it acts as an aphrodisiac. • Burn it as incense or place a bag of seeds under your pillow to induce prophetic dreams. • Hide a bag of seeds near a pet's bed or in a lover's home (or where they keep their computer/smartphone) to stop them straying.

CAUTION

If consumed in larger quantities, cumin can lower testosterone; it should not be ingested to excess during pregnancy.

Cumin, Black

(*Bunium bulbocastanum*)

MAGICAL FORMS

also known as great pignut or earthnut • native to the Mediterranean, including Turkey, Greece, and Iran • sometimes its seed oil form is sold as black seed oil (*Nigella sativa*) though the two are different botanically • now grows in the USA and elsewhere • reaches three feet • wispy foliage and frilly leaves with small pale, often white, flowers in umbrella-like clusters • blooms from May to July, followed by fruit pods filled with seeds • magically use the root, seed, or essential oil

PLANET AND ELEMENT

Saturn • Earth

MAGICAL USES

the prophet Mohammed said that black cumin heals all diseases except death • the pure seed carrier oil can be used as massage or for anointing your brow alone or with fennel, oregano, tea tree, or thyme essential oil for asserting your identity and to overcome body image issues if you have been discouraged by spite or jealousy • add to or buy hair and beauty products containing the oil to enhance your charisma • honeymooners should eat these or *Nigella sativa* seeds as an aphrodisiac • seeds left in the full moon for fertility

HOW TO USE

If you can obtain a round taproot (once eaten as a vegetable; tastes like sweet chestnuts), chop it and hide a piece in a bag in your kitchen so that you will always have sufficient resources, replacing it when it withers. • Hang a net of the seeds above and just inside the front door to repel evil spirits or thieves who, it is said, are forced to count the seeds and give up.

CAUTION

Do not ingest the plant during pregnancy, and only use the oil topically in later trimesters on medical advice. • The leaves may be slightly toxic.

Cup and Saucer Vine

(*Cobaea scandens*)

MAGICAL FORMS

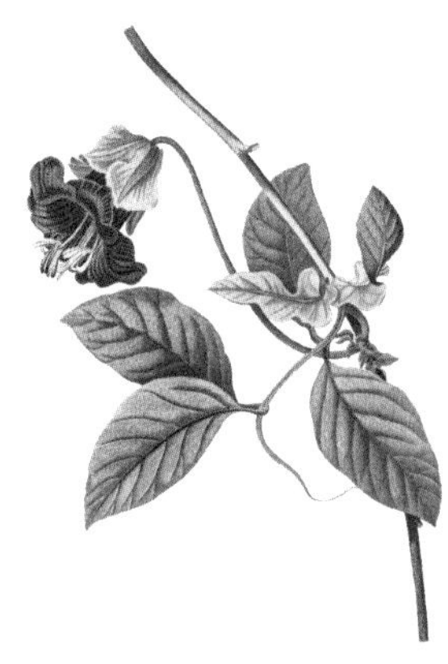

also called Mexican ivy or cathedral bells • a flowering vine, so called because of the large cup and saucer or bell shape of the purple flowers and long curling white stamens that look like bell ropes • though native to Mexico and tropical North America, the fast-growing vine is frequently cultivated in gardens in temperate areas of many regions and flowers in late summer • in the wild it will reach thirty to forty feet high • the honey fragrance appears once the flower opens • flourishes also in a large container but needs support to climb • magically use the growing vine, the cut flowers in bouquets or flower arrangements, and the flowers, dried or fresh

PLANET AND ELEMENT

Jupiter • Air

MAGICAL USES

an Inca offering flower • decorate a celebration venue with the flowers, especially if a formal occasion or exotic setting

HOW TO USE

Bury a written ambition beneath the vine before flowering so that fulfillment will grow upward and bloom like the vine. • Hold a fresh or dried flower where you can hear church bells, cathedral bells, or chanting, and let the sounds answer what you need to know most. • Whisper a secret burden you cannot share close to the vine and level with a flower cup and leave it there. • Anonymously send the cut flower to a secret or desired love, or leave it on their doorstep or workspace, filling the cup or bell flower with love and asking that you will have a sign that the love is returned.

CAUTION

Always be wary when handling if you have sensitive skin. • Do not ingest or inhale too deeply.

Curry Plant

(*Helichrysum italicum*)

MAGICAL FORMS

also called Italian strawflower • the curry plant can be grown in pots and containers as well as in the garden • has the same magical properties as the larger curry tree • unlike, and not to be confused with, the huge tropical curry tree (*Murraya koenigii*), also called the curry leaf plant, whose leaves are used in making curries (see "Curry Tree," p. 148) • magically use the whole, growing plant; leaves; dried flowers; and oil

PLANET AND ELEMENT

Mars • Fire

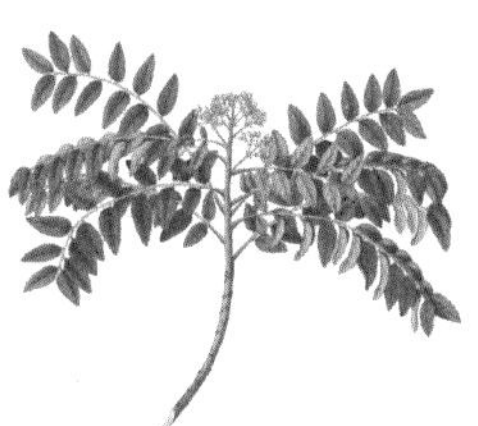

MAGICAL USES

drives away evil influences and entities • protects against emotional vampires • potency • magical tea from the flowerheads, or the leaves as a flavor in cooking, to inflame passion and wake up a hesitant lover • similar flavor to licorice when cooked • especially helpful if there are gender issues

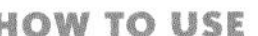

HOW TO USE

Burn the leaves on a bonfire, any Tuesday (the day of Mars), to keep malevolent spirits away from your home. • Alternatively, use the oil, which has a rich, sweet, spicy smell, diluted in a diffuser or burner to remove a troublesome ghost, poltergeist, or sexual demon from a room or building, opening all the windows afterward for the spirit to leave. • Grow in the garden or kitchen to draw abundance and prosperity to your home. • Keep the dried yellow flowers with three small pieces of gold, such as earrings, in a gold-colored bag to draw abundance and prosperity. • Hang it from a tree or shrub in your garden, or on a large plant on your balcony, to create a boundary. • Even a single pot will act as a boundary for all who would cheat you online and offline in your home.

CAUTION

The curry plant is considered safe, but the oil must be well diluted or used as a cream to prevent allergies. • Do not ingest. • Avoid during pregnancy.

Curry Tree

(*Murraya koenigii*)

MAGICAL FORMS

also called the curry leaf plant or sweet neem • a small tropical and subtropical tree or bush from India and Sri Lanka • can grow in tropical areas in the USA or as an indoor plant • the fresh leaves are aromatic, spicy, and used in curries, dahl, rice, and chutneys • leaves are fried or ground or, like bay leaves, added whole for flavor and removed before serving • can be bought from Asian stores and very popular in southern Indian cuisine • white fragrant star-shaped flowers that appear throughout the year, followed by red or black berries • curry powder is different, consisting of turmeric, cumin, coriander, and chili powder • magically use the curry tree leaves, fresh and dried, and the berries

PLANET AND ELEMENT

Mars • Fire

MAGICAL USES

protects against mind control and emotional vampires • speeds any magical workings • gives impetus for dynamic action and change

HOW TO USE

Empower a fresh leaf or leaves, using the quantity specified by the recipe, with the protective or proactive purpose you need. After cooking, wash and dry the favoring leaf or leaves and burn them on a fire. • Collect berries or leaves (you can also use dead leaves), wait until they are dry, and grind them while naming the mind control or the manipulative person from whom you wish to be free, then put them in a small container and tip away at a crossroads.

CAUTION

The berries are not toxic but should not be eaten raw. They can be used in cookery like peppercorns or in making jam. • They may upset animal digestion. • The leaves are safe to ingest during pregnancy when cooked and in moderation.

Cyclamen

(*Cyclamen* spp.)

MAGICAL FORMS

especially *Cyclamen persicum*, also known as Persian cyclamen; *Cyclamen hederifolium*, also known as ivy-leaved cyclamen; and *Cyclamen pupurascens*, also known as purple cyclamen • magically use the whole, growing plant in gardens or indoors in pots; fresh and dried flowers; and oil

PLANETS AND ELEMENTS

Mars/Moon • Fire/Water

MAGICAL USES

protection, especially against ill-wishing and malevolent spirits • endings leading to beginnings • fertility • passion • mending broken hearts

HOW TO USE

Keep the plant in the bedroom to increase libido and also to drive away any harmful spirits. • Called the incense of Mary, cyclamen are placed on altars dedicated to the Virgin Mary, especially white ones with red inner circles, often with petitions for a child. • White cyclamen are also placed on graves on All Saints' Day, one of the days of the ancestors, on November 1, calling on the saints for protection at a time when spirits were believed to roam freely. • Purple cyclamens are given for good luck to someone relocating or changing jobs. • Anoint white candles with the essential oil diluted in olive or almond carrier oil on full moon night before lovemaking for successful conception and a joyous pregnancy. • Anoint yellow candles, or give a bouquet after the birth, to send blessings to new parents and their infant. • Scatter the pink blossoms into still water to end the pain of betrayal and restore self-love and confidence.

CAUTION

Cyclamen is toxic to dogs and cats. • The tubers are especially toxic in large quantities to both humans and pets. • Though ivy-leaved cyclamen (*Cyclamen hederifolium*) and European purple cyclamen (*Cyclamen pupurascens*) are sometimes used medicinally, generally avoid ingesting cyclamen. • Do not use the oil during pregnancy or if you have very sensitive skin.

Cymbidium

(*Cymbidium lowianum*)

MAGICAL FORMS

also known as Low's boat orchid because of the shape of the flower lip • magically use the whole, growing plant; as long-lasting cut flowers; and the petals, fresh and dried

PLANET AND ELEMENT

Moon • Water

MAGICAL USES

an exotic colorful flower popular throughout the world • to brighten fall and winter weddings as well as spring • a flower of lasting friendship, making new friends, and getting to know a new partner's friends if they seem resistant • for travel overseas • a lovely gift delivered to the cabin for someone going on a cruise, especially to a tropical destination

HOW TO USE

Because the Low's boat orchid can attach itself to other plants, though not necessarily parasitic, on the waning moon hold two flowers growing closely together and separate one from the main plant. Place it in a vase of water to represent loosening codependency ties with a partner or parent. When the separated plant fades, release the petals on a windy day, or from a hilltop, on any waning moon. • Considered to be the oldest cultivated orchid dating back to the sage Confucius in ancient China, set orchid flowers on a table or altar where you practice I Ching. • Meditate on it for a glimpse of past worlds, especially if you feel connections with its origins in the Far East. • Since these orchids can grow wild on rock surfaces, keep one in a bottle garden grown on stones in your home or workplace to cultivate and preserve friendly interactions. • Give a potted plant as a housewarming or new-job gift to a friend who is moving away so that they will rapidly make new friends and to preserve the existing friendship between you despite the distance.

Cypress Tree

(*Cupressaceae* family)

MAGICAL FORMS

Monterey cypress (*Hesperocyparis macrocarpa*) is native to California • also in Europe, New Zealand, and some African countries • lemon cypress (*Hesperocyparis macrocarpa* 'Goldcrest') has a citrus fragrance • dwarf lemon cypress (*Hesperocyparis macrocarpa* 'Goldcrest Wilma') • Lawson cypress (*Chamaecyparis lawsoniana*), also called Port Orford cedar, is native to California, where it is used by Karuk Indigenous people to build sweat lodges • magically use the growing trees; branches; wood; leaves, fresh and dried; and essential oil from Italian cypress (*Cupressus sempervirens*)

PLANET AND ELEMENT

Saturn • Earth

MAGICAL USES

cypress is associated with mourning rituals • branches were placed on graves to assist the journey to paradise • Persian legend says cypress was the first tree to grow in paradise • rituals to move on from grief and loss or after a period of stagnation

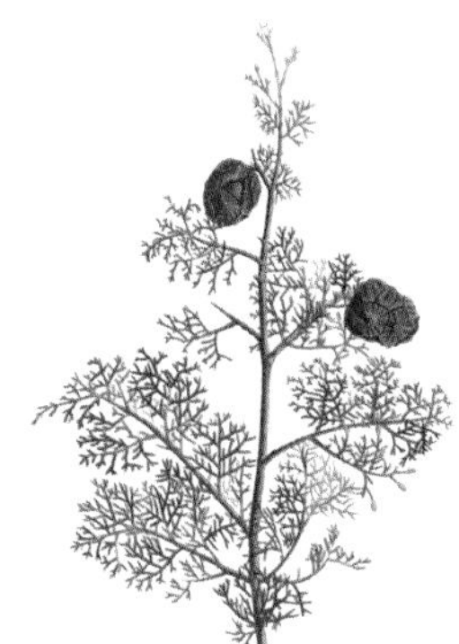

HOW TO USE

At Halloween, and the ensuing Samhain and Days of the Dead, restless spirits roaming free are kept away from celebrations of the wise ancestors by burning the dried fragranced leaves as incense or casting the fallen branches on bonfires. • Rub a drop of the oil diluted in olive oil into a purple candle to reverse curses.

CAUTION

Most cypress is nontoxic to humans or animals, though it is not edible. • Lemon cypress is child and pet friendly. • Cypress should not be used medicinally or as oil by people with high blood pressure or during pregnancy. • The oil should always be very well diluted and not ingested. • Beware of the Leland cypress (*Cupressus × leylandii*) as it can cause skin irritations.

Daffodil

(*Narcissus* spp.)

MAGICAL FORMS

also known as jonquil • the common yellow daffodil, *Narcissus pseudonarcissus*, is found both cultivated and in the wild in New England • the white with yellow center daffodil, poet's daffodil (*Narcissus poeticus*), is naturalized over the eastern USA since it was brought by the colonists • daffodils are believed to grow in profusion in the wild on what was once regarded as sacred land • according to legend, daffodils sprang up in the Garden of Gethsemane to console Jesus and through the ages have become a symbol of Easter/spring rebirth • see "Narcissus" (p. 305) and "Jonquil" (p. 240), which share biological roots but have different magical properties • magically use the growing plant, wild, cultivated, and cut; and flowers, fresh and dried

PLANETS AND ELEMENTS

Mercury/Venus • Air/Water

MAGICAL USES

forgiveness • finding one true love • good luck • fertility • the daffodil spreads its goodwill, optimism, and friendship to all who see daffodils growing or have it in pots or in a vase • starting again when things go wrong • flower of spring equinox, marking the end of winter • the emblem of Wales and symbolic of their roots to those of Gaelic heritage worldwide

HOW TO USE

Bring the first daffodils of spring into the home for good luck, blessings, and new beginnings, and to ensure abundance in the home throughout the year. • Collect, pick, or buy yellow daffodils on a Wednesday, the day of Mercury, for good fortune and white and yellow on Venus's day, Friday, to attract and keep love. • Have a bunch in the bedroom to enhance fertility. • Grow them in the garden or keep in a vase on an outfacing window to drive away all harm and repel negative spells. • Sprinkle dried petals to attract benign spirits to your rituals. • Mix dried daffodil flowers with rose petals around a photo of a lover to bring him or her back or for unrequited love to be fulfilled.

CAUTION

All daffodil bulbs are highly toxic to humans and pets.

Dahlia

(*Dahlia* spp.)

MAGICAL FORMS

especially *Dahlia pinnata*, Mexico's national flower and the official flower of Seattle and San Francisco • magically use the growing and cut flowers; petals, fresh and dried; and edible bulbs and petals

PLANET AND ELEMENT

Moon • Water

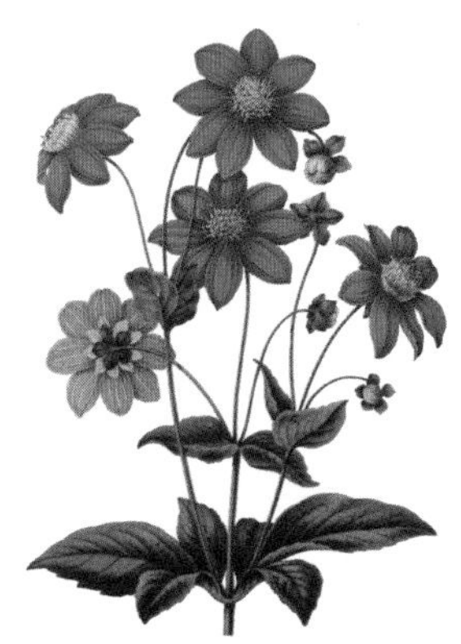

MAGICAL USES

travel • eternal love • flowing with the changes of life • all moon magick • pink or purple for enhancing beauty, as a token or renewal of lasting commitment, anniversaries, or Valentine's Day • white for birth, new life, and the renewal of trust • red for a new career, to stand out positively, and make an impression • burgundy (often called black) for moon magick on the wane to remove pain and sorrow

HOW TO USE

The dried petals in a sleep pillow bring astral travel, lucid dreaming (knowing you are dreaming while asleep and so able to change a dream), and dream recall. • Petals in a sleep pillow can also be used to connect with angels, guides, deceased relatives, or a dream lover, maybe yet unknown, on the sleep plane. • Scatter dark purple or burgundy petals to the winds to let go of what is no longer needed or to free yourself from guilt concerning a living or deceased person.

CAUTION

Dahlias are nontoxic to humans but mildly toxic to dogs and cats. • They may cause mild skin irritation for some people, so wash after arranging the flowers in a vase if there is a problem.

Dahlia, Hamari Gold

(*Dahlia pinnata* 'Hamari Gold')

MAGICAL FORMS

a huge, powerful dahlia with magical properties • deep gold with light bronze highlights that sparkle in sunlight • dahlias originate in Mexico and South America, but the Hamari dahlia, like many others, is sold and grown in the USA, the UK, and Europe • blooms mid to late summer and fall • a good substitute, and almost as impressive, is the bright yellow dahlia Karma • magically use the gold dahlia as a growing plant or cut flowers, fresh or dried

PLANET AND ELEMENT

Sun • Fire

MAGICAL USES

a flower of the sun, as well as of the sun gods, such as the ancient Greek Helios, Japanese Amaterasu, and the Celtic mother and daughter solar goddesses Grainne and Aine • also used for petitions and offerings to Michael, archangel of the sun • a recommended flower for the seventy-fifth wedding anniversary, the original diamond anniversary • for all wedding, birthday, and congratulatory bouquets, where two or three of the huge flowers provide a dramatic centerpiece to recognize achievement and to offer wishes for prosperity, health, and joy

HOW TO USE

Because it is associated with the inner Solar Plexus chakra energy center in the middle of the base of the rib cage, press gently on this area while focusing or meditating on a growing or cut 'Hamari Gold' for personal power and confidence. • Carry the petals with you in a sachet and touch them whenever you need to take center stage or assert your personal power and communication skills or recall necessary facts, especially if you are facing a critical audience or individual who has discouraged you.

CAUTION

Avoid if pregnant. • Toxic to dogs and cats.

Daisy

(*Bellis perennis*)

MAGICAL FORMS

also known as lawn daisy or English daisy, includes several varieties • flowering plant often considered the archetypal representation of a daisy, although *Leucanthemum vulgare*, the ox-eye daisy or marguerite, has similar magical properties • magically use the whole, growing plant; cut flowers; petals, fresh or dried; and essential oil

PLANET AND ELEMENT

Venus • Water

MAGICAL USES

for romance • love divination • luck in love • connection with the fey, especially on Beltane • protection of children • linking the seen and unseen worlds, making anything possible • guarding against the evil eye of envy

HOW TO USE

Give the larger daisies as a gift to a lover with a promise to return as made by medieval knights whose lovers gave them a daisy to wear as they rode away to slay their dragons. • Pluck the petals from a daisy to answer if the diviner is loved with a *yes* or *no*. • Pick a handful of daisies with eyes closed to answer how many weeks or months before she or he returns. • Bury a silver dollar beneath a daisy root for money on Friday, the day of Venus. • Hide a daisy chain high in small children's rooms to keep them safe from accidents, illness, and fey enchantment, replacing the chain when the daisies wilt. • Use the leaves and flowers in magical cookery to bring or to bring back gentle love and affection. • Place a daisy chain under your pillow to rekindle love, one flower for each day, week, or month apart. • Speed an urgent spell made when the daisy opens in the morning for fulfillment by the time it closes. • On Beltane morning, anoint white candles with infused daisy oil and light to call romance.

CAUTION

Do not use the oil or ingest if you suffer with blood clots or anemia or if pregnant or breastfeeding.

Daisy, African

(*Arctotis* spp.)

MAGICAL FORMS

also known as the cape daisy • a genus of flowering plants often grown ornamentally • native to southern Africa • magically use the growing plant, buds, and petals

PLANET AND ELEMENT

Moon • Water

MAGICAL USES

for joy • celebrations of all kinds • transformations and makeovers • creating a link between the everyday world and the celestial • opening spiritual healing energy channels, especially Reiki, acupuncture, and massage • flower psychometry

HOW TO USE

Meditate on the growing flowers, in sunlight as they open, to attune to your higher self and plant spirit messages. • If you are teaching a class, mist around your aura or the room with the essence or flower water mixed with rose or lavender water both before and after yoga or the energy transference. • Place the dried blossoms in a white silk charm bag along with a selenite and empower in full moonlight to increase your psychic powers and to protect against fears, especially those of the night. • Place the dried buds in a lilac bag along with a small creamy or pink moonstone and empower on the crescent moon for attracting love. This can also be used for modest money ventures to be fulfilled within the month, after which the contents of the bag should be cast into flowing water.

CAUTION

While there is no reported toxicity, it should be avoided with pregnancy.

Damiana

(*Turnera diffusa*)

MAGICAL FORMS

member of the passionflower family • a shrub native to Texas, Mexico, Central and South America, and the Caribbean • found in southern parts of the USA • magically use the growing plant; flowers; leaves, dried or fresh (especially dried in teas and sweetened with honey or stevia); and as incense

PLANETS AND ELEMENTS

Moon/Venus • Water/Fire

MAGICAL USES

the ultimate love and lust herb, as an aphrodisiac tea • for rituals, meditation, connecting with spirits and higher dimensions • in magical cookery to enchant a desired lover • to relax workaholics • to induce sleep in chronic insomniacs • a herb of women's rites of passage

HOW TO USE

Burn the dried yellow flowers, especially on a Friday as in traditional Mayan, Aztec, and Mexican practice. • Carry them in a sachet to increase passionate lovemaking. • Use with sex magic or to draw a passionate lover if you are alone. • Use the tea before divination to enhance clairvoyance. • See visions of the future in the incense smoke. • Use for astral travel during sleep or meditation either by drinking the tea or burning incense. • Use for lucid dreaming, the awareness you are dreaming during the sleep process and so able to change or influence dreams while experiencing them.

CAUTION

Avoid if you have blood sugar problems or are on medication, as damiana can lower blood sugar levels. • Do not use during pregnancy, if trying to become pregnant, or if breastfeeding. • Beware of the smoke, as directly inhaling it or using it to excess can cause a high; always use in moderation.

Dammar Gum Resin

from (*Shorea weisneri*) or (*Agathis australis*)

MAGICAL FORMS

from coniferous evergreen trees, mainly known for their aromatic light white or pale yellow milky gum resin with lemon fragrance • also known as cat's eye resin • the gum oozes from the Southeast Asian *Shorea weisneri* coniferous, which stands tall above the forest canopy • also sourced from the North Island New Zealand coniferous evergreen *Agathis australis* tree • magically use as incense, obtainable worldwide • magically burn with nonresinous flowers or leaves to enhance their properties or on its own on charcoal

PLANET AND ELEMENT

Sun • Fire

MAGICAL USES

connecting with light beings, angels, and archangels • relieves sadness and the dark night of the soul • brings protection from self-destructive thoughts and serenity to accept life as it is

HOW TO USE

Add a crushed or powdered layer of dammar to a wish jar with lavender heads, rose petals, and dried chamomile flowers, plus a layer of mixed amethyst/rose quartz chippings, and keep it sealed in the center of your home if there has been sadness, loss, or quarrels. Shake it every morning and evening, and ask for blessings on your home and family present and absent. • Burn dammar resin before and during meditation, prayer, divination, or ritual to create a barrier between yourself and the everyday world if you have a frantic life or have only a small private space and little time to connect with your spiritual work.

Dandelion

(*Taraxacum officinale*)

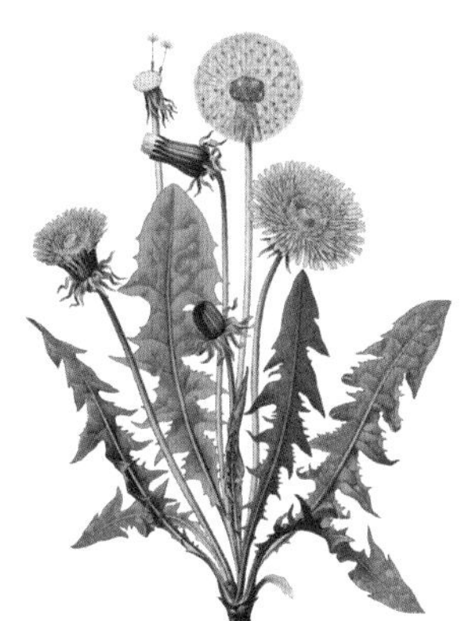

MAGICAL FORMS

leaves can be gathered all through the year • magically use the whole plant, petals, spores, leaves, and root

PLANET AND ELEMENT

Jupiter • Air

MAGICAL USES

spores for wish magick and wind magick • abundance • ability to understand dreams in a sleep pillow • to possess the nobility and courage of the lion/ess as king/queen of the animals if one lacks actual power or status in present life • fast regrowth for regeneration spells

HOW TO USE

Traditionally, the dandelion is a form taken by sun fairies to prevent careless humans treading on them. The fey travel on dandelion spores, and if you send fairies on their way by blowing on a dandelion, facing each direction in turn starting with north and turning clockwise, then you may have a wish. • Create a wishing jar filled with dandelion spores, to be released at times you need good luck, and add more spores when the jar is empty. • Dandelions act as transmitters of love; blow the seeds from a ripened dandelion head in the direction of a lover to carry your thoughts. • As a tea made from the leaves or dandelion root, it increases psychic awareness and can be enchanted by stirring with a stick of cinnamon, especially for love. • Burn the dried flowerheads in an incense mix to increase clairvoyance. • As used in traditional folk love divination, pluck the petals to answer questions with alternate *yes* or *no* answers concerning a lover's fidelity and intentions.

CAUTION

While generally considered safe to consume, it may interfere with antibiotics, anticoagulants, and blood sugar medications. • It is not advised for people with serious bile duct or gallbladder issues or allergies to the ragweed/daisy plant family.

Date Palm

(*Phoenix* spp.)

MAGICAL FORMS

includes *Phoenix dactylifera*, *Phoenix roebelenii* (the pygmy or dwarf date palm), and *Phoenix canariensis* (Canary Island date palm) • a tall tree up to a hundred feet high, topped with 100 to 120 feathery fronds, each ten to sixteen feet long as a canopy • native in North Africa and the Middle East and grown in tropical and semitropical areas of North and South America, southern Europe, and lands such as Australia • dwarf palms or the Canary Islands date palms can grow in pots but tend to not produce fruit indoors • magically use the whole, growing tree; palm fronds, which are often found fallen beneath a tree; fresh and dried date fruit; and pits/stones

PLANET AND ELEMENT

Sun • Fire

MAGICAL USES

magical cookery or the fruit eaten fresh or dried to generate fertility before lovemaking • rolled in powdered sugar before eating, to attract romance and increase libido • pits/stones carried in a charm bag to restore virility (extra powerful if the fruit is shared by a couple) • place a fresh palm frond or part of one over the door to attract prosperity and repel earthly malice and paranormal threats; replace it when it withers

HOW TO USE

A symbol of immortality and renewal, dates have been discovered in the tombs of pharaohs, and mummies were sometimes wrapped in date palm fronds. • The date tree's botanical name is *Phoenix* after the mythical bird of rebirth, because new shoots spring from the stump of an old decaying tree, taking the place of the parent tree. • Wrap nine decaying dates in a small or partially cut date palm frond (being careful of sharp edges), and tie in red thread while naming the new beginnings you need to grow from a recent loss or setback. Bury this at or near a three-way crossroads for the transition of past, present, and future and go home a different way. • Meditate beneath a date palm or a dwarf one to receive visions of past worlds, your own and ancient lands where the tree grew, that hold insights into your present life.

Davana

(*Artemisia pallens*)

MAGICAL FORMS

the plant rather than the oil is prized and grown in India mainly for religious ceremonies, but the oil is used worldwide and valued in perfumes and Ayurveda • many small yellow flowers and silver/white/gray silky foliage • magically use the essential oil made from the flowers and leaves or incense sticks (occasionally found on the internet) • you may even be lucky enough to discover an Asian supplier or Ayurvedic center that will sell you the dried flowers to bless your home as a bouquet or woven into a circlet

PLANET AND ELEMENT

Mercury • Air

MAGICAL USES

traditionally the flowers are an offering to Lord Shiva • anoint the Third Eye in the center of the brow and your inner wrist pulse points before meditation, yoga, prayers, chanting, or breathwork

HOW TO USE

Burn incense sticks or diffuse or burn the oil for protection against the effects of trauma and attack, whether psychological, physical, or psychic. • As an aphrodisiac, use the diluted oil for mutual massage with your partner. • Add a few drops to your bath to bring romance and tenderness to your lovemaking if you are always in a hurry or too tired. • Add a drop or two of davana oil to an aroma bracelet; the best kind have two or three porous lava stones, clay or wooden beads, plus crystals of your choice. Anoint the lava or wooden beads to absorb the oil, leaving the bracelet to dry. Be sparing with the oil, and always wear the bracelet with the oil facing away from your wrist. It will release its fragrance throughout the day. Your davana bracelet will allow you to rise above pettiness and spite and attract not just romance but new friendships and deepen existing ones.

CAUTION

There is insufficient research to know if davana is safe during pregnancy or lactation. • Davana is phototoxic. • You may be allergic to it, even when well diluted, if you are allergic to ragweed, marigolds, or daisies.

Daylily

(*Hemerocallis* spp.)

MAGICAL FORMS

most commonly grown as the yellow 'Stella d'oro' or the orange *Hemerocallis fulva* • native to China, Japan, and Korea and naturalized in temperate parts of North America and Europe • resembling a lily but related to aloe and red-hot pokers with bushy grasslike foliage from which grow the tall stems of the trumpetlike flowers • *Hemerocallis* means "beauty for a day," for the flowers last only twenty-four hours, though are rapidly replaced by other flowers • some like the yellow 'Stella d'oro' and the 'Purple d'oro' rebloom in the fall • magically use the growing flowers in a garden or pot/container before blooms appear, with some just coming into bloom, and with buds attached, so that your plants will keep producing new flowers as one dies

PLANET AND ELEMENT

Sun • Fire

MAGICAL USES

a twentieth wedding anniversary flower that talks about making plans for enjoying every moment of every day and not worrying about past or future • give as a growing bouquet with flowers at different stages of growth or as a potted plant with several flowers that can be cultivated in the garden afterward • a gift for mothers from sons on Mother's Day

HOW TO USE

Because the individual flower lasts only a day but others replace it, place a cut newly blooming flower in a shallow dish of water in your bedroom if you are seeking a flirtation but not a serious relationship. • This can also deter overly serious lovers or enliven a partner who has lost their spontaneity. • As it fades, carry the fading petals in a sachet for a fun evening or social event without strings or angst, and scatter the petals before entering the venue or meeting a new date. • Throw faded petals where nothing grows as a way of forgetting a bad experience or relationship, and then buy or cultivate new buds.

CAUTION

Daylilies are toxic to cats but not to dogs, and humans can eat most parts of the plant.

Deadly Nightshade

(*Atropa belladonna*)

MAGICAL FORMS

also known as belladonna • a flowering shrub growing wild in North America, Europe, North Africa, and western Asia • up to five feet tall with purple flowers and inky sweet berries • magically use the plant and berries with the utmost care as it is highly poisonous, even on contact

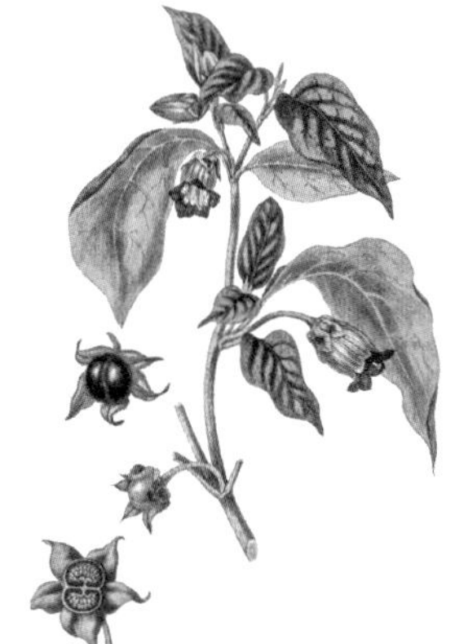

PLANET AND ELEMENT

Saturn • Earth

MAGICAL USES

in the past *belladonna*, meaning "beautiful woman" in Italian, formed part of enchantment and glamour spells, and Italian women applied the juice to dilate their eyes to add to their mystique (highly dangerous) • for centuries belladonna was mixed with fat for astral projection and as an infusion drunk by the priests of Roman Bellon, the goddess of war, to invoke her courage and victory in battle • the flowers and leaves are still occasionally added to incense mixed with peppermint, vervain, and thistle to give courage for a major challenge • there are many safer substitutes (some listed in this book)

HOW TO USE

With incredible caution, the whole chopped plant with berries can be added to a protective bottle along with rusty iron nails, a black onyx crystal, and sour red wine. Seal and keep in a safe place for powerful defense against curses.

CAUTION

The roots are most lethal of all, and the sweet berries, even one or two, pose a great danger to children. • Belladonna should never be ingested or used medicinally except with permission of an experienced physician as part of an accredited mix, exactly as prescribed, where it may be used for illnesses as varied as asthma, diverticulitis, and Parkinson's diseases. • On the whole, it is not worth the risk magically.

Deer Brush

(*Ceanothus integerrimus*)

MAGICAL FORMS

a leafy bush up to thirteen feet tall with fragrant, fluffy white, blue-lilac, or occasionally pink clustered blossoms • blooming in late spring to early summer or late summer to fall depending on the kind • ideal for midsummer and fall equinox celebrations • native to the forests or cultivated in gardens in the western USA, Arizona, New Mexico, Oregon, Washington, and in the UK and Europe • loved by deer • deer brush provides nitrogen for the soil for regeneration after fires • magically use the flower water, the growing or dried blossoms, and the essence

PLANET AND ELEMENT

Mercury • Air

MAGICAL USES

lessening conformity to society's expectations and norms • reducing the need to fit in and seek approval from those who have influence in your life • traditionally, the flowers were crushed in water by the Indigenous people and mixed to create lather for washing hands/bodies and for purification • also as soap by early settlers

HOW TO USE

Wash nonporous artifacts, or sprinkle the crushed flower water round jewelry you have inherited, acquired at a garage sale, or that have unhappy memories to make them your own. • Take the essence regularly if you have strong feelings but fear speaking out or going against convention. • Anoint your inner wrist points for your heart and the soles of your feet with the diluted essence in order to shape-shift in your mind into a deer or astrally travel on the back of a deer to experience freedom and escape from convention.

CAUTION

Deer brush is not considered toxic. • Tea from the leaves and extracts from the bark are used for a variety of conditions, including improving digestion and boosting the immune system. • However, deer brush has not been officially approved, and so care and expert advice should be sought, especially if taking regular medication and or if pregnant.

Deertongue

(*Dichanthelium clandestinum*)

MAGICAL FORMS

deertongue grass is a relative of *Panicum capillare* (see "Witchgrass," p. 477) • native to Chicago region • grows in eastern North America and eastern Canada, basal deertongue-shaped clusters of leaves, with up to five foot tall flower stem with purple flowers • can be bought as chopped, dried leaves online or from magick stores • magically use aromatic fresh or dried leaves

PLANET AND ELEMENT

Mars • Fire

MAGICAL USES

used by settlers in bundles to freshen clothes and rooms and as a cure-all tea by both the Native North Americans and the settlers • awakens psychic powers • for persuasiveness in court cases or tribunals to obtain a verdict in your favor • in love incense or sachets to call a gentle, loving partner, especially in LGBTQ relationships • for encouraging a marriage proposal in a hesitant partner

HOW TO USE

Carry the dried chopped leaves in a sachet if you are involved in negotiations or legal or official matters. • Whisper the desired result into a closed and sealed bag of dried leaves before any major meetings or confrontations. • Since *clandestinum* refers to the seeds/unformed flowers that remain hidden in the stem ready for the second seed-shedding in the fall, tape the seeds beneath a copy of documents concerning secret financial negotiations, private deals, and correspondence, or where evidence must be concealed until the right time, then lock it in a drawer.

CAUTION

Deertongue is currently considered unsafe in food in the USA and not generally taken medicinally, except under expert advice, as it has been suggested that it may thin the blood and cause liver damage.

Delphinium

(*Delphinium* spp.)

MAGICAL FORMS

also dwarf delphiniums and the related similar and magically interchangeable larkspur (*Consolida ajacis*), a smaller annual flower less stately than the perennial delphinium • larkspur resembles the claw of a meadowlark while delphinium buds look like the bottle nose of a dolphin (*delphis* is the Greek word for "dolphin") • magically use the whole delphinium or larkspur flower, growing or cut, and the dried flowers

PLANET AND ELEMENT

Jupiter • Air

MAGICAL USES

reaching goals • achieving ambitions • expansion of opportunity, especially in career and business • optimism • altruism • to bring lasting happiness in love • naturally protective against spite and jealousy (traditionally against snakes and scorpions) • magically they are powerfully protective and empowering flowers • larkspur's magical name recalls the Greek mythological hero Ajax the Greater • mythologically, the delphinium originated from the blood of Ajax

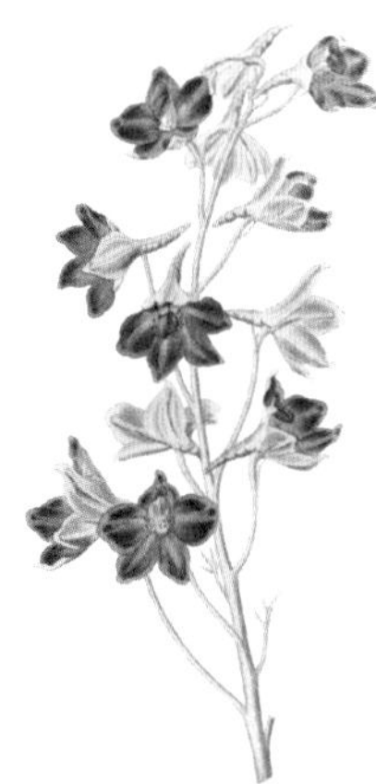

HOW TO USE

The cut delphinium flowers, especially the taller varieties in blue, increase connection with the goddess and angelic energies when in arrangements on the altar. • Both plants are grown in the gardens to keep away malicious ghosts. • Keep any printouts of career applications near a vase of tall cut delphinium flowers in order to stand out above other applicants and obtain the employment you desire.

CAUTION

Both plant species are poisonous if the plant is ingested, and many practitioners suggest washing your hands after handling them as a precaution. • These plants are not suitable where children or pets play.

Devil's-Bit Scabious

(*Succisa pratensis*)

MAGICAL FORMS

called devil's-bit scabious to distinguish it from similar but botanically different scabious plants • slender root with hairy stem and few leaves, globular pale to deep blue-purple pincushion flowerheads, each petal the same size, blooming July to October • root looks as if it has been bitten off at the end • native wildflower to the UK, western and central Europe, and western and central Asia • grows in eastern North America and can be cultivated in gardens in temperate zones in most regions • magically use mainly the root

PLANETS AND ELEMENTS

Mercury/Venus • Air/Water

MAGICAL USES

according to legend, the devil, upon seeing the plant, was angry at the good it might do for humankind and so bit off the end of the root to destroy it • despite that it flourished • use devil's-bit to remove and prevent curses, hexes, and jinxes • drives away spirit attack • brings good fortune • awareness of illusion, false friends, and false lovers • draws the right partner

HOW TO USE

Because it survived the devil's attack in the legend and by association, carry the whole root in an amulet bag when you know you will be facing confrontation, spite, or jealousy from neighbors, family, or work colleagues. If the amulet bag is sturdy, bury the root after a week or two and replace it. • Burn the chopped root in an incense mix or keep under the doorstep with rue if you suspect a psychic attack against you or your home, whether earthly or a malevolent spirit. • Grown in the garden or dried in a cut flower arrangement, devil's-bit will protect the home from all who would deceive you, offer false friendship, or seek to steal your partner and will attract or maintain true love.

CAUTION

Although not regarded as toxic to humans or pets, it has not been used medicinally since 1900, except in a decoction.

Devil's Claw

(*Harpagophytum procumbens*) or (*Martynia annua*)

MAGICAL FORMS

flowering shrubs, with hooklike fruits resembling claws that cling to clothing or animals' fur • *Harpagophytum procumbens*, native to the Kalahari Desert in South Africa and the floral emblem of Botswana, will grow almost anywhere • its trumpet-shaped flowers are often purple-pink with yellow throats • introduced into Europe during the early 1900s and the kind most used medicinally • the name devil's claw is also the name given to the North American plant *Martynia annua,* indigenous to the southern USA with white to pink or yellow flowers • can be grown indoors as well as in warm climates • magically use the roots and claws of either species with care and the tea/decoction of the dried crushed roots, mainly sold in the *Harpagophytum procumbens* variety

PLANET AND ELEMENT

Mars • Fire

MAGICAL USES

the tough black fiber of *Martynia annua* was woven into baskets by Native North Americans of California and the Southwest and the fiber is used in knot and binding magick • both kinds are so called because if animals eat the plant, they starve if the claws attach to their jaw • the claws of either species are used as amulets to stop gossip, spite, and rumor • the roots are crushed in incense for protection and to banish malevolent forces

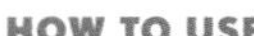

HOW TO USE

Add the tea/decoction of either plant to a floor or doorstep wash to remove lingering misfortune. • When moving to a new home, burn the incense mixed with frankincense and rosemary before moving furniture into the new house.

CAUTION

Martynia annua is nontoxic but can cause photosensitivity if applied to the skin and lowers blood pressure, so not suitable if suffering from hypotension (low blood pressure).

Devil's Club

(*Oplopanax horridus*)

MAGICAL FORMS

also known as devil's walking stick or Alaskan ginseng • a relative of ginseng, but not a true ginseng • grows between three and five feet, sometimes even higher, on the Alaskan coast, adjacent regions of Canada, and northwestern North America • will grow in other parts of the world • densely thorned stems that can become thickets • wide branching leaves also with spines • red berries • magically use, but handle with care, the thorny stems and the dried root bark and inner stem bark, which can both be bought online already chopped and prepared

PLANET AND ELEMENT

Mars • Fire

MAGICAL USES

considered sacred by Indigenous people • in ritual and amulet bags use the inner root and bark to remove spiritual blockages

HOW TO USE

With a great care, thick gloves, and a sharp implement, cut off the thorns and spikes and place them in a defensive bottle, adding apple cider vinegar, to remove and keep away curses, hexes, and threatening callers if you live in a potentially dangerous area or are being harassed by unscrupulous debt collectors or street gangs. • Tie one or two stems, with thorns attached, creating a handle of thick cloth and twine to make a broom, and use this outdoors to sweep away misfortune from your home. • Light protective dragon's blood or frankincense incense and prop up your devil's club broom so that you can see it dimly through the smoke to use as a focus for meditation or chanting to astrally travel and break through the barriers of everyday life. • You should only work with devil's club when in a calm frame of mind, asking your guides that your work be for the highest good, harming no one.

CAUTION

Though traditionally used for centuries in folk medicine and still obtainable in decoctions and salves, research on its safety is limited, so avoid ingesting during pregnancy and breastfeeding or if you have diabetes. • Keep children and pets away from the thorns. • The berries are poisonous: do not eat under any circumstance.

Devil's Shoestring

(*Tephrosia virginiana*)

MAGICAL FORMS

also known as goat's rue or catgut • related to honeysuckle • name refers to long stringy roots • magically use mainly as roots made into oil (place root in grape-seed or almond oil, steep for two weeks, and shake gently each day—or buy commercially)

PLANET AND ELEMENTS

Saturn • Earth/Water

MAGICAL USES

devil's shoestring is an important root in Hoodoo but has become popular in magick generally in its defensive and luck-bringing qualities • so named because the stringy root was believed to trip up the devil or evil spirits trying to approach or indeed to tangle up any earthly ill-wisher • protective knot magick with tangled root in spells to bind others from harm • to preserve good fortune and money

HOW TO USE

Place a few drops of oil on outer window ledges and doorframes to keep away malicious spirits and misfortune. • Place a drop of oil on a copy printout of job applications or apply while sealing the application envelope to bring a favorable response. • Knotted dried roots above a doorway deter unwelcome visitors and prevent any who do enter from spreading gossip or confidentialities. • Carry a small twisted root in a red bag with powdered cinnamon for gambling. • To attract business, tie a root around a green dollar note or silver dollar and keep where you deal with finances to preserve or restore resources if there are money or business difficulties.

CAUTION

Devil's shoestring is poisonous to fish. • Humans and pets should not ingest.

Dianthus

(*Dianthus* spp.)

MAGICAL FORMS

including pinks (*Dianthus plumarius*), China pinks (*Dianthus chinensis*), and sweet William (*Dianthus barbatus*); also the related *Dianthus caryophyllus* (see "Carnation," p. 102) • mentioned in Thomas Jefferson's garden in Monticello as *Dianthus plumarius* • magically use whole plants in the garden, flowers, leaves (with care), and essential oil (mainly found as carnation)

PLANET AND ELEMENT

Moon • Water

MAGICAL USES

twin soul love • considered a divine flower bringing connection with personal deities from ancient Greek and Roman times • enhancing beauty and radiance inside and out • in wedding bouquets for lasting happiness • in Victorian times promised lasting devotion

HOW TO USE

Plant dianthus in your Moon garden to bring family affection, harmony between couples, and admiration of the self by others and also to attract wealth and love. • In Japan, dianthus is picked and allowed to fly away to remove troubles, especially in love.

CAUTION

Sweet William flowers are edible and used as garnish in magical cookery, but the leaves can cause gastroenteritis in humans and pets. • *Dianthus chinensis* stimulates contractions and should not be eaten raw by humans or pets and in some people may cause skin irritation. • For precautionary reasons, dianthus plants generally should be avoided medicinally during pregnancy and the weeks after giving birth.

Dill

(*Anethum graveolens*)

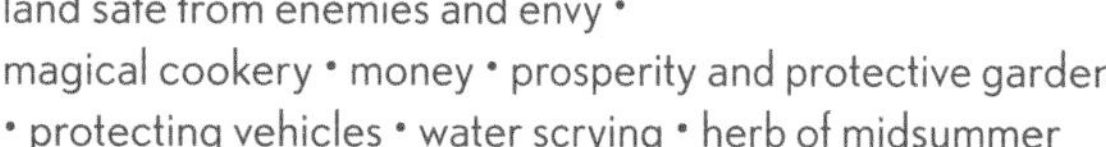

MAGICAL FORMS

magically use the herb, fresh and dried; seeds; and oil, but not in excess

PLANET AND ELEMENTS

Mercury • Air/Earth/Fire

MAGICAL USES

against negative magick, curses, jinxes, and ill-wishing • against unfair taxation and officialdom • charm bags against misfortune • keeping home, loved ones, and land safe from enemies and envy • magical cookery • money • prosperity and protective garden • protecting vehicles • water scrying • herb of midsummer

HOW TO USE

Add dill seeds daily to a growing prosperity jar. • Bound dried seed heads, stalks, or fresh herb hung over entrances, outside children's rooms, or dried and scattered around boundaries repel sickness, misfortune, and all danger. • Add an infusion to car wash water for safe journeys and anti-theft. • Place seeds or fresh chopped herb in a bath sachet to increase charisma or libido, or to attract a lover. • Protect pets by burying some of their hair along with dill seeds. • Place the seeds inside a shiny witch ball, large bauble, or glass fishing float and hang on tree to protect premises. • Soak iron nails with a dill infusion to make defensive warrior water.

CAUTION

Generally safe, dill juice may make you more sensitive to the sun. • Avoid oil if pregnant. • Avoid taking dill internally if allergic to carrots.

Dittany of Crete

(*Origanum dictamnus*)

MAGICAL FORMS

rare, but one of the most remarkable and ancient magical and medicinal herbs, dedicated in ancient Greece to Eros and Aphrodite (the Roman Venus), deities of love • the wild plant is protected in Crete, but the plant is grown in the USA and parts of Europe and the UK in herb gardens • well worth searching for • magically use the whole plant, leaves, and oil

PLANET AND ELEMENT

Venus • Water

MAGICAL USES

ultimate herb for striving after love however difficult the circumstances, because lovers in Greece for centuries have climbed inaccessible rock faces to pick dittany as a token of risking all for love • manifests spirits • said to be protective against venom, human and reptilian • for labyrinth work • higher spiritual awareness

HOW TO USE

Mix with vanilla, benzoin, and sandalwood or with frankincense and burn as incense to aid astral projection. • Burn as part of a love incense before sleep to meet lovers on the dream plane. • Use the oil in a diffuser to encounter past Minoan worlds and the Neolithic deities, heroes, and heroines of the Cretan labyrinth, such as Ariadne and King Minos, and to connect or commune with beings of other ancient worlds. • Use the herb in magical cookery to make the spellcaster irresistible in love and as an aphrodisiac. • Use the leaves to flavor vermouth, wines, spirits, soups, sauces, and salads.

CAUTION

Avoid if pregnant or breastfeeding and if allergic to basil, lavender, or oregano. • Dilute the oil well, and stop using dittany if skin irritation occurs.

Dittany, White

(*Dictamnus albus*) or (*Dictamnus fraxinella albus*)

MAGICAL FORMS

also called fraxinella • belonging to the rue family • a cousin of the less obtainable Dittany of Crete from the oregano family; sometimes they are confused • elegant white flowers (can be pink or tinged with purple) standing as spikes on top of branched, round, thick stalks with leathery, aromatic leaves • magically use the whole flower, growing in the garden or cut; roots collected in the fall; flowering tops in late summer (can be dried); and seed pods

PLANETS AND ELEMENTS

Venus/Sun • Earth/Fire

MAGICAL USES

an alternative to the crystal rose bush for a fifteenth anniversary bouquet or another milestone in a long-lasting relationship (can be given with a miniature ornamental tree of crystals) • the cut flowers in the bedroom are considered an aphrodisiac, a creator or restorer of passion and romance in a long-standing relationship where family responsibilities may have dulled romance • white dittany is very volatile, as it exudes an aromatic, flammable vapor in hot, dry weather and can easily be ignited by an open flame (possibly a similar plant, if not this one, may have been the origin of Moses's burning bush) • not suitable for incense or around candles

HOW TO USE

White dittany is considered in traditional European folklore to protect against bites of venomous snakes, infectious diseases, and poison. • In the modern world, the dried flowers or chopped roots can be kept in an amulet bag well away from combustible sources in the home or workplace to guard against human spite and vicious words or actions. • Make wishes on the seed pods that are carried on the wind for the increase of passion in your life, not just for love but if you have lost sight of your dreams. • If they do not fly, collect them carefully in a disposable paper bag as the plant can be toxic to the skin, especially in sunlight, and tip them into running water to carry your desires to fruition.

CAUTION

White dittany is toxic.

Dock

(*Rumex obtusifolius*)

MAGICAL FORMS

also known as bitter dock or broad-leaved dock • best in wildflower areas and kept cut back • magically use the whole, growing plant; leaves; flowers; and seeds

PLANET AND ELEMENT

Jupiter • Air

MAGICAL USES

usually found growing close to nettles in the wild as an antidote to nettle stings and so both plants used together for anticurse, ill-wishing, antibullying, or against spite • attracting prosperity to a business and new source of income to the home • fertility and potency • healing

HOW TO USE

The seeds are an important ingredient in incense mixes to attract money. • A seed pouch or chopped dried leaves and flowers, hidden near the payment collection point or financial computer in a business, encourages potential customers to make a purchase. • Place nine seeds as a fertility symbol in a small pouch to be worn around the waist from dawn on the day of the full moon by each of the partners when trying for a child. Then tip both sets of seeds together into a larger pouch, set on an indoor window ledge, and pierce with a long silver pin on full moon night before lovemaking.

CAUTION

Avoid medicinally if you have kidney stones. • Generally safe, but do not eat the leaves in excess. • Do not use with preexisting gastrointestinal illnesses, during pregnancy, or while breastfeeding.

Dock, Yellow

(*Rumex crispus*)

MAGICAL FORMS

a flowering plant native to Europe and western Asia • naturalized across North America as far north as Alaska and considered invasive in California and Oregon • magically use the dried deep-yellow root, whole or chopped

PLANETS AND ELEMENT

Mercury/Jupiter • Air

MAGICAL USES

abundance • prosperity • increasing business acumen and awareness of financial advantage • dried, very finely chopped root can be bought commercially from herbal stores and burned on a bonfire or as part of incense to break ties with the past and clear away fears, doubts, and resentments holding back progress

HOW TO USE

Sprinkle the powdered root outside your business premises or workplace to increase sales. • Drink the tea (which may need sweetening) before visiting a bank for a loan, especially connected with business and before financial speculation or making investments that may involve a risk but offer potential great gain. • Keep a root in a yellow charm bag with the amount of money you seek to acquire etched on the side. Whenever finances change or the root withers, replace the bag and root. Tie the old bag and root to a thriving tree to prevent loss of what has been gained or promised.

CAUTION

Avoid dock if pregnant or breastfeeding. • Do not ingest the raw plant or root. • Do not use if you have gastrointestinal problems, blood clotting disorders, kidney stones, or an allergy to ragweed.

Dogwood

(*Cornus* spp.)

MAGICAL FORMS

also called cornels • magically use the growing tree; leaves, especially in vibrant fall colors; spring flowers, fresh and dried; bark; berries; and sap

PLANET AND ELEMENT

Mars • Fire

MAGICAL USES

wishes • protection against cruelty since it is told that because the flowers were cross-shaped and the wood among the hardest, dogwood was used in the crucifixion • Jesus made the tree so it would never grow large enough to be used for execution crosses again • keeping secrets • for dog rituals to find the right pet • flowering dogwood is the state flower of North Carolina • flowering dogwood (*Cornus florida*) has exotic pink, white, or red bracts and is used as an ornamental display • some superstitious folk insist the flowers should not be brought into the house or burned on an indoor fire

HOW TO USE

Add the dried flowers or bark to love sachets for fidelity. • To prevent pets fighting or to deter your dog from attacking other dogs, add a hair clipping from the aggressive animal (or from both, if your pets are equally to blame) to sugared water and dogwood sap, placing all in a sealed jar and shaking nightly or before a walk. • Dried or pressed dogwood leaves set between pages prevent the curious from prying into your journal or love letters; use this technique also in a set of meeting papers to ensure confidentiality. • Engrave a dog or cat's name on a piece of dogwood and sharpen it, facing the point inward to the room to protect your pets from illness, getting lost, straying, being stolen, or involved in accident.

CAUTION

Most dogwoods like the common dogwood (*Cornus sanguinea*) are nontoxic. • A few species do have mildly toxic berries, but the unpleasant taste deters children and pets. • If in doubt, check the dogwood species with a garden center or botanist. • Some people find the leaves and bark can cause skin irritation.

Dong Quai

(*Angelica sinensis*)

MAGICAL FORMS

also called Chinese angelica or female ginseng • honey-fragranced plant with umbrella-like clusters of small, white flowers from August to September • indigenous to China, its long roots have been used for medicinal purposes for thousands of years in China, Korea, and Japan • considered an all-healer • related to carrots and celery • grows in moist, well-drained soils and is also increasingly popular as a garden ornamental in the USA, Europe, the UK, Iceland, and Lapland • magically use the decoction, powdered root, leaves, stems, and growing plant

PLANET AND ELEMENT

Moon • Water

MAGICAL USES

health and happiness • for specific wishes and needs

HOW TO USE

In magical cookery, empower the leaves (similar to celery), the roots (like sweet potato), or stems (that taste of licorice) with your desire, such as health, happiness, or good fortune, as you chop the plant and stir the pot. Stand any sealed health supplements—not just dong quai—in a container half filled with the powdered root. Leave the container overnight to strengthen the healing powers of the chosen remedy—on the waxing moon for gradual returning of strength, the full moon for resolving a major crisis or slow-to-heal illness, and the waning moon to take away pain. • Drink or eat in a pre-lovemaking meal as an aphrodisiac, for older couples especially, or those who have been celibate for a while and want to rediscover their sexuality. • Meditate on the blossoming flowers to connect with past worlds if you suspect you were once a healer.

CAUTION

Do not use dong quai during pregnancy, as it may bring on contractions. • Do not use within two weeks of elective surgery or if menstruation is very heavy. • Avoid use if taking blood thinners, hormone medications, or going in sunlight immediately after taking a dong quai supplement. • Men should not use in excess, as it can cause breast enlargement.

Downy Avens

(*Geum triflorum*)

MAGICAL FORMS

also known as old man's whiskers or prairie smoke (see "Avens," p. 42) • bowl-shaped wildflower pointing downward with pink-red sepals clasped around its petals and a small opening in the base for bees to enter after pollination • long, creamy to pink-purple feathery seedheads open to the sky, resembling puffs of smoke • fine hairs or down cover the flowers, leaves, and stems • native to many states of central and northern USA and southern Canada, as well as the UK in relatively mild coastal areas • can be grown in the garden • open, wispy, pink seedheads turn golden and seeds are dispersed by the wind

PLANET AND ELEMENT

Mercury • Air

MAGICAL USES

the flower essence calms adults with hyperactive tendencies, and children and teens diagnosed with socially challenged syndromes • for those who are workaholics or work in a fast, pressurized environment to avoid burnout • the whole aerial plant can be used for dried flower arrangements

HOW TO USE

Meditate on the growing, open, wispy flowers to connect with Air spirits. • Use the dried flowers in the center of the home to create gentle unfolding energies and measured expression. • Use the essence regularly with overactive, impulsive, or autistic children who react angrily to sudden change. • If they are resistant to taking the essence, add a few drops to a nightly bath or put a little on the underside of the pillow to center emotions and bring relaxed sleep.

CAUTION

The flower essence is safe. • Native North Americans used the roots as a decoction against coughs and fevers and the crushed seed pods for menstrual cramps. • However, modern research has not confirmed the safety of ingestion or topical use. • In pregnancy or if taking regular medication, expert advice should be sought.

Dragon Fruit

(*Selenicereus undatus*) or (*Hylocereus undatus*)

MAGICAL FORMS

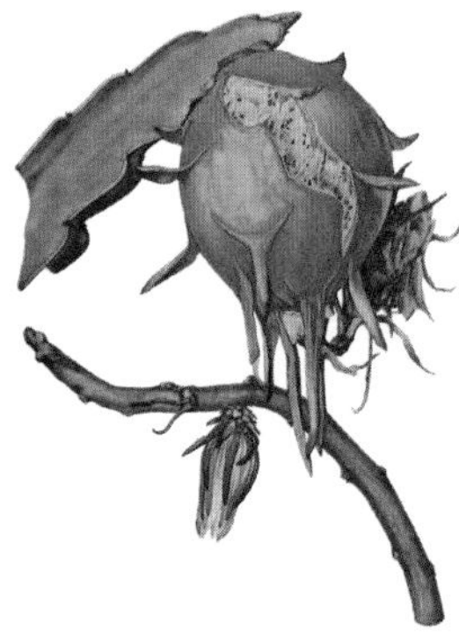

also called pitaya • bright pink fruit from the *Hylocereus* cactus, clinging to trees for support and to reach sunlight, but with its own root system • dragon-like leathery skin and scaly spikes • native to the area between southwestern USA and Mexico, and South America • naturalized in Hawaii, Vietnam, southern China, and Australia • magically use the whole fruit, the pink or white flesh, the blooming flowers for night and moon magick, and the seeds

PLANETS AND ELEMENTS

Moon/Mars • Water/Fire

MAGICAL USES

linked to the moon and as part of a shared feast on the full moon • used in Vietnam on New Year celebrations for good fortune • as a focus for all forms of dragon magick • eaten for protection because of its strong outer skin • tastes like a combination of a pear and a kiwi with a hint of lemon

HOW TO USE

On a full moon and eclipses, on your altar or outdoors, make an offering of the open flowers to the dragon goddess and call your dragon guardian, asking for the strength and courage of the dragon. • Eat the fruit before dowsing, connecting with the ancestors or meditation, anointing your brow with a little juice. • Wash and dry the seeds as a fertility charm, placing them beneath your mattress or pillow in a biodegradable bag. Make love on the full moon. In the morning, hang the bag on a thriving fertility tree or a fruit tree—apple for a boy, pear for a girl.

CAUTION

Dragon fruit is popularly considered nutritious and healing in moderation, as it is filled with iron and magnesium and is hydrating. • It is safe in pregnancy, but inform your midwife or physician.

Dragon Tree

(*Daemonorops draco*) and (*Dracaena draco*)

MAGICAL FORMS

a fast-growing rainforest tree, dragon tree is found in the Amazon basin • large heart-shaped leaves and greenish white flowers • magically use its deep-red resin, fresh or dried (the most common magical form); bark; dried as powder; in chunks; as long reeds (resins are needed to make non-combustible incense burn well); and as essential oil

PLANET AND ELEMENT

Mars • Fire

MAGICAL USES

love rituals • protection • dispels negativity and fear of spirits • increases male potency • courage • self-esteem • overcoming intimidation and fears of the unknown • for all dragon magick rituals • the red color of the powder gave rise to the medieval belief that it was made from the blood of slain dragons

HOW TO USE

Burn dragon's blood incense facing an open window in total darkness to call an estranged lover back. • It increases the power of other incenses, especially to drive away all malevolence, earthly and paranormal. • Set a long strand of dried dragon's blood resin beneath the mattress to overcome impotence. • Make a magical ink using dragon's blood powder, alcohol, and gum arabic for writing magical symbols or making talismans and charms. • Cast a little frankincense, myrrh, and dragon's blood on to a safely guarded bonfire or hearth fire to drive away restless spirits or neutralize disturbing earth energies beneath the home or land. • Pass ritual tools through dragon's blood incense smoke to consecrate them. • Inhale the diffused oil or incense fragrance to induce shape-shifting.

CAUTION

If you have a latex allergy, care should be taken with dragon's blood. • Oil should be well-diluted. • As a precaution, avoid if pregnant. • Even if you use a commercial dragon's-blood skin product, do a patch test if you have sensitive skin.

Dulse

(*Palmaria palmata*) or (*Rhodymenia palmata*)

MAGICAL FORMS

translucent brownish red/purple seaweed with forked, hand-shaped tendrils resembling torn paper • found in rockpools, on rocks, and growing from larger seaweeds, picked during June and September in the mid to low intertidal interlude of the tides • grows on shores in Scotland, Ireland, France, Canada, and parts of the North American Atlantic coast • magically use whole, fresh, dried in sunshine, or purchased in powder form

PLANETS AND ELEMENT

Jupiter/Moon • Water

MAGICAL USES

in magical cookery to increase sexual passion as the meal is empowered and shared • more mundanely recorded as a health-bringing ingredient to food and medicinally as early as 600 CE by St. Columba and his monks • in the far north of Scotland as late as the nineteenth century, lines of "dulse wives" sat on wooden stools along the harbor, selling dulse for frying (tasting like bacon) in soups or stews or for making into flour • for all ocean or inland water rituals • dried and powdered/chopped to be sprinkled around the boundaries of the home or a business for protection and continual flowing healing and harmony energies with the tides, no matter how far away the ocean

HOW TO USE

A single handful of dulse preserved in a jar of alcohol such as whiskey or brandy, facing the front door, welcomes in health, harmony, and abundance to the home or workplace. Replace with a new jar of preserved dulse every New Year's Eve. • Throw it into the outgoing tide to take away misfortune and replace it with good luck when the tide turns. • Cast a frond into the air from a high place or tie it to a bush on a cliff edge for the blessings of the air spirits on any future plane journeys or for successful international internet ventures.

CAUTION

Avoid dulse without medical advice if suffering from thyroid or kidney problems.

Dwarf Boxwood

(*Buxus sempervirens*)

MAGICAL FORMS

tightly packed glossy evergreen green leaves • grows to no more than three feet • the even smaller *Buxus sinica* var. *insularis* grows to two feet • both are cultivated as border hedges in ornamental gardens and as miniature bonsai trees, especially the *sempervirens* variety • the boxwood bonsai is a miniature complete version of the full-grown pompom-shaped tree, and its branches and versatile trunk are wired to give the shape of the full-grown tree • boxwood bonsai trees thrive all over the world, inside as part of a miniature garden and outdoors in warmer climes and in summer • magically clip your dwarf boxwood into different animals and birds as guardians of the home • make the bonsai tree the central focus of the life force in your home or workplace

PLANET AND ELEMENT

Saturn • Earth

MAGICAL USES

attracting money and good luck • weaving a protective barrier around the home or workplace • an ideal fifty-sixth wedding anniversary gift, representing lasting love and long life • attracting new sources of income • inspiring forgotten or undeveloped talents

HOW TO USE

Set your boxwood bonsai in the center of a miniature garden with crystals, pebbles, water, and small growing plants to spread the life force through the home and keep away malign spirits, especially in an old house. • Meditate or chant to astrally travel beyond the bonsai to the old worlds of the Far East and connect with ancestors who saw boxwood hedges in Europe, where the plant is native, or the USA, where boxwood hedging arrived in the 1650s.

CAUTION

The boxwood is rarely used medicinally in the modern world because of recently discovered side effects.

Early Stachyurus

(*Stachyurus praecox*)

MAGICAL FORMS

a flowering plant, native to Japan, that grows in cool temperate zones around the world • ten to twenty catkin-like flowers on drooping flower spikes or racemes resembling strings of pearls, appear on each plant before the leaves fall during the late winter or early spring, hanging from polished-looking arching chestnut-colored branches • the flower buds open to reveal small bell-shaped yellow blooms • leaves are red and yellow in the fall • magically use the growing plant or a branch with flowers or fall leaves attached

PLANET AND ELEMENT

Jupiter • Air

MAGICAL USES

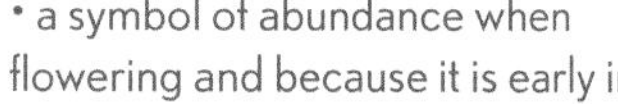

associated with the links between earth and the heavens, the pearl-like flowers form ladders between the dimensions, ideal for meditation • a symbol of abundance when flowering and because it is early in the year, of rapidly advancing prosperity through climbing the ladder to success • its Latin name referring to ears of corn makes this a fertility and sexual prowess charm, especially for men with impotence or premature ejaculation

HOW TO USE

Focus on a taller, growing, flowering plant that can reach up to ten feet, with its pearl-like strings. • As you do so, hold a dish of separate pearls (they need not be real ones, but pale yellow are useful), gently moving them continuously so that they become a background swish to induce a light trance. • Ascend the pearly ladder in your mind until you enter a realm of light where you will become aware of light beings within the shimmer. • You will experience a sense of calm and renewal and the answers to questions you did not know you needed to ask will flow into your mind. • As the experience fades, continue to shake the pearls ever slower until you are aware of the daily world again.

CAUTION

Early stachyurus is not toxic to humans or pets.

Ebony Tree

(*Ebenaceae* family)

MAGICAL FORMS

includes Ceylon ebony (*Diospyros ebenum*), Gabon ebony (*Diospyros crassiflora*), Queensland (Australia) ebony (*Diospyros humilis*), and the Texas ebony tree (*Ebenopsis ebano*) • dark brown/black trunks and often black inner heartwood, the Ceylon and Gabon species grow in Sri Lanka, West Africa, and India • the Texas ebony, the only exotic hardwood in the USA, is found in the brushlands in southwestern USA and Mexico (can in early stages be grown in a pot) • *Diospyros* wood has been shaped in the past as chess pieces, small statues, and tuning pegs from the inner heartwood that polishes like a dark mirror • can still be obtained and ethically used as previously created artifacts (see caution below) if cleansed with hyssop or pine incense smoke • magically use the edible seeds from the Texas tree • Texan wood is available in small quantities through a licensed hobbyist or craft outlet and can be used in magick bags

PLANET AND ELEMENT

Saturn • Earth

MAGICAL USES

for musical gifts and success • for clarity of mind and persuasive communication • creating lasting harmony • as a small antique magick mirror surface (hard to find and expensive but worthwhile) for contacting the ancestors • the empowered Texan seeds as lucky charm jewelry (you can make your own) or cooked and the inner part eaten to enhance psychic powers

HOW TO USE

Precious and expensive because of its scarcity, ebony is considered one of the most protective woods if a small quantity of legally obtained Texan wood or a pre-used *Diospyros* small artifact is carried in a dark-colored amulet bag. • The Texan wood and Texan dried evergreen leaves and/or flowers can be put in a charm bag for worthwhile causes, desires, and genuine needs, but should never be used to seek an unfair advantage or negative purposes, as the power rebounds on the user.

CAUTION

While Texan ebony is not considered toxic, *Diospyros* is possibly an irritant as wood dust.

Echinacea

(*Echinacea angustifolia*)

MAGICAL FORMS

also known as purple coneflower • magically use whole, growing plant; flowers; roots; and oil

PLANETS AND ELEMENTS

Mars/Jupiter • Fire/Air

MAGICAL USES

known as an all-healer and strengthens immunity to destructive pressures, physical and emotional • amplifies the power of other spell ingredients and magical tools • for all who must be warriors for their cause • offered to the cosmos or higher self to strengthen a ritual • used by Native North Americans for connection with the Great Spirit • an herb of spiritual growth and awareness where altruism and idealism are at the fore • for wisewoman and wise man initiation ceremonies

HOW TO USE

Keep a sachet of petals in your purse or wallet to attract health and prosperity. • Meditate on cut or growing echinacea flowers to induce a sense of peace and well-being. • Use a few drops of oil with eucalyptus oil diluted in water as a spray mist to banish recurring minor illnesses and petty quarrels from the home and around your workspace. This creates a protective barrier if others are lethargic or negative. • In a diffuser or burner, echinacea oil promotes spiritual dreams, enhances personal intuitive powers, helps resisting, and encourages trust.

CAUTION

Echinacea is generally considered safe, but do not use medicinally if you have an autoimmune condition or plant allergies. • If pregnant, consult a physician or midwife. • Do not take in excess or in several different forms at once as a remedy.

Edamame

(*Glycine max*)

MAGICAL FORMS

immature, unripened green soy beans still inside the pod • consumed for thousands of years in China as a nutritious snack • spread to Japan and Korea in the eighth century • first produced in the USA in 1855 and Europe by 2008, especially in Japanese cuisine • bunches of pods on the upright bushy two- to three-foot-tall plant are harvested from July through mid-October • boiled and removed from the pod, which can be tough even after cooking • magically use the raw pods containing the beans and the cooked beans (see "Soybean," p. 420).

PLANETS AND ELEMENTS

Mercury/Mars • Air/Fire

MAGICAL USES

for new ventures that will take time to develop • for seizing opportunities that present risk but potential success • to attract backing for an embryonic business • for magical cookery to develop a sideline or second business, especially with a love partner • feed peeled and cooked to immature teens and adults to hasten progress in maturity

HOW TO USE

Keep the beans still in their pods in a basket in the kitchen. • Empower them before cooking to attract additional income from a number of small sources. • Pierce holes in the tops of the raw pods and string them across the kitchen ceiling if you are hesitating over determining the right moment for a venture. • Cut one end of the string before the event and catch as many of the pods as you can in a big basket or cloth to indicate how easy early attempts will be.

Edelweiss

(*Leontopodium nivale* subsp. *alpinum*)

MAGICAL FORMS

a short-living plant growing naturally high in mountains • magically use the whole, growing plant and flowers, fresh and dried

PLANET AND ELEMENT

Jupiter • Air

MAGICAL USES

consists of fifty to five hundred small flowers that form into two to twelve flowerheads with five to fifteen white velvety leaves, creating a double star shape • favored for star magick, air magick, winter rituals, snow rites, mountain magick, and ceremonies to call air and mountain spirits • the flower of overcoming all odds, no matter how stacked they seem against you • its short life is a reminder to enjoy the present and not worry about past or future • ideal for resisting pressures and intimidation, magically and psychologically

HOW TO USE

Carry the dried flowers if moving far from home to keep connection with your roots and your ancestors if they came from the other side of the world. • The dried flowers are traditionally carried in an amulet bag to lower psychological, psychic, and physical profile in times of danger or potential confrontation, and against physical or emotional attack and mind manipulation (it was once believed to be bulletproof). • Growing the plant or meditating on it is said to attract the blessings of the plant spirits to grant wishes. • If you see edelweiss growing wild while on vacation, while it is not permitted in many lands to pick the flowers, merge your aura with the edelweiss through breathing to fill yourself with pure healing and the flowing life force. • Various myths exist of lovers who risked their lives climbing to reach this inaccessible plant to offer to a lover as a sign of total devotion. • Burn the dried flowers as incense to keep away bad spirits and illness from the home, family, and animals.

Eggplant

(*Solanum melongena*)

MAGICAL FORMS

known as eggplant in the USA and Australia because the white variety in its early stages resembles a swan's egg; called aubergine in other parts of the world • an erect herbaceous plant, with edible fruit that is harvested from August onward and eaten as a vegetable • reaching two feet tall, with hairy prickly leaves and stems, deep roots, violet flowers succeeded by a large purple, green, black/very dark purple or white fruit • shiny smooth skin enclosing the abundant flesh that is filled with seeds • native to India and Southeast Asia, eggplant grows both in tropical and some temperate climates worldwide, including regions of the USA and southern parts of the UK • magically use the seeds, the whole fruit (sold in supermarkets worldwide), and sliced and prepared for magical cookery

PLANETS AND ELEMENT

Saturn/Venus • Earth

MAGICAL USES

attracts abundance • brings gradual regrowth after loss or setback • gives insight into indecision • when cooked in any way and eaten, the purple plant brings courage, the white protection, the green understanding of the motives of others, and black easing through natural endings to beginnings

HOW TO USE

Set a whole eggplant in the center of your kitchen table to prevent accidents and spills and to deter all who come with ill intentions from lingering (replace regularly). • Peel (as many folks do) and slice an eggplant, adding a little salt, spice, or cooking oil on top of the slices, to take away sickness and misfortune and attract health, wealth, and happiness to those eating the meal. • Scoop out the seeds of an aubergine before cooking. Wash and dry them outdoors or where the air circulates. Place them in a charm bag to hold whenever you need to make a fast or important decision. Afterward, bury or scatter them outdoors.

CAUTION

The leaves are toxic and should not be ingested. • Though medicinally used to boost immunity and digestion, avoid excessive quantities if you suffer from kidney problems or are pregnant. • Avoid if taking medication for Parkinson's disease.

Eglantine

(*Rosa rubiginosa*)

MAGICAL FORMS

known as sweet briar or sweetbriar rose • eglantine describes wild, brambly roses increasingly introduced to wildlife or larger gardens or hybrids suitable for smaller gardens, but the true briar rose is pink and white • magically use blossoms, leaves, thorns, and rose hips

PLANET AND ELEMENT

Mercury • Air

MAGICAL USES

developing talents especially connected with words and poetry • protective against spite and envy and those who would deceive • for secret or unconventional love where there is strong opposition • overcoming hurt and betrayal • encountering the fey • used in Shakespeare's *Cymbeline* for truth in love and in *A Midsummer Night's Dream* for fragrant enchantment • the flower of Elizabeth I

HOW TO USE

The crushed blossoms release an apple scent that is an aphrodisiac. • Leaves and blossoms crushed with almonds make a powerful love sachet to help get you positively noticed by your desired love who seems unaware. • Briar rose refers to its fierce spindly thorns that are added to defensive bottles to counteract a curse or hexing and used against danger from a stalker or ex who will not let go. • Briar rose is used in flower waters and essences, especially by those seeking first love or who have been deeply wounded or rejected in love.

CAUTION

Remove the bitter white base from the petals and the hairs just below the fruit hips before cooking and eating, as these can cause digestive and mouth problems. • Avoid the hips if you are allergic to ordinary rose hips and consult a physician or midwife before using if pregnant. • Beware of the thorns if there are small children or pets.

Elder Tree

(*Sambucus nigra*) or (*Sambuca canadensis*)

MAGICAL FORMS

black elder tree (*Sambucus nigra*) is found in the UK, Europe, and the USA • the American black elderberry (*Sambuca canadensis*), or common elder, is native to large areas of North America east of the Rockies and south to Bolivia in South America • elderblossom and elderberry are famous as teas, especially for ceremonial gatherings and nature spirit rites and for good luck, wealth, and happiness shared by a newly committed couple • fragrant flowers, creamy colored, bloom in late May • purple-black sour berries grow late summer to the fall • as a wand, elder is used for exorcism rituals • magically use the whole, growing tree; leaves and branches; and berries, fresh or dried

PLANET AND ELEMENT

Venus • Water

MAGICAL USES

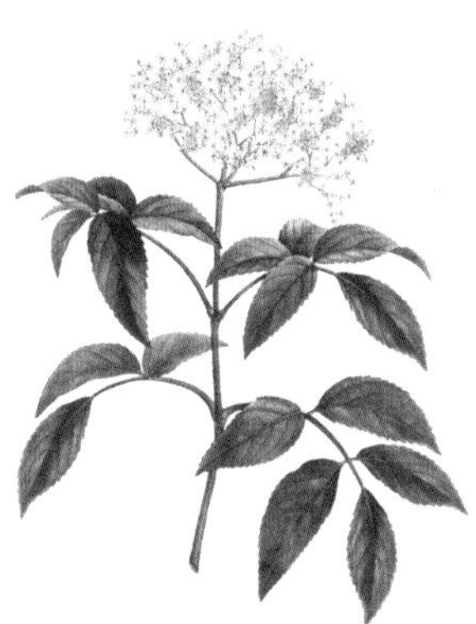

it is said that if you wear a crown of elder twigs on May Eve (April 30), you will be able to see magical creatures and ghosts • elder trees offer a doorway to the Otherworld beneath their roots on this evening, if one sits beneath the branches, but those who fall asleep under them might not return for years

HOW TO USE

Leaves of elder scattered in the direction of the four winds give protection from hostility and from storm damage and other extremes of weather. • Dried elderberries as part of an incense mix attract benign faeries. • Branches or wreaths from the tree would be hung on the outside of houses on May Eve to drive away malevolent spirits.

CAUTION

The elder is not to be cut without permission of the Elder Mother tree guardian. • Uncooked berries and other parts of the *Sambucus* are poisonous.

Elecampane

(*Inula helenium*)

MAGICAL FORMS

flowering plant from the sunflower family • magically use the whole, growing plant; dried and fresh roots; and flowering stem/leaves

PLANET AND ELEMENTS

Mercury • Air/Water

MAGICAL USES

calls home what or who is lost • fast acting and amplifies spells against trickery • protects against mischievous nature essences • named after Helen of Troy, whose tears were transformed into the herb

HOW TO USE

Add dried leaves and flowers to love charms. • The dried whole herb and flowers should be added to a spell jar while reciting the purpose of the jar, as elecampane strengthens the power of other herbs, flowers, symbols, and crystals within the jar. • Pass your hands in front of the growing plants, naming a person, animal, or item that has been lost, has gone away, or has been taken from you as a continuous chant—the writing hand clockwise and the other counterclockwise. Build up the speed of words and movement and then, when you have reached full power, clap and say, *Come home to me*. Repeat this practice nightly at sunset.

CAUTION

Do not take if pregnant or breastfeeding, or internally in large quantities at any time, as excess may cause diarrhea and vomiting or spasms. • Elecampane can cause skin chafing, so before applying the decoction directly to the skin, do a patch test.

Elemi Gum Tree

(*Canarium luzonicum*)

MAGICAL FORMS

the *Canarium ovatum*, often called the pili tree, has similar magical properties, though some see this as a separate resin-bearing tree and source for elemi oil • large tropical trees growing up to ninety-eight feet, with profuse resin and essential oil • native to the Philippines, the Moluccas, and Southeast Asia • related to the trees producing frankincense and myrrh • the resin can be messy to burn and does not work well on charcoal • magically use the essential oil produced from the oily resin, often known as an economical version of frankincense, but with far more spiritual and emotional balancing

PLANET AND ELEMENT

Sun • Fire

MAGICAL USES

an oil of inner radiance • diffuse before and during meditation, yoga, and breathwork and to encourage mindfulness • increases youthfulness • removes stress • for rites of passage • to let go of preconceived limitations

HOW TO USE

Use the oil regularly in baths, inhalation, and diffusing/burning, or on a saucer near a radiator at work (do not let it run dry) to prevent burnout in an overdemanding life and to overcome restlessness for attaining the next goal. • Dilute the oil to anoint the third psychic brow energy center and the center of the forehead to connect with higher spiritual realms and beings and for mystical experiences. • Wear an aroma bracelet or necklace, with lava beads infused with the oil, when walking or staying in nature to connect with nature essences and the higher devas.

Eleuthero

(*Eleutherococcus senticosus*)

MAGICAL FORMS

popularly called Siberian ginseng, though it is not botanically a ginseng • small, woody shrub, growing in Russian forests and the northern regions of China, Japan, and Korea • the roots are used dried and chopped for tea decoctions • roots often cover vast distances underground • a bush can be twenty feet high • the root is the main part used in magick and can easily be obtained online or as tea in health stores for rituals, charms, and amulets • powdered root and occasionally bark can also be found

PLANET AND ELEMENT

Mars • Fire

MAGICAL USES

in rituals against stress and exhaustion • to bring concentration before examinations if you have other commitments that take your attention • for motivation in overcoming obstacles

HOW TO USE

Following the Russian tradition, hang a bag of the chopped root over the doorway to bar the entrance to restless spirits, especially those remaining on the land if a bad experience occurred nearby even centuries earlier. • Carry a root in an amulet bag if you are traveling, especially to unknown or potentially hazardous places. • Burn chopped ground roots or powder in incense to purify the home and guard against accidents before any renovation or decorating. • If possible, seal a root behind a fireplace in a new or newly renovated home for protection. • Keep a root in your car for safe journeys, particularly long ones.

CAUTION

Eleuthero is generally considered safe but may raise blood pressure. • Not enough is known about effects during pregnancy and breastfeeding, so refrain from using it during those times. • Do not use if suffering from diabetes or if taking hormone therapy or anticoagulants, as the plant has not been fully researched medically in these cases.

Elm Tree

(*Ulmus* spp.)

MAGICAL FORMS

American elm (*Ulmus americana*) grows in eastern North America • English elm (*Ulmus procera*) was introduced to the UK from Spain by Bronze Age ancestors, probably reaching the USA with fifteenth-century explorers and sixteenth-century settlers • slippery elm (*Ulmus rubra*) is found on both sides of the Atlantic • magically work with the living trees, wood, dried leaves, and bark, particularly the fragrant inner bark of slippery elm

PLANETS AND ELEMENTS

Saturn/Moon • Earth/Water

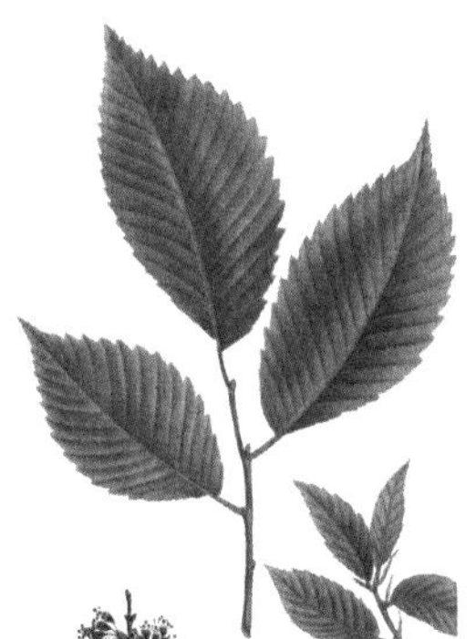

MAGICAL USES

the wood as a charm for communication and clear speech • to make connection with elves • protection if a branch is hung over an outside door • female magick and rites of passage • water resistant, making elm a powerful dowsing rod for finding water, oil, and minerals

HOW TO USE

At dawn, sit beneath an elm, fashion a fallen small branch into a wand, and sing to attract the wood elves who will bring good fortune. • To contact the higher nature spirits/devas, meditate regularly beneath your special tree and leave offerings beneath it. • Bind a slippery elm bark twig or another sharp twig with yellow thread, burning it on a hearth or bonfire to prevent malicious gossip, false flattery, and spite from jealous friends, family members, or colleagues. • Also burn dried leaves or bark as part of an incense mix to increase psychic powers before divination. • Create an amulet bag of dried leaves. Hold it while practicing a speech or necessary communication. One by one, scatter the leaves on the path you take to the venue, keeping one as your *aide mémoire* during the event.

CAUTION

Avoid during pregnancy.

Elm Tree, Chinese

(*Ulmus parvifolia*)

MAGICAL FORMS

also known as lacebark elm • the full-sized tree with mahogany-colored bark, small glossy green leaves that turn yellow and red in the fall and fall off in midwinter • growing to eighty feet • native to China, Japan, and Korea but growing worldwide • resistant to Dutch elm disease • also grown as the dwarf Chinese elm (*Ulmus geisha*), which will thrive in a container • most prized as the miniature bonsai tree that flourishes indoors and outdoors in the summer • magically use the growing tree and especially the bonsai, which is the easiest bonsai to maintain and represents the perfection of nature written small

PLANET AND ELEMENT

Moon • Water

MAGICAL USES

as a bonsai, brings good fortune and protection • in meditation, gives insight into the future • also for harmony in the workplace • the full-grown tree blowing in the wind will reveal answer to questions and concerns, in their rustling leaves • the bonsai for children old before their time to stimulate their imagination

HOW TO USE

Make your Chinese elm bonsai the center of a miniature garden with rocks, small pools, winding paths, tiny plants, and flowers near the center of your home so that good fortune and abundance energies can circulate. • A dwarf Chinese elm in a container either side of the front entrance acts as a shield against misfortune and illness and filters stress and negativity from those returning home after a challenging day. • Meditate on your bonsai and enter the miniature world via its pathways to lands of fantasy, especially before sleep, ensuring magical dreams.

CAUTION

Dogs and cats may react badly to eating the leaves and bark of the larger trees.

Empress Tree

(*Paulownia tomentosa*)

MAGICAL FORMS

also called princess or foxglove tree because its purple gemlike flowers resemble foxgloves • native to the mountains of central China, named after the daughter of Czar Paul I of Russia • also grows in Japan • naturalized in western Europe and large areas of the eastern USA • magically use the growing tree in situ, its fresh or dried flowers, and foliage containing flowers displayed ornamentally

PLANETS AND ELEMENT

Moon/Venus • Water

MAGICAL USES

increases wealth, success, popularity, expertise • for women's power rites • planted in China for the birth of a girl, and when the tree is grown, it is used to carve into her marriage chest • because it spreads seeds extensively, it takes water from other plants and is a pioneer, one of the first trees to take hold in a damaged ecosystem and regenerate after a fire • for business expansion plans in a ruthless market or to resist a takeover

HOW TO USE

Set a small flowering branch on your altar for rituals where survival is essential, if you are in danger of losing a home, career, love, or finances, especially for single mothers or anyone denied a justifiable promotion, compensation, or recognition. • Meditate beneath the tree for inspirational ideas and to attract opportunities to move up to the next level. • Keep a fallen flower, dried if in bloom, or dried leaves in a gold charm bag to transfer new motivation into your working life.

CAUTION

Empress is considered invasive and is banned in some states of the USA because of its rapid spread, but it is not toxic to humans or animals.

Endive

(*Cichorium endivia*)

MAGICAL FORMS

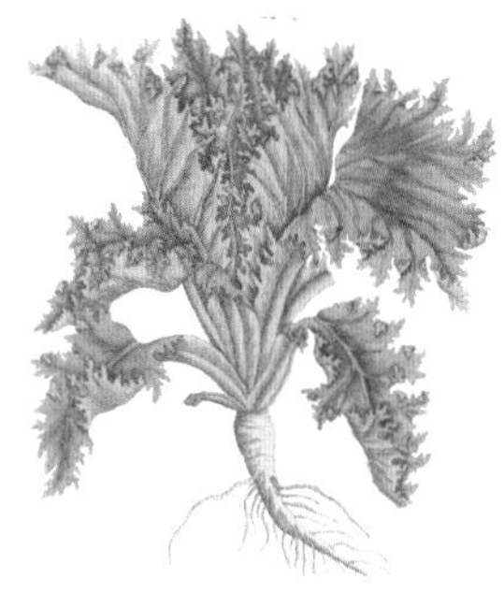

varieties include curly endive (var. *crispum*), with narrow leaves, and escarole (var. *latifolium*), with broader leaves • whole plant, growing or cut, as a vegetable or salad ingredient, leaves, stem • traditionally, the cut plant should be replaced every three days, and harvested with a piece of gold (tie an earring around a trowel) or antler kept for the purpose, to bring money and add passion to love • best days of the year for harvesting are considered to be June 27 and July 25 for ultimate power

PLANET AND ELEMENT

Jupiter • Air

MAGICAL USES

for domestic and folk magick rather than ritual (could be part of a culinary garden) • magical cookery • increases and maintains wealth • to facilitate smooth house moves, an endive plant with roots taken from the old garden and replanted, if possible, in the new garden or, if not, eaten in the first meal

HOW TO USE

Eat an endive raw (some are quite bitter) to increase prosperity. • Steam the whole plant and share it with a partner to take sex magick to new heights. • If single, enchant your endive before cooking to bring confidence at social events and to attract love, so you will not need to eat your endive alone in future. • Chop an endive and put it in a love bottle or jar spell, preserved with virgin olive oil and rose petals, to keep a long-term love faithful and drive away rivals and temptation.

CAUTION

As a culinary plant, the endive is generally safe cooked or raw, but avoid if allergic to birch tree pollen.

Eryngo

(*Eryngium* spp.)

MAGICAL FORMS

also known as sea holly, with more than 230 varieties/cultivars • blue cap sea holly (*Eryngium planum*) has numerous tiny silver-blue flowers in a tight cluster • most eryngo species grow in the USA • the rattlesnake master eryngo (*Eryngium yuccifolium*) is native to the eastern USA, with button-like chartreuse-colored flowers, taller than many other species • grows in gardens, cultivated especially but not exclusively in coastal regions • magically use the whole growing plant of the big blue sea holly (*Eryngium zabelii*), with steel-blue thistlelike flowers on top of a mound of silvery-blue leaves, and the dried or fresh flowers and root of any eryngo

PLANETS AND ELEMENTS

Jupiter/Moon • Air/Water

MAGICAL USES

the root can be carried in a charm bag to increase male virility • the root was eaten in sixteenth-century England, candied as a sweetmeat as a male aphrodisiac • the whole flowers, especially the blue and silver kinds, are often cut and dried in a wedding bouquet for love that will withstand any opposition and remain united throughout the years • the master rattlesnake flowers dried in a sachet or a flower arrangement protect against spite at work or socially

HOW TO USE

Burn the dried flowers in an incense mix to restore peace after a quarrel. • Tape a small bag of the powdered or dried, crumbled herb beneath the doormat if a family member always comes home from work (or school) in a bad mood. • Place a tall vase of Miss Willmott's ghost (*Eryngium giganteum*) with silver leaves in a haunted room or house for a week and then cast the flowers into flowing water.

CAUTION

Do not use eryngo if you are allergic to celery, fennel, or dill. • Exercise caution if using during pregnancy.

Eucalyptus

(*Eucalyptus* spp.)

MAGICAL FORMS

silvery-blue leaves that release menthol fragrance when bruised and create a blue haze in heat • yellow to cream fluffy flowers • eucalyptus is most popular as oil, powdered, and in numerous healing remedies • native to Australia • a healing tree among the Indigenous people • grows in suitable climates throughout the world, including warmer parts of the USA • can flourish in containers in cooler regions if brought under cover when cold • magically use the whole, growing tree or shrub; dried flowers; leaves, fresh or dried; and oil

PLANET AND ELEMENT

Moon • Water

MAGICAL USES

the ultimate health and healing tree • called the tree of adaptability because of its power to rapidly regenerate after bushfires • freedom • cleanses and banishes negativity and anger • moves longstanding problems toward resolution by offering a fresh perspective • clear communication • job opportunities • travel

HOW TO USE

Eucalyptus rituals are best when the sun and moon are both in the sky. • Add the oil to a floor wash to remove sickness, misfortune, or inertia, or after a quarrel. The water cast out of the front door afterward opens the home and family to an ongoing flow of health-bringing, optimistic energies. • Fill a sleep pillow or poppet/doll with dried eucalyptus flowers, dried rose petals, and lavender heads to which a drop or two of eucalyptus oil has been added for refreshing nights if you always wake tired. • Burn a green candle surrounded by the leaves to send healing through the light to someone in hospital or far away. • If possible, add eucalyptus leaves to any healing bouquet you send.

CAUTION

The bark, leaves, and sap are toxic to humans and pets if ingested. • If you have a heart condition, epilepsy, or high blood pressure, limit or avoid eucalyptus remedies. • Dilute the oil well if applying to the skin. • If you are pregnant, check with a medical professional before use.

European Spindle Tree

(*Euonymus europaeus*)

MAGICAL FORMS

also called the common spindle • small long-living tree found throughout Europe and western Asia • native to the UK from Celtic times as one of the divinatory tree staves • grows in the USA, invasive in Oregon, New Hampshire, and New Jersey • though largely wild, it is planted in parks and gardens for its beauty in the fall when the leaves turn purple, red, and yellow, and its pink and orange nonedible fruits ripen from September to October (see "Burning Bush," p. 86) • magically use the dried leaves and fruits in the fall (with care), the growing tree, or the wood made into spindles, skewers, charcoal, and clothes pegs, especially if you can find antique spindle-wood objects at a garage sale or market, or new from traditional crafting stores

PLANET AND ELEMENT

Mars • Fire

MAGICAL USES

small spindle-wood artifacts as an amulet assist you in any creative work or business, especially the charcoal if you are artistically inclined • for finishing tasks and fulfilling obligations • questioning authority if it is unjust or corrupt

HOW TO USE

Carefully fill a small bag of dried, chopped fall leaves and fruit to bring a court case that is lingering to be resolved in your favor. • Take white paper and spindle-wood charcoal, allowing your hand to draw an image of your spirit guardian. • Obtain an old spindle-wood or traditionally crafted peg or spindle and visit an industrial or farming museum or reconstructed village to connect with the old worlds.

CAUTION

The bark, leaves, and fruit are poisonous to humans, pets, and livestock, though beloved by birds, especially the robin. • In the nineteenth century, the powdered bark was used to remove headlice and as an emetic and diuretic, but it has been discovered to share properties of digitalis (foxglove).

Eyebright

(*Euphrasia officinalis*) and (*Euphrasia rostkoviana*)

MAGICAL FORMS

native to and grows wild in western and central Europe and parts of southern Europe • naturalized in the USA • small, scallop-edged, white- or purple-veined petals with a yellow center and black spot resembling an eye • magically use the fresh and dried aerial parts and the dried, chopped leaves, which can be bought online or used in tea bags that can be made into a magical infusion or split and used in spell bags

PLANET AND ELEMENT

Mercury • Air

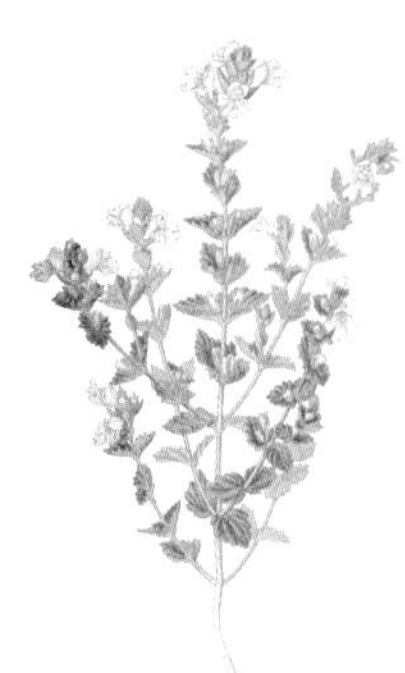

MAGICAL USES

named after one of the Greek Charities, Euphrasia, spirit of joy and celebrations • increases clairvoyance • brings awareness of what is hidden or untrue • according to legend, the linnet bird used eyebright to give her young clear vision and shared the secret with humankind

HOW TO USE

Drink the tea or go where the plant grows for visions of the fey. • Burn in incense or hold a charm bag of the dried herb over a document or photo of a person to know instinctively what is true and what is illusion or falsehood. • Take the bag along to auctions and yard sales to alert you to a good bargain or a fake as you hold it in your dominant hand or the pocket on that side of your body, and allow the other hand to pass over the item. • Add to a sleep pillow or put a bag under your pillow for prophetic dreams and to keep away nightmares.

CAUTION

Eyebright is thought to be unsafe to use directly on the eyes unless using a sterilized version, and only then with medical approval. • Do not use if pregnant or suffering from diabetes, and never use in excess.

False Sandalwood

(*Eremophila mitchellii*)

MAGICAL FORMS

small to medium tree with flaky bark, pale-green leaves, and usually white, bell-shaped flowers • sticky leaves and branches because of the resin • native to the grazing lands of the warm temperate zone of New South Wales, Australia, and the tropics of Australia's northern Queensland, growing wild • the oil is made from the heartwood and bark • magically use primarily as essential oil (a substitute for sandalwood), as fallen leaves or branches, or as a powder

PLANET AND ELEMENT

Mercury • Air

MAGICAL USES

the oil stabilizes thoughts to remain in the present moment for mindfulness, meditation, yoga, and breathwork • brings healing to your home and aura when the oil is burned or diffused • diluted for anointing candles before spiritual work (makes candle extra flammable, so use in safe place) • for working with animus energies in either sex

HOW TO USE

The tree is part of the Indigenous tradition, with the leaves and wood ceremonially burned and the smoke used to welcome the ancestors, celebrate coming-of-age rites, say goodbye to the departed, remove negative spirits, and cleanse an area. • Burn incense after adding a drop or two of the oil, or include a little of the powdered Buddha wood to incense on charcoal, for any rites of passage. • Alternatively, fan smoke from the diffused oil to contact other dimensions. • If you are lucky enough to find a source of the dried leaves or wood, burn them outdoors in ceremonies to welcome the seasons and the ancestors by walking through the smoke.

CAUTION

Nontoxic, but there is insufficient data on the safety of the oil with pregnancy or breastfeeding. • Generally dilute the oil well, and do not ingest. • Never apply flames directly to the essential oil, and always use small amounts of oil if adding to unlit wood, leaves, or incense. • If outdoors, burn away from trees as Buddha wood is very flammable.

Fennel

(*Foeniculum vulgare*)

MAGICAL FORMS

flowering plant related to the carrot • magically use herb, fresh and dried; roots; and seeds

PLANET AND ELEMENT

Mercury • Air

MAGICAL USES

all forms of travel, vacation, relocation, commuting, and long journeys • the safety and sleep of babies and small children • diminishes jealousy and possessiveness and disarms hidden enemies • domestic protection against unwelcome neighbors, evil spirits, and intruders • fertility and preconception to bring body into alignment with its natural cycles • good luck in gambling • perseverance to win despite any obstacles • unites people or situations that are pulling in opposite directions • water scrying, especially for questions about fertility and families • herb of midsummer

HOW TO USE

Carry a charm bag with a silver dollar for luck in gambling. • To aid conception, add seeds to a charm bag and empower on the crescent moon and again on each full moon, gently pricking with a silver pin. Replace the bag on the last night of the wane and bury it under a thriving fennel plant. • For home protection, gather seeds in a net over the main entrance to your home so unwelcome visitors or thieves magically have to count them before entering. • Create a protective garden against all external hostility. • Sprinkle root decoctions and infusions along boundaries with difficult neighbors to deter complaints. • Anoint an egg buried during the full moon under fennel plants to call a baby into the womb.

CAUTION

They should not be ingested while actually trying to conceive, in pregnancy itself, or during IVF, as they can bring on menstruation.

Fenugreek

(*Trigonella foenum-graecum*)

MAGICAL FORMS

an annual plant popularly incorporated into cooking • magically use the whole, growing plant; seeds (most generally used in magick and healing); and the fresh and dried leaves or powdered seeds as a spice in magical cooking

PLANETS AND ELEMENTS

Saturn/Mercury • Earth/Air

MAGICAL USES

called the plant of growth in every way, especially increasing prosperity over a period of time through a series of rituals • protects during astral travel and mediumship • an herb of Lughnassadh (a Gaelic festival) or Lammas (a Christian holiday), marking the first harvest at the beginning of August in the northern hemisphere, attracting abundance and deserved financial rewards

HOW TO USE

Fenugreek is exceptionally good in prosperity pouches and money spells. • Sprinkle the seeds across thresholds of business premises to attract customers. • Burn as incense to enhance meditation and psychic powers. • Excess fenugreek should always be buried after a ritual. • Add a fenugreek infusion, made by boiling and steeping seeds in water and draining, to floor washes to bring blessings to the home, banish poverty, and attract abundance. • Empower the seeds by leaving them in a sachet on the full moon and the next morning placing them under the mattress until the next full moon to enhance fertility, replacing the sachet each full moon.

CAUTION

Excess fenugreek can cause skin allergies and upset stomach. • Fenugreek is not to be taken with diabetes medicine. • It is not recommended in pregnancy.

Fern, Boston

(*Nephrolepis exaltata*)

MAGICAL FORMS

also as Delta maidenhair fern (*Adiantum raddianum*) • Boston ferns (indoor or in warmer climates) and Delta maidenhair ferns are nontoxic • unlike male fern (*Dryopteris filix-mas*), which is poisonous • magically use the seeds and the cut or whole, growing plant, fresh or dried

PLANETS AND ELEMENTS

Mercury/Saturn • Air/Earth

MAGICAL USES

associated with increasing prosperity • unexpected money or gifts and a sudden boost to business • good luck • offering gateways to otherworlds, especially the realms of the fey • highly protective • travel opportunities • a plant of the midsummer solstice

HOW TO USE

Keep Boston fern in a pot in a bathroom or kitchen to prevent money draining away down water outlets. • Ferns planted near the doorstep bring protection to the home. • Burn as incense to connect with spirits or the world of nature essences. • If golden fern pollen is scattered to the winds at midsummer or on a map, it is said to reveal the location of hidden treasure or where a golden opportunity lies. • Added to a bouquet, fern enhances the energies of the other flowers. • If the seeds are gathered on a white cloth, a pewter dish, or a Bible then shaken on the ground with a hazel rod, they confer invisibility or a low profile in future times of danger. • Dried ferns thrown on hot coals exorcise evil spirits and, when burned outdoors, are traditionally said to cause rain to fall.

CAUTION

Delta maidenhair fern should not be taken internally during pregnancy. • Check before buying that the chosen ferns are nontoxic to humans or animals.

Feverfew

(*Tanacetum parthenium*)

MAGICAL FORMS

flowering plant that is part of the daisy family • grown ornamentally and for use in medicine • magically use the whole, growing plant, as well as aerial parts harvested in summer, including flowers and leaves, both fresh and dried

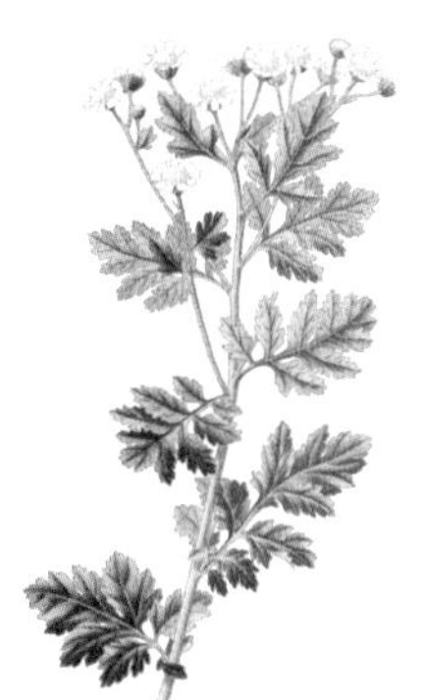

PLANET AND ELEMENT

Venus • Water

MAGICAL USES

reduces addictions and bad habits • removes the hold of destructive lovers • warns of false love online • keeps away illness, accidents, and stinging insects from the dwelling and family • for a peaceful home • guards travelers and all who must go to unfamiliar or hostile environments • herb of the Midwinter Solstice • traditionally believed to guard against *elfshot*, flying fey arrows attacking and causing sudden pain and ill fortune

HOW TO USE

In protective rituals, add to a sachet or plant in the garden. • Can be included in mojo bags, alone or with hyssop and rosemary, to prevent accidents while traveling, or sealed in a bag with a St. Christopher medal and comfrey root for the same purpose. • Add to a bath as a tea or part of a sachet to break hexes and jinxes that make you accident-prone. • Mix with red nettle and plantain as a protective amulet against malevolent spirits.

CAUTION

Do not take during pregnancy. • May disturb digestion if excess is taken internally. • Eat on bread to prevent mouth ulcers. • Avoid if taking blood thinners.

Fig Tree

(*Ficus carica*)

MAGICAL FORMS

known as the common fig, a tree with edible fruit • cultivated for thousands of years • excavated from 5000 BCE in Neolithic sites • recorded from around 1560 CE in the New World • grown in its miniature form as a houseplant • dwarf fig trees are as magically powerful as larger ones • the tree is sacred to the Roman mother goddess Juno, to the ancient Egyptian Isis, and to all goddesses who bring fertility to women, as well as to the ecstatic and unbridled passion of Dionysus if a man has potency issues • it is also said that the Buddha received enlightenment beneath a fig tree • magically use fruit and seeds

PLANET AND ELEMENTS

Jupiter • Air/Fire

MAGICAL USES

brings wealth • abundance • luxury acquisitions and vacations • considered by many to be the Tree of Knowledge of Good and Evil in the Garden of Eden, and so is a symbol of necessary knowledge attained at a cost

HOW TO USE

When grown as a houseplant or dwarf tree in the garden or in a container if short of space, the plant guards against poverty and lack of resources. • Eat the fruit as a fertility and potency symbol before lovemaking to conceive a child, or carve a small piece of the wood into a phallic symbol, placing it under the mattress. • Cast the wood into flowing water the morning after lovemaking to aid conception. • A fig tree or a single branch over the door on the outside of the house ensures travelers will return safely. • Using a pin, etch a symbol of what you most desire on a fig leaf. • As it dries out, the wish will be granted—the slower the drying, the better the omen. • Enchant fig fruits and share them with a lover to strengthen the attraction between you.

CAUTION

The milky sap can cause skin irritation. • Figs may interfere with the effect of blood thinners.

Figwort

(*Scrophularia* spp.)

MAGICAL FORMS

Scrophularia lanceolata (early figwort) spans most states in the USA except the Deep South • *Scrophularia californica*, known as the Californian bee plant, is found in California • *Scrophularia nodosa* is known as the common or knotted figwort, which grows in the UK, Europe, the USA, and Asia • *Scrophularia marilandica*, called late or eastern figwort, grows throughout the eastern and central USA and parts of Canada • called "the good leaf" in Wales • magically use leaves, root, and flowers

PLANET AND ELEMENT

Venus • Earth

MAGICAL USES

protects against jealousy and spite • brings health to the user • the herb of midsummer: smoked over the solstice fires and hung in the home for health and prosperity • beloved by bees and so brings messages from the ancestors

HOW TO USE

The leaves can be burned in smudging ceremonies for cleansing a sacred outdoor area or an indoor space where there has been anger, sorrow, sickness, or misfortune. • To protect against the evil eye, add a chopped root to a red bag. • Using a sage or thyme incense stick like a pen, draw an eye in the air with its smoke in front of the closed bag. • Make a weak decoction from the chopped root, or a tea from the dried leaves and flowers and anoint door handles and window latches indoors and out to cleanse the home at midsummer or any other seasonal change point.

CAUTION

Do not use if suffering from a heart condition. • Check with your midwife before using the herb internally or on skin during pregnancy or while breastfeeding.

Fir Tree

(*Abies* spp.)

MAGICAL FORMS

numerous varieties growing wild and cultivated from China to Spain and in North America, including the noble fir (*Abies procera*), native to the northwestern Pacific coast ranges • the most popular Christmas tree in the world • the California red fir (*Abies magnifica*) grows in the Sierra Nevada and Cascade mountains, the Fraser fir (*Abies fraseri*) in the southeastern Appalachian Mountains, and the European silver fir (*Abie alba*) throughout Europe and the UK • large trees are closely related to the *Pinaceae* family (including cedar, pine, and spruce trees) • unlike the pine or spruce, the fir needles attach singly to the branches with a suction-like cap • magically work with the growing tree, cones, or needles

PLANETS AND ELEMENTS

Jupiter/Mars • Air/Fire

MAGICAL USES

birth and rebirth • new beginnings • cleansing • unexpected gifts and money • those using the tree can call on the blessings of Druantia, the Celtic fir tree goddess—goddess of fire and protectress of mothers and newborn children

HOW TO USE

Collect the soft cones or fallen needles and create good-luck charms by carrying in a green bag. • Sit in a fir grove against a fir tree, asking your questions when there is a lull in the wind. • Listen to the answer as the wind picks up and shakes the needles. • Buy a fir with roots or potted in soil for Christmas. • After the Christmas holiday, plant it in your garden and decorate it with solar lights to use it as your wish tree throughout the year.

CAUTION

The foliage and green berries are mildly toxic if ingested raw.

Fir Tree, Douglas

(*Pseudotsuga menziesii*)

MAGICAL FORMS

found throughout the northwestern seaboard from Mexico through the USA to Canada, including Vancouver Island; also in Europe, Australia, New Zealand, and the UK, especially Scotland • introduced into Europe by botanist David Douglas in 1827 • heights in excess of 245 feet, branches may not begin until over a hundred feet • magically use the tree in situ and the citrusy bright green tips of the needles in protective and healing brews

PLANET AND ELEMENT

Jupiter • Air

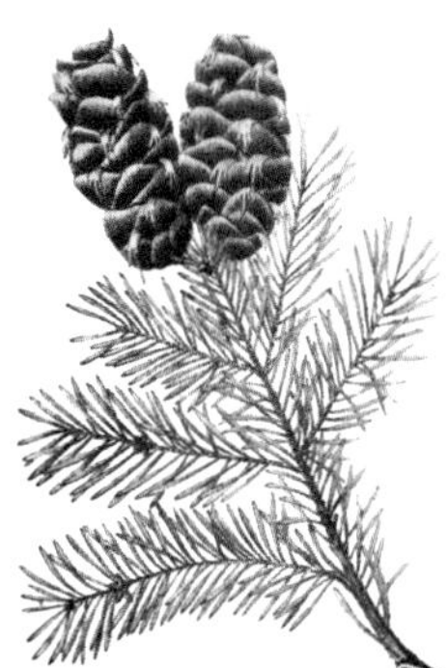

MAGICAL USES

related pairs of trees recognize and feed carbon to the root tips of their own kind through underground networks • Douglas needles and cones are used in rituals for strengthening family ties • cones kept in the home in an amulet bag near the food store ensure that there will always be a roof over your head and sufficient resources

HOW TO USE

An Indigenous story tells of a mouse that was offered shelter in a tree during a forest fire (the trees are largely fire resistant because of the thick bark and high branches). The mouse's hind paws and tail can still be seen sticking out of the cones, where he burrowed for safety and fed on the seeds within the cones until the fire had passed. • Traditionally, the evergreen branches are decorated as Yule trees and wreaths. • Meditate gazing upward, holding the base of the tree, to travel astrally to higher dimensions. • Sprinkle an infusion made from the green tips on your doorstep or add to a kitchen-floor wash to prevent accidents from fire, electrical faults, or natural disasters.

CAUTION

The leaves and bark can occasionally cause irritation.

Fir Tree, Siberian

(*Abies sibirica*)

MAGICAL FORMS

native to Siberia and northern China • an evergreen conifer with a pyramid shape, very aromatic leaves or needles, and silvery bark • grows in many northern habitats including northern Europe and the USA • smaller ones are used for Christmas trees • magically use the essential oil extracted from all green parts of the tree, especially from old mature leaves or needles; the growing tree or fallen branches; and loose tea as *Pinus sibirica* (white pine), available online or from specialty herbalists

PLANET AND ELEMENT

Jupiter • Air

MAGICAL USES

maintaining or restoring harmony • helps overcome exhaustion • defuses anger at home and confrontation in the workplace • aids in acceptance of what cannot be changed • helps with the courage to leave a toxic relationship • overcoming self-doubt

HOW TO USE

Burn or diffuse the oil from Thanksgiving through Yule and at any part of the year when gloom descends and a celebration seems far away. • Use a personal inhaler or aroma beads when you feel panic rising if you suffer from compulsions or obsessions such as OCD. • Drink the tea (make sure it is from a reputable Siberian fir source) if you work or live where you feel constantly on trial. • If worried about ingesting the tea (check the product with your physician or herbalist), sprinkle the infusion around a tablet, your home or workplace computer, or a mobile phone if they are a route of psychological attack. • Drink the tea only in moderation.

CAUTION

The oil is not recommended for use during pregnancy or while breastfeeding, and some experts suggest not to use it in baths or on the face if you have sensitive skin or chronic health problems. • Avoid if you have kidney issues, ulcers, or gastritis.

Fireweed

(*Chamaenerion angustifolium*)

MAGICAL FORMS

an herbaceous wild flowering plant • called fireweed in North America; in some parts of Canada called the great willowherb; and in the UK, Europe, Asia, and Ireland called rosebay willowherb • a profusion of bright, tall, pink flower spikes, blooming in late summer • the white alba form is cultivated in gardens • opening first at the bottom, in Russia the top flowers welcome the fall • for centuries fermented in Russia to make herbal tea and used in folk medicine • leaves, shoots, and stems are usually considered edible if cooked • this plant sprang up in bombed cities such as Liverpool in the northwest UK after World War II and after the Great Fire of London in 1666, defiantly covering the devastation and uniting people in hope • fireweed honey is greatly prized though rare • magically use the aerial parts and honey

PLANETS AND ELEMENTS

Venus/Mars • Earth/Water/Fire

MAGICAL USES

rituals for the end of summer, welcoming the fall • rebirth, bringing life to stagnant situations and what has been abandoned because of its ability to regenerate spoiled land • through its specially adapted seeds with cottony fibers acting as tiny parachutes, it disperses over long distances and germinates immediately after fire

HOW TO USE

Collect the dried top flowers, especially around the fall, for charm sachets to ensure that better times will return after sickness, sorrow, or natural disasters. • Tie together the dried long stems in knot magick to bind families, communities, and companies together after a major reversal.

CAUTION

Avoid fireweed in pregnancy without expert advice.

Fireweed, Dwarf

(*Chamerion latifolium*)

MAGICAL FORMS

also called river beauty willowherb • purple or violet-pink, four-petal flowers with white stamens, flowering July to August • erect stems and willowy leaves • grows wild in the north of the northern hemisphere in river gravels after snow melts and at the edges of streams, including northern Europe, parts of the UK, northern North America, the Arctic and subarctic regions, and northern India • can be cultivated in moist places in gardens in cool climes • magically use the whole, growing plant; dried flowers; and flower essence

PLANET AND ELEMENT

Moon • Water

MAGICAL USES

the national flower of Greenland representing, like the land, survival even in the harshest times • as the flower and flower essence, for relieving shock, grief after loss, trauma after emotional or sexual abuse • gives strength to leave an abusive situation • to use after a major setback or emotional pain to move forward

HOW TO USE

Sip the essence in water or drink the tea made with leaves (avoid those leaves that are hairy) when memories threaten to overwhelm. • Shred the fading flowers and float them downstream from a bridge to let go of grief, anger, and a sense of loss. If they get stuck, accept that healing will take time. Go down to the actual water and drop them in. • Add the essence to a spritzer water bottle and spray around your head and shoulders to clear your aura of stuck or cloudy thoughts, especially if you must see people or visit situations that are connected to a loss or betrayal or from which you do not feel entirely free.

CAUTION

Consult a doctor before ingesting, even as a tea, if pregnant.

Five-Flower Rescue Cream

MAGICAL FORMS

cream made from the Five-Flower Rescue Remedy developed by Dr. Edward Bach, with the addition of essence of crab apple (*Malus sylvestris*), a fruit that is native to the USA • made by combining four drops of the rescue remedy that consists of Cherry Plum, Clematis, Impatiens, Rock Rose (also called Labdanum), and Star of Bethlehem (see p. 427) with five drops of crab apple • blended with shea butter

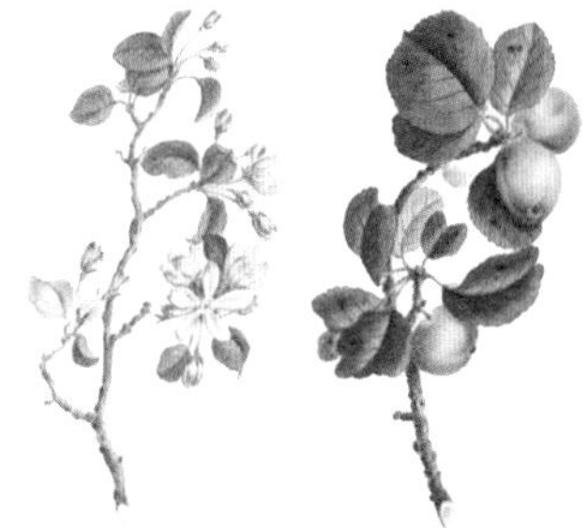

PLANETS AND ELEMENT

Moon/Venus • Water

MAGICAL USES

to protect hands, face, and body against environmental pollution • removing the stresses that are reflected in poor skin tone and rashes increased by anxiety • crab apple brings relief for those who dislike their appearance or personality • for counteracting obsessive-compulsive disorder, especially fear of germs and catching diseases without excessive hand washing

HOW TO USE

In massage, mix the cream with a few drops of gentle oils, such as lavender or rose, to improve your self-image before lovemaking if you fear you are unattractive and are unable to relax. • Rub into the skin to ease bruises and sites of muscle pain or tension, easing physical ailments by honing the body's restorative energies. • Considered effective for diaper rash.

Five-Flower Rescue Remedy

MAGICAL FORMS

developed by Dr. Edward Bach, the most famous flower remedy • combines essences of Cherry Plum, Clematis, Impatiens (also called Labdanum), and Star of Bethlehem • as liquid with a yellow dropper • gummies to chew at times of crisis

PLANETS AND ELEMENT

Moon, Venus/Water

MAGICAL USES

relieves anxiety • physical and emotional stress • panic attacks and hyperventilation • fears, especially when confronted with a phobia trigger • protects against shock from trauma, accidents, and abuse

HOW TO USE

Take the nighttime remedy, which adds white chestnut to the mix (see "Chestnut Tree," p. 118), under the tongue before bed to relieve insomnia caused by thoughts, worries, and nightmares. • Administer the remedy to defuse confrontational situations, both by those experiencing the crisis and those helping. • Cherry Plum (*Prunus cerasifera*) is used for controlling anger. • Clematis (*Clematis vitalba*) helps express suppressed emotions calmly. • Impatiens (*Impatiens glandulifera*) quells impatience and is helpful for ADHD children.

Flax

(*Linum usitatissimum*)

MAGICAL FORMS

a flowering plant cultivated as food and for its fibers • flax dates back to Neolithic times and is sacred to Holda, the wisewoman form of Frigg, the Norse Mother Goddess, who gave flax to humankind, teaching them to weave and also caring for unborn children • magically use the whole, growing plant; seeds; and oil

PLANET AND ELEMENT

Mercury • Air

MAGICAL USES

attracts money through sudden business opportunities • for luck in enterprise • brings happy, healthy, and quick-witted children • for increased awareness of household, workplace, and nature spirits

HOW TO USE

Use in rune rituals and Asatru magick. • Add a few flax seeds to a lidded ceramic pot each day, along with a coin, to incubate wealth. • Flax flowers or a sachet of flax and mustard seeds near the home entrance guard against hexes and malign magick. • Add flax and red pepper to a sachet kept under the mattress, which will protect you from predatory spirits of the night. • Encourage children to dance around these Mercury-ruled flowers on their seventh, fourteenth, and twenty-first birthdays, or do it on their behalf for their ongoing health, happiness, and exposure to fortuitous opportunities. • Use strong flax stems for knot magick. • Eat ground seeds to improve employment prospects. • Hide the whole seeds in corners on business premises to attract unexpected business.

CAUTION

In excess, flaxseed can cause bloating and stomachaches. • Stop ingesting flax two weeks before surgery because it acts as as estrogen, which can stimulate clotting. • Avoid in pregnancy or if you are having treatment for hormone-related cancers. • Seek advice if taking regular blood sugar, blood pressure, or blood clotting medications.

Fleabane

(*Erigeron* spp.)

MAGICAL FORMS

including common fleabane (*Erigeron annuus*), Mexican fleabane (*Erigeron karvinskianus*), and Philadelphia fleabane (*Erigeron philadelphicus*) • 390 varieties worldwide, 170 in the USA • *Erigeron annuus* is native to North America and found in almost every state in the USA • short white to pinkish petals surrounding a yellow center • loose clustered flowers on top of a single stem • blooms late spring through fall • may become seeds before the flowers fade • magically use the growing, flowering plant or the dried leaves and flowers

PLANET AND ELEMENT

Mars • Fire

MAGICAL USES

removes malevolent spirits from the home and prevents them from reentering • traditionally added to rushes on the floor of medieval houses or planted outside doors to kill fleas • still a deterrent to bugs, mice, and rats

HOW TO USE

Tie a sachet of dried fleabane mixed with capers and St. John's wort above the lintel of the front door. • Burn fleabane in incense or grow in a pot to remove low-level malicious spirits you may have unwittingly called up during a séance or spirit board session. • Carry a sachet of fleabane if you suffer from sexual inuendo or harassment at work or socially.

CAUTION

Common fleabane is mildly toxic to humans and pets if ingested.

Flour

MAGICAL FORMS

the result of an alchemical process converting grain to a refined product • one of the earliest staples, representing security and sustenance • magical substance that can increase resources and provide stabilizing energy in an uncertain money situation (see "Bread," p. 79, as well as the individual grains from which flour is created, such as "Wheat," p. 470) • magically use flour from your chosen source, especially if indigenous to your home or ancestral region, or from a local flour mill that sells to visitors where you can watch the process of its creation.

PLANET AND ELEMENT

Saturn • Earth

MAGICAL USES

for developing an idea into a viable financial form, as flour represents the staple ingredient of pancakes, bread, cookies, and pastry • mixing flour in a bowl fills it with your desires and needs, and adding other ingredients refines them; cooking creates a magical spell that conveys these energies and all those who consume the product absorb the results • for ventures that may take time and effort to fulfill

HOW TO USE

With a knife, write your intention into flour that you are mixing to add it to what you are baking. • Sprinkle a rough-grain flour on the floor of a new home, business, or workspace and sweep or vacuum it up to attract resources, especially if the previous owner or renter experienced misfortune or financial troubles. • Cook with refined white flour for conventional progress or unrefined flour for financial and property stability through creative or craft-based endeavors. • Put flour in the double pans of scales, one side with very little, and transfer from the full side to balance and therefore restore good fortune. • Take flour heaped in a single-pan scale and place it in a container to reduce debt, making sure you use the transferred flour in baking projects as soon as possible.

Flowering Currant

(*Ribes sanguineum*)

MAGICAL FORMS

including the cultivar 'Pulborough Scarlet' • flowering ornamental shrub with sweet-smelling clusters of dark-red or rose-pink tubular flowers (believed to house the fey before their summer location change) that cover the bush in April and May • native to western North America as far south as California • introduced into parks and gardens in the UK in 1817 • aromatic leaves • small black or dark-purple, edible, but not sweet, berries can be made into preserves and cordial • magically use the leaves and flowers in tea that can be purchased as teabags online, the growing plant in bloom, and the flower essence

PLANET AND ELEMENTS

Venus • Earth/Water

MAGICAL USES

to overcome inertia, despair, or lethargy • to treat seasonal affective disorder • to give purpose and the will to continue even if odds against you seem overwhelming • for healing the body that may be suffering as a result of mental pressures and opposition • the blossoming flowers should not be picked and taken indoors

HOW TO USE

In winter, during the brightest part of the day, take the essence or drink the tea brewed from the flowering currant to defeat seasonal blues and fill your body with the life force of the vibrant flowers. • Add the essence to water, shake well, and spritz around your aura energy field to fill yourself with the confidence to face and overcome problems head-on. • Meditate on the flowering plants, breathing in the rich color and aroma to connect with the fey world.

CAUTION

The essence is safe in pregnancy, as well as for children, pets, and other plants. • The plant is not toxic, but seek medical advice before ingesting the tea if pregnant.

Flowering Spurge

(*Euphorbia corollata*)

MAGICAL FORMS

wild flowering plant from an extensive genus of plants, not all of which are dangerous, though the sap tends to be toxic • blue-green leaves that redden with age • can grow to three feet • found in central and eastern North America, except for the northern areas of Canada; south and east Africa; southeastern Australia; New Zealand; and Europe • blooms June to October as five white, glandular appendages surrounding small, yellow flowers • an attractive ornamental plant in gardens, and a magnet for pollinators • magically use the flowering plant in situ without touching it and the dried flowers

PLANET AND ELEMENT

Saturn • Earth

MAGICAL USES

like many toxic plants, traditionally used as a boundary outside the home to protect against all harm, set where visitors will not brush against the sap • make an image of flowering spurge a screen saver or lock screen on a computer, tablet, or phone to repel hackers, viruses, malicious emails, and malevolent social media

HOW TO USE

Many experienced practitioners have a locked box in a high place with different labeled compartments for various toxic dried flowers and leaves to be used only for defensive magick against particularly vicious spirits and humans, not to harm but to repel. • Keep the flowers in a small dark bottle with thorns or tangled plants and sour milk or vinegar to be washed away under hot water down an outside drain or faucet and the drain washed out with an organic cleaning product and masses of water.

CAUTION

All parts of the plant are poisonous, particularly the sap. • Flowering spurge should not be ingested. • Handle only while wearing gloves. • Great care is needed around children, pets, and unwary visitors.

Forget-Me-Not

(*Myosotis sylvatica*)

MAGICAL FORMS
perennial plant with intensely blue blossoms • magically use growing plant and flowers

PLANET AND ELEMENT
Venus • Water

MAGICAL USES
for an absent, estranged, or undemonstrative lover, especially if your love is now with someone else and you still love them • to bring on dreams of lovers from past lives • in love spells meant to provoke a commitment, especially if you or your love must travel away • for positive experiences in online dating • to improve your memory for an examination, test, or assignment

HOW TO USE
Send to a love, ex-love, or desired lover on Valentine's Day to telepathically call you to their mind. • Hold the flowers before sending them, saying *Forget me not* nine times. • Grow in the garden and, when the flowers bloom, make a wish on the crescent moon for a past lover to return. • Keep a vase of the flowers indoors and grow living plants outside the front and back doors to enable chi to find its natural path. • Place near a photograph of a deceased family member to bring on happy memories and stay spiritually connected. • Keep in a love sachet including locks of hair from you and your love when you must be apart. • Carry in a bouquet at a wedding as "something blue" for lasting love.

CAUTION
Forget-me-nots are not to be used in pregnancy or while breastfeeding because of the potential for liver damage. • Check with a pharmacist or reputable herbalist and use only commercial products, if at all.

Forsythia

(*Forsythia* spp.)

MAGICAL FORMS
magically use the whole, growing plant when in golden bloom; the dried flowers; and the leaves

PLANET AND ELEMENTS
Sun • Fire/Air

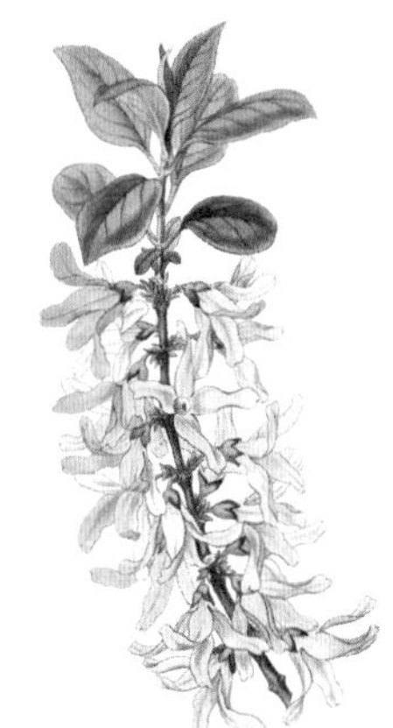

MAGICAL USES
increases self-confidence and improves self-image • provokes joy after sorrow • brings light and hope to any situation • abundance • wealth • excellent for forecasting long-term plans • health • beauty • use to mark the coming of spring and new beginnings when forsythia first blossoms, particularly if dark days or negative emotions seem endless

HOW TO USE
In love, confidence, and prosperity rituals, use forsythia to represent the four elements, four directions, and the four seasons. • Meditating on the yellow flowers, whether using the cut or live plant or while burning incense, fulfills long-term desires. • The flower represents the spring equinox and can be woven into trees or crowns to amplify its power. • In magical cookery, use as a syrup or in a gelatin for increasing radiance and charisma and enchanting a lover or would-be lover.

CAUTION
Forsythia may slow blood clotting, so avoid in pregnancy.

Foxglove

(*Digitalis purpurea*)

MAGICAL FORMS

native to western Europe • grows wild in many states of the USA and in gardens worldwide if there is a cool, moist climate • where it grows wild is said to mark a fey place • *Digitalis purpurea*, the most common kind of foxglove, is purple, pink, and white • the large yellow foxglove is found as *Digitalis grandiflora* • comes in other colors as there are numerous cultivars and hybrids • tall, upright stem with bell-shaped flowers • flowering season between June and September • the nontoxic flower essence amplifies the meaning of the flowers • magically use the growing flower in situ

PLANET AND ELEMENT

Moon • Water

MAGICAL USES

for bringing clarity to thoughts and decision-making • the "fox" in foxglove is a corruption of *folk*, meaning "the little people" in Celtic lands • flowers are called *fairy gloves* in Wales and *fairy bells* in Ireland • the flowers should not be picked, a wise precaution in view of its toxicity, and because it acts as shelter for tiny nature spirits and disturbing it will bring misfortune • when grown in the garden or an outdoor tub, it was believed to ward off evil spirits • in the language of flowers, foxglove represents the keeping of secrets

HOW TO USE

The flower essence is taken to prevent muddled thinking, offering a sense of direction to those who have lost their bearings in life. • Add the essence to baths, or mix it in massage oil and in sprays to help let go of old patterns, relationships, and free-floating anger. • Meditate or chant a mantra near the growing wild or cultivated flower to bring solutions to complex problems, which may appear in a prophetic dream the night after you do so (and to supercharge this process, anoint your brow with the essence before beginning meditation and before sleep).

CAUTION

The leaves, flowers, and seeds are highly toxic if eaten. Handle with care and keep the flowers away from children and pets.

Fragonia Shrub

(*Agonis fragrans*)

MAGICAL FORMS

found wild in Western Australia • grown commercially for the oil on large plantations in southwestern Australia • a shrub with white, tightly clustered flowers • magically use the essential oil, produced from the stems, twigs, and leaves

PLANET AND ELEMENT

Moon • Water

MAGICAL USES

releases emotional blockages, unwarranted guilt, and fears • increases ability to communicate feelings • boosts memory and focus • the white flowers used in bouquets, whether fresh or dried, can help to express what is hard to convey in words

HOW TO USE

For promoting harmony after a busy or stressful period, add a few drops of the oil to the bath, on a pillow, or diluted for a massage. • Create a spray for your room or workspace by diluting oil with water to create an oasis of calm even while the world is turning too fast. • Take a small stoppered bottle of fragonia mixed with lemon, lavender, and a gentle carrier oil to work or a social occasion and rub a drop onto pulse points to alleviate anxiety. • Inhale a little of the pure oil if you are worried about a meeting that may prove confrontational or before encountering people who make you feel insecure and inadequate.

CAUTION

Avoid fragonia in pregnancy and during lactation or if taking blood thinners or blood pressure medication. • Dilute before applying to the skin, and do not ingest.

Frankincense

(*Boswellia sacra*)

MAGICAL FORMS

from the incised bases of one of three Boswellia trees native to Saudi Arabia, Ethiopia, Somalia, India, and the East Indian islands • related to other fragrant gum trees, including myrrh • this huge tree can be grown in dry climates such as Arizona, southern California, and Nevada • magically use the sap—the gum resin of the tree, once hardened into a red glassy substance—as crystals for incense or as an essential oil

PLANET AND ELEMENT

Sun • Fire

MAGICAL USES

known from biblical times as a costly sacred incense • the ultimate Sun incense, for ceremonial magick • use in rituals relating to ambition, authority, expansion of business interests, travel, creative ventures, the performing arts, prosperity, and contact with Light Beings and those from other dimensions • use for help overcoming addictions • drives away bad influences and malicious spirits who may masquerade as beloved relatives

HOW TO USE

Burn the incense or diffuse the oil for past-life visions and dreams. • Use well-diluted oil for anointing chakra energy centers, especially the Crown and the Third Eye for power and protection. • Add a drop to pure sunflower or virgin olive oil (both Sun carrier oils) to anoint a white candle for success, wealth, or leadership. • Burn with bistort for increasing psychic powers and before divination. • On the midsummer solstice, use a lighted frankincense incense stick to write in the air over a gold candle, as it is the color of the sun, empowering fame, fortune, luck for those seeking to reach a desired travel destination, or confidence to imprint your wish on the ether. • Use in a bath with lavender and sandalwood oils for a sense of well-being and to restore your self-image if others have denigrated you or if you feel unloved or unlovely.

CAUTION

Do not use frankincense during pregnancy. • It can be a skin irritant, so dilute well.

Freesia

(*Freesia* spp.)

MAGICAL FORMS

including *Freesia refracta*, common freesia • magically use the whole, growing plant; cut flowers; and petals

PLANET AND ELEMENT

Venus • Water

MAGICAL USES

clarity where there is confusion • overcoming blockages and fears of change • for increasing trust • for friendship • increases belief in inner beauty so others admire you • corresponds with maternal love, especially in pink flower shades • to overcome opposition • happiness • astral projection • past lives • communication with angels • flower psychometry

HOW TO USE

Freesia can be used in potpourri combined with two or three of the following: chamomile, jasmine, honeysuckle, lavender, lilac, lilies, or roses to create a sense of well-being and attract abundance into the home. • Keep a pot near your home or work computer, or any location in which you do banking. • Add freesia blossoms to a bath or carry the dried petals in a pink sachet to ease anxiety due to change and transition, scattering them when you reach your destination or goal. • Freesia is excellent for wedding bouquets and is the seventh anniversary flower, which is a natural time for a couple to be planning the next seven years and is also traditionally a time of restlessness in a relationship (sometimes called the seven-year itch). • Inhale the scent from freesia flowers or potpourri to awaken the psychic senses, which can help you explore the past, future, and even other dimensions.

CAUTION

Freesia can cause skin irritation.

Fuchsia

(*Fuchsia* spp.)

MAGICAL FORMS

the *Fuchsia* genus has over a hundred different species, including *Fuchsia triphylla* and *Fuchsia magellanica* • can be grown indoors or out • magically use the whole, growing plant; berries; leaves; and flowers

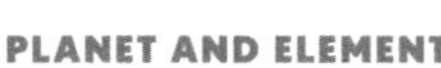

PLANET AND ELEMENT

Mercury • Air

MAGICAL USES

to promote honest dealings • aligns with the energy of following one's own path and rejoicing in uniqueness, spontaneity, and allowing the inner child to come out to play • brings deep love and trust and heals sorrow and abuse

HOW TO USE

The flowers are favored in folklore as a home for the fey. • Fuchsia's tubular flowers, flaring petals, and long white sepals act as ladders for fairies. • Leave crystal offerings and honey to keep their influence in home and garden benign. • All parts of the plant are edible, so they are ideal for magical cookery such as cakes. • Use the flowers and berries in jams, chutneys, and cookies, and the flowers and leaves as decorations to bring everlasting love, enchantment, and happiness to your family. • Hold a flower to reveal when someone is lying or unfaithful. • Make a chain of fuchsia, using string if necessary, each flower representing a wish, and hang the chain on a tree to blow away in order for those wishes to come true.

Fumitory

(*Fumaria officinalis*)

MAGICAL FORMS

also called Earth Smoke because it was believed the first plant rose from the vapors deep within the earth • magically use the growing plant and all parts except the root

PLANET AND ELEMENT

Saturn • Earth

MAGICAL USES

traditionally used to drive away bad spirits growing close to your home • fumitory will reverse bad fortune and attract money, both personally and in the workplace • used to purify ritual tools and ritual spaces, especially before major ceremonies • described from Roman times as a medicinal and protective plant

HOW TO USE

Fumitory is burned on bonfires, especially at Halloween, as the smoke drives away evil spirits and bad spells. • It can also be used as incense in the home to remove poltergeists, sexual demons, and restless ghosts from the land on which your home is built. • Sprinkle a trail of the dried, chopped herb downstairs around a new home, starting with the front door and moving out through the back door to banish evil spirits. • Alternately, sprinkle the herb front to back then vacuum front to back to remove all unlucky or sorrowful vibes left over from a previous owner. • Keep dried flowers and leaves with a tiger's eye or citrine crystal in a magic bag close to a source of heat to attract money into your home, or hidden where you handle money for business purposes.

CAUTION

Use in moderate quantities only with the advice of a doctor; some question its safety if ingested. • Avoid if pregnant or breastfeeding.

Galangal, Lesser and Greater

(*Alpinia officinarum*) and (*Alpinia galanga*)

MAGICAL FORMS

also known as Low John the Conqueror • magically use the growing plant, mainly the root

PLANET AND ELEMENT

Mars • Fire

MAGICAL USES

both lesser and greater galangal have the same magical properties • justice and resistance against intimidation by officialdom especially if corrupt • in charm bags, the root is used as a substitute for High John the Conqueror root, which is very toxic • success in all official matters • for good results in examinations and on tests • called "the spice of life" given by God to keep away illness by the twelfth-century German mystic Hildegard von Bingen

HOW TO USE

Worn or carried, the root brings good luck in legal matters. • Galangal increases favorable outcomes in court cases or official hearings. • For fortunate outcomes, put galangal on top of summonses. • A sachet containing the root and three pieces of silver attracts lasting prosperity. • The powdered root in an incense mix removes curses, hexes, jinxes, and ill wishes. • To increase passion, sprinkle under the bed.

CAUTION

Galangal root is mildly hallucinogenic, so apart from quantities taken in food, it is best to avoid ingesting or inhaling. • If in doubt, use ginger instead.

Galbanum

(*Ferula galbaniflua*) and (*Ferula gummosa*)

MAGICAL FORMS

amber-colored gum resin extracted from the roots and lower stem of this wild plant, now mainly grown on the northern slopes of the mountains of Iran, in Turkey, and in parts of the Mediterranean • it can grow to be four or more feet tall • from the fennel family • available worldwide from specialty magical stores and online • traditionally, the resin is magically used in incense and oil

PLANETS AND ELEMENT

Jupiter/Sun • Fire

MAGICAL USES

a ceremonial oil and incense dating back to ancient Egyptian times, when it could only be used by royalty, as mentioned in ancient Egyptian papyri • in the book of Exodus, galbanum is one of the main ingredients in the sacred incense burned in the temple of Solomon that also included frankincense and myrrh • galbanum remains a significant part of formal ritual magick for incense burning and anointing sacred artifacts • lifts the soul magically and spiritually to new heights

HOW TO USE

Burn the woody, earthy incense or diffuse the oil during meditation to receive visions of ancient temples and ceremonies. • Galbanum can also reprogram old ideas and attitudes by allowing you to step temporarily beyond the physical world and commune with spirit guardians. • Dilute the oil and anoint your Third Eye, located in the center of your brow, with the shape of an eye to remove the evil eye of envy from your life and seal it against future attack and all harm, both paranormal and earthly. • Anoint candles with a drop of the oil for rituals of blessing, connecting with all who have practiced and sometimes suffered for their spiritual beliefs.

CAUTION

Though cited medicinally in the writings of Hippocrates, the ancient Greek father of Western medicine, and the Roman philosopher Pliny the Elder, it is not certain if galbanum oil is safe to ingest. • It may react with medications such as blood thinners and diabetes regulators. • Avoid the oil and inhaling the incense during pregnancy.

Gardenia

(*Gardenia jasminoides*)

MAGICAL FORMS

also known as the cape jasmine • magically use mainly the flower petals, whether fresh or dried

PLANET AND ELEMENT

Moon • Water

MAGICAL USES

healing • bringing peace • attracting new friends, love, and lovers • increasing meditative and spiritual powers • use in the garden or home to call good spirits and for nature spirit magick • enhances radiance and charisma

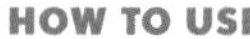

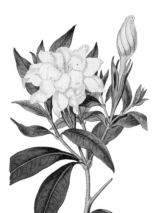

HOW TO USE

Fresh blossoms increase healing, so give to those who are ill. • If dried, use in an incense mix, especially on the full moon. • Dried gardenia scattered over thresholds brings and maintains domestic and workplace peace. • Use the diluted oil in baths. • Wearing a blossom will attract love like a magnet. • In perfumes, gardenia has an aphrodisiac quality. • The flower speaks to harmony in the years ahead when used as a bouquet in wedding or handfasting ceremonies. • Give a properly empowered pot as a housewarming gift for a happy home. • Gift one to a secret love or admirer.

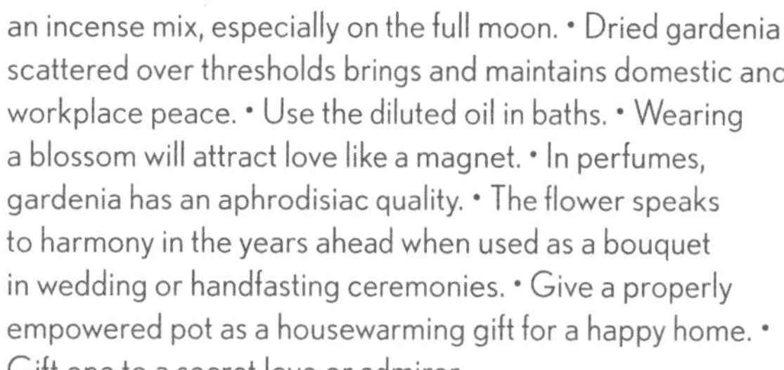

CAUTION

The oil is not recommended for pregnancy, during breastfeeding, or for children. • Use with a carrier oil.

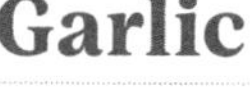

Garlic

(*Allium sativum*)

MAGICAL FORMS

magically use the growing plant, mainly the harvested clove

PLANET AND ELEMENT

Mars • Fire

MAGICAL USES

the ultimate domestic protection • psychic defense, especially against unfriendly spirits, envy, and emotional vampires • for calling the wise ancestors • increases passion • for use in magical cookery (as long as both parties eat the enchanted meal)

HOW TO USE

Traditionally, garlic is left at crossroads on All Hallows Eve in honor of Hecate, the ancient Greek crone goddess who signifies the intersection of past, present, and future. • Set on west-facing window ledges, also on All Hallows Eve, to welcome the ancestors and keep out malicious ghosts roaming free at this time and in the two days following. • A string of garlic on the kitchen ceiling keeps away all danger from the home, guards against accidents in the kitchen, and should be replaced when the cloves begin to shrivel (but they should not be eaten!). • To remove warts or skin blemishes, a clove should be rubbed on the afflicted place and then buried.

CAUTION

Avoid eating garlic in excess if pregnant or when using blood thinners, or when about to undergo surgery.

Garlic, Wild

(*Allium ursinum*)

MAGICAL FORMS

shoots of the broad, spear-like leaves appear in mid-February • a profusion of starry, white flowers appears in March or April, and seeds by June • magically use the cut or whole, growing plant

PLANET AND ELEMENTS

Mars • Fire/Earth

MAGICAL USES

Allium ursinum means "bear's garlic" because traditionally bears ate wild garlic to regain their strength after hibernation; it was also sought by boars and badgers, so it is linked with magical strength and courage • for discovering power animals and, as dried flowers, for spontaneous as opposed to formal ritual magick for recalling past lives because blooms invariably grow in ancient woodlands • repels malevolent spirits • for healing, especially when the flowers are in bloom

HOW TO USE

Wild garlic is planted in the thatch of Irish cottages to ward off bad luck and the enchantment of malevolent faeries; when planted in gardens, it is similarly protective against earthly and paranormal harm and garden and external house repair accidents. • Roman soldiers and the Celts ate wild garlic to bring them victory, and so wild garlic, especially for spells cast among the flowers, has strong attracting properties for success involving action and facing difficult odds.

CAUTION

Their leaves are similar to lily of the valley, which is poisonous, so crush to test for garlicky smell and still exercise care if harvesting wild. • Wild garlic can cause allergic reactions, especially if someone is allergic to onions or leeks. • Avoid using if you are taking anticoagulants.

Gentian

(*Gentiana* spp.)

MAGICAL FORMS

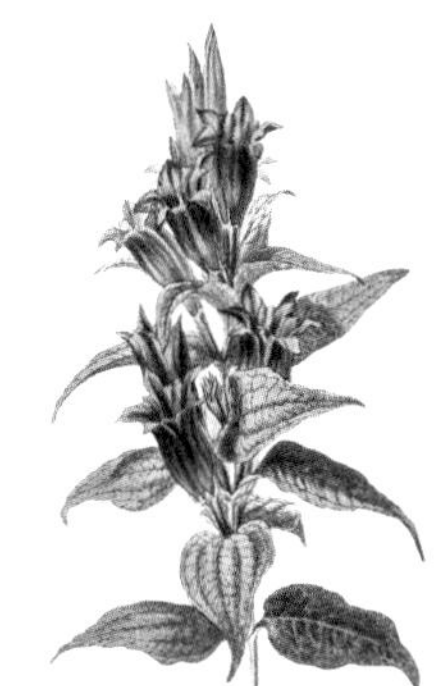

grows in all sizes • among the smallest is the spring gentian, *Gentiana verna* • frequently cultivated in gardens, especially rock gardens, as well as in containers • magically use the whole, growing plant, as well as the seeds and flowers, which are famed for their many hues of blue

PLANET AND ELEMENT

Mars • Fire

MAGICAL USES

adds power to any spells or incense mixes • gives courage to resist and overcome human snakes and those who betray • used in color magick and flower psychometry • enables connection with higher realms, especially angels and Beings of Light, through meditating on particularly beautiful blue flowers in sunlight, outdoors, against a blue sky

HOW TO USE

Add the flowers to love bath sachets to increase radiance and attract love. • Draw a particular lover to you by writing their name with the index finger of your writing hand over and over in the bathwater. • Include dried flowers or dried, chopped root in an incense mix to break a curse, hex, jinx, or ill wishes. • If you want to magically uncross an obstacle someone has put in your way, cross two sticks, uncross them, declare yourself free, and cast them into a bonfire or bury them along with dried gentian root, then walk away—you're free. • Know that you have harmed no one, just merely removed ill wishes. • Alternatively, scatter the seeds to the four winds, releasing yourself by calling out loud from whom or what you seek to be freed.

CAUTION

Medicinally, avoid in pregnancy, when breastfeeding, and while taking medication for blood pressure or ulcers.

Geranium

(*Pelargonium* spp.)

MAGICAL FORMS

many varieties, including the fragrant *Pelargonium odoratissimum* • magically use the whole, growing plant; flower petals, either fresh or dried; leaves; and essential oil

PLANETS AND ELEMENTS

Moon/Venus • Water/Earth

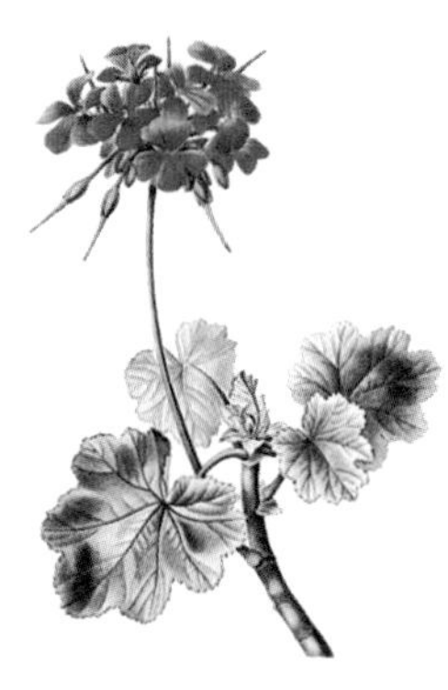

MAGICAL USES

amplifies happiness and friendship • a catalyst for reunions with old friends • brings or restores love • for harmony in the home and workplace • heals coldness and indifference • diminishes self-doubt and fear of failure, and discourages overcritical people • deters intruders • increases fertility

HOW TO USE

Pink or red geraniums planted in the garden or indoors as potted plants create protective barriers and keep away snakes, both reptilian and human. • White geranium petals added to incense bring fertility and confidence while socializing. • In magical cookery, include in a tea or cake to call love in. • Use fresh red or pink geranium leaves to anoint doorknobs and windows in order to protect the home. • Add a few drops of oil to a protective floor wash.

CAUTION

Geraniums are nontoxic for pets or humans, but the oil may occasionally cause skin irritation if not well diluted.

Gerbera Daisy

(*Gerbera jamesonii*)

MAGICAL FORMS

also known as the Transvaal daisy • closely related to the African daisy (a cultivar), but they are different species • similar also to gazania, called the treasure flower • gerbera is the national flower of Eritrea in Africa • use the growing plant in vivid colors • cut flowers, especially in white for weddings (the White Queen is an appropriate variety), are also potent magically • fresh and dried petals work as well

PLANET AND ELEMENT

Sun • Fire

MAGICAL USES

gift white varieties to express love between generations • a bouquet, pot, or growing patch of gerbera releases the inner child and generates spontaneous joy, especially in its orange form • use the red variety for falling head over heels in love • gerbera is more proactive than the African daisy and less materially oriented than the treasure flower • send red flowers for a partner's birthday, particularly if life has become routine • pink is good for celebrating a newborn baby, whether at a naming ceremony or baptism

HOW TO USE

Since the flower will always turn toward the sun, use gerbera in yellow, red, or orange for sun magick on any Sunday. • Place in the center of your altar or, if a live plant, wherever it is growing, for rituals related to success, new ventures, leadership bids, and hopes of fame and fortune. • Meditate or practice pranic breathing or any form of focused breathwork in the evening when the flowers naturally release oxygen, expelling darkness and fears. • Inhale the golden life force to incubate during your sleep. • Manifest in the morning as pure energy. • Binding the flower in gold ribbon attracts your twin soul. • When the flower fades, carry the dried petals in a gold bag to any social event or interview, audition, or performance for confidence and double the luck.

Gerbera Daisy, Orange Germini

cultivar of (*Gerbera* spp.)

MAGICAL FORMS

the sunshine flower is a miniature form of the large gerbera or Transvaal daisy • part of the sunflower family • a concentrated source of sunshine and light • there are several equally vibrant orange varieties you can choose, including allure and baila • magically use the whole, growing plant; cut fresh or dried flowers; or fresh or dried petals

PLANET AND ELEMENT

Sun • Fire

MAGICAL USES

though available in many colors (pink, purple, red, yellow, and white), the brilliant mini-orange gerbera offers a powerful sun connection, and with Michael, archangel of the sun • a suggested flower for the forty-first wedding anniversary, sometimes called the land anniversary because a couple may be thinking of buying a vacation home, relocating upmarket, downsizing, or even buying a patch of land • for weddings in sunny places as bouquets, or centerpieces for engagement parties and baby showers

HOW TO USE

Display three flowers in a vase in the bedroom as the ultimate fertility symbol, the middle flower's stem cut shorter to represent a baby, the flowers loosely tied with orange ribbons. • Pluck petals from flowers (a dozen or more), fill a basket, and then ask everyone present at a party where family or friends have not met for a while to take a handful and scatter them outdoors, making wishes for the happiness of everyone present and the occasion being celebrated. • Keep three small, orange, dried flowers with three orange crystals in a sunshine bag, hanging it on a suncatcher where the morning sun enters and the breeze circulates to keep joy, health, harmony, and enthusiasm flowing through the home or workplace. Replace the contents on Midsummer Day at noon.

CAUTION

Use with care if pregnant.

Ghost Plant

(*Monotropa uniflora*)

MAGICAL FORMS

also known as Native American ghost pipe • a rare wild parasitic plant with white stems and flowers • three to nine inches high • native to temperate zones of North America, northern South America, and Asia • white because it does not contain chlorophyll, but feeds off particular fungi attached to trees and does not need light • a bell-like single flower that appears between late spring and fall • can be grown in gardens, but it is difficult as there must be a host tree—often a beech—and the correct fungus and shade • magically work with the growing plant in the wild or in a woodland area of a botanical garden

PLANETS AND ELEMENT

Moon/Venus • Earth

MAGICAL USES

use the growing flowers at twilight or in the dark for connection with the wise ancestors and woodland nature spirits • a symbol of making peace with the past and those who have passed over • protection against malevolent spirits

HOW TO USE

Sit close to the plants to send and receive messages from beloved deceased relatives. • Hang to keep away nighttime specters, especially incubi and succubi, sexual spirit predators. • Hang an enlarged print of the flowering ghost plants facing the front door, and then burn a white candle on special anniversaries, Halloween, and the following two days (the Days of the Dead) to welcome the wise ancestors.

CAUTION

Though the whole dried plant was traditionally favored for pain relief, as well as to treat respiratory and digestive disorders, and is still used in tinctures and teas, the plant is considered slightly toxic and also mildly hallucinogenic. • It is not recommended to ingest except on medical advice.

Ghost Tree

(*Davidia involucrata*)

MAGICAL FORMS

also known as handkerchief tree • a tree native to the woodlands of southwestern China • introduced into Europe, the UK, and North America in 1904 • grown as an ornamental tree • upwards of forty feet tall with a single, small, bisexual red or purple flower held between a pair of huge, showy, creamy, oval, white bracts in April and May, that appear like handkerchiefs or the archetypal ghost in a white sheet • the bracts wave in the slightest breeze and so the tree is also known as the dove tree • magically use the dried or fresh bracts, or the growing tree

PLANET AND ELEMENT

Mercury • Air

MAGICAL USES

helps in speaking telepathically to an absent loved one you may not have seen for some time • for bringing peace if there has been an estrangement • for recalling loved ones who have departed this life, as it can send and receive messages on the breeze • in the world-famous Kew Botanical Gardens in London, the flowering of the Kew handkerchief tree was at one time announced every May in *The Times* journal

HOW TO USE

Sit in the wind below the waving bracts (you may need to find your tree in a botanical garden or park). Gaze up at the "handkerchiefs," allowing their rhythm to lull you into other dimensions so you feel close to someone no longer with you either temporarily or permanently. • Dry two or three fallen bracts and put them, with or without the enclosed flower, in a white charm bag to carry to work or hang on a wall in the area where family and visitors are most likely to relax for ongoing peace and harmony. • It can also be used to reunite LGBTQ couples.

Giant Honey Flower

(*Melianthus major*)

MAGICAL FORMS

bush grows in hotter parts of North America, notably in southern California and seasonally as an ornamental in cooler zones of the continent and around the world • fresh and dried bluish-green to silvery foliage • leaves and flowers are brewed as teas • magically use the fresh and dried honey-scented, brownish-crimson to maroon flowers; the whole, growing plant; and the papery seed pods after flowering, holding black hard-shelled seeds

PLANET AND ELEMENT

Sun • Fire

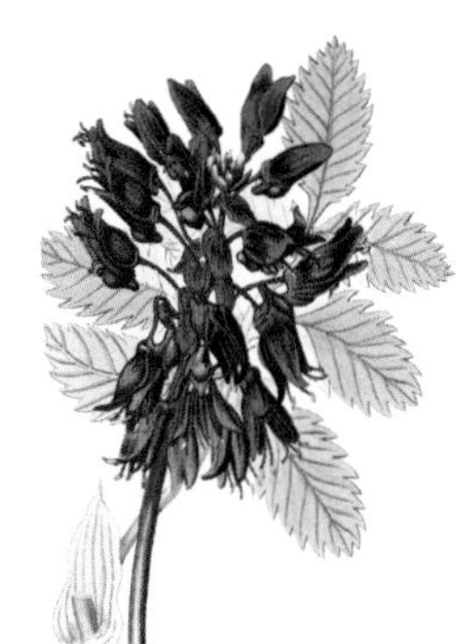

MAGICAL USES

attracts fertility, abundance, happiness, and sunshine energies whatever the time of the year or weather • a good base red tea like rooibos but sweeter and lifts the energies of other herbs and flowers used in teas

HOW TO USE

Grow the bush outside the door or in patio or conservatory containers to bring fun and laughter into the home. • Offer tea at informal celebrations and share to spread cheer with gloomy folk or in unpromising situations. • Place the seeds in a charm bag to carry for successful money transactions or negotiations, and afterward scatter the seeds to the winds. • Break open the seed pods and cast them into water to bring fertility during the waxing moon.

Giant Redwood Tree

(*Sequoiadendron giganteum*)

MAGICAL FORMS

enormous tree growing on the western slopes of the Sierra Nevada • relatedly, coast redwood (*Sequoia sempervirens*), grows on the narrow coastal band of five hundred miles from Monterey, California, to the Oregon border • the qualities of these gigantic trees are reflected in their magical properties • redwoods may be more than 330 feet high and up to 3,500 years old, with intertwining shallow roots that spread outward, intertwining and even fusing with other redwoods in their community • magically use the whole, growing tree and fresh and dried leaves

PLANET AND ELEMENT

Sun • Fire

MAGICAL USES

for rituals for family, community, workplace, or more global unity • for lofty ambitions that may take time to fulfill • for regeneration, since the new tree shoots grow from the roots of a dead tree • for networking and extending influence rituals • for entering or advancing in politics • creating or joining a franchise • turning around an ailing business • establishing companies involved in beauty and luxury • starting a dating or recruitment agency on- or offline

HOW TO USE

Link the earth with the heavenly realms by traveling the tree's great height by sitting on the ground next to one, gazing up to the top of the tree, or adding the dried leaves to an incense mix. • Create or buy a wand or staff to use in ritual or hold in front of you for connecting with personal past worlds. • Obtain an opalized redwood or redwood opal, petrified wood from an ancient extinct redwood forest in Mexico, similar in color and banded formation to living redwood. Carry this as a lucky charm for long life, the growth of ventures, and for making connection with a past love, estranged family member, or close friend with whom you have lost touch. • Meditate on the fossilized redwood stone for visions of ancient lands, especially those indigenous to the tree.

Gillyflower

(*Matthiola incana*)

MAGICAL FORMS

also known as stock flower or hoary stock • magically use the whole, growing plant, or as cut or dried flowers

PLANET AND ELEMENT

Venus • Earth

MAGICAL USES

dedicated to the ancient Greek Aphrodite, goddess of love (the Romans linked Aphrodite with Venus) • brings family joy • for gentleness • the ultimate celebration gift flower • in China, a symbol of good fortune, often given at Chinese New Year

HOW TO USE

The white gillyflower is used in bouquets at weddings and for new parents. • On an altar, this flower brings connection with angels and Beings of Light and can form the centerpiece of a love altar or ritual. • Red flowers are a gift for Valentine's Day and special anniversaries and are offered as a token of lasting love. • Pink flowers are for Mother's Day and friendship; white are for when your mother is no longer on earth or in your life. • Purple flowers express congratulations for a major success. • Meditate on gillyflowers and the scent will connect you with higher realms and call the blessings of the house and family guardians. • Added to potpourri, dried pink blossoms increase happiness at home and at informal parties with friends and family, especially if there are newcomers to the family present. • In magical cookery, the flowers are edible and offer special adornments to celebratory cakes and desserts according to their color. • Carry the dried, white blossoms in a sachet to keep away ill-wishers socially and at work. • Hang a large bag of dried flowers of mixed colors over the front door to keep away malicious spirits and all who would threaten domestic happiness, and also to attract wealth and abundance.

Ginger

(*Zingiber officinale*)

MAGICAL FORMS

best but not exclusively grown in warm climates or indoors in pots • used for three thousand years in China • believed to have originated in the Garden of Eden • magically use rhizomes or growing plant

PLANET AND ELEMENT

Mars • Fire

MAGICAL USES

perfect for all money-making enterprises, especially speculative, and to reverse the outflow of money • used when a new, bold financial approach is needed • for exploration, energy, and health • brings or renews passion • good for travel, as well as new ventures and enterprises • brings success, power, promotion, and leadership • for adding speed to any urgent need • use root as substitute for galangal • a spice for Lughnasadh and Lammas, as well as Thanksgiving

HOW TO USE

Add to a charm bag with three small pieces of gold to attract wealth or a wealthy, passionate lover. • Make ginger and honey tea for someone you would like to know better in the workplace and stir in the energy of your power of attraction. • Burn ginger and other spice incense sticks if business or the stock market is not in your favor. • Empower your jar of ginger in magical cooking for whatever you need urgently. • For protection, place in a protective bottle with sour milk and iron nails and then bury the bottle.

Gingko Biloba

(*Gingko biloba*)

MAGICAL FORMS

also commonly called the maidenhair tree (different botanically, but has leaves that are visually similar to the maidenhair fern) • its genus first appeared 290 million years ago, and its form is virtually unchanged • magically use the growing tree, with large fanlike leaves that are rich yellow in the fall, but do not flower, and the individual leaves, dried or preferably fresh, for tea

PLANET AND ELEMENT

Saturn • Earth

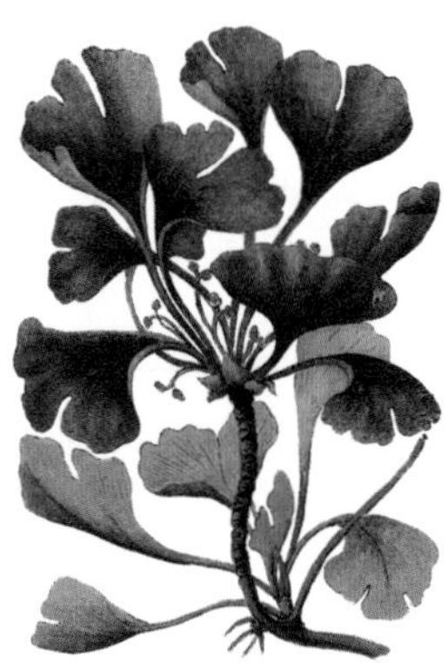

MAGICAL USES

because of its age (the oldest existing tree is 3,500 years old, growing in China), use for an amulet or tea for long life and against illnesses linked to aging • for past-life meditation • keeps long-term partners faithful • for male potency • cultivated since ancient times in Chinese and Japanese temples • often called a Tree of Life • gingko tolerates cold weather • though widely cultivated throughout the world, it is endangered • the national tree of China

HOW TO USE

The yellow fall leaves can be dried for a long-term money-attracting charm bag. Add eight Chinese divinatory coins, then keep inside a cash register if you have a business, or where you do your banking at home or work. • Surround a golden candle with a circle of the dried herb, sprinkle a little of the dried herb in the flame, or roll the candle in the herb before lighting for abundance in all things. • Plant a small tree for a newborn baby to ensure a long, healthy life and that the infant will become wise.

CAUTION

If you take regular medication such as anticoagulants, check with your physician or an experienced herbalist before using gingko biloba.

Ginseng

(*Panax ginseng*)

MAGICAL FORMS

this is the true ginseng, though other herbs adopt its name • also American ginseng (*Panax quinquefolius*), which is endangered in the wild • called the "Wonder of the World" plant • grows in a number of regions in North America as well as its original home in China, Korea, and other Asian countries • use the sturdy roots in various forms: whole, chopped, or powdered are the part of the plant mainly used in magick and for making the healing and empowering tea • white ginseng is made using the dried root, and red ginseng by drying and steaming the root • both are equally potent in healing and magick

PLANETS AND ELEMENT

Mars/Sun • Fire

MAGICAL USES

to call forth protection, love, and charisma • to acquire things of beauty and worth • to fulfill wishes through visualization and ritual chanting • for male potency and renewed energy

HOW TO USE

The root is an all-purpose charm to attract whatever it is you want when carried in a bag or placed in the home or workplace. • Alternatively, make an intention to attract all good things and to keep away harm through your enchanted root. • Some practitioners etch wishes, whether specific or all-purpose, on the side of the root and then cast it into flowing water. • Burn the powdered root in incense to break a curse or ill wishes. • Endow the tea with whatever strengths or healing you most need as you stir it. • Share the brew with a lover to experience passionate lovemaking, especially if one of you has inhibitions.

CAUTION

Because it is a stimulant, don't ingest ginseng if you drink a lot of coffee. • Avoid if pregnant or breastfeeding, or if you have diabetes.

Ginseng Ficus

(*Ficus macrocarpa*) or (*Ficus retusa*)

MAGICAL FORMS

a popular species of tree used in producing bonsai miniature trees: the two kinds often are grafted together • also called the Chinese banyan • member of the fig family and native to China, tropical Asia, and Australia, where it is known as the Moreton Bay fig • the ficus ginseng bonsai shares many of the characteristics of its big sister in compact form • mainly grown indoors with many elevated visible roots, making the belly-shaped, often red, trunk appear as though on legs, resembling a ginseng root • hence the name but not the medicinal properties • can live up to a hundred years • magically use the whole miniature tree

PLANET AND ELEMENT

Sun • Fire

MAGICAL USES

often gifted for a seventy-third anniversary or a house-warming • place the tree where air can circulate to attract abundance, health, fertility, wealth, and positive energies • filters out whatever is physically, psychologically, or spiritually toxic • use your bonsai as a focus for family unity-building sessions and to peacefully iron out differences • strongly linked with the Chinese wood element, the ginseng ficus bonsai encourages creativity, growth, and springtime energies all year long

HOW TO USE

In Chinese style and in the spirit of Japanese Zen, create a miniature garden around your tree with rocks, greenery, crystals, and a small water feature as an oasis of calm and for meditation. • Traditionally believed to house spirits, your ginseng ficus will welcome your house and workplace guardians to ensure continuing blessings on your home and/or workspace and to keep away all harm.

CAUTION

The ginseng ficus is toxic if ingested, so keep away from children and pets. • In tropical conditions, your bonsai may produce berrylike figs, but these are not good to eat. • If you have a latex allergy, take care around the sap.

Gladiolus

(*Gladiolus* spp.)

MAGICAL FORMS

called the sword flower because of its tall, spiky flower and long, grasslike foliage resembling the base of a sword • magically use the growing plant, cut flowers, and fresh and dried blossoms

PLANET AND ELEMENT

Mars • Fire

MAGICAL USES

promotes strength, especially of character • courage • generosity • integrity • soothes the pain of unrequited love • was the flower of Roman gladiators because the winner would be showered with gladioli; therefore it represents the idea of never giving up • gladiolus is the flower of Friendship Day on the first Sunday in August

HOW TO USE

The gladiolus flower is used instead of a wand in rituals for courage. • In Victorian times, a single red gladiolus was sent as a sign of undying love with the message "You pierce my heart with your sword." • Traditionally, the leaves of cut plants are tied together facing down in protection spells or hung over the bed. • Red gladioli are a Valentine's Day gift or can be sent on anniversaries. • White gladioli are added to wedding bouquets for eternal happiness and fidelity and also sent to funerals if the deceased had lived a distinguished, honorable life. • Purple flowers signify congratulations on a new job or a major success. • Yellow wishes a speedy recovery from illness, positive energy for a housewarming, or appreciation for coworkers. • Pink flowers are great for a date night, Mother's Day, or to celebrate the birth of a baby.

CAUTION

Gladioli are toxic if ingested by pets. While traditionally used in healing, the root is poisonous to humans and pets. • Though cooking the root may remove the toxicity, the sap can cause irritation to sensitive skin, so take care when handling.

Gladiolus, Byzantine

(*Gladiolus communis* subsp. *byzantinus*)

MAGICAL FORMS

called the heirloom flower of the gladiolus family, a traditional form of this elegant-colored, orchidlike, funnel-shaped wildflower, blooming from late May to mid-June • native to southern Europe and northern Africa, it grows in the wild in England having escaped from gardens • grown in the south of the USA for hundreds of years • thrives in thirty-nine states from coastal Maine to southern California, notably in Georgia, Alabama, and South Carolina • found growing in old cemeteries and the land and boundaries of abandoned homes blooming from late spring to early summer • first mentioned in the USA in 1629 • magically use the growing flowers in situ, and cut or dried flowers

PLANET AND ELEMENT

Saturn • Earth

MAGICAL USES

act as a detective, find Byzantine gladiolus in old abandoned settings, sit among the flowers and let them carry you back to the place as it used to be and those who brought flowers to now abandoned cemeteries or grew them in their gardens • for planting, if necessary in a container, to restore tradition to a modern or impersonal home

HOW TO USE

Surround a lit purple candle with the dried flowers, scenting them with a timeless fragrance, such as lavender or rose, to travel back to fields of wildflowers where once you walked and maybe encounter people or situations that will offer answers to the present. • Use the cut flowers in a bouquet or venue decoration for people getting married or remarried later in life, for renewal of vows, and as a substitute for ordinary gladiolus as the fortieth wedding flower as a pledge of timeless love.

CAUTION

The roots are toxic to dogs, cats, and horses. • Avoid during pregnancy as a precaution.

Glastonbury Thorn Tree

(*Crataegus monogyna biflora*)

MAGICAL FORMS

originated in the Middle East • biennial flowering, with white blossoms at Christmas and Easter • grows mainly around the Glastonbury area in southwestern England • the plant is said to come from an original tree planted in 64 CE • a Glastonbury thorn may be found in the New York Botanic Gardens • to grow one yourself you will need to graft a cutting from a Glastonbury thorn (ask for help from a specialty tree center) on to an ordinary hawthorn rootstock • magically use the growing tree and the essence

PLANETS AND ELEMENTS

Mercury/Mars • Air/Fire

MAGICAL USES

acts as a center for outdoor ritual and meditation • the original holy thorn was said to have appeared when Joseph of Arimathea arrived in Glastonbury in southwestern England carrying the Holy Grail after the crucifixion • Joseph's staff, set on the ground, burst into flower • the essence, like all thorns, has a reputation for courage and staying power, as well as repelling negative influences • the essence supports the user through transitions, especially unwilling ones to bring peace and acceptance • cleanses and purifies troubled energies, restoring a harmonious inner self

HOW TO USE

Wherever you live in the world, you can call in meditation from the Guardian of the Glastonbury Thorn to take you back to the ancient worlds of the Holy Grail, King Arthur, and the misty Isle of Avalon. • Anoint your Third Eye and the middle of your hairline for your Crown energy spiritual center. • Add a drop or two to a warm bath for children who are afraid of the dark or ghosts, telling them stories of brave King Arthur and his knights (probably the fifth-century Celtic king who defended England against the Anglo-Saxons).

CAUTION

The essence is quite safe, but the tree is not intended for consumption, though hawthorn trees generally are not considered toxic.

Gnocchi

MAGICAL FORMS

potato based, parcel-like dumplings, introduced by the Romans into Europe and by Italian settlers into North America, Canada, Australia, and New Zealand • potatoes bring security and stability and any chosen plant-based additions increase this food's magical properties • for example, tomatoes used in the sauce add the energy of wealth, health, and fertility; garlic adds protection; semolina or wheat flour produces abundance; basil adds passion and is a money bringer

PLANETS AND ELEMENTS

Saturn/Mercury • Earth/Air

MAGICAL USES

incorporate all the strengths of the ingredients in a chant as you add and combine them to make gnocchi, or as you place the ready-to-cook gnocchi in the pan, maybe adding extra significant herbs • use the preparation (making, mixing, rolling, shaping, filling, sealing, and stirring) of your creation (or ready-prepared gnocchi) in the pan, as well as the serving of your dish, as you would a magick spell: raise the power, release it in the cooking, and absorb it as you and others eat

HOW TO USE

Place any natural peelings or eggshells in a compost or food bin so no resources will be wasted throughout the days ahead. • Gnocchi is traditionally eaten on the twenty-ninth day of the month to enable you to have the money to pay what you owe and need in the coming month. • On a non-leap year, bury a small portion of gnocchi in the earth on the twenty-eighth day of the month before sharing. • For luck in personal finance, put a green dollar or note (any currency) beneath your plate of gnocchi before eating; afterward keep it in your wallet or purse, or store or business cash register, and do not spend it.

Goat's Beard

(*Aruncus dioicus*)

MAGICAL FORMS

also known as buck's beard or bride's feathers • also *Aruncus dioicus* 'Zweiweltenkind', translated as "child of two worlds," a smaller form of the plant particularly adaptable to growth in moist and dry conditions alike • a number of plants have been given this folk name • this version has upright ferny foliage with arching plumes of creamy-white, feathery flowers resembling a goat's beard • native to temperate parts of Europe, Asia, and eastern and western USA, both wild and in gardens • magically use the fresh or dried flowers, as well as the growing plant or cuttings from it

PLANET AND ELEMENT

Saturn • Earth

MAGICAL USES

as an amulet for matters where caution is needed • for talismans with specific timeframes connected with relationships where two people from very different worlds come happily together • to bring luck to older marriages or commitments • meditate on the growing plant for visions of the fey

HOW TO USE

For harmony, set the cut (dried or fresh) plant around a room in vases, in places where relatives, friends, or neighbors with very differing world views come together. • In the same way, it's helpful to have the plant nearby when resolving a boundary dispute or community matter. • Since the male and female flowers grow on different plants (the males are showier with numerous stamens while the female has three), use the individual feathers from each mixed in a charm bag on a full-moon night for fertility. • Use at any time of the month for IVF appointments or any other medical intervention for fertility, especially for same-sex couples.

CAUTION

Seeds of female plants are toxic to humans and pets.

Golden Alexander

(*Zizia aurea*)

MAGICAL FORMS

also including *Smyrnium olusatrum*, commonly referred to as alexanders • both golden alexander and alexanders are members of the Apiaceae (celery, carrot, or parsley) family but bloom on different sides of the Atlantic • golden alexander is a mainly wild plant growing across North America for thousands of years • the only food for the swallowtail butterfly • alexanders, with their less showy yellow or lime-green flowers, were introduced into Britain by the Romans from Mediterranean coastal areas • magically use the growing or cut plants, fruits, seeds, or yellow, flat-topped starburst flowers

PLANET AND ELEMENTS

Saturn • Earth/Air

MAGICAL USES

The UK and European alexanders were grown in monastery gardens in medieval times as vegetables and for medicinal usage and are still found in abandoned monastery or abbey gardens • use the growing alexander plant's flowers, fruits, and seeds magically for abundance and healing rituals • add the golden alexander flowers, which blossom in the spring for about four weeks (UK and European alexander flowers bloom April to June) to sachets for money rituals and charms • the seeds of both kinds of alexanders are good additions to fertility charm bags

HOW TO USE

If you can find UK and European alexanders growing in an old monastery, abbey, or church garden, meditate with them to connect with old worlds. • Sit among UK and European alexanders growing near the sea to get in touch with the tides of your own inner rhythms. • If you have a garden, track down and grow golden alexanders to connect with the original land on which your home stands, or if you are restless to put down roots. • Practice butterfly magick near golden alexanders, as the butterfly is a form frequently taken by beloved ancestors.

CAUTION

Golden alexander is nontoxic, but beware to not mistake it for the later-blooming wild parsnip, which can cause skin irritation.

Golden Eardrops

(*Ehrendorferia chrysantha*) or (*Dicentra chrysantha*)

MAGICAL FORMS

flowering aromatic wildflower, sometimes included in the poppy family • native to California and Baja California • has clusters of bright-yellow flowers, each resembling the shape of an ear • grows in dry brushy areas, especially burned ground a few years after a bushfire • can grow to reach between one and a half and five feet tall • you may find the dried flowers online or buy the plants from a specialty garden center to grow in a dry, warm garden (but this is not easy) • it is easier to magically use the flower essence, which contains the same strengths and can be obtained widely online

PLANET AND ELEMENT

Mars • Fire

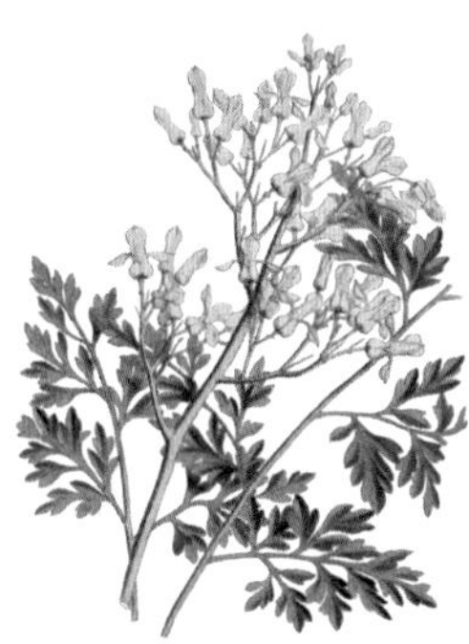

MAGICAL USES

both the dried flowers and the flower essence increase the ability to take what is of value in the past, present, and future and shed the rest • helps to overcome toxic and abusive childhood experiences

HOW TO USE

Anoint the Third Eye, the energy center located on your brow, with a drop of the essence to increase clairaudience or enhanced psychic hearing before mediumship or when reading the tarot if seeking help of a spirit guide. • In meditation, place two drops of the essence on each inner wrist point for the Heart and another for the Crown center, located in the middle of the hairline, to experience past worlds, especially your own childhood. • The insight you gain may explain present fears and phobias. • Add a few drops of the essence to the water of a vase of flowers to revive old memories. • When the flowers fade, wash the water away under a running tap and cast the plucked petals off a bridge, saying *Water under the bridge, I let go and so I am free to be me.*

CAUTION

It is not recommended to ingest dicentra plants, but the flower essence is safe.

Golden Rain Tree

(*Koelreuteria paniculata*)

MAGICAL FORMS

also known as the Pride of India and China Tree • native to China, Japan, and Korea, introduced to Europe in 1743 and the USA in 1763 • in the USA, this tree flowers in midsummer with clusters of canary yellow flowers • when the flowers are finished blooming, the petals cascade to the ground like golden rain, with the fruit replacing the flowers, each piece of fruit containing three large, hard, black seeds • each season brings forth new parts of the tree that can be used in rituals

PLANET AND ELEMENT

Jupiter • Air

MAGICAL USES

for remembering deceased relatives • the seeds make wonderful protective necklaces; create after the fruit spills open in November • use the fruits on small branches in dried flower displays for bringing abundance to the home

HOW TO USE

Stand beneath the tree, among the falling petals, circling the tree while making wishes for happiness and fulfillment. • Dry some of the fallen petals and keep them in a charm bag if you are seeking success and recognition. • Use the fallen petals in money pouches for unexpected sources of wealth. • Preserve and dry the flower clusters, the golden fall leaves, and the fruit and seeds collected in their own season, and place them in a charm bag as a reminder to follow your own unique destiny and stay in harmony with the seasons, especially if you work in a city.

CAUTION

No part of the golden rain tree should be ingested raw by pets or humans, though it is used medicinally under expert advice. • Its leaves and shoots should always be cooked, but first check for contraindications. • Avoid in pregnancy. • In parts of the eastern USA, the golden rain tree is considered invasive.

Goldenrod

(*Solidago* spp.)

MAGICAL FORMS

consists of about eight species still native to North America that can be cultivated in gardens and have powerful magick • once considered invasive, goldenrod is increasingly valued for its many esoteric powers • *Solidago altissima* is also known as late or tall goldenrod • blue stemmed goldenrod (*Solidago caesia*) is not aggressive and offers magical cut flowers • sweet goldenrod (*Solidago odora*) is a two- to four-foot nonaggressive plant with anise-scented leaves and yellow flowerheads • showy goldenrod (*Solidago speciosa*) grows to be one to three feet tall, with dense clusters of tiny yellow flowers • autumn goldenrod (*Solidago sphacelate*) is a twelve- to twenty-four-inch species holding plumes of yellow flowers • a notable cultivar, produced by special breeding, is golden torch goldenrod, also known as Wichita Mountains solidago, a thirty-inch plant with rich gold flowers • little lemon (*Solidago hybrid dansolitlem*) is an excellent magical compact variety (eight to twelve inches), with pale-lemon-colored flowers, and keeps away spite • magically use the plant (cuttings or a growing plant), as well as the flowers

PLANET AND ELEMENTS

Venus • Water/Air

MAGICAL USES

especially good if you do a lot of flower, love, and prosperity magick

HOW TO USE

Use the dried flowers in meditation for guidance in ways to make money. • Carried in the purse, the dried flowers in a sachet ensure unexpected money and success coming in and not going out. • Use goldenrod for finding water or treasure by dowsing with the plant. • Tie a stalk to your dowsing rod for increased success. • Use for butterfly magick and for bringing dreams of a future love.

CAUTION

Can cause gastrointestinal problems, dehydration, kidney problems, and gallstones if ingested. • Do not use if pregnant.

Goldenseal

(*Hydrastis canadensis*)

MAGICAL FORMS

also called yellow puccoon • related to the buttercup and native to southeastern Canada and eastern USA • a sacred herb among the Cherokee nation and other wise Indigenous healers • first brought to England in 1760 • a small herb producing a single flower in spring that becomes a cluster of inedible bright-red berries • magically use the dried (especially) and fresh rhizome and the powdered rhizome to make a decoction tea or an infusion for rituals

PLANET AND ELEMENT

Sun • Fire

MAGICAL USES

used in prosperity spells and for protection against money loss, as well as in rituals to counteract fraud and promote healing • regarded as a cure-all in the nineteenth century • restores energy and health after a long or serious illness or an epidemic

HOW TO USE

Drink and offer the tea at work if there is a cliquey or gossipy atmosphere, or if people are suffering from sick building syndrome. • Keep a rhizome hidden inside the front door to filter out unfriendly energies, both earthly and paranormal, and to welcome in good fortune, health, and prosperity. • If you have a back door, hang a rhizome there to prevent money flowing out. • If you don't have a back door, tie two rhizomes together with red thread at the front door and replace them when they wither.

CAUTION

Goldenseal is toxic if taken in excess. • Avoid this plant if you have high blood pressure or if you are pregnant or breastfeeding.

Gorse

(*Ulex europaeus*)

MAGICAL FORMS

also called furze or whin • prickly evergreen shrub, growing to ten feet tall • native to western Europe, especially the UK and Ireland, on heaths, open woodlands, and wastelands • also popular as garden hedging • introduced to North and South America, South Africa, and New Zealand • aromatic yellow spiky flowers that bloom from January to June • in summer when seeds spread, it can become invasive • magically use the growing flowers, the dried yellow flowerheads, and the flower essence and remedy

PLANETS AND ELEMENT

Mars/Sun • Fire

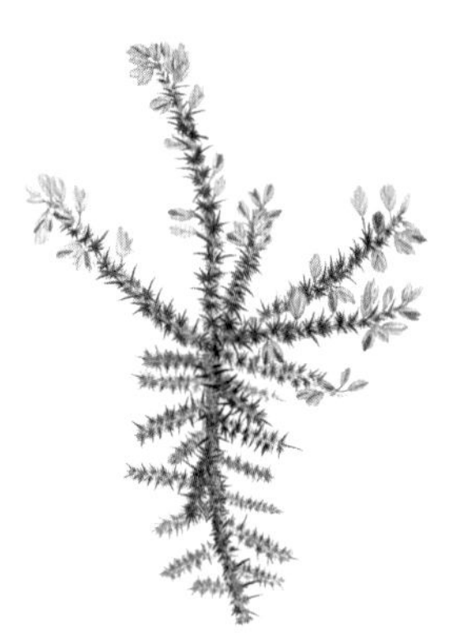

MAGICAL USES

one of the Celtic divinatory tree staves • golden gorse blooming at the spring equinox heralds the return of life and enthusiasm • coins can be tossed into the growing plants for prosperity and luck • adding shredded golden flowers to a sachet at any time of the year will attract financial wealth • gorse is a flower for mothers and grandmothers

HOW TO USE

Keep a vase of dried gorse in your kitchen for health and happiness and encourage inert family members to make an effort. • Add a few drops of the flower essence to a warm bath if you or a family member has lost hope, is suffering a chronic illness you fear will never improve, or wants to overcome the "glass half empty" approach to life. • Add the flower remedy to meals or drinks if you constantly reject the help of others. • In Irish folklore, gorse flower tea is drunk as a general tonic and for colds, coughs, and sore throats. • Sprinkle it around as flea repellent, but not on animal sleeping places.

CAUTION

Do not use if pregnant or breastfeeding.

Grains of Paradise

(*Aframomum melegueta*) and (*Amomum melegueta* 'Roscoe')

MAGICAL FORMS

a spice belonging to the ginger family, originally from West Africa and brought to the USA by European explorers and traders, maybe as early as the fifteenth century • have recently become more popular in the USA as a culinary spice • can be grown outside in a warm climate or in cooler conditions as an annual, or inside • used in hoodoo root work as a luck-bringer • magically use the whole plant, especially the seeds

PLANETS AND ELEMENTS

Mars/Jupiter • Fire/Air

MAGICAL USES

known as a wish herb • to bring blessings and remove curses and hexes • brings success in legal, employment, and financial challenges • called grains of paradise because early spice traders said they came from peppers grown in the Garden of Eden that floated down the river from paradise, giving the plant divine power to bring blessings and right wrongs

HOW TO USE

To make a wish, crumble the seeds within your hands, then cast them in all four directions, beginning with north and repeating the wish at each direction. • Afterward, rub your hands together so any grains left will fall on the earth to be absorbed or blown away. • The seeds can be burned in an incense mix for protection and to increase psychic senses. • Carry the seeds, whether loose or within a pod, in a green bag with three green aventurine or amazonite crystals for successful gambling, speculation, or even buying a lottery ticket. As you hold it, the right information or numbers will come into your mind. However, if you draw a blank, do not gamble. • Place the seeds in a blue bag when you need justice, and before entering an official building sprinkle them on the threshold. If that's not possible, place in a plant pot near the door to leave all unfair judgments outside.

CAUTION

Avoid if pregnant or breastfeeding.

Grape

(*Vitis vinifera*)

MAGICAL FORMS

the European grape is native to the Mediterranean, central Europe, and southwestern Asia • grape vines are grown in warm, temperate places around the world • there are twenty-five species in the USA in addition to the European grape, including the summer grape (*Vitis aestivalis*), native to the eastern USA; and the Arizona grape (*Vitis arizonica*), native to Arizona, Utah, Nevada, New Mexico, California, Texas, and Mexico • the grape plant is a fast-growing vine with tendrils lifting it from the ground • magically use the grapes on the vine, tendrils, and picked or purchased fruit

PLANET AND ELEMENT

Moon • Water

MAGICAL USES

rebirth and renewal • joy • ecstasy • passion • good luck in games of chance

HOW TO USE

Grow or buy, then eat green grapes for an ongoing inflow of money and success in speculation of all kinds. • Red grapes bring love, romance, and fertility, especially when shared with a lover. • Eat purple for power and psychic insights when you need luck and confidence in your own decisions. • Cut off lengths of the tendrils with black or purple grapes attached, then burn or cast them out to cut off negative or unwise influences, addictions, indulgences, and persistent psychological and psychic attacks. • Use the fruitless and flowerless vine (remove leaves) for knot magick to bind a specific person or situation from harming you. Tie the severed vine strand to a tree or shrub well away from the vine, then bind your name and a lover's name (written on a strip of paper attached to the vine with red twine), so that as the vine grows, so will the love.

CAUTION

Beware of plants such as Canadian moonseed (*Menispermum canadense*) that look similar but are poisonous.

Grapefruit

(*Citrus × paradisi*)

MAGICAL FORMS

this plant was created in the eighteenth century by crossing the pomelo tree (*Citrus maximus*) with sweet orange (*Citrus sinensis*) • large, yellow fruit • native to tropical Asia • now cultivated in Brazil, California, Florida, and Israel • the oil that is extracted from the peel is made mainly in California • magically use the fruit, including the peel, and the essential oil

PLANET AND ELEMENT

Moon • Water

MAGICAL USES

for new beginnings • reduces food cravings and other addictions • balances mood swings • enhances psychic abilities, especially psychometry and clairsentience • purification • manifesting needs

HOW TO USE

When the moon can no longer be seen in the sky, peel the grapefruit and hang the skin over the door until it dries. Then grind and powder the skin. Sprinkle the powder around thresholds and outside the front and back door to give psychological and psychic protection against adversaries, especially secret ones and malevolent entities. • To restore your energies after a loss or setback, cut a grapefruit in half and anoint each half with grapefruit essential oil. Tie the two halves together with red ribbon and, holding the grapefruit to your psychic Third Eye in the center of your brow, allow its life-giving powers to pass into you, and then cast the grapefruit into running water. • Cut a grapefruit in half and on one half use your index finger to write invisibly on the flesh what you wish to lose from your life. On the other half, write invisibly what or who you most want to gain or attain. Eat the fruit of the wishing half and press the other half of the fruit down into a bowl of salt, leaving it until it dries out, then bury it.

CAUTION

Dilute the oil well before applying to skin. • As it is a phototoxic oil, avoid direct sunlight after use.

Grape-Seed Oil

(*Vitis vinifera*)

MAGICAL FORMS

a product made from the grapes used in making wine • light, odorless, easily absorbed, and inexpensive both for cooking and in a more refined form as a carrier oil for essential oils or used alone on the skin • magically use the oil topically (can be used undiluted), as a carrier oil to enhance other essential oils, or in cookery

PLANET AND ELEMENT

Moon • Water

MAGICAL USES

called the oil of pure joy, it can be used for personal and family happiness if included in magical cooking • used as a carrier oil, it acts as a neutral agent when combined with other essential oils, adding to the specific power of the oil with which it mixes • use in massage and ritual burning • can take on the power of other heavier carrier oils, such as almond for increasing fertility, evening primrose for new beginnings and regeneration, and hazel for justice • grape-seed oil is named in the Bible as being part of a dish called pulse eaten by Daniel to give him strength and courage

HOW TO USE

When used in massage, grape-seed oil reduces stress. • Incorporate in rituals, empowerments, and chants. • Use to anoint the Third Eye and nonporous statues, and to bless ritual objects. • Grape-seed oil, when used alone, can be imprinted with any magical purpose. • When used as a beauty product on skin and hair or to diminish blemishes and stretch marks, it can be empowered to bring inner and outer radiance and restore or preserve youthfulness.

CAUTION

The carrier oil should not be ingested. • Avoid all grape seeds if you are taking blood thinners or medication to lower blood pressure or cholesterol. • Carry out a patch test if you have very sensitive skin.

Grass-of-Parnassus

(*Parnassia palustris*)

MAGICAL FORMS

white, five-petaled wildflower with heart-shaped leaves around the base and translucent green stripes, surrounding the flower's gold stigma and stamens • not a grass • less than ten inches high • each beautiful flower grows singly • can be used to create a flower essence, but due to loss of wetlands in Scotland, northern England, and northern Wales, it can be hard to find • blooms between June and September, heralding the harvest • four main kinds of northern grass-of-Parnassus are found in the USA, especially in Alaska, Washington, Missouri, North and South Carolina, and as far south as Arizona and New Mexico • in folk medicine, it has been used as an infusion against indigestion, as a mouthwash for a sore throat, and dried and powdered to treat wounds • magically work with the flower essence, in situ or as a living plant grown in a damp patch of the garden

PLANETS AND ELEMENT

Moon/Venus • Water

MAGICAL USES

breaks down emotional barriers and opens the heart to trust and love • releases fears • the nineteenth-century Scottish poet Andrew Lang celebrated its beauty • as such, the herb has become associated with artistic, creative, and musical ventures, as well as prophetic abilities

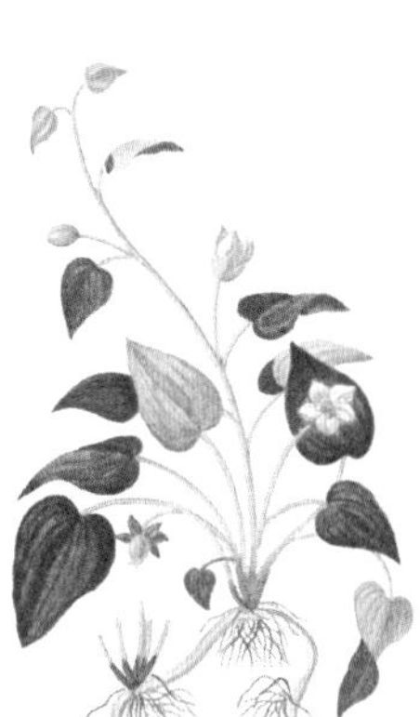

HOW TO USE

Add a few drops of the essence to a glass of water, sipping it through the day if you find it hard to show vulnerability or openly express yourself creatively. • Add a little bit of the essence to a rose or chamomile massage oil if your partner finds it hard to show tenderness in lovemaking. • Put a drop or two under your pillow for prophetic dreams.

CAUTION

Since scientific research has not yet demonstrated its safety, be cautious ingesting except for accredited remedies. • Avoid if pregnant.

Grass-Widow

(*Olsynium douglasii*)

MAGICAL FORMS

flowering wildflower from the iris family, native to the Pacific Northwest • found in southern British Columbia, Washington, Oregon, the Rocky Mountains, Nevada, Utah, and Idaho as far as the northern end of California • intense, reddish-purple bowl- or bell-shaped satiny flowers on upright stems with clumps of grasslike leaves clinging to the base of the stem • blooms in early spring for three or four days • can grow in gardens and containers • traditionally, a remedy for digestion problems and food intolerances, as well as coughs and colds • magically use the growing foliage and the flower essence

PLANET AND ELEMENT

Saturn • Earth

MAGICAL USES

overcomes fears of all kinds, especially fear of being judged by others • releases old patterns and self-imposed limitations • changes beliefs if you feel they are no longer valid • calls back a lover who is neglectful or frequently absent, hence the name, though it may refer to the fact that grass-widow blooms earlier than many plants and therefore stands alone

HOW TO USE

The grasslike leaves can be shaped into a ball, a witch's ladder, or tied in knots for protection and binding spells, as well as for good luck. • Tie the leaves in a cross shape, then cut and bury them at a crossroads or outside the home of someone who has cursed or hexed you. • Add a few drops of the flower essence to your water bottle if you are in a work or social situation where you are being assessed or you fear you are being thought inadequate.

CAUTION

There is insufficient research to prove its safety. • Avoid if pregnant.

Grasses

(*Poaceae* family)

MAGICAL FORMS

a very large family of over ten thousand species, cultivated as ornamental plants, on lawns, or as cereal crops • examples include Kentucky bluegrass (*Poa pratensis*), which grows in the northern, eastern, and Pacific Northwest USA and also in Europe • Zoysia grass (*Zoysia* spp.), one of most popular lawn grasses in the southern USA, is found from the Carolinas to Missouri • in the UK, feathery meadow foxtail (*Alopecurus pratensis*) resembles a fox's tail • Bermuda grass (*Cynodon dactylon*), a common lawn grass in the USA, is an Ayurvedic herb • English ryegrass (*lolium perenne*) is plentiful in the UK • in practice almost any grass can be used in rituals and spells

PLANET AND ELEMENT

Saturn • Earth

MAGICAL USES

for protection • fertility (especially sweet fragrant vernal grass, which is found in the southeastern USA and in continental Europe, mainly north from Switzerland) • knot magick • money spells (any of the cereal grasses) • bouquets of ornamental grasses such as feathertop grass (*Pennisetum villosum*) can be dried for display in the home or planted for abundance, health, and wealth • for past-life visions, sit alone in a tall grass meadow • for growth in any area of your life, use in poppets, spell bags, and bottles

HOW TO USE

Weave a grass ball and hang it inside a front window to keep away all harm, unfriendly visitors, and malicious entities. • Make and leave a grass baby under the full moon outdoors if you wish to conceive a child, replacing it when the grass begins to wither. • Use long grass strands for tying knots to bind those who would harm you. • Couch grass (*Elymus repens*) will remove restless spirits, jinxes, and hexes if you tie a knot in it and then cut the knot. • Tie bundles of long dried grasses and then invert them to sweep a doorstep, removing misfortune, illness, or quarrels from the home. • After sweeping, burn the bundle.

CAUTION

If using lawn or wild meadow grasses, check that they have not been sprayed with chemicals.

Green Champa Incense

MAGICAL FORMS

incense sticks made from various white champa flowers, such as from the Kanak tree (*Pterospermum acerifolium*), also called the Muchakunda or Karnikar tree • also incorporates fragrant oils from the Indian fir tree (*Monoon longifolium*), which only flowers for three weeks a year with green, star-shaped blossoms • green champa may also be infused with tropical honeysuckle, citrus, and sandalwood for fragrance, and, to make the sticks burn well, with halmaddi, a semi-liquid resin from the *Ailanthus malabarica* tree • earthy, highly fragrant, and spicy • green champa is sourced from Southeast Asia from Burma to India, much sold worldwide from India • can be rolled and burned in charcoal • use in meditation, ritual, and for astral travel • check that your green champa is made from pure plant ingredients, as the cheaper kind may contain chemicals and affect its efficacy for magical purposes

PLANETS AND ELEMENTS

Venus/Moon • Earth/Water

MAGICAL USES

to balance inner energy points for meditation, yoga, and relaxation • for nature rituals to connect with the devas • allows love to grow in its own time and way

HOW TO USE

Light twin green champa incense sticks set in individual holders so the sticks cross, with a squat red candle in front of them. • Gaze through the flame into the swirling smoke for visions of ancient worlds that you may visit through astral travel. • Set a lighted green champa stick in a holder in front of a mirror. • Ask questions and symbols will appear in the smoke, reflected in the mirror.

Green Tea

(*Camellia sinensis*)

MAGICAL FORMS

originally from eastern Asia, first grown in the USA from the late eighteenth century by South Carolina planters and found in many lands, including Australia • green tea is made from the leaves and buds of the shrub, like black, white, oolong, and pu'erh tea • green tea is the unoxidized form, one of the least processed kinds of tea and low in caffeine • magically use brewed green tea or teabags alone or mixed with other herbal, floral, and fruit teas as a base and to enhance their qualities

PLANETS AND ELEMENTS

Moon/Venus • Water/Earth

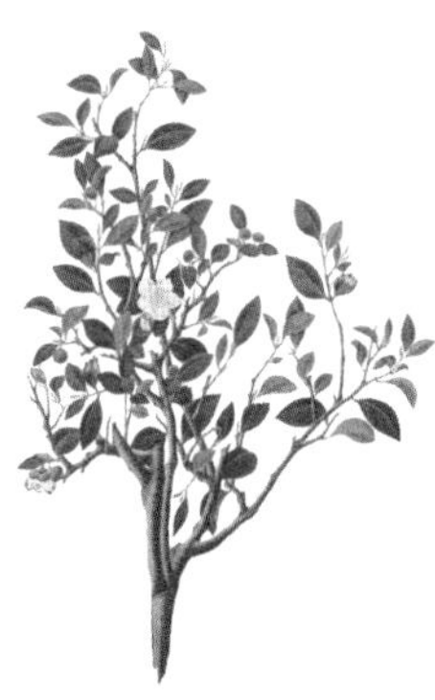

MAGICAL USES

for tea ceremonies, with the making, pouring, and drinking following a slow, measured, contemplative pace • drink to move away from the rushing world • brings health, cleansing, passion, and money • loose leaves can be used for tea leaf reading and tasseomancy

HOW TO USE

To make your green tea drinking experience into a spell, add the ingredients—the leaves for Earth, then the water (hot, but not scalding), allowing the heat (the element Fire) to empower the mix. The steam and fragrance rising is the Air element, which can carry your petitions to the cosmos. Finally, to absorb the combined elemental strengths within you, sip the green tea. • Add other flowers or herbs to the tea, such as lemon balm for opening psychic awareness or jasmine for love. • Note that many commercial floral teas already contain green tea.

CAUTION

Green tea should not be consumed in excess, especially in pregnancy, nor taken with stimulant drugs, beta blockers, or blood thinners.

Grove Sandwort

(*Moehringia lateriflora*)

MAGICAL FORMS

also called bluntleaf sandwort • a white, five-petaled, delicate woodland wildflower, from the carpetweed family • two to eight inches high • grows in the north and northwestern USA, Canada, Europe, and Asia • magically use in situ (can be cultivated in wildflower gardens) and as a flower essence

PLANET AND ELEMENT

Moon • Water

MAGICAL USES

encourages positive parent/child relationships, especially maternal • overcomes lack of physical and emotional nurturing and bonding between mother or father and child of any age, particularly in a situation in which a parent was absent or found parenting difficult • the growing plants can be used to connect with the earth and earth energies • for animal mothers who reject their newborns

HOW TO USE

Add a few drops to your bath, humidifier, or massage oil, or sip the essence in water if you find it hard to bond with a baby, especially for women after a traumatic birth or when there was major surgical intervention. • Add to the water of a mother animal who is finding it hard to feed her offspring. • If your own mother is emotionally distant, spritz the house before she visits or put a little under your tongue before meeting her away from your home or speaking on the phone. • Take the essence in the weeks before meeting a birth parent for the first time if you sense their reluctance.

Guava

(*Psidium guajava*)

MAGICAL FORMS

small tropical tree or shrub with edible fruit • the fruit is increasingly grown in tropical and subtropical regions throughout the world, though native to the tropical Americas and the Caribbean • can be cultivated as an indoor potted plant in more temperate regions. • drink the fresh or dried leaves as tea (the dried leaves can be purchased in many health food stores) • magically use the fruit or flowers, fresh or dried

PLANET AND ELEMENT

Venus • Water

MAGICAL USES

cleanses negative or redundant feelings, as well as bad atmospheres at home and in the workplace • in India, the tree is considered sacred, especially when growing near water, and represents health, happiness, beauty, and well-being

HOW TO USE

Cast the fruit into running water or the ocean during a full moon to conceive a child. • Drink the tea or eat the fruit regularly to generate creativity and prosperity, offering a small portion to Mother Earth. • Share the fruit or tea with an undemonstrative lover to kindle romance, or as a sign of enduring love if love cannot be openly expressed. • Carry a sachet of the dried flowers for ongoing wealth, fertility, the generosity of others, and abundance in your life in the way most sought or needed.

CAUTION

The fruit is considered safe for humans, but the tea and leaves should be treated with caution in pregnancy, while breastfeeding, or if taking regular prescribed medication.

Guggul Resin

(*Commiphora wightii*)

MAGICAL FORMS

from the Indian bdellium tree, also known as the guggul, gugal, or mukul myrrh tree • a relative of the Indian myrrh tree, though it smells differently, guggul is mentioned in Ayurvedic texts dating back to 600 BCE and praised for its medicinal properties • currently threatened by overharvesting, the fragrant, soft brown resin, native to southern Pakistan and western India, comes additionally from northern Africa to central Asia and in parts of the USA • magically, it is mainly purchased as incense for magick rituals and burning in the home as resin or a powder • guggul superior resin comes from the *Commiphora mukul* tree from Pakistan, and has a higher concentration of oil than the Indian tree, allowing the incense to burn longer and more richly for prolonged rituals

PLANET AND ELEMENT

Mars • Fire

MAGICAL USES

for rebirth and rejuvenation • as an aphrodisiac and to win love against rivals and opposition • frequently mixed in other incenses • slightly sweet and earthy, with a balsamic fragrance • a natural choice for earth rituals including blessing land if you are building or renovating a property, clearing troublesome energies from a home you have recently purchased, and for war-torn or despoiled regions

HOW TO USE

An everyday version of ceremonial myrrh, *guggula* means "protects from disease" in Sanskrit. • It prevents the cares of the day from spilling over into the evening and night. • In India, it is burned for a quiet end to the day, to resolve all disagreements or ill feelings, bringing peaceful sleep. • Because the tree is thorny, the incense is burned around doorways and window frames to repel psychic attacks at home or around the workplace.

CAUTION

Avoid ingesting or inhaling guggal resin deeply when trying to become pregnant, during pregnancy, and if taking hypoglycemic medication or anticoagulants.

Gum Arabic Resin

mainly from (*Acacia senegal*)

MAGICAL FORMS

a resin obtained by removing part of the tree's bark and tapping the gum that oozes out • the resin dries on the branches as it is released, so it can be collected without damaging the tree • the tree is grown south of the Sahara from Senegal in the west to Somalia in the east • used in ancient Egypt for embalming and for creating paints • magically use resin or powdered resin

PLANET AND ELEMENT

Sun • Fire

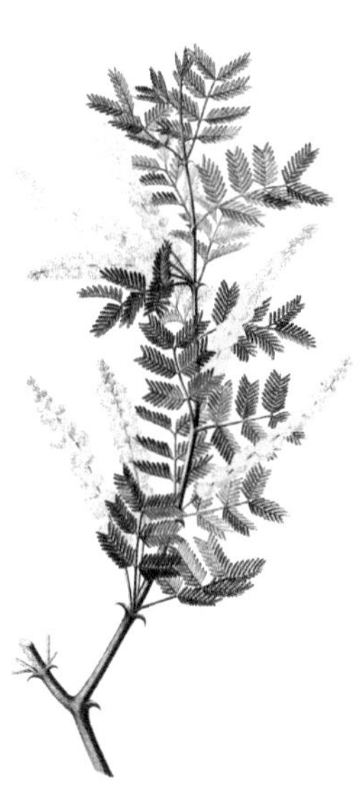

MAGICAL USES

for secrets and secret love • making friends • attracting new love • family matters • love under difficult circumstances • finding what has been lost or taken

HOW TO USE

Burn resin to carry prayers and petitions to the deities or Higher Beings of Light • Gum arabic resin will strengthen the magical properties of other herbs and flowers by enabling them to burn more easily, thereby supporting their qualities.

Gypsophila

(*Gypsophila paniculata*)

MAGICAL FORMS

also known as baby's breath • tiny, delicate, white or pink button-like blossoms • often grown as ground cover • is considered invasive in parts of the USA • magically use cut or dried flowers, or growing plant

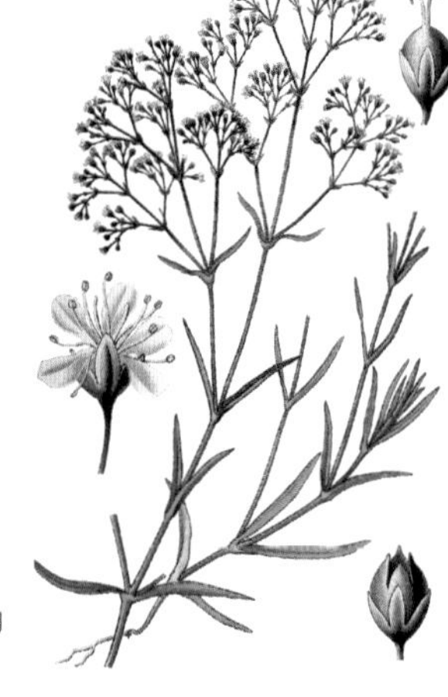

PLANET AND ELEMENT

Venus • Water

MAGICAL USES

popular at weddings as part of a traditional bouquet along with white roses, especially if a couple already has children together or one of the couple is pregnant at the time • take a bunch wrapped in white ribbons as a gift to baby showers or on a first date • attracts nature spirits to the garden • the flowers are often dried and preserved for early spring festivals to call back the growth of the year at the beginning of February: Candlemas (a Christian feast festival) or Imbolc (a Gaelic festival) in the old seasonal year

HOW TO USE

Use gypsophila in water rituals since it resembles the sea, with frothy-looking flowers and narrow gray-green or green-blue leaves. • Add a little of the dried, powdered flower petals into the rolled wax of a candle being made for Candlemas at the beginning of February or a pinch of the powder dropped into the flame of the first candle lit at the festival. • Place the dried flowers into a blue or turquoise bag with an aquamarine, ocean jasper, or any green crystal and tie the bag with blue twine before casting it into flowing water as a tribute to ask for the return of what or who is lost or has gone away. • To create a love charm, carry a green cloth with baby's breath, rose and carnation petals, and a silver heart.

CAUTION

Gypsophila is toxic to humans and pets.

Hackberry Tree

(*Celtis occidentalis*)

MAGICAL FORMS

also European Hackberry Tree (*Celtis australis*) • the hackberry tree is native to North Dakota and flourishes throughout the USA • the European hackberry is indigenous to southern Europe, North Africa, and Asia Minor, and was introduced to the UK in 1796 • magically use the tree wood, leaves, berries, or whole, growing tree in situ

PLANETS AND ELEMENTS

Moon/Mars • Water/Fire

MAGICAL USES

use as a wand for protection from malicious spirits and to call positive change into your life, as well as success for creative ventures • use the dried or fresh leaves, pale yellow in the fall, to help with money matters • in the Middle East, the red or purple berries are believed to grow only in moonlight, so they can be used to decorate an altar or magical special place for full moon celebrations

HOW TO USE

Combine finely powdered wood chippings or powdered bark with full moon incense and burn with lunar myrrh resin, or burn the wood cast with prayers and wishes on full moon fires. • Add the cooled ash with a little unburned wood or powder to a silver amulet bag to keep away all harm, both earthly enemies and predators and malevolent spirits, until the next full moon, when it can be replaced. • The migratory hackberry butterfly, with its orange and white wings, uses the hackberry as a host tree for its caterpillars. • When seen flying or feeding on sap around the hackberry tree, the hackberry butterfly symbolizes transformation, regeneration, and rebirth, and is a lucky omen.

Harebell

(*Campanula rotundifolia*)

MAGICAL FORMS

though blue like the bluebell and with multiple flowered bell cups, it is an unrelated plant • if growing wild, harebell covers open meadows, mountain slopes, and the edges of shores whereas the bluebell chooses sheltered woodlands • the harebell is larger than the bluebell and blooms later in the summer, between July and September as opposed to the bluebell's spring flowering • harebells grow in gardens and wild through North America and Eurasia • named after the hare, harebells are called witches' bells or witches' thimbles • witches were believed to change themselves into hares and hide among the harebells to avoid detection • magically use the growing plant, flower essence, or cut flowers, fresh or dried (ask permission before picking in case they are sheltering the essence of a witch)

PLANET AND ELEMENT

Moon • Water

MAGICAL USES

hope • restoration of trust • used in Celtic magick and, for those of Celtic descent, to recall Celtic ancestors • since hares are the sacred creatures of Andraste, the Celtic moon goddess whose High Priestess was the warrior queen Boadicea, harebells are a magical symbol of courage • moon magick • butterfly and bee magick for shape-shifting

HOW TO USE

Use flower essence to open a heart closed by fear or vulnerability and to align with love from all sources. • Add the flower essence to water as a spray to apply before critical visitors arrive, or use around your workspace. Meditate on the growing flowers for inspiration when the odds seem against you. • Set the flowers in the center of an outdoor altar or grow a circle of harebells around the altar. • In rituals, use harebells to send strength to all who are facing persecution or prejudice. • Turn around nine times counterclockwise on a full moon night among growing harebells or circle a vase of harebells set between you and the moon counterclockwise to ask for a swift resolution of any slow-moving matter.

Hawthorn Tree

(*Crataegus monogyna*)

MAGICAL FORMS

also known as common hawthorn • magically use the whole, growing tree, as well as blossoms (especially fresh), and either fresh or dried leaves

PLANETS AND ELEMENTS

Mercury/Mars • Air/Fire

MAGICAL USES

the ultimate magick and fairy tree • believed to form a protective hedge around the homes of wisewomen and to be the division between the worlds, hence the term *hedgewitch* • Olwen the Welsh White Goddess crossed the universe, shedding hawthorn blossoms that became the Milky Way • hawthorn is crafted for creativity, fertility, and star magick • for male potency • banishing harm • good luck • protection of property against bad weather, especially storms • considered unlucky to bring the blossoms in the house except on the morning of May 1

HOW TO USE

Following an old tradition, pick hawthorn blossoms on the morning of May 1 with a partner to hasten the conception of a child, and for abundance. • Only cut wood from the tree when it is in blossom. • Carefully add the thorns to a protective bottle with sour red wine and hawthorn leaves, then bury it near your home to repel curses and ill wishes from those who must visit. • To see nature spirits, sit beneath a hawthorn tree at twilight. • Do not shelter under one on the fairy festivals, Midsummer Eve, or Halloween, or you will become enchanted by the fairies. • Oak, ash, and thorn growing together offer a doorway to other worlds, especially those of the fey. • Consume hawthorn berries as a tea to increase psychic abilities.

Hazel Tree

(*Corylus* spp.)

MAGICAL FORMS

plants of the genus *Corylus*, including the common hazel (*Corylus avellana*), which is found in the UK and Europe, and also cultivated in the USA, and *Corylus americana*, the American hazel, which is native to eastern and central USA and Canada • magically use the whole tree, including its wood and nuts, and from the *Corylus avellana* specifically, the oil as a carrier oil

PLANET AND ELEMENTS

Venus • Water/Earth

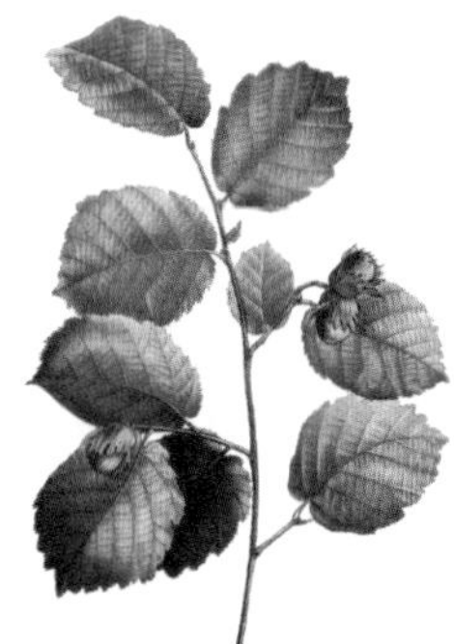

MAGICAL USES

the traditional single-forked dowsing stick is cut from a living hazel and is used for finding water, lost items, and subterranean psychic energy lines • one of the Celtic sacred trees • for use in rituals for wisdom, justice, creative writing, success in all official matters, good luck, and fertility • good for developing psychic powers

HOW TO USE

Hazel is associated with the number nine because of the nine poetic nuts of inspiration, in myth described as hanging on the tree over Connla's Well in Tipperary that was believed to stand at the center of the Otherworld or the Land of Eternal Youth. • Keep nine nuts in a bowl in the space you use for writing or creating. • A hazel rod was handed to a petitioner or defendant in a Druid court to allow them to state their cause without interruption. To channel this capability, make a charm bag with nine small, smooth, identical hazel sticks; nine matching leaves; and, if you can obtain them, nine dried blossoms with just a single drop of the oil each. Before closing the bag, say nine times, *So justice shall be done*. Take the closed bag to a court case or official hearing where you are being unfairly treated or to your workplace if your opinions are overlooked or overridden.

Hearts of Palm

MAGICAL FORMS

from *Euterpe edulis*, jussara or palmtieiro palm, as well as its relative the acai palm (*Euterpe oleracea*) and the coconut palm (*Cocos nucifera*) • a vegetable with edible stalks, inner heart, and buds from certain palm trees including the cabbage palm (*Sabal palmetto*), which is native to the southern USA, the Yucatan Peninsula, and the West Indies • very nutritious source of fiber and minerals such as iron, potassium, and zinc • mainly sold canned • buy hearts that are from multistemmed trees (some grown specially), like the acai palm (see p. 15) so that harvesting the heart does not destroy the whole tree • magically use the environmentally harvested raw or cooked palm heart

PLANETS AND ELEMENT

Moon/Venus • Water

MAGICAL USES

in magical cookery, the ultimate aphrodisiac • to summon a love that seems unattainable • to share with someone you would like to know better, emotionally as well as sexually

HOW TO USE

Find a growing tree, touch your heart, and then use your wedding ring finger to trace the initials of the person you love or desire to love, entwined with your initials, on the tree. Enclose the two sets of initials in an invisible heart. • Share hearts of palm as part of a Valentine's Day meal or on Sundays and Fridays to increase your sexual magnetism and make yourself irresistible to a hesitant or uptight lover.

Heather

(*Calluna vulgaris*)

MAGICAL FORMS

colorful perennial found in Europe and Asia Minor • magically use the whole plant, especially the flowers, dried or fresh; the leaves; and as incense

PLANETS AND ELEMENTS

Sun/Venus • Fire/Earth

MAGICAL USES

pink heather can be used for good luck, loyalty in love, friendship, and if love is going wrong • white, for immense good fortune, the granting of wishes, and love after loss • purple, for faithfulness when lovers must be apart, when talking to spirits, and for attracting money and successful gambling • any color can help increase fertility • to increase passion between committed lovers or devotion to any cause • creativity

HOW TO USE

In the workplace, a small pot of heather reduces bullying and conflict. • Grown in the garden, it encourages a loving, united household. • If you add heather flowers to a bath sachet or as an infusion in bathwater, you can prevent a relationship from progressing too fast sexually. • Burning incense traditionally attracts rain and frees blocked emotions. • Bind long strands of heather as a broom for clearing sacred space, or add the flowers to a floor wash to protect the home. • Sitting close to heather opens the door to the world of fey and aids shape-shifting.

Heather, Bell

(*Erica cinerea*)

MAGICAL FORMS

heathland plant • dark purple-pink bell-shaped flowers, blooming between July and September • grows wild on heathlands • also cultivated in gardens throughout the UK (except the East Midlands), in western and central Europe, and naturalized in Nantucket, Massachusetts • attracts bees, producing dark fragrant honey that rivals manuka honey for its health-giving properties • magically use the growing plant, the honey, and the flower essence

PLANET AND ELEMENT

Sun • Fire

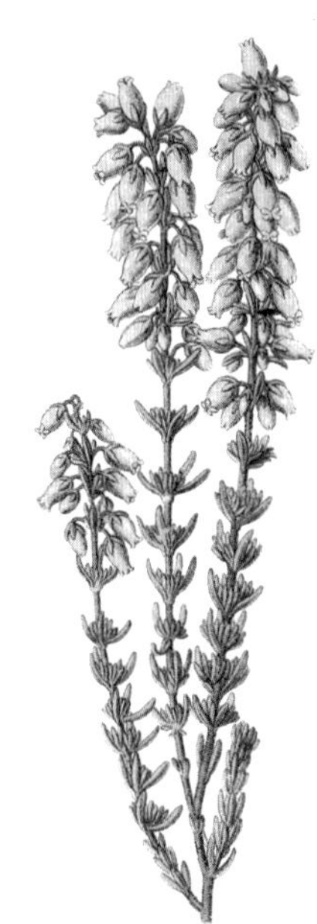

MAGICAL USES

heals a loss of personal confidence, anxiety, and lack of self-esteem that may be manifest as mood swings • being too easily influenced for fear of giving offense • for children and pets, the essence is sold mixed with vegetable glycerin instead of brandy • mix a drop or two in pet food for animals who hide when strangers call • sacred to the Breton Heather goddess who was called Uroica, to Grainne, the Celtic solar crone goddess, and to the maiden goddess Brigid, the goddess of healing, fertility, all crafts, and inspiration

HOW TO USE

Use it to connect with ancestors in meditation. • Sip the essence in a glass of water, or apply a few drops of the essence under the tongue if you find it hard to stand against emotional pressures and guilt trips by others.

CAUTION

More evidence is needed to rate the effectiveness and safety of bell heather for use during pregnancy or by breastfeeding moms.

Helichrysum

(*Helichrysum* spp.)

MAGICAL FORMS

also known as everlasting flower or strawflower • a flowering shrub native to the Mediterranean and southern Europe, reaching up to two feet high, with gray, hairy foliage and papery, bright-yellow flowerheads that survive long after they are cut • also grows in sunny, dry areas in the USA and the UK • can be grown potted almost anywhere indoors • used to create an essential oil that is extracted from all green parts, stems, and leaves • though frequently called the curry plant because of its distinctive fragrance, the oil is earthy and herbaceous, and the actual flowers are quite resinous and spicy • magically use the oil and the cut, dried flowerheads

PLANETS AND ELEMENTS

Sun/Jupiter • Fire/Air

MAGICAL USES

for overcoming writers' or any creative block • enhances intuition • brings heightened spiritual awareness of other dimensions • often called "the spiritual warrior" because the oil, if inhaled, kick-starts the courage to speak out or act

HOW TO USE

The oil, when diffused, removes sad memories, even those from past lives that hold back future love and life. • Grow the flowers in the garden or crush a few dried flowerheads with oil added for fragrance into potpourri. • If you wish, augment potpourri with extra-fragrant dried flowers like lavender, rose petals, or jasmine for different magical effects. • Keep a potted plant in the kitchen with other spicy-smelling potted herbs to give the home a calm and spiritual—but lively!—atmosphere at mealtimes, and to call the household guardians and angels.

CAUTION

Do not use flower or oil if pregnant or breastfeeding.

Hellebore

(*Helleborus* spp.)

MAGICAL FORMS

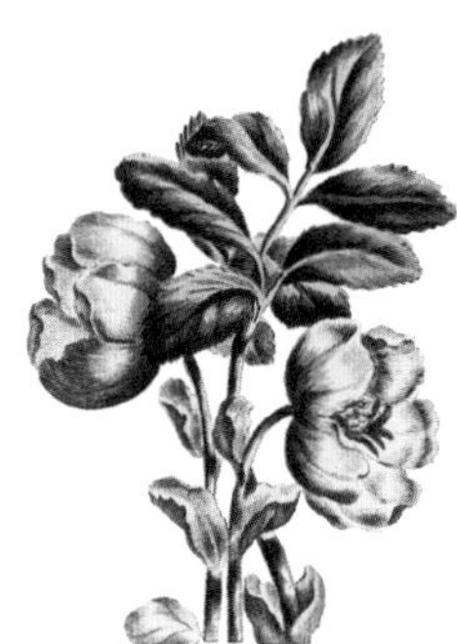

in modern times, the flower is often used in wedding bouquets • its ancient meaning was less benign, as it was often implicated in deliberate poisonings (Alexander the Great was said to be poisoned with white or false hellebore) • magically use the whole, growing, cut, or dried plant; dried powdered root; and cut flowers, fresh and dried

PLANET AND ELEMENTS

Saturn • Earth/Water

MAGICAL USES

in all its forms, hellebore represents long-lasting love through the years • for second- or third-time-around weddings or rededication of vows • *Helleborus niger*, the Christmas rose, is particularly lovely in white with golden stamens and *Helleborus orientalis*, the Lenten rose, is often plum or deep purple and associated with restraint and thoughtfulness

HOW TO USE

The powdered dried plant or root has been traditionally used in banishing and protection spells and to create a circle of invisibility to lower one's profile if entering a potentially confrontational situation. • Float the dying plant or petals in water, especially in Lent or during the waning moon, to remove addictions, curses, and fears. • Burn a plant that has faded on a bonfire or hearth fire or make into incense in order to stop gossip and slander.

CAUTION

The whole plant is very toxic to humans and pets so it is no longer used medicinally for safety reasons. • Hellebore can also be a skin irritant. • Often, roses are substituted magically for these reasons, though hellebore belongs to the buttercup family, not to the rose family.

Hemlock Tree

(*Tsuga* spp.)

MAGICAL FORMS

including eastern hemlock (*Tsuga canadensis*) and western hemlock (*Tsuga heterophylla*)• shady conifers • eastern hemlock is native to southern Canada and northeastern USA through the Appalachian Mountains down to Georgia and beyond • the western hemlock grows in the Pacific Northwest and western Canada and was introduced into Britain in 1852, where it is one of the most prolific conifers • thrives also in northwestern Europe and southern New Zealand • magically use the growing tree, cones, needles, and dense foliage

PLANET AND ELEMENT

Saturn • Earth

MAGICAL USES

a woman's tree among Canada's Kwakwaka'wakw people; female warriors made headdresses from the tree for ceremonial dances • beloved by Queen Victoria, who changed its name to *Tsuga albertiana* to honor her husband, Albert (though it was changed back) • for tough love, as well as for nurturing and protection of the vulnerable, because new trees grow in the protective shade of the parent tree • for secret love and love trysts • supports change, travel, and long-term plans

HOW TO USE

Shelter in the dense foliage of the tree or where multiple trees grow, holding the trunk and allowing it to fill you with acceptance of inevitable change, to mourn what can be no more, and to experience visions of past worlds in other forests that you have visited. • Tie a dried large sprig of the tree around copies of travel documents or brochures so that future travel may be safe and you will be protected from last-minute setbacks or delays. • Leave the bundle at home until you return.

Henbane

(*Hyoscyamus niger*)

MAGICAL FORMS

also known as black henbane or stinking nightshade • flowering herb • highly toxic member of the nightshade family • native to temperate Europe, Siberia, Great Britain, and Ireland • naturalized through much of the world • introduced into the USA in the 1600s for medicinal and ornamental purposes, but escaped cultivation and now grows wild in northeastern, midwestern, and western North America, reaching between one and two feet tall, sometimes higher • funnel-shaped flowers with five cream or pale- to dark-yellow petals with purple veins and dark centers • magically use the chopped root or dried plant only with extreme caution and for defensive magick against extreme threats

PLANETS AND ELEMENTS

Moon/Saturn • Water/Earth

MAGICAL USES

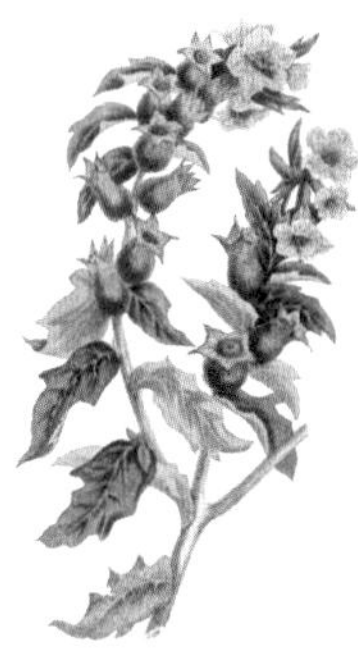

hundreds of seeds have been found in Viking graves, probably used by the *berserkers,* Norse warriors who wore bearskins and were totally fearless, some said in a state of divine madness in battle • a hallucinogenic, henbane was added to fat from dubious sources in medieval times and rubbed on the body for astral projection and flying magick

HOW TO USE

The henbane plant is still added to defensive bottles and in rituals during the dark of the moon to confuse persecutors. • Once popular as a protective incense and to call spirits, now you should substitute dried ferns, as the smoke of henbane is toxic and may create false terrors. • Mugwort is safer for visions.

CAUTION

Henbane is a narcotic and can kill you if wrongly ingested; only take under strict medical supervision. • It is poisonous to the touch, so handle with gloves and keep it away from children and pets.

Herb-Robert

(*Geranium robertianum*)

MAGICAL FORMS

also known as Roberts geranium • a relative of cranesbill, native to Europe, Ireland, northwestern USA, British Columbia, parts of Asia, and North Africa • with crane-shaped pods that eject their seeds in different directions over great distances • flowers are white and blue-violet, May to September, with five petals • the leaves have a spicy, acrid smell when rubbed, and a short stalk that is close to the ground • the herb mixture can be purchased online, as can the tea bags • magically use the dried leaves, stems, and flowers, and the bird-beak-like seed pods

PLANETS AND ELEMENTS

Mercury/Venus • Air/Water

MAGICAL USES

for seeing nature spirits if you grow the plant in your garden or find it wild • named after Robin Goodfellow, the ancient British mischievous house goblin, also known as Puck, famous in Shakespeare's *A Midsummer Night's Dream* • brings fun and spontaneity to life and releases the inner child, especially in overserious partners or solemn children • keep in a purse or wallet to attract prosperity

HOW TO USE

Burn the ground herb as part of an incense mix for good fortune, making wishes in the rising smoke. • Carry the dried flowers in a sachet and place under your pillow to bring fertility. • Alternatively, keep five seed pods in an open dish for the three nights before and the night of the full moon. On the following day, the fifth in your cycle, scatter four of the seeds from the pods in the four directions and the fifth upward. • Drink a tea made from the leaves, flowers, and stems of the plant, or use commercially available tea bags, sprinkling the dregs outside your front door to attract abundance and to remove any worries holding you back from happiness.

Herb Salts

MAGICAL FORMS

culinary herbs, magically blended with salt and symbolizing health, prosperity, fertility, and protection, amplified by whatever herbs are in the mix • this combination gives a concentrated burst of power and/or protection greater than the individual separate ingredients • since salt comes from the earth and sea, it is a natural partner in plant magick • magically, you can empower ready-made herb salts, on sale in almost every grocery store, or devise a whole range of home-created salts for your magical work

PLANET AND ELEMENT

Saturn • Earth

MAGICAL USES

add to magical cookery, a charm, an amulet, a spell bag, or a wish powder • basil salt brings courage, fidelity, and prosperity • caraway attracts love and guards against theft • use celery for money and fertility • garlic is used for protection and domestic happiness • parsley is for good fortune after loss and for learning • use rosemary for heightened passion and the return of a lover • sage is used to reach career goals and brings justice • use thyme for health and knowledge

HOW TO USE

To make your salt, grind together 350 grams (12 ounces) of the best-quality sea salt you can get with 2 teaspoons of very finely chopped fresh herbs (you can use more than one kind) or 1 teaspoon of chosen dried herbs, chanting the purpose of the herb salt continuously as you mix and grind. • Sprinkle a few empowered grains of herb salt into the flame of a candle, naming what it is you desire to increase or, alternatively, cleanse from your life. • Carry a twist of empowered mint or tarragon herb salt in silver foil or greaseproof paper when traveling to avoid accidents and dangers, especially at night. • The salt also protects against bullying. • Sprinkle chopped nettle salt outside doors and along boundaries to deter intruders, whether earthly or restless spirits.

Hibiscus

(*Hibiscus* spp.)

MAGICAL FORMS

grows well in tropical, semitropical, and warmer climates or as a potted plant indoors • as common or hardy hibiscus (*Hibiscus syriacus*), and rose mallow (*Hibiscus moscheutos*), can grow outdoors in containers to be brought indoors when it gets cold • found still fragrant as a wreath when Tutankhamun's tomb was opened in 1922 • magically use the whole, growing plant; calyces (protective layer around the flower bud); fresh and dried petals; and roots

PLANETS AND ELEMENT

Saturn/Venus • Earth

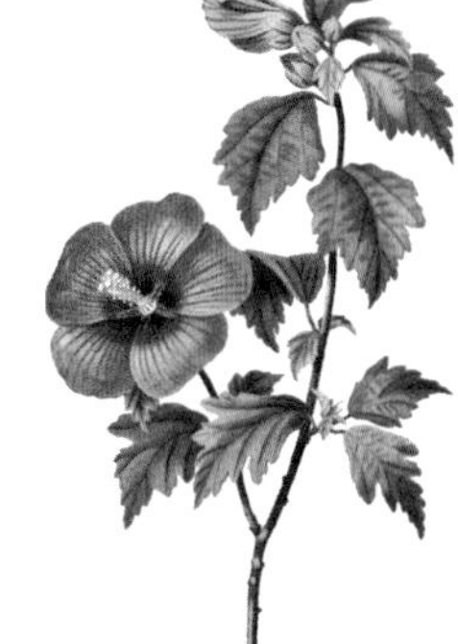

MAGICAL USES

fragrance increases psychic powers by awakening clairsentient powers • increases family love and happiness • increases libido • brings love and passion later in life • use for attracting twin soul love • increases self-esteem and promotes loving yourself as you are • attracts the fey • sacred to the Hindu goddess Kali, and so a powerful token for women who have been abused, as well as for sex magick rites

HOW TO USE

For increased fertility, make a small poppet filled with dried hibiscus flowers and set it in a woven cradle, keeping it hidden somewhere in the space where you make love, to call your infant into your life. • Perform meditation while burning hibiscus incense or inhaling the scent of the fragrant flowers to link with past lives, especially those in ancient Egypt. • Use the flower in love sachets or offer to your intended as tea to make yourself irresistible in a desired lover's eyes, especially if they are hesitant. • Add hibiscus to a dream pillow for prophetic dreams. • For a natural aphrodisiac, keep red hibiscus plants in the bedroom or add red petals to incense.

CAUTION

Excess hibiscus may cause liver problems.

Hickory Tree

(*Carya* spp.)

MAGICAL FORMS

at least eighteen different species of this tree exist, including shagbark hickory (*Carya ovata*), which is native to the eastern and midwestern USA and southern Canada, and shellbark (*Carya laciniosa*), which mainly flourishes in Ohio and the Mississippi River valleys • twelve different hickory varieties grow throughout North America • the hickory tree is also found in European and UK forests • magically use the large edible nuts, hickory leaves (especially those from the shagbark that turn golden yellow in fall), the wood, and the roots

PLANETS AND ELEMENT

Jupiter/Mercury • Air

MAGICAL USES

for use in earth, fire, and wind magick • for finding or changing direction • the wood works well as a travel amulet • in the Carolinas, traditionally driven into a doorpost to ensure a faithful partner • for perseverance, add to an incense mix

HOW TO USE

Burn a chopped hickory root and mix the ashes with cinquefoil herb (see p. 124), then add as an amulet to a blue justice bag to take to court or keep with summonses or official papers for success in legal matters. • Burn the bark in or near the home to attract good fortune and keep or drive away malevolent and restless spirits. • Use hickory wands where strong willpower is needed for the manifestation of results over time.

High John the Conqueror Root

(*Ipomoea purga*) or (*Ipomoea jalapa*)

MAGICAL FORMS

an Impomoea species related to the sweet potato and morning glory • expensive and rare root that is therefore often added in small pieces to spells or oils • the original John was reputedly the son of an African king; after being sold into slavery, he married the devil's daughter, Lilith • John defeated the devil through magick • High John is popularly considered the most powerful multipurpose magical root • magically use the cut fresh or dried root and the oil

PLANET AND ELEMENT

Mars • Fire

MAGICAL USES

in hoodoo magick, it is carried in a bag as a talisman for luck, success, attracting love, money, male sexual prowess, and as an amulet of protection against all evil

HOW TO USE

Add a piece of High John to oils for money, love, success or protection. • High John is often added to blends in which herbs or flowers are steeped in olive oil. • High John strengthens the purpose of any oil. • To make pure High John oil, cut the base of three small roots, then seal and steep the jar for a few weeks, shaking daily. • To use the root for gaining money or success in gambling or business, wrap a green dollar bill (preferably from a leap year) around a silver dime and a small root, folding the dollar inward. Seal in a green or red flannel bag, then anoint the bag every day with three drops of High John oil. Keep this bag with you 24/7 to allow the money to come in.

CAUTION

High John is poisonous if ingested. • Handle it with care and use gloves or wash hands afterward. • Keep High John in all its forms away from children and pets.

Hinoki Tree

(*Chamaecyparis obtusa*)

MAGICAL FORMS

also known as false or Japanese cypress • evergreen tree with horizontal spreading branches that is native to southern Japan • considered sacred in the Shinto religion • the wood was used to construct Shinto temples • also grows across the USA, the UK, and globally • magically work with the growing tree, incense, and essential oil

PLANET AND ELEMENT

Moon • Water

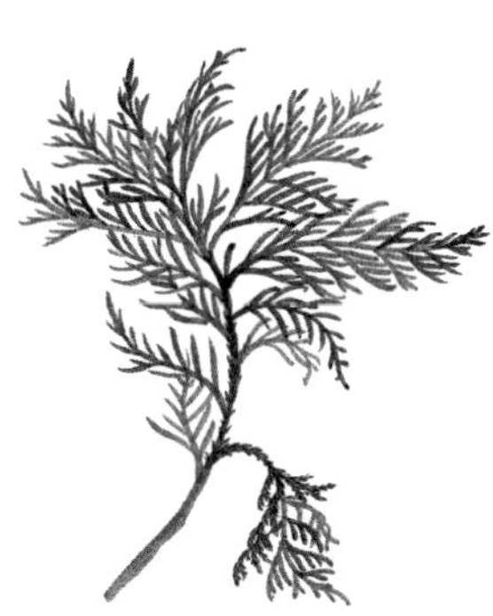

MAGICAL USES

signifies sacred connections, rituals, meditation, and ceremonies to open spiritual pathways, to explore past worlds, and more mundanely, to defuse anger

HOW TO USE

Burn or diffuse the oil or burn the incense sticks to receive messages from your ancestors, most easily through images in the smoke or words and images in your mind that surface as you hear your ancestors' voices within you. • Sit beneath the tree with your back against the trunk to make connection with higher nature beings who live within these ancient trees, which can live hundreds of years and grow up to seventy-five feet tall. • Use the oil or incense before meditation to make the transition from the everyday world and sense your spirit guides coming closer.

CAUTION

Do not use oil or incense during the first trimester of pregnancy.

Holly

(*Ilex* spp.)

MAGICAL FORMS

a genus consisting of over 570 species of plants, including American holly (*Ilex opaca*) and common holly (*Ilex aquifolium*) • will grow as a bush or small tree, but can become very tall • is made into wreaths most used around Yule • magically use the cut or whole, growing plant; berries; and leaves

PLANETS AND ELEMENTS

Saturn/Mars • Earth/Fire

MAGICAL USES

sacred to the Celts as one of the seven magical trees • one of the Ogham tree staves and also one of the nine woods used in ceremonial fires • wreaths have been put on doors at Yule since time immemorial to offer winter shelter for the fae and wood spirits • a holly wand consecrates ritual knives • decorating the home at Yule with holly brings luck for the year ahead • grown around the property, holly protects against lightning, sorcerers, bad weather, damage to the home, and restless spirits who are active around the seasonal change points

HOW TO USE

At sunset on the shortest day of the year, silently gather nine holly leaves from a nonspiny tree, tie in a white cloth with nine red knots, and place beneath your pillow to make dreams come true. To dream of a future love, especially later in life, add nine ivy leaves, which are the symbol of the Yule Ivy Queen, alter ego of the Holly King. • Three berries cast into flowing water after the light has faded on the shortest day of the year promise new life will return, whether fertility for a desired child or new beginnings generally, with the dawn. • Pick nine more leaves and berries as the Yule light returns and place in a sealed sachet to carry until midsummer in order to bring courage, the power to overcome seemingly impossible odds, and money owed or that was unfairly lost.

CAUTION

The berries are highly poisonous, so remove them from holly used for indoor decorations if you have curious pets or small children.

Hollyhock

(*Alcea rosea*)

MAGICAL FORMS

Neanderthal man was found buried with hollyhocks • hollyhocks were also discovered in the tomb of the ancient Egyptian pharaoh Tutankhamun • hollyhocks were brought back to Europe by the Crusaders from the Holy Land, where the plant had been introduced from Asia • one of the earliest flowers to reach the New World • extensively used medicinally in medieval Europe • magically work with the growing or cut flowers, fresh and dried blossoms, seeds, and flower essence

PLANETS AND ELEMENTS

Mars/Jupiter • Fire/Air

MAGICAL USES

a flower of Lammas, the first harvest, celebrated in early August, when traditionally children would carry a single long hollyhock around the fields in procession, symbolizing abundance and fertility • also considered a fertility icon because of the number of seeds hollyhocks shed year after year • its height signifies leadership, and the purple and white represent nobility and ambition to do good for others, as well as personal elevation • a fey flower believed to shelter flower spirits and faeries • in the seventeenth century, superstition told that drinking a tea including hollyhocks, thyme, marigold, and hazel buds would not only give sight of the fey, but also make it possible to communicate with them so that they would grant wishes

HOW TO USE

Because of its long history dating back to antiquity, it is an ideal flower for meditation, with the growing flowers in situ or cut flowers placed on an altar. • Hollyhock offers visions of past worlds, both personal past lives and visions of ancient times. • The seed pods can be used as a charm to bring money or possessions when most needed. • Releasing the seeds from a pod on the full moon calls a baby; if the seeds stick together there may be twins or births of subsequent children in close succession in the future, and a large family close in age. • Infuse fresh blossoms in cold water overnight, then add two or three drops of the flower essence before drinking to restore or create confidence when dealing with authority or those with big egos.

Honesty

(*Lunaria annua* var. *albiflora*)

MAGICAL FORMS

also known as silver dollar or moon plant • its purple flowers are said to glow in the moonlight • translucent, papery seed pods shaped like silver discs • honesty was used as a fifteenth-century ingredient for astral projection • magically work with the growing plant, its flowers (fresh and dried), and the pods and membranes

PLANET AND ELEMENT

Moon • Earth

MAGICAL USES

inspires integrity • use for financial advantage, especially acquiring money through luck • dispels inner fears and malevolent spirits of the night • for use in moon magick • for identifying thieves and liars • the pods or membranes, as part of a dried flower arrangement, offer assurance that the truth will always be spoken in your home or relationship

HOW TO USE

Place three seed pods or three silver pod membranes along with a silver dollar in a small silver bag or purse on a Monday, the Moon night, or two nights before full moon. Burn a silver candle over the closed bag for three consecutive nights and carry it with you or keep it where you do your finances to bring short- and long-term prosperity, or in your workspace to gain recognition at your job. Every month, replace the seed pods (but not the coin), throwing them into flowing water. • Keep a silver membrane or pod in your purse or wallet and you will never be short of resources or good fortune. • Scatter a trail of dried or fresh flowers from your boundary to your front door to call wealth and keep away both on- and offline cheats. • Place nine dried flowers under your mattress to keep away specters of the night. • Listen to the rustling papery pods of the growing plant in the wind for messages from Earth and Air spirits, especially close to the full moon; ask what you most need to know, and you will hear the answer in the rustling or your inner voice. • Gaze at the flowery or silvery plant through a semicircle of three jasmine or myrrh incense sticks during the waxing moon. Allow your mind to follow the smoke trail for visions of other realms.

Honey

MAGICAL FORMS

unique substance, made incredibly powerful by the transformational process of the nectar of plants chosen by the bees which predate humanity • each type of honey is different, but shares the collective energies of the alchemical formation • magically work at a safe distance from where bees are collecting the nectar • cooking with and eating a flower honey absorbs the flower's sweetness and abundance

PLANETS AND ELEMENT

Sun/Venus • Fire

MAGICAL USES

in magical cookery, any type of honey softens critical or discouraging attitudes and promotes family unity • eating your chosen honey brings fertility and abundance in money and resources • many types have a distinctive aroma, especially if made locally by hand

HOW TO USE

When observing bees collecting nectar for honey, close your eyes and allow the buzzing to carry you back to old worlds when perhaps you made your own honey. • Acacia honey, from a plant called American acacia in the USA, is produced from the black locust tree (see p. 269) and should be eaten for a favorable result in court cases. • American sourwood tree blossom honey (see p. 419) should be consumed during rites of passage, especially entering the wisewoman phase. • Called "the honey of the angels," sourwood honey should be eaten or used to sweeten a drink before meditation or bedtime to connect with your guardian angels. • Tupelo honey (see p. 65) added to rose tea calls romance, and if added to a bedtime drink, brings dream plane love visions. • Manuka and bell heather honey are considered healers, while clover honey calls good luck and can be added to a wish tea with rosemary and thyme. • Following Chinese tradition, beehives set in orange tree orchards produce orange blossom honey for fertility and attract abundance to the home. • Wildflower honey is darker and stronger than many other varieties. • Buy a local wildflower mix to connect with the indigenous earth spirits and fey.

Honeydew Melon

(*Cucumis melo*)

MAGICAL FORMS

plant produces large round or oval pale-green fruit with smooth greenish to yellow skin • native to North Africa, southern France, and Spain • grown worldwide in sunny semiarid climates including China, Turkey, and the USA, especially California and Arizona • magically use the whole and sliced melons and the seeds

PLANET AND ELEMENT

Moon • Water

MAGICAL USES

a symbol of the belly of the Mother Goddess • set in the center of an altar, with a hole in the top for a candle, to call fertility, especially on the full moon • for triggering self-healing powers if you experience chronic minor, but debilitating, illness

HOW TO USE

On full moon night, if a relationship has lost its spark, cut your melon in half. • Scoop out the flesh of one half to share later. • Fill the empty half with spices, herbs, and flower petals of your choice. • Sail it on a lake or river, making a wish that the love connection may grow strong once more. • Drill or pierce a hole in the seeds to make triple bracelets (paint and varnish them if you wish). • Wear them on your writing hand to attract abundance in the form of money, health, charisma, and positive results every time you spontaneously move your hand outward. • Cast a bag of melon seeds to the wind to launch a new idea or project. • Scatter a handful of seeds on a map and see where most fall to indicate a good vacation or relocation area.

Honeysuckle

(*Lonicera periclymenum*)

MAGICAL FORMS

also known as woodbine • a highly scented flower, popular in Elizabethan gardens, signified by its use in hidden arbors as a secret love tryst flower • flower of spring equinox • one of the most magical Druidic plants • magically use flowers, fresh and dried; flower essence; and oil, though it can be hard to obtain pure honeysuckle oil

PLANETS AND ELEMENTS

Jupiter/Venus • Fire/Earth

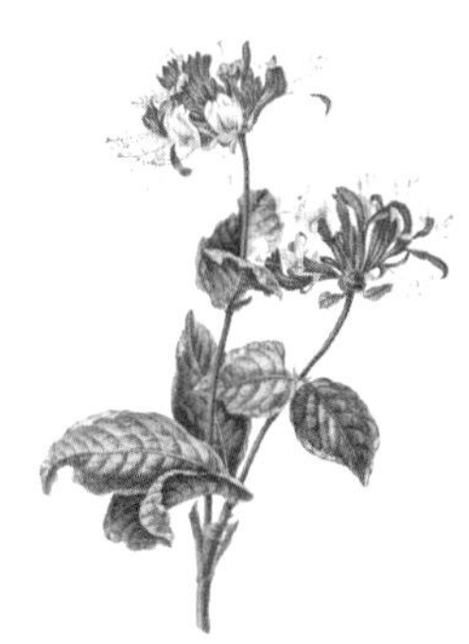

MAGICAL USES

as a doorkeeper, turns away doubts and fears • keeps family members who feel vulnerable safe within the home (good against teenagers' friends who may wield an undesirable influence) • improves psychic powers • grows wealth and promotes career opportunity • encourages benign nature spirits

HOW TO USE

Growing honeysuckle outside your door or up external walls keeps domestic happiness within the home. • The plant brings good luck and repels all whose envy would spoil it. • Burn incense or diffuse oil while meditating on the journey to self-discovery. • Honeysuckle can be used in commitment rituals instead of ivy to prevent possessiveness. • Diffuse the oil as a room cleanser to clean out quarrels, misfortune, and sorrow. • The flower essence can be used to let old, sad memories go. • Burn a green candle with honeysuckle to attract money.

CAUTION

Avoid the berries, as most are poisonous. • Honeysuckle can sometimes cause digestive problems, skin irritation, and photosensitivity, so ingest at your own risk and, when using topically, do a patch test.

Honeysuckle, Japanese

(*Lonicera japonica*)

MAGICAL FORMS

a trailing shrub with fragrant white flowers • called *jin yin hua* in traditional Chinese medicine, "the gold-silver flower," because flowers of different ages on the same plant change from white to yellow • magically use fresh and dried leaves as tea, vine lengths with leaves and flowers, the whole growing plant, and black berries

PLANET AND ELEMENTS

Jupiter • Air/Earth

MAGICAL USES

cuts ties with destructive influences, situations, and people • for spreading your influence and networking • as tea or cut flowers, sweetens sour people (see "Honeysuckle," p. 221) • use the dried berries as a talisman for winning votes, increasing status, getting a promotion to a position of influence, or for any takeover bid

HOW TO USE

Place the early white and later yellow stages of flower with a piece of silver and gold in a gold charm bag for business, workplace, or personal money-making enterprises, to represent the acquisition and growth of wealth. • Because it is an especially pervasive, clinging form of honeysuckle, resistant to destruction and regarded as invasive in some states in the USA, cut, knot, and bury pieces of the vine, first removing the flowers and leaves, naming them as you do so with whom or what you wish to remove from your life. If what you wish to remove is a bad habit or fear, knot the vine around a symbol of the problem, such as a cigarette or gambling chip, before burying.

CAUTION

Check with a doctor before ingesting if pregnant or taking regular medication.

Honeysuckle, Orange

(*Lonicera ciliosa*)

MAGICAL FORMS

also known as western trumpet honeysuckle • large, climbing, twining plant with numerous tubular, bright-orange, non-fragrant flowers • produced late spring to midsummer, the flowers become translucent, red-orange berries • the vine needs support, often trained up fences, in arbors and walls, becoming twenty to thirty feet high and thirty feet wide • attracts hummingbirds, bees, and butterflies • native wild to the forests of western North America, but also cultivated in gardens in the USA and other lands • found in cold remedies and as a sedative and contraceptive, especially in the 1800s, but not used anymore • magically use the growing plant and flower essence

PLANET AND ELEMENT

Jupiter • Air

MAGICAL USES

especially as flower essence, use for flowing creativity and focus, to become less disturbed by outside disruptions, interruptions, and distractions • ideal for centering those who work or create from home • also calms inner frustration and irritability within the artist, writer, or creator caused by creative blocks

HOW TO USE

Grown on the outside of the home wall or boundary fences, honeysuckle attracts prosperity, health, and happiness, and insulates against anger and tantrums from tots, teens, and drama kings and queens of all ages. • Sit facing the climbing plant with half-closed eyes and use it as a shamanic ladder to climb to other realms. • Anoint your throat and brow with a drop of the essence to open creative channels and take away frustration and irritability when ideas will not come. • Anoint door handles and inner window locks with the essence added to water or spritz the room where you work at home to exclude timewasters and unnecessary interruptions on- and offline.

CAUTION

Avoid in pregnancy, as not enough is known about the safety or otherwise of honeysuckle.

Hops

(*Humulus lupulus*)

MAGICAL FORMS
native to North America, South America, Europe, and Asia • grown commercially in northern Europe, the UK, and the northern states of the USA • the branching stem allows the plant to climb from fifteen to twenty-five feet tall • magically use the dried strobiles, the fragrant female flower, the small seed cones or cone-like catkins that grow on the end of the tall brines, the stem, the dried leaves, and the dried or powdered herb (obtainable online)

PLANET AND ELEMENT
Saturn • Earth

MAGICAL USES
fresh or dried garlands can be used as luck-bringing decorations that can be used at celebrations or to protect the home • promotes healing • attracts money • for recovery from loss or debt • an offering at the autumn equinox celebrations, a symbol of regeneration • first brewed as beer in the eleventh century

HOW TO USE
Traditionally, a pinch of hops, a pinch of dried lavender, and three bay leaves are tied in a white cloth with three knots and sewn or secured inside a pillow to bring peaceful sleep and dreams. • Sprinkle the dried leaves to create a protective circle for outdoor rituals. • Rub the dried leaves on the forehead to enhance divinatory abilities, and keep a sachet with tarot cards or runes.

CAUTION
Hops are highly toxic to dogs. • They should not be ingested if taking blood thinners or hormone therapies, or during pregnancy and breastfeeding. • Hops may cause skin allergies, so handle with care.

Horehound

(*Marrubium vulgare*)

MAGICAL FORMS
named after Horus, the hawk-headed Egyptian sky god, and burned in incense in ancient Egyptian rituals dedicated to Horus, his mother Isis, and his father Osiris, the latter in regeneration rituals • blooms through summer • magically use the cut or whole, growing plant; the aerial parts, tops, and leaves, dried and chopped; and the flowers, fresh and dried

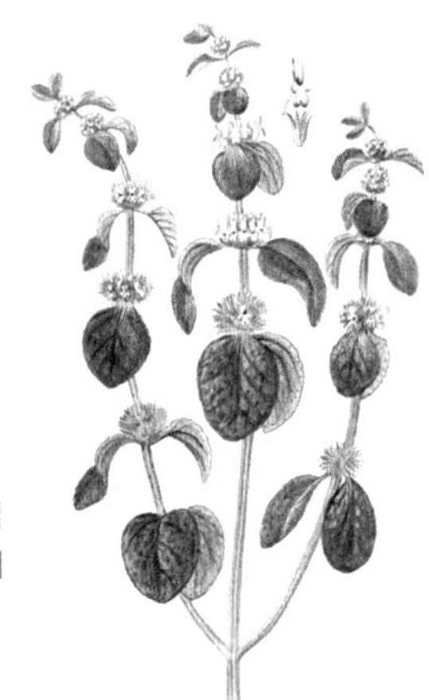

PLANETS AND ELEMENTS
Mars/Mercury • Fire/Air

MAGICAL USES
use in protective sachets against ill wishes and illusory enchantment by fleeting pleasures and unwise influences • meditate on plants for creative awakening if you are feeling blocked

HOW TO USE
Sprinkle a circle of the dried herb as a magick circle of protection before a defensive ritual or if you are contacting the spirit world. • Use the dried herb to mark out a magical space within which magick can occur without the intrusion of earthly influences and thoughts. • When horehound is in flower, it can be gathered, dried, and tied with red ribbon, then hung in the home to bring peace and balance and for keeping away specters of the night.

CAUTION
Avoid during pregnancy or if trying to get pregnant.

Hornbeam

(*Carpinus* spp.)

MAGICAL FORMS

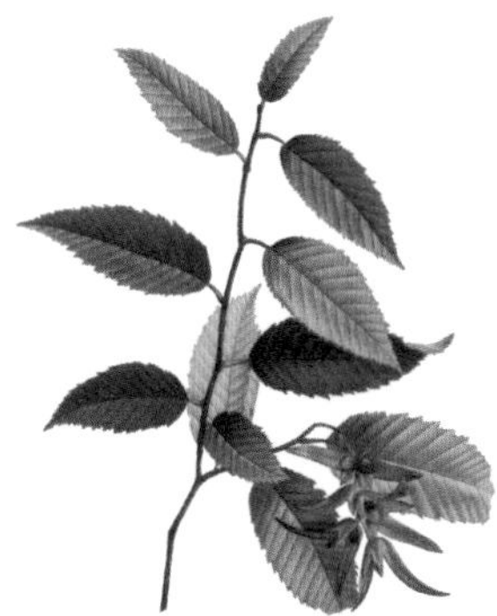

includes American hornbeam (*Carpinus caroliniana*), also known as ironwood; European hornbeam (*Carpinus betulus*); and American hophornbeam (*Ostrya virginiana*), also known as hardtack or ironwood • the American hornbeam grows wild down the eastern coast of North America • more widely cultivated as hophornbeam throughout the temperate USA and southern Europe • common hornbeam flourishes in southern England, central Europe, and southwestern Asia, and increasingly in the USA • an incredibly hard wood whose embers glow for a long time, so use hornbeam fires with great care in an outdoor or hearth fire vigil that may last many hours • magically use the wood or growing tree

PLANETS AND ELEMENTS

Saturn/Mars • Earth/Fire

MAGICAL USES

wish magick • following dreams • determination, ethics, and facing challenges with courage • going it alone away from the comfort zone

HOW TO USE

Burn hornbeam wood in an outdoor or hearth fire before a long, difficult journey alone or when leaving home, family, or a safe career and venturing into uncharted territory. Once the charcoal or ashes cool, scoop a little into a small, sealed jar. Carry it, or alternately a small hornbeam artifact, with you for reassurance during long, dark nights. • A wand made from common hornbeam should be for personal use and its spell purposes never named aloud.

Horseradish

(*Armoracia rusticana*)

MAGICAL FORMS

plant in the Brassicaceae family, along with broccoli and cauliflower • deep tap-like root, unearthed in fall, has a powerful flavor • magically use the cut or whole, growing plant, fresh or dried; the dock-like leaves; the white flowers, fresh and dried; and the root

PLANET AND ELEMENT

Mars • Fire

MAGICAL USES

for purification • banishing negativity • winning competitions • magical cookery • virility, sexual satisfaction, conception

HOW TO USE

The dried and powdered root should be sprinkled on doorsteps, entrances, and any dark corners, basements, or attics to remove the presence of malevolent or restless spirit energies. • Hang the dried plant over doorways to repel curses, jinxes, and hexes of the past, present, and future. • Planted in the four corners of a garden or potted in a kitchen, horseradish attracts prosperity and good fortune. • Stir horseradish sauce, either while making it or when opening a commercially purchased jar, to soften critical relatives or friends during a meal. • Burn horseradish in an incense mix if you find it hard to concentrate while meditating. • Women should place the root on their womb for sexual ecstasy while lovemaking. • Men prevented from achieving an erection through anxiety should set the root over their genitals, especially if conceiving a child is proving problematic. • Carry the chopped root in a green bag for luck when gambling and place the bag on top of lottery tickets.

CAUTION

Do not ingest if you have thyroid issues.

Horsetail

(*Equisetum arvense*)

MAGICAL FORMS

produced by spores, not seeds • does not flower • found as fossils descended from huge trees, dating from the Paleolithic Age • native to Europe, North Africa, northern Asia, and North and South America • the fir-tree-like shoots grow between ten and twenty inches tall in summer, resembling horses' tails • the fertile light-brown spring stems have a spore on top and become sterile while growing • magically use the aerial parts, especially the leaves and the stems, as well as the shoots

PLANETS AND ELEMENT

Venus/Saturn • Earth

MAGICAL USES

use in fertility incense mixes, though horsetail is not fragrant, and in rituals to conceive a baby • trimmed, crossed, dried spring stems, sometimes with red thread knotted in the center, were believed to aid fertility if hung on the wall behind the bed • a charm bag of the dried leaves is still carried to horse and dog racing and competitions for good luck

HOW TO USE

The growing plant, with its deep roots, represents secure travel and returning safely home, whether daily or a long journey, in which case an amulet of the chopped fir-like shoots should be carried. • Made into whistles, the spring stems were traditionally played to command snakes. • The cut, dried, crushed, and sometimes powdered stems have become an amulet to protect against human snakes, often with dried lemongrass herbs added. • Tea made from the leaves, with raw honey added, gives strength, courage, and determination to succeed in any venture, and the tea or tea bags are readily available online (use the leaves in a resinous incense mix).

CAUTION

Avoid if pregnant or breastfeeding.

Houndstongue

(*Cynoglossum* spp.)

MAGICAL FORMS

includes *Cynoglossum officinale*; *Cynoglossum creticum*, also called blue houndstongue; and *Cynoglossum virginianum*, also called wild comfrey • long, grayish, hairy leaves, and a stem resembling a dog's tongue • once used for dog bites • tongue of dog was one of the ingredients in the witches' cauldron in Shakespeare's *Macbeth* • *Cynoglossum officinale* has either maroon or reddish-purple funnel-shaped forget-me-not-type flowers or flowers in shades of blue-purple to white • *Cynoglossum virginianum* is native to the USA, *Cynoglossum officinale* to the UK and Europe • both have hairy seed clusters like nuts, with a seed that clings to clothing • magically use (with care) any of the hairy parts of the plant that stick

PLANET AND ELEMENT

Saturn • Earth

MAGICAL USES

prevents problems with other people's dogs • stops lies about you from being believed, especially legally or officially

HOW TO USE

Grow houndstongue against a fence or in a pot on an adjoining wall if you are disturbed by a neighbor's constantly barking dog. • Slip a small amount of the dried leaves into a sealed hollow metal tube on your dog's collar to protect them on walks if they are afraid of other dogs. • The herb has a noxious smell, so add a small amount of the dried leaves, chopped stems, or nutlets to a sealed amulet bag, sweetened with lavender or rose petals. • Take the bag with you if you are facing a court case or a line of questioning, or are seeking compensation. • Any lies and slander will cling to the perpetrator of the untruths or evasions against you.

CAUTION

Houndstongue plant may cause skin irritation: handle with care. • It is dangerous to cattle, horses, and goats.

Huckleberry

(*Vaccinium ovatum*)

MAGICAL FORMS

also known as evergreen huckleberry or California huckleberry • cousin of the bilberry and blueberry (see p. 72) • related to the eastern and southeastern *Gaylussacia huckleberry* varieties • huckleberry is a spreading flowering shrub, blossoming with pale-pink urn-shaped flowers that blossom between April and May, which become highly edible black or purple berries • native to western North America from British Columbia to northern California • bronze-red leaves become glossy-green in summer months • magically use the cut flowers and leaves (these last about three weeks), dried flowers, and fresh berries

PLANETS AND ELEMENT

Moon/Venus • Water

MAGICAL USES

in magical cookery, use for family happiness and a sense of well-being, especially after a berry-picking outing • huckleberries bring good luck, psychic protection, magical dreams, and a strong connection with nature and nature spirits • increase intuition and awareness of the previously unseen • Mark Twain's fictional character, the happy-go-lucky, resourceful Huckleberry Finn, captures the spontaneous power of the berries when eaten to make anything possible if chances are taken and disbelief suspended

HOW TO USE

Use the fresh-cut, blossoming sprigs, particularly if attached to ripening berries, in wedding bouquets to bring fertility and abundance. • Burn the dried leaves in a heatproof container in well-ventilated rooms as smudge or in incense, spreading the smoke with a feather or your hand to remove poltergeist activity, malicious spirits, and hexes or curses known or unknown.

CAUTION

Avoid if pregnant or breastfeeding.

Hyacinth

(*Hyacinthus orientalis*)

MAGICAL FORMS

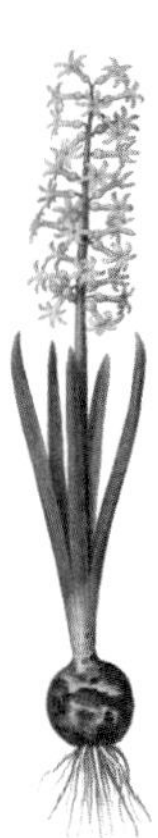

flowering plant with fragrant flowers that bloom in the spring • flower of the spring equinox • the young Hyacinthus was killed by the Greek father god Zeus, who became jealous of his love for Apollo, the god of light; Apollo transformed Hyacinthus into the beautiful, fragrant flower so the young man might live eternally and renew the promise of joy returning every spring • magically use whole growing or cut plant, petals, or essential oil (as it is very rare and expensive, it is more often sold as fragrance oil)

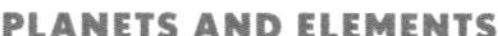

PLANETS AND ELEMENTS

Venus/Saturn • Water/Earth

MAGICAL USES

for healing self-esteem issues and rebuilding trust after betrayal • new beginnings • regaining lost love • creating a happy home • mending quarrels with or between friends or family • flower psychometry

HOW TO USE

Use in dream pillows for peaceful sleep, to prevent nightmares, and to bring on psychic dreams of past worlds, twin souls, or dream lovers. • Spray a mist containing a few drops of essential or the more diluted fragrance oil in water where you will be carrying out psychic work to enhance meditation, visualization, and spell casting. • Carry the petals in a sachet for happy sex while single, as well as trans and gender-fluid relationships. Carry the sachet to meet the right person and when you are afraid your partnership will encounter prejudice from narrow-minded family members or friends. • Burn the dried flowers to remove hexes and curses and in passing-over ceremonies if you sense a departed loved one is holding back.

CAUTION

The bulbs are toxic if eaten. • Hyacinths can cause skin irritation if the bulbs are handled or if a person's skin is very sensitive to the stem, so use with care.

Hyacinth, Grape

(*Muscari armeniacum*)

MAGICAL FORMS

also called muscari, for its genus • smaller than true hyacinths, with upturned flower cups clustered together resembling grapes • magically use the growing plant, fresh and dried cut flowers, and flower essence

PLANETS AND ELEMENTS

Saturn/Moon • Earth/Water

MAGICAL USES

popular for weddings, especially in nosegays, in its clear-blue, white-and-blue, and white bicolor varieties • features in different religions and forms of spiritual celebrations as a symbol of blessings on the union • grape hyacinths have been grown for thousands of years • in the ancient Greek myth, Hyacinthus was loved by Apollo and Zephyrus, god of the West Wind • Zephyrus, in a fit of jealousy, caused Hyacinthus's death, but his slain blood became the grape hyacinth; in some versions, the tears of Apollo mingling with the blood caused the colorful blooms • especially the yellow flower is used in anti-envy and -jealousy rituals, against the Evil Eye • at the bottom of the plant, the flowers wither as the top ones come into bloom, allowing a ritual to release power over days and run its course

HOW TO USE

Plant grape hyacinths along any pathway from your home to carry their harmony into your daily life. • Add dried flowers to a sleep pillow to protect against nightmares. • Plant in your garden or display cut flowers to guard against hostile energies from whatever source. • Each day, add a few drops of the flower essence to potpourri containing the dried flowers, plus dried rose petals and lavender. Keep at home or in your workspace if you feel excluded, undervalued, or isolated from family or colleagues' social events. Inhale the potpourri to give others positive awareness of your presence and opinions. • Ingest a little of the essence yourself any morning you need to network face to face, online, or by phone, and keep your potpourri near while you are interacting with others.

Hydrangea

(*Hydrangea* spp.)

MAGICAL FORMS

numerous species of many-petalled deciduous shrubs • the most common cultivated kind, *Hydrangea macrophylla*, thrives in the USA and worldwide • the wild *Hydrangea arborescens* is found growing in the eastern USA from Boston to Florida and in many other places • used medicinally by Native North Americans, including the Cherokee nation • magically use the whole plant growing in a garden or in the wild, cut fresh and dried flowers, and bark

PLANETS AND ELEMENTS

Jupiter/Moon • Air/Water

MAGICAL USES

for changing career, retirement, redundancy, or when resigning from the workplace for a new life • breaking curses and hexes • in Japan the blue flower is an expression of regret • purple hydrangeas represent mystery, wealth, and spiritual links with higher realms • pink represents appreciation • white is aligned with weddings and formal celebrations • green is for renewal, rebirth, and health • yellow is for loyalty and friendship • as bouquets or centerpieces, hydrangeas in any color draw people of different ages and backgrounds together and spread blessings

HOW TO USE

Burn the bark in an incense mix to remove a curse. Alternatively, add the flowers to a floor wash or bath to break a curse. If the source of the curse is unknown, on any waning moon night, hold a single hydrangea to a mirror so you are not reflected and say, *Reflected be, back to the source of whoever sent this hex to me.* Set the mirror on an outward-facing wall outdoors until the moon disappears, and tie the flower to a tree away from your home. • Hydrangeas planted on either side of the door or along a fence act as guardians against earthly intrusions or paranormal influences and shield against ill wishes and harm, accidental or deliberate, as well as attract good fortune. • Bless and send a pot of yellow or pink hydrangeas as a housewarming gift.

CAUTION

Hydrangeas are toxic to humans and pets, so do not ingest.

Hyssop

(*Hyssopus officinalis*)

MAGICAL FORMS

a small shrub that flowers during the summer • hyssop is mentioned many times in the Bible for its power to cleanse the body of illness • magically use the growing plant; the dried aerial parts of the flowering herb, especially the dried leaves; and the oil extracted from flowers and leaves

PLANET AND ELEMENTS

Jupiter • Air/Fire

MAGICAL USES

the ultimate cleansing and purification herb • removes negative influences from property, precious artifacts, places, and people • banishes self-defeating thoughts and doubts, leaving positivity

HOW TO USE

Burn hyssop mixed with eucalyptus, thyme, and lavender as part of a sacred incense to lift energies in any place or situation. • Hyssop is the ultimate infusion, to be sprinkled over areas of negativity in the home and objects that have unwelcoming or sorrowful vibrations, as well as for consecrating ritual tools. • Anoint a white candle with the oil, which was considered sacred in ancient Egypt, and burn the candle in a room needing cleansing, or use a diffuser to cleanse the room. • Hang the dried herb over windows to keep away negative energies, thieves, and intruders. • Use the herb, tied to a leather or wooden handle and dipped in water, to asperge a ritual area before ceremonies.

CAUTION

Do not use if pregnant or breastfeeding.

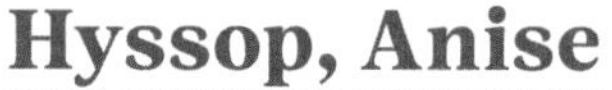

Hyssop, Anise

(*Agastache foeniculum*)

MAGICAL FORMS

related to, but different from, hyssop • of the mint family • native to northern North America • wild and cultivated, grows in the Midwest, the Great Plains, and Canada • flowers have a long blooming season, from June to September • magically use the whole, growing plant; the cut, spiky flowers; the fragrant leaves and flowers, fresh and dried, especially in blue to lavender purple, the colors of harmony

PLANET AND ELEMENT

Mars • Fire

MAGICAL USES

in dream pillows to drive away nightmares and sad thoughts • used traditionally in medicine bundles for protection, to attract positive energies, and uplift the energies • a purifier of people and situations as a tea and sprinkled to clear sacred spaces • overcomes trauma • magical cookery for parties and celebrations

HOW TO USE

Dried, the flowers are long-lasting and protect the home, especially if you are frequently absent, if you call into them the power of the house guardian. • In the garden, anise hyssop attracts bees and butterflies and so may be used for all Air magick, to attract abundance and for connecting with deceased relatives who may take the form of butterflies. • The flower of happiness, fill an area of the garden with them or keep the cut flowers where the breeze will carry the uplifting sensations through the home or workspace. • Use the dried flowers in crafts to decorate the home and potpourri (a delicate licorice scent) if you have moody teenagers or grumpy relatives visit or stay. • Offer as a cheering gift to natural pessimists.

Illawarra Flame Tree

(*Brachychiton acerifolius*)

MAGICAL FORMS

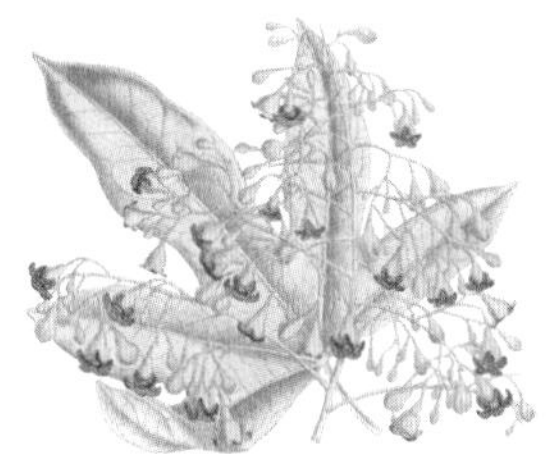

native to Queensland and New South Wales, Australia (Illawarra derives from the indigenous name for the coastal region of New South Wales) • can be forty to sixty feet high, but half that height when grown in California • numerous bright-red, bell-shaped flowers and a swollen trunk where water is stored • the inner bark is a traditional Australian Aboriginal medicine, used for food and to make fishing nets and string • not to be confused with the red flowering royal poinciana (*Delonix regia*), the tropical tree native to Madagascar and also found in Australia and parts of the USA • the tree can be grown on patios or as an indoor potted plant in cooler regions as a focus for magick • magically use the fallen blossoms and the growing tree in situ

PLANETS AND ELEMENT

Mars/Sun • Fire

MAGICAL USES

protection against accidents, loss of identity, and codependency • for courage to speak and act against the status quo or bullies

HOW TO USE

Set a dish of the fallen blossoms in water for an instant energy boost, enthusiasm, and inspiration in a lethargic office or home environment. • Set the flowers on your altar or special place to represent the Fire element in more formal magick rituals. • Meditate beneath the tree or with your potted plant, especially when the flowers are in bloom, to awaken your true self if you seek to be free but are emotionally, financially, or physically reliant on or controlled by another.

CAUTION

The seeds, though edible, are covered in hairs that are hard to remove and may cause an allergy. • The seeds are also toxic to animals and birds.

Impatiens

(*Impatiens walleriana*)

MAGICAL FORMS

a component of the Five-Flower Rescue Remedy (see p. 181) • also known as busy Lizzie • an antidote to poison ivy, which in the wild often grows near impatiens • magically use the growing flower, including its petals

PLANET AND ELEMENTS

Mercury • Air/Water

MAGICAL USES

for flower psychometry • enjoying the moment • leisure and sports activities • discovering the best time to act or wait • overcoming impatience with life and others and acting impulsively • maternal devotion and patience because traditionally impatiens were planted in gardens dedicated to the Virgin Mary and considered sacred • possesses the valuable dual capacities to generate focus and the patience to see tasks through

HOW TO USE

Add the flower essence or the rescue remedy of which it is a part to water in a room spray to calm impatient family members or work colleagues. • Carry the dried petals in a small sachet pinned to your clothes if competing in races or athletic pursuits to prevent distractions. • Take the seeds in a small, orange bag to protect yourself against any situation where you may face spite, jealousy, or venomous words. • Keep a pot of busy Lizzie in your home if you are an overworked parent or caregiver trying to juggle work and home and you seem always to run out of time. • A pot of impatiens in a yoga or meditation studio stills the minds of clients rushing in after a busy day.

Indian Paintbrush

(*Castilleja linariifolia*)

MAGICAL FORMS

native mainly but not exclusively to the western Americas from Alaska south to the Andes, northern Asia, northwestern Russia, Mongolia, and Kazakhstan • *Castilleja linariifolia* has been the state plant of Wyoming since 1917 • brightly colored, spiked bracts are red, yellow, pinkish white, pink, orange, and purple, resembling a paintbrush overflowing with paint • the origin of the paintbrush plant is as follows: a homesick Blackfoot woman fell in love with a prisoner of her people and ran away with him • she used her own blood to paint an image of the village to which she could never return • the first paintbrush flower grew where she dropped the bloodstained stick that she used to paint it • magically use the growing plant or individual bracts, fresh or dried

PLANET AND ELEMENTS

Venus • Water/Earth

MAGICAL USES

a magical symbol in rituals for those far from home who cannot return • used in rites and meditation on the growing or cut plant for happiness, creativity (especially artistry) • yellow for a career or location change • orange for striking out alone and doing things your own way • red for a desired love or much-wanted baby • multicolored for launching a creative career • magenta, pink, or purple for building a spiritual path

HOW TO USE

Choose a number of red and orange paintbrush flowers, whether growing in nature or cut, to keep on your altar. Name each as you touch it with an identical red and orange Indian paintbrush serving as a wand, specifying a wish or plan you desire to put into practice. • Write the name of a current project that has come to a halt or is not working out by tracing it invisibly on a piece of fallen bark. Afterward, burn the bark.

Inmortal

(*Asclepias asperula*)

MAGICAL FORMS

also called antelope horns, milkweed, or spider milkweed • a flowering plant often called antelope horns because its seed pods curve like horns • very intricate green-and-white flowers with maroon centers and bright-green leaves • native to southwestern and midwestern USA and northern Mexico • grows wild and in flower gardens • they are remarkably adaptable and can be cultivated in the UK and Europe as well as other states in the USA, though they especially love dry, sandy soils • magically use the growing plant and flower essence

PLANET AND ELEMENT

Venus • Earth

MAGICAL USES

overcomes a lack of self-esteem and feelings of inadequacy and inferiority that may manifest as depression, inertia, lethargy, or a victim mentality and instead creates a sense of personal worth • for teenagers with poor self-image that may, in extremes, manifest as eating disorders or self-harm

HOW TO USE

Take the flower essence in water or add to massage oil the week before PMS. Continue until the onset of menstruation. • If teenagers have become hermits, add a few drops of essence to a bath, add to room spray and spritz their bedrooms, or use oil in a humidifier. • As this plant is a host to the Monarch butterfly and other pollinators, meditate on the growing flowers as butterflies (often regarded as spirits of the departed) settle, sending and receiving messages to and from relatives no longer with you. • Alternatively, visualize a herd of antelopes moving swiftly across the plains outrunning all fears and dangers.

CAUTION

The plant is toxic to humans, grazing animals, and pets.

Iris

(*Iris* spp.)

MAGICAL FORMS

numerous varieties; best known as purple and yellow flowers, for example *Iris hollandica* • named after Iris, the goddess of the rainbow, who traveled via the rainbow between the heavens and earth • symbol of reincarnation in ancient Egypt; irises were placed in Egyptian funeral temples and tombs to grant safe passage to the afterlife • the Orris (often from *Iris germanica* or *florentina*) is used extensively in magick as incense and as a potpourri fixative but is difficult to obtain as it is one of the world's most expensive perfume ingredients • the iris seems most effective magically when the whole flower is used, but dried petals can substitute in spells and for enhancing magical and spiritual energies when it is not flowering • magically use the growing plant, dried or fresh cut flowers, and the dried root

PLANETS AND ELEMENTS

Mercury/Moon • Air/Water

MAGICAL USES

a sacred flower bringing communication with deceased relatives, and for receiving long-awaited news • mending quarrels • moon magick for love and romance • the three upper petals represent faith, wisdom, and valor in many lands

HOW TO USE

Traditionally, the iris is placed on women's graves so that the goddess Iris will guide them to the afterlife. • A small patch of iris should be planted or a pot of bulbs or the cut flowers sent on the day of a baby's birth, baptism, or naming ceremony as a blessing on the health and happiness of the growing child. • The iris has signified purification since Roman times, a custom continued in modern magick by placing cut flowers overnight in the center of an altar before a major ceremony or in an area to be ritually cleansed. • Keep a sachet of the dried flowers, a vase of the cut flowers, or bulbs growing in a pot in your workspace or the center of your home to defuse free-floating irritability, flare-ups of anger, and misunderstandings.

CAUTION

Toxic to pets and can be toxic to humans, especially the bulbs/rhizomes.

Iris, Northern Blue Flag

(*Iris versicolor*)

MAGICAL FORMS

water-loving form of Dutch iris (see "Iris, Yellow Flag," p. 232), growing around water features in gardens in Europe, the UK, and North America (the latter where it is native), as well as wild in wetlands and shores • each stalk has three to five blue-violet flowers with white veining on the petals • also found as the water flag iris (*Iris pseudacorus*), the wild iris (*Dietes grandiflora*), the lighter-colored southern blue flag (*Iris virginica*) in eastern USA, and the sky-blue and white Rocky Mountain iris (*Iris missouriensis*) • magically use mainly the root, but also the whole plant growing by water and the powdered root, which can be bought online from magick stores

PLANET AND ELEMENT

Venus • Water

MAGICAL USES

as the root, a lucky charm for financial gain, especially for business, in cash registers and near charge card machines • it is said that as long as you carry the root in a green bag on your person, you will never lack money

HOW TO USE

Mix the powdered root with powdered nutmeg and cinnamon in a charm bag to attract a partner who is wealthy or, more ethically, rich in love and kindness. • Burn the powdered root in an incense mix with a money-drawing resin, such as frankincense or copal, whenever you need an urgent infusion of money. • Use for all water rituals, casting as an offering silver coins into the water where the plant grows, asking for the growth of what is most needed.

CAUTION

All parts are considered poisonous, especially when blue flag is ingested raw, though it is traditionally used medicinally. • Handle with care and use medicinally only with expert advice and preparation.

Iris, Yellow Flag

(*Iris pseudacorus*)

MAGICAL FORMS

also the Dutch iris, *Iris × hollandica* • two varieties of yellow irises: the water-loving yellow flag iris, and the land-based hybrid, the Dutch iris, in forms such as the Yellow Queen • sunshine semiaquatic yellow flag iris, flowering May to August, grows wild in watery places or can be cultivated along garden ponds or in a container of shallow water • flourishes in the USA, Asia, Europe, and North Africa • considered invasive in forty US states • the Dutch iris flowers late spring to early summer • the Dutch iris is mostly found in bouquets or the cut flower for vases • magically use the yellow flag iris in situ or its fresh or dried petals and flowerheads, the whole plant growing in a garden, and fresh or dried petals or flowerheads

PLANETS AND ELEMENT

Sun/Moon • Water

MAGICAL USES

flag iris is often gifted as a plant for the fifty-seventh anniversary for a couple who have a wildlife garden with a pond or the Dutch yellow iris as a bouquet or cut flowers for the same occasion • the Dutch iris is also sent for a friend's birthday, as a get-well-soon wish, or to express loyalty to someone close who is facing injustice or loss • cast yellow flag iris petals in their own water source to make wishes and to name creative ventures you wish to launch

HOW TO USE

Yellow flag iris is a natural water purifier. • Float flowerheads in a bowl or in the center of your altar, divination table, or meditation space to keep the energies pure. • Display in the middle of the home to remove confrontation or resentment, or if you know difficult visitors will soon be arriving. • Keep mixed, dried, water- and land-based yellow petals in a yellow charm bag near your computer if you are hoping for a reunion with a lost love or friendship that ended badly. • Take the bag along to the first meeting for the all-essential blend of head and heart.

CAUTION

All parts of the iris are toxic to some degree to humans, cats, dogs, and horses. • Ingestion should be avoided and the flower handled with care.

Ivy

(*Hedera helix*)

MAGICAL FORMS

common or English ivy is a climbing or ground plant that also grows in the USA, Europe, and western Asia, mainly in temperate zones • a climbing plant that clings to trees and structures • ivy can be grown as a trailing plant indoors • at midwinter solstice celebrations such as Saturnalia or Misrule in ancient Rome, ivy was worn as a crown as a symbol of female fertile power • magically use the whole plant, trailing pieces of vine, fresh and dried leaves, and its white flowers that bloom in fall or early winter, whether fresh or dried

PLANETS AND ELEMENTS

Mercury/Saturn • Air/Earth

MAGICAL USES

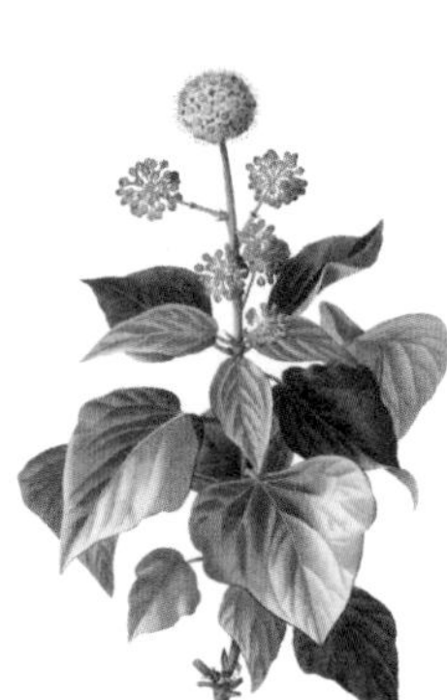

for magical protection • houses covered in ivy are believed to be safe from psychic attack • use in rituals for committed love and fidelity • use ivy in binding spells and as a wreath indoors to attract love and abundance

HOW TO USE

Cut the tendrils and cast them to the wind to free yourself of unwanted attachments. • Use in Goddess rituals, with holly for the God, especially outdoors in places where both plants grow close. • Keep ivy flowers, if possible on a tendril, in a white bag with holly berries for fertility. • Burn ivy incense that is very fragrant in the bedroom on the night of a full moon before lovemaking and place your fertility bag where the moon shines on it, the rest of the month hiding it beneath your mattress. • Ivy wreaths were worn in ancient rites of Bacchus, the Roman god of wine, to minimize drunkenness. • So entwined, fronds of ivy in a purple amulet bag reduce the power of alcohol abuse and should be carried on social occasions where there is a chance of overindulgence.

CAUTION

English ivy is toxic to humans and pets if ingested. • Fresh leaves can be a skin irritant.

Jacaranda Tree

(Jacaranda mimosifolia)

MAGICAL FORMS

considered by many to be one of the most beautiful trees on the planet • originating in South America, jacaranda flourishes in the subtropical and tropical zones of North America including California, Florida, and the southwestern USA • bright-green fernlike leaves become dark green and fade to yellow in the fall • purple or blue flowers appear from spring through summer • in Mexico, its blossoming is celebrated • Pretoria, South Africa, is named Jacaranda City as it is transformed every spring by the abundance of trees • flourishes in Australia and through the world where the climate is sufficiently warm • magically use the growing tree, as well as the blossoms and leaves, whether fresh or dried

PLANETS AND ELEMENT

Mercury/Jupiter • Air

MAGICAL USES

acts as a powerful natural absorber of carbon dioxide • jacaranda is used in Air rituals and especially clean air and global warming rites • associated with the wise Amazonian moon goddess who descended via the jacaranda tree to teach women her knowledge and wisdom • some myths say she endowed the tree with its ethereal blossoms • the blossoms are believed to herald and carry the spring for springtime festivals and the rebirth of any situation or relationship

HOW TO USE

Sit beneath a blossoming Jacaranda tree—if a flower falls upon you, it will bring good luck and money (the more that fall, the luckier you will be). • The jacaranda tree also promises success in examinations, tests, or where money input is needed (it is popular on university campuses). • Use as a talisman for a new job or business venture. • If you come across jacaranda trees in an unexpected location, it is reassurance that you are on the right path, so persevere. • Scatter the fallen leaves to remove all regrets for what did not work out. • Make promises to yourself you will fulfill by the time the tree blossoms again.

CAUTION

All parts of the tree are toxic.

Jackfruit Tree

(Artocarpus heterophyllus)

MAGICAL FORMS

large tropical tree, native to India, related to the breadfruit tree • the largest tree-borne fruit in the world, with huge banana-pineapple-melon-tasting fruits when ripe • greenish-yellow or yellow when ripe, a jackfruit can weigh up to forty pounds • in 1915, Arthur V. Dias, a Sri Lankan freedom fighter, planted up to a million jackfruit seeds after the destruction of the rice crop and saved the people from long-term starvation • grows in tropical zones of Southeast Asia and Brazil • in southern Florida and Hawaii, grows naturally outdoors • it can be cultivated in hothouses almost anywhere • magically use the fruit and the seeds, whole or cooked; the whole tree; and the large, green leaves

PLANET AND ELEMENT

Sun • Fire

MAGICAL USES

for fertility, health, prosperity, protection, family stability, and creativity • supports any major undertaking or huge task that is of importance

HOW TO USE

Set an unripe, green jackfruit on your altar or special place (it will take around seven days to ripen). On the outer unripe skin, trace what you need or desire to be fulfilled or attained by the time the jackfruit ripens by writing the desire invisibly with the index finger of your writing hand. Each night, light a yellow candle, repeat the wish, and then blow out the candle, continuing until your jackfruit ripens. If it is ripening on a tree, select your jackfruit and invisibly write your wish on the growing fruit every day. • Pick, prepare, and eat the fruit (note that jackfruit can be sticky with its latex or sap, so wear gloves). • To conceive a child, remove seeds on the full moon night and leave them open to full moonlight before lovemaking. • On the next morning, cast them into running water or from a high place. Leave the uncooked plant outdoors after a full moon night, available to birds or animals.

Jack-in-the-Pulpit

(*Arisaema triphyllum*)

MAGICAL FORMS

one of the most intriguing plants, its shape resembling a preacher (Jack) standing in his pulpit • possibly named after an actual minister who came over to the USA with the Pilgrims, though the plant is indigenous to eastern North America • an inner spadix or spike (the preacher) contains the flowers, surrounded by a hooded spathe (the pulpit) that is striped or tinged with purple • bright-red berries follow the flowers • Jack-in-the-pulpit traps insects within its hood • magically work with the whole plant in situ or the cut root

PLANET AND ELEMENT

Mercury • Air

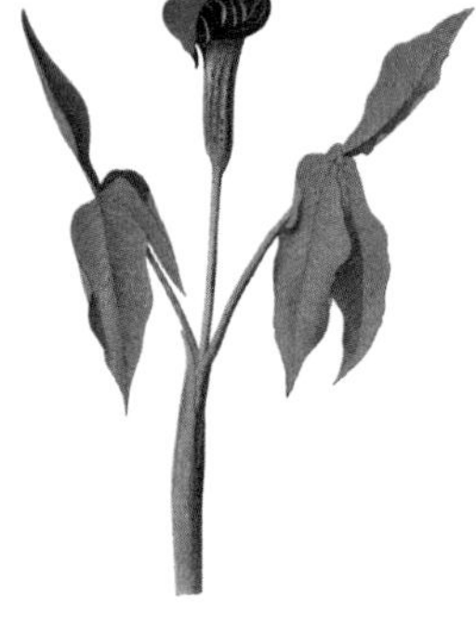

MAGICAL USES

a seventh-anniversary flower for reassessing and listening to inner wisdom and each other • in love magick, the hooded spathe and spiky spadix represent the union of yin and yang • a talisman for gender fluid individuals and those in LGBTQ relationships who encounter opposition, because the plant has both male and female reproductive organs within the single plant and can change its gender from year to year

HOW TO USE

The dried root, carried in a charm bag, protects against predators of all kinds and those who seek to lead others astray. • Bury earthy agate crystals with Jack in winter, saying goodbye to hyperactivity and situations and people that no longer make you happy. • Use the winter for reassessing, and as Jack regrows in the spring, dig up your crystals and launch new beginnings.

CAUTION

Jack-in-the-pulpit is very toxic to people and animals if consumed raw, though known as Indian turnip because Native Americans cook the bulbous roots. • It can also cause skin irritation.

Jacob's Ladder

(*Polemonium caeruleum*)

MAGICAL FORMS

member of the phlox family • ladderlike leaves with blue (and rarely, pink or white) flowers • the biblical Jacob was driven out of the Promised Land by his mother because his brother, Esau, intended to kill him • on his journey, Jacob had a dream of angels ascending and descending a ladder from heaven and was given divine reassurance he would one day return to the place where he had the dream and he and his offspring would create a great race • magically use the growing plant, leaves, and flowers

PLANET AND ELEMENT

Jupiter • Air

MAGICAL USES

promises the end of an involuntary absence or relocation • a sacred flower for spiritual and psychic development • use for messages from angels, guides, ancestors, and plant devas • for butterfly and bee magick • flower psychometry

HOW TO USE

Seal the dried flowers in a sachet or as part of a dream pillow for prophetic dreams and connection with angels, ancestors, and spirit guides in sleep. • Grow the plant in the garden to connect with plant spirits and keep away the negative effects of disloyal family members, also debt collectors and bailiffs. • The leaf ladders can be chopped, dried, and carried in a blue or yellow bag to examinations, tests, and interviews as a charm for rising in the world. • Burn Jacob's ladder in an incense mix to open channels for automatic writing through Metatron, the scribe archangel who will guide your hand to write what you most need to know.

Jade

(*Crassula ovata*)

MAGICAL FORMS

often called the dollar, money, or lucky plant • native to South Africa • grown throughout the world as an indoor potted plant, except in tropical regions • its jade-green, fleshy leaves resemble coins • star-shaped pink or white flowers may bloom in winter or early spring • magically use the whole, growing potted plant or the fresh leaves and flowers

PLANET AND ELEMENT

Venus • Earth

MAGICAL USES

a twelfth-anniversary plant, often given with a piece of jade jewelry or crystals • because it is so long living, fifty to seventy years or more, it represents a long-lasting marriage or friendship and can be passed down when an adult child moves into their own home to transfer some of the happiness and good fortune

HOW TO USE

Set your jade plant in the center of a room so that the chi can flow around it, increasing health and harmony in the home. • Also place one on an inner window ledge in the workplace to call in good fortune and prevent it from leaving, and to generate enthusiasm and increased productivity. • Bury a circle of nine small jade crystals in the soil of the plant to increase the luck, money, and love potential being released by the plant (a natural air detoxifier) if there are relationship or financial problems or if bad luck from external factors seems to be piling up. • Make a talisman, taking a green bag and placing three leaves that have either fallen off the plant or have been carefully cut from it inside, along with fresh jade flowers if available. Take the bag when asking for a loan, a new job, or when luck will play a major factor in launching an enterprise or opportunity. Release the contents afterward.

CAUTION

Jade is mildly toxic to humans and pets. • No parts should be ingested.

Jade, Dwarf

(*Crassula ovata*) or (*Portulacaria afra*)

MAGICAL FORMS

grown as a houseplant • thick trunk, fine branches, and green oval-shaped leaves • in its natural environment can reach ten to fifteen feet high • shaped like a complete tree with wire • native to South Africa, but can be cultivated in warmer climates in the USA and other tropical/subtropical lands as an ornamental • the bonsai can also be taken outdoors in more temperate regions in the summer

PLANET AND ELEMENT

Venus • Earth

MAGICAL USES

money and good luck • symbol of abundance and can be part of a miniature bonsai garden with other species or set in the center of a room or home to enable the ch'i life force to circulate • like the jade plant, the bonsai can be given as a twelfth anniversary gift • set on the main table to make business events and housewarming a success

HOW TO USE

If you are worried about money and you find a dwarf jade tree growing in situ, place your arms around the tree facing it; if you have a potted plant, place your arms around the pot to receive abundance. • If you are anxious about your health or mortality or that of a loved one, whatever your age, walk around the plant ten times in a clockwise circle, counting in tens to represent long life and strength. • Set your bonsai surrounded by small jade crystals in a newly built home to connect with the traditional guardians of the land.

CAUTION

The dwarf jade is mildly toxic to humans and pets. • No parts should be ingested, though it is used in some homeopathic remedies.

Japanese Andromeda

(*Pieris japonica*)

MAGICAL FORMS

exceptionally beautiful ornamental evergreen flowering shrub or small tree • native and wild in Japan and eastern China in mountainous areas • also an ornamental in parts of the USA, Canada, Europe, and the UK, growing up to fifteen feet high • new foliage is initially bronze-pink, becoming and remaining glossy green throughout the year • lightly fragrant white or pink hanging bell-shaped flowers, blooming late winter to early spring • after flowering ends, the dried flowers remain on the plant throughout the season, so ideal for flower decorations and arrangements • many cultivars, including the mountain fire, have red foliage and white blooms • magically use the flowering plant in situ and the fresh and dried flowers

PLANET AND ELEMENT

Jupiter • Air

MAGICAL USES

in feng shui, Japanese andromeda growing in a garden increases the flow of the life force in a gentle, harmonious way to bring a sense of well-being to all who sit or meditate in the garden • the mythical Greek princess Andromeda was chained to a rock in the sea because her mother boasted she was more beautiful than the sea god Poseidon's daughters—a reminder to look below the surface with people and situations rather than taking them at face value (and in the same way, remember that this plant is toxic)

HOW TO USE

Use the growing plant in situ as a focus for meditation and contemplation or for sharing quiet times with loved ones, especially if your life is frantic and keeps you apart. • Add the dried flowers to an arrangement and display indoors to calm energies if family members are constantly rushing in and out or if you or your partner are workaholics.

CAUTION

Japanese andromeda leaves and nectar are toxic to humans and pets. • Gloves should be worn when handling the plant, and caution should be used around children and animals, especially if the plant is taken indoors.

Japanese Cryptomeria

(*Cryptomeria japonica*)

MAGICAL FORMS

also known as Japanese cedar or sugi • a conifer, not a cedar • native to Japan and China for more than two thousand years, the tree in the Japanese tradition contains the sacred life force • often forming the central pillar of temples and sacred shrines so that the indwelling power of the nature deity might bless the site • grows in the USA and also in the UK • can be potted when young and trained as a bonsai • magically use the growing tree, dried and fresh needles, and cones

PLANET AND ELEMENT

Jupiter • Air

MAGICAL USES

a sacred tree that links one with the Higher Self, nature spirits, and devas • lives over two thousand years, and it is thought a specimen in Japan may be seven thousand years old • used to explore past lives • also used for detoxing and quitting bad habits

HOW TO USE

Burn Japanese cryptomeria in incense during ceremonies to contact ancestors and guides. • In the forest, use it in situ for *Shinrin-yoku*, or forest therapy, involving meditation and immersing oneself in nature to create a deep sense of calm and oneness with nature. • According to an old Japanese gentleman I knew well, if you see a *kodama*, an ancient Japanese tree spirit (typically spotted as an old woman or man that seems part of the foliage that dwells in sacred Japanese cedars and other sacred trees), ask their blessing and then depart. Return with an offering (you will no longer see them), ask for nothing, and you will be rewarded in the weeks ahead.

Japanese Sakaki Tree

(*Cleyera japonica*)

MAGICAL FORMS

sacred flowering evergreen tree in the Shinto religion • native to warm parts of Japan, China, Myanmar, and northern India • traditionally used in sacred buildings as the indwelling spirit of the Mononoke, the magical life force • sakaki signifies the boundaries between deities and humankind • can grow in the USA, including in the Northwest, along the West Coast, in the South and the Southwest, and in North and South Carolina • there are two special sakaki trees hidden in the Seattle Japanese Garden and other specialty Japanese gardens worldwide • magically use the growing tree; the large, shiny leaves (too large for bonsai); the wood; the flower essence (often called the shrine offering essence); and as part of a cleansing mist, used traditionally before entering a sacred place

PLANET AND ELEMENT

Jupiter • Air

MAGICAL USES

said to be the sacred tree against which the bronze mirror of Amaterasu, the Japanese sun goddess, was propped, which revealed her beauty and persuaded her to leave the cave that had plunged the world into darkness, so it is seen as a symbol of self-appreciation • used as offerings or for aligning the body, mind, and spirit • for connection with nature, forest spirits, and devas • for all natural magical rituals

HOW TO USE

Use the tree essence or the mist to induce a state of meditation to move into harmony with the higher self and create spiritual calm. • Buy a small sakaki artifact such as a comb or a *tamagushi*, a formal offering of a leaf attached to paper on a hemp string, to use if you cannot work directly with the tree or its leaves. Respectfully place the artifact, surrounded by greenery, on your household altar (combs, tamagushi, and even dried or powdered leaves are obtainable from online Southeast Asian specialty stores).

CAUTION

Do not ingest if pregnant or breastfeeding.

Jasmine

(*Jasminum* spp.)

MAGICAL FORMS

a genus of flowering shrubs that contains over two hundred varieties, including *Jasminum rex*, royal jasmine; *Jasminum officinale*, common jasmine; *Jasminum sambac*, Arabian jasmine; and *Jasminum polyanthum*, pink or white jasmine • magically use the whole, growing plant outdoors or as a potted plant; the fresh or dried flowers; and the oil

PLANET AND ELEMENT

Moon • Water

MAGICAL USES

increases love • wealth • prophetic dreams and enhanced intuition • self-confidence • radiance and charisma • to attract good fortune and the right people into your life • use in full-moon baths and rituals • an aphrodisiac • for secret lovemaking desires to come true • enhances male potency and female fertility • protects against emotional vampires and love rivals • melts emotional blockages and fears

HOW TO USE

Wear as a perfume or use diluted oil as a fragrance to attract spiritual twin soul love. • Use jasmine oil to anoint a white candle for prophecy and to discover the identity of a secret admirer. • Anoint a red candle for increasing passion or a green candle for money, or encircle the candle with fresh flowers for a similar effect. • Burn as incense, diffuse during meditation or while reciting mantras, or anoint the Third Eye with the diluted oil for connections with the spirit world. • Grow jasmine in the home and garden to remove negativity and for continuing peace, family happiness, and abundance.

CAUTION

Do not make tea with Confederate jasmine (*Trachelospermum jasminoides*) or Carolina or yellow jessmamine (*Gelsemium sempervirens*), as both are toxic.

Jewelweed

(*Impatiens capensis*) and (*Impatiens pallida*)

MAGICAL FORMS

found through most of the USA except for Montana, Wyoming, California, and the Southwest • naturalized in England, France, and parts of central and northern Europe in the 1800s and 1900s • *Impatiens capensis*, called orange flowering jewelweed or spotted touch-me-not, has trumpet-shaped orange and yellow flowers with mottled, reddish-brown spots inside the trumpet and bluish-green leaves • Native Americans called *Impatiens capensis* jewelweed because of its bright colors; it's also known as common jewelweed or orange balsam • in *Impatiens pallida*, or pale yellow jewelweed, the petal-free flower remains closed and produces most of the seed pods, which, when touched, explode, releasing their seeds, hence the nickname "pale touch-me-not" • because of its shape as it blooms, jewelweed is sometimes called the open heart • often grows near poison ivy and stinging nettles • magically use the unpopped pods, the seeds, the leaves, and the trumpet flowers, fresh and dried

PLANET AND ELEMENT

Mercury • Air

MAGICAL USES

keeps away stalkers, intruders, and those who interfere, as well as any kind of paranormal attack • linked with the fey • jewelweed leaves are an antidote to spiteful words and actions

HOW TO USE

The whole plant, given in a pot for the garden of a beloved or in an arrangement with either fresh or dried cut flowers and leaves, offers love without conditions. • Drop water on a leaf or go to your growing plant after a rainfall and make a wish on the sparkling jewel drop before it disappears. • Alternately, hold the leaf underwater so it glistens with water jewels, make your wish, and allow the leaf to float or sink to the water sprites, who may grant your wish. • Pop a seed pod in the open air and allow the seeds to fly where they will to let go of restrictions, prohibitions, and obstacles in your life.

CAUTION

Avoid if you have kidney problems.

Jezebel Root

from (*Iris* spp.)

MAGICAL FORMS

the root of irises native to Louisiana, including *Iris fulva*, *Iris hexagona*, *Iris brevicaulis*, and *Iris foliosa* • also grown in other temperate regions • the original Phoenician ninth-century BCE Jezebel was a temptress queen who used sexuality for power • magically use the root, whole and chopped, or in an essential oil (root and oil available from magical or other specialty herbal and occult stores)

PLANETS AND ELEMENTS

Venus/Mercury • Earth/Air

MAGICAL USES

a defensive and empowering herb, especially for women • it should never be used in anger, for revenge, or to bind or dominate someone against their will for love or for unfair gain at the expense of others • associated with success in gambling and speculation, as well as business success, especially for a woman setting up a business • use in wish magick • all positive love magick • for female ambitions if there are unfair factors

HOW TO USE

Unless you are experienced in magick, hoodoo, or voodoo, stick to simpler but effective use in spell bags. • Wrap a green dollar around a single small root in a green bag for financial success, adding a gambling chip or lotto ticket if you are gambling. • Carve your initials and those of your love or a desired lover on a root, then place it in a sealed red bag while saying, *Let love grow if right it is to be and willingly*. • Write a wish or petition to Venus in green for love or to Mercury in yellow for money or business (don't use unfamiliar spirit names), placing the note with the chopped root and a drop or two of Jezebel oil in a blue bag, keeping it hidden for a month, then burning the petition and roots outdoors.

CAUTION

Jezebel roots are poisonous, so do not ingest. • Handle with care, and if in doubt substitute another iris root (see p. 231) in your spell bags.

Jimsonweed

(*Datura stramonium*)

MAGICAL FORMS

also called thornapple or devil's trumpet • erect flowering plant, part of the nightshade family • grows to three feet high • long white or violet trumpet-shaped flowers and spiny fruit capsules • native to Central America • grows in the USA and throughout the northern hemisphere and can be invasive • considered highly toxic but cultivated for medicinal purposes • magically, not used much in the modern world, except as the datura flower essence (which is sometimes also derived from *Datura wrightii*)

PLANET AND ELEMENT

Saturn • Water

MAGICAL USES

of ancient origin, jimsonweed was once used by the Inca priesthood to induce prophecy and in medieval European flying potions • the datura flower ironically acts homeopathically in its flower essence form for removal of toxins from the mind and to bring light at the end of the tunnel • though not stated by suppliers, the essence is said by magical practitioners to be an aid to astral travel if taken before sleep and to bring prophetic dreams

HOW TO USE

Add a blossom, dried very carefully away from people and pets, into a sealed, white bag with three iron-based stones, tied securely. • Use more safely as a single drop of datura essence sprinkled on three iron pyrites, iron stones, or hematite, which can be set near a computer when you need to discover if a person or offer online is genuine. • Alternatively, keep the bag as an amulet in a safe place if others are intruding on your privacy or unduly spotlighting you for blame.

CAUTION

Use jimsonweed under strict medical supervision only. • All parts of the plant are poisonous if ingested and should be handled with care.

Job's Tears

(*Coix-lacryma-jobi* var. *lacryma-jobi*)

MAGICAL FORMS

also called tear grass • pearly grains of the wild grass grown throughout Asia • hard-shelled, shiny, tear-like seeds are used in rosaries, prayer beads, and other jewelry • plant is grown as an ornamental • naturalized in the southern USA and other warm parts of North America • dating back thousands of years in China and more than a thousand years in India • also still prized among the Eastern Cherokee people • magically use the seeds, obtainable from craft stores and online, as well as in magick stores • there is a softer cultivated form that is commonly used for cooking and eating, *Coix lacryma-jobi* var. *lacryma-yuen*, but it is not as good magically

PLANETS AND ELEMENT

Mercury/Jupiter • Air

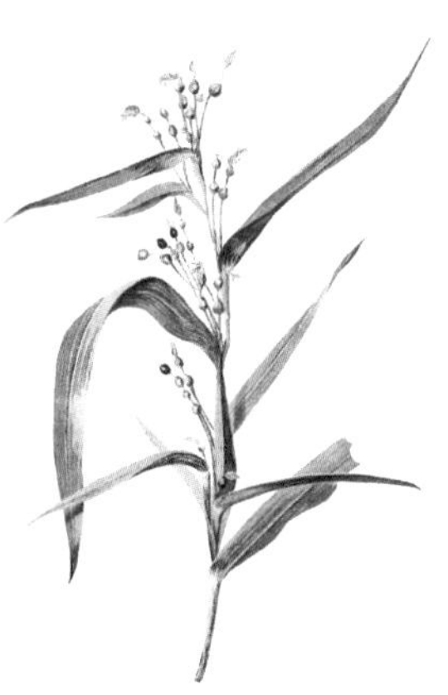

MAGICAL USES

offer protection against any sorrow and are said to absorb pain, bad luck, or sickness • named after the biblical Job, who endured many sorrows with stoicism • an amulet, necklace, or bracelet of beads created from the seeds can be a reminder of better times ahead that can be reached through patience

HOW TO USE

Three seeds in a bag brings good luck, especially in gaining new or more lucrative employment. • Carry five in a bag for rapid growth of what is desired, such as love, fertility, or money. • Seven will grant wishes: seal the bag and carry it for a week, naming your intention every day, then cast the seeds into running water, throwing them over your left shoulder. • Place an amulet bag with nine seeds over your front door to keep or drive away malevolent spirits, misfortune, ill-health, and troublemakers.

CAUTION

Avoid any Job's tears while pregnant.

Jojoba

(*Simmondsia chinensis*)

MAGICAL FORMS

the jojoba shrub is native to the deserts and woodlands of the southwestern USA and Mexico • also found in desert areas in the southern hemisphere • can grow three and a half to six feet tall with small, green-yellow flowers without petals, which become an acorn-shaped fruit capsule containing a hard seed, from which the carrier oil is extracted • cultivated for the oil • more of a wax than an oil, as it is solid at room temperature • warm or slightly dilute it with another carrier oil such as almond to use • valuable because it requires little or no refining and is long lasting • magically use the carrier oil

PLANET AND ELEMENT

Moon • Water

MAGICAL USES

called the oil of versatility because its composition is close to the skin's own oil • is used in skincare, as well as in rituals for beauty, radiance, and youthfulness • use for anointing purposes, especially on the Third Eye for opening the self to spiritual energies as well as earthly possibilities and aligning mind, body, and spirit

HOW TO USE

For enhancing love and healing after a relationship rift, use jojoba oil in mutual massage by combining with a few drops of another gentle essential oil or alone before lovemaking. • If mutual massage is not possible, massage your inner pulse points for your heart center to make psychic connection with an absent or estranged lover while speaking words of reconciliation. • Use before Reiki and meditation and in ceremonies of purification on the inner wrist point, the Third Eye, and middle of the hairline for the Crown energy to open the self or a client to the healing of spirit guides and angels and to transmit and receive messages from wise ancestors.

Jonquil

(*Narcissus jonquilla*)

MAGICAL FORMS

a close cousin of the daffodil, sometimes called the rush daffodil because of its rushlike foliage • the most aromatic of the narcissus family • white or pale-yellow flowers, although can be pink or orange or sometimes brighter yellow • originally native to southern Europe and Africa but now grows extensively in many parts of the USA, Canada, and Europe • magically use the whole plant growing in the garden or wild; the flowers, cut, dried, or fresh; and the essential oil

PLANET AND ELEMENT

Mercury • Air

MAGICAL USES

encourages mutual love and family unity, especially if adding to a family through remarriage, adoption, or fostering, or trying for a child, because it has four or five flowers on the same stem • justice, especially personal • clearing up misunderstandings • for young love or finding love after betrayal • use instead of daffodil if you want more subtle energies or a slower-building result • for new beginnings in love, career, or life after a setback

HOW TO USE

Inhale the oil from a diffuser or oil burner to lift depression, anxiety, or stress, or to enhance psychic senses, especially clairsentience. • If you have been wrongly accused by a friend, family member, or colleague, surround a magical circle with the dried petals to enclose yourself in protection and afterward scatter the flowers along with the accusations to the winds. • Use as part of a wedding bouquet if the relationship has had earlier difficulties or has overcome opposition. • Also gift or display to celebrate a newborn baby or multiple births, especially after problems.

CAUTION

Toxic for pets and humans, especially bulb and flowers. • Do not ingest the plant or use the oil internally or undiluted. • Avoid if pregnant or breastfeeding.

Judas Tree

(*Cercis siliquastrum*)

MAGICAL FORMS

a variation of the redbud tree with a religious myth attached to its name that has passed beyond its specific religious significance, entering folk tradition and magick • as such, has attracted magical properties not found in other redbuds • called the Judas tree because it was said that it was a tree of this species on which Judas Iscariot hanged himself after betraying Jesus • thereafter the tree became short and spindly and its white flowers became stained blood red or magenta, appearing around Easter • native to western Asia and southeastern Europe, also growing on the hillsides of Israel and Palestine (some say the name is a corruption of the tree of Judea) • brought to France and the northern Mediterranean by the Crusaders and also in milder parts of the UK, where it was introduced in the 1600s • closely related to the Chinese redbud (*Cercis chinensis*) and the North American eastern redbud (*Cercis canadensis*) and so may be found in the eastern USA, but needs care in growing there • magically use the whole tree, especially in flower; the dried flowers and leaves; and the seeds, which can be used for artwork and crafts

PLANETS AND ELEMENTS

Mercury/Saturn • Air/Earth

MAGICAL USES

flowers and leaves are used in rituals for forgiveness, especially self-forgiveness, after betrayal • for the healing of unresolved anger, regrets, or bitterness with someone who has died

HOW TO USE

Shred the flowers from a bridge over running water to wash away sorrows, guilt, and regrets when you know you have made a mistake, been unfair, or wronged someone and can't put it right. • Use the Judas tree to hide luggage labels on which you have written messages to someone with whom you are not yet—or maybe never will be—able to openly express love.

CAUTION

The leaves, pods, and seeds are mildly toxic.

Juniper

(*Juniperus communis*)

MAGICAL FORMS

a small shrub or tree in the cypress family • plant of the midwinter solstice • grows wild or in a container • magically use the full tree in situ, cut leaves, berries (fresh and dried are considered especially magical), and oil

PLANET AND ELEMENT

Sun • Fire

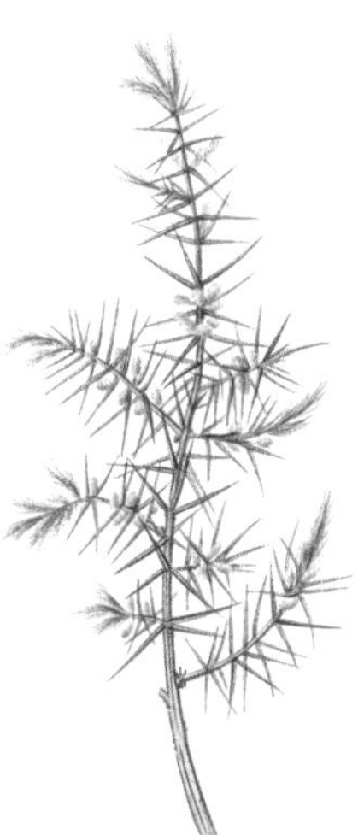

MAGICAL USES

for banishing negativity • male potency • new beginnings • money • luck, especially in lotteries or gambling • purifying homes and protecting against accidents, thieves, and all forms of illness • for justice

HOW TO USE

Cleanse the home on New Year's Eve by burning the incense, made from leaves and dried crushed berries. • Burning or diffusing the oil heightens psychic awareness. • A few drops of the oil in water act as a floor wash to remove bad atmospheres from the home. • Carry a sprig as an amulet to protect against accidents, theft, and illness. • Increase male potency by carrying the berries in a sachet. • Grow juniper outside your door to protect the home against misfortune. • As an amulet, the dried berries guard against malevolent ghosts.

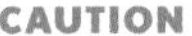

CAUTION

Avoid if pregnant or breastfeeding, or if you have kidney disease.

Kale

(*Brassica oleracea* var. *acephala*)

MAGICAL FORMS

loose-leafed vegetable from the cabbage family • cultivated for at least two thousand years in the eastern Mediterranean, including what is now Turkey • with blue-green, light-green, red, or purple leaves depending on the kind • harvested mainly in the winter, from September to May • most popular as crinkly, curly kale • known through Europe since the Middle Ages • thrives in cold weather • had been falling out of favor in the UK for several centuries, but was revived as a superfood in 2008 in the USA, where it has its own day on the first Wednesday in October • made into smoothies and juices as well as eaten as a vegetable because of its high nutritional value • some kinds with pink leaves are also grown as an ornamental • magically use the vegetable in cooking and growing

PLANETS AND ELEMENT

Sun/Mars • Fire

MAGICAL USES

in magical cookery, use the empowered kale for courage, determination, and fighting against injustice • eat during periods of training for increased sports prowess and stamina

HOW TO USE

Like its cousin the cabbage (see p. 88), kale was used for love divination on Halloween in Ireland, a custom immortalized by the poet Robert Burns in Scotland and taken to the USA by settlers. Kale was picked directly from the fields by blindfolded participants to identify their future lover. • Lots of dirt on the leaves and stalk indicated wealth and status. The shape and size of the kale foretold the appearance and height of the intended. The participant then nibbled the raw heart, its flavor and sweetness revealing a future love's disposition and generosity. They then took the stalk home and put it behind the outer door. The first person encountered in the morning would, it is said, either be or lead to meeting the future spouse. • Grow kale in different colors in the garden so you will never be short of food, money, or love, especially throughout the winter.

Kapok Tree

(*Ceiba pentandra*)

MAGICAL FORMS

also called silk-cotton tree • grows in Central and South America, the Caribbean, parts of West Africa, in southern Florida, and occasionally in central Florida • leaves, roots, and gum are used in Ayurvedic medicine • its relative, the red cotton tree (*Bombax ceiba*), is found in southern California, Tampa, and more rarely in Orlando • magically use the whole, growing tree, as well as the wood, bark, fiber, and seed pods

PLANET AND ELEMENT

Jupiter • Air

MAGICAL USES

use fiber to fill peaceful dream pillows and protective magical healing poppet dolls for those who are vulnerable or sorrowful • sacred tree of the Mayans and Aztecs, for linking with spiritual higher energies • as a world tree, connecting the dimensions • astral projection • communication with the ancestors and wise guides • fiber is a long-lasting buoyancy aid, supporting thirty times its own weight in water

HOW TO USE

Add a small piece of the fiber to an amulet bag for safety at sea or while traveling overseas. • Wrap a sharp knife and scissors in layers of kapok, secured with white thread. • Keep the parcel on a high shelf to prevent accidents, especially in the kitchen. • Enclose tiny clay figures in kapok fiber to represent noisy neighbors and dogs, then add a small rose quartz in each mouth. • Hold the bundle whenever your neighbors or dogs become overly loud, saying softly and continuously, *Quieter be, that we may live in harmony*. • The bark, a small piece of the tree, or an artifact made from its wood shields against paranormal harm, since in the folklore of Trinidad and Tobago a huge kapok tree is said to imprison the Demon of Death.

CAUTION

Kapok seeds contain toxic compounds that can cause vomiting, diarrhea, and even death if ingested in larger amounts.

Kava

(*Piper methysticum*)

MAGICAL FORMS

indigenous vine native to the Hawaiian islands and Polynesia, commercially cultivated in tropical areas of the USA and Australia • used ceremonially, at celebrations such as weddings, and socially for relaxation • magically use the fresh or dried powdered root, customarily made into a tea • if you cannot get fresh root to pulverize, chop and powder dried root to make the infusion

PLANET AND ELEMENT

Saturn • Earth

MAGICAL USES

provides psychic, psychological, and physical protection • good fortune • physical and emotional calm • quiet sleep • family unity and sealing friendship bonds especially in kava ceremonies where the drink is brewed communally and shared

HOW TO USE

Drink as an infusion, or sprinkle the dried powdered roots around boundaries, window ledges, and thresholds to protect against evil and bring good luck. • Hang dried roots or leaves in a tied bundle over the bed to prevent harm from any source while you sleep, especially if you have paranormal dreams or night terrors. • Drink or scatter the infusion as part of a ritual before, during, or after a group or private rite to welcome the wise ones, enhance psychic powers, and raise magical energies.

CAUTION

Do not ingest if you have a liver disorder or take blood thinners. • Check with a physician prior to ingesting if you receive regular medication for chronic conditions.

Kelp

MAGICAL FORMS

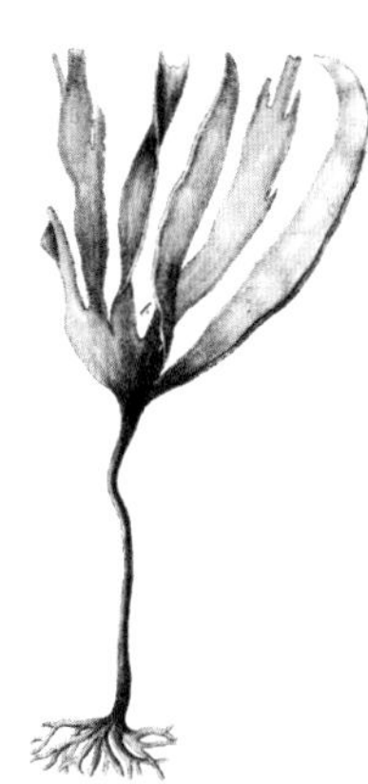

common name for multiple species, including *Laminaria digitata*, large brown algae seaweed, also called oakweed; and *Nereocystis luetkiana*, an American form of kelp also called edible kelp or bullwhip kelp (see "Bladderwrack," p. 68) • grows in shallow oceans as forests • the whole giant plant can be found washed up on shore or broken into pieces • purchased as edible seaweed • dried, powdered kelp sold commercially • magically use fresh or dried kelp

PLANET AND ELEMENT

Moon • Water

MAGICAL USES

for sea rituals, used from Celtic times • wind rituals • brings action after stagnation • good for wishes • magical cookery

HOW TO USE

Add powdered kelp or a dried and chopped piece of kelp (in which case, replace when it crumbles), to a green amulet bag for protection against accidents or illness, especially at sea. • The same amulet bag is good for safe travel overseas, especially on long journeys. • For growing and ongoing prosperity, add powdered kelp or a small piece of kelp to a glass jar. Cover with whiskey on the night before the full moon, then seal the jar and place it on an indoor window ledge. Shake the jar weekly. Every New Year's Eve, bury the unopened jar near your home before midnight, and replace with a new one on New Year's Day. • Cast a piece of kelp found on the shore into the waves at the turn of the tide to invoke the powers of the ocean for successful change or to call home a lost or estranged love who is overseas.

CAUTION

Avoid ingesting kelp if you are taking blood thinners. • Take care to avoid using kelp from polluted waters.

Kentucky Coffee Tree

(*Gymnocladus dioicus*)

MAGICAL FORMS

at one time was the state tree of Kentucky • considered rare • grows throughout the state and in eastern and central USA • its seeds were boiled by pioneers as a substitute for coffee, which was a skill taught to them by the Indigenous people of the area • magically use the leaves: bronze-pink in late spring for new beginnings, bluish-green when mature for all matters needing resolution, and butter-yellow in the fall for money rituals • use also the growing tree, which is beautiful in all seasons, and its seeds (including coffee made from the seeds) and pods

PLANET AND ELEMENT

Mercury • Air

MAGICAL USES

for adapting to all circumstances • for overcoming toxic people and environments • use the small, starlike, white flowers of early summer for star and wish magick

HOW TO USE

Listen to the pods on the trees rattling in the wind for warnings that should be heeded. • Fill rattles or gourds with the seeds to accompany magical chants and dancing. • Create a protective and lucky charm by hanging a seed on a necklace. • Cast a large handful of the seeds on the ground and count them individually to answer a binary question—yes–no; go–stay; wait–act now; speak–be silent—until you run out of seeds (add a new random handful each time you ask a question). • A bagful of seeds, shaken before gaming, can bring good luck. • They can assist in determining when to gamble and when to hold back.

CAUTION

Pods and seeds are poisonous if not cooked well or boiled, so avoid ingesting, and handle all parts of the tree with care.

Kiss-Me-over-the-Garden-Gate

(*Persicaria orientalis*)

MAGICAL FORMS

native to China or Uzbekistan (there's confusion as to which), the flowering plant became popular cultivated in the USA after President Thomas Jefferson favored it in his famous Monticello garden • also grows in England and Europe • long, pink, soft arching floral spikes, also in dark pink or white, growing more than seven feet tall • the name describes the tall plant invitingly leaning over a garden fence or gate • blooms between midsummer and fall • beloved by hummingbirds • magically use the plant growing over gates or fences, as cut flowers in bouquets, or dried in flower arrangements and crafts

PLANET AND ELEMENT

Jupiter • Air

MAGICAL USES

in its cut form, as a token of romance sent to a would-be love • protective when planted in the garden, near the entrance, to welcome those with good intent but to deter those who come to spoil happiness • because it reseeds itself, it is a natural symbol of fertility and of increasing abundance • a Victorian love flower, it is romantic but restrained, typical of the wooing of that era

HOW TO USE

Display the cut flower as an indication of willingness to be approached but that the would-be lover should take their time in advancing the romance. • Gift cut flowers to those who have been hurt in love or have left a relationship and need to regain trust, or display them yourself if this applies to you. • Make the flowers the centerpiece of a dried flower arrangement to preserve love in the home throughout the years, and as a promise of lasting love by the giver.

Kiwi

(*Actinidia deliciosa*)

MAGICAL FORMS

a sweet, tangy, egg-sized and -shaped fruit with a light-brown skin and edible pale-green or golden flesh filled with rows of edible black seeds • grows on a woody vine • native to central and eastern China, where it was once an offering to nature spirits for a good fruit harvest • now exported worldwide and cultivated most notably in New Zealand where its name is shared by the national flightless bird • also grows in California, Italy, and Chile • made popular by USA and British service personnel in New Zealand during World War II, reaching the UK and later California • rich in vitamins and believed to regulate blood pressure if eaten • magically use the fruit and the seeds

PLANETS AND ELEMENTS

Moon/Venus • Water/Earth

MAGICAL USES

for unconditional love and opening the heart to new family members • tolerance • forgiveness of self as well as others • associated with the inflow of money and with heightened sexuality and sensuality, especially if eaten on Fridays, Venus's day

HOW TO USE

Wash and dry the seeds, counting them for answering yes–no, go–stay, act now–wait questions. • Eat the fruit and seeds before lovemaking to heighten fertility. • Keep dried kiwi seeds in a net with dried apple pips (do not eat) over the door for protection against harm to the home and family and to draw in abundance, health, and wealth. Replace the seeds when they are withered.

Knotweed

(*Polygonum aviculare*)

MAGICAL FORMS

known as knotgrass and, in Eastern medicine, as Bian Xu • widespread and considered invasive in many temperate areas • beware the related Japanese knotweed (*Polygonum cuspidatum*), which can choke gardens and structures • magically use the aerial parts, including the fresh or dried leaves

PLANETS AND ELEMENT

Moon/Saturn • Earth

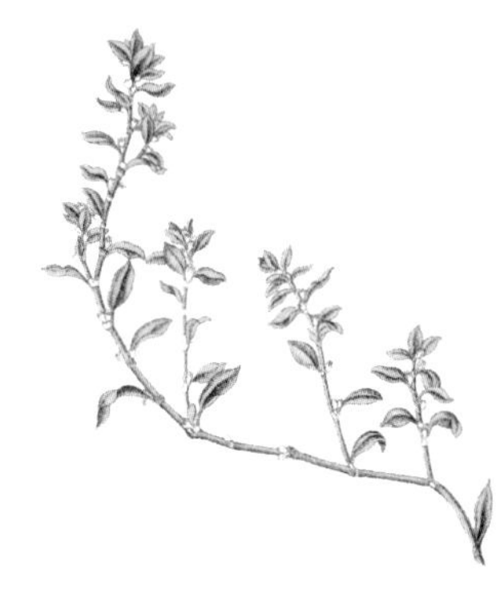

MAGICAL USES

for all binding spells against the actions of those who would damage a relationship through jealousy • to encourage loyalty in lovers or friends • for keeping promises in love • for uniting your own and your partner's existing children • important to keep the magick positive and bind behavior, not people, as knotweed has been used in the past in spells to harm others

HOW TO USE

To remove sorrows, hold knotweed in your nondominant hand, pointing to the earth and naming what troubles you; afterward, drop it into a patch of knotweed or bury it. • Use in knot spells instead of thread to bind bad habits, illnesses, undesirable influences, and fears until the knotweed breaks. • More positively, loosely bind love poppets filled with dried lavender for fidelity between willing lovers.

Kola Nut Tree

(*Cola acuminata*)

MAGICAL FORMS

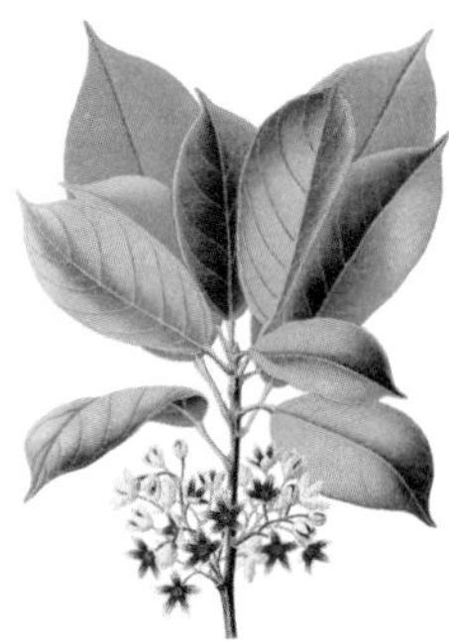

tropical tree that can be sixty-five feet high • dark-green leaves, yellowish-white flowers • needs a lot of rainfall to thrive • large, woody seed pods, with five to ten red or white seeds that are the nuts, the part used magically and medicinally • the powdered nuts can be made into a tea, after their creamy outer skin is removed • also used in making commercial cola • native to West Africa and grown in the tropics, Nigeria, the West Indies, and Brazil • magically use the nuts, as well as tea or infusions made from them

PLANET AND ELEMENT

Mercury • Air

MAGICAL USES

useful for charm bags for good fortune • protects against malice at work and in the community • nuts with up to three lines are regarded as sacred to the gods • with four lines they bring good fortune and blessings to the user • five for fertility, protection of the home, and against the evil eye • six lines to call upon the wisdom of the ancestors • seven or more, rarely found, as an omen of prosperity and luck

HOW TO USE

Drink the Bissy tea, as it is called in Jamaica, made from fresh kola nuts that are powdered and dried after grinding. • Chew the nut to improve memory for study—it is sometimes called "the actor's friend" because of its power in aiding the memorization of lines, and also for public speaking. • Carry half a nut, having previously eaten the other half, to protect against accidents if in a hazardous situation. • Traditionally, the nuts are handled with a knife, not fingers.

CAUTION

Do not ingest the nut if you have high blood pressure, peptic ulcers, or heart palpitations. • The nut/powder is not considered safe while pregnant or breastfeeding.

Kunzea

(*Kunzea ambigua*)

MAGICAL FORMS

shrub or small tree, also called white cloud • sometimes also called poverty bush because it will grow in poor soils and after disturbance of the land by natural phenomena or human destruction • white or pink (in cultivation) fragrant, fluffy flowers • left to its own devices, this lovely bush can appear sparse and neglected and may not flower • member of the myrtle family • the shrub can be endemic in parts of Australia and Asia and has been introduced to England • the oil is extracted from leaves, twigs, and green branches • magically use the essential oil, which is as yet relatively unknown, but increasingly sold worldwide

PLANET AND ELEMENT

Mercury • Air

MAGICAL USES

for regeneration • seeking new possibilities • to overcome restrictions imposed by others or by personal fears • cleansing the home after illness, misfortune, or quarrels • banishing troublesome folk from your life without harming them

HOW TO USE

The dried plant, especially leaves (it was suggested to me by a local source) were traditionally burned for stamina, as well as consumed as a tea. • Essential oil is known as the runners' oil. • In modern times the diluted, empowered oil is massaged into the soles of the feet and leg muscles (both areas connected with the root action energy or action center of the body), not only for physical relief of pain and stiffness, but to speed up situations and give the stamina to chase after opportunities when they seem to move further away. • Burn or diffuse the oil while planning an adventure or wilderness vacation or if you run into opposition for freedom to follow your dreams, when others say you are taking too many risks. Inhale whenever you feel claustrophobic and hemmed in by life, especially in the city, or when you are suffering from petty gossip or narrow-minded people.

CAUTION

Perform a patch test before using the oil if you have sensitive skin.

Kyphi

MAGICAL FORMS

kyphi is a compound composed of sixteen ingredients • many practitioners keep the precise formula secret • often may include aloeswood, cinnamon, frankincense, galangal root, juniper berries, mastic gum, lemongrass, myrrh, mint, sandalwood, and storax bark • separately, after steeping for several days, add raisins and either dates or sweet red wine and tupelo honey • everything is then combined while naming the intention of the incense and rolled into pellets • there are many recipes online or it can be bought from reputable online or local magick stores • when burned, kyphi produces a lot of smoke • as it is a wet incense, it should be placed on tin foil on a healing plate

PLANET AND ELEMENT

Sun • Fire

MAGICAL USES

burned in ancient Egyptian temples in the evening to close the day • the oldest recipe appeared in *The Papyrus Ebers* from around 1500 BCE • used in ritual magick and for reaching higher realms • one of the most sacred and mystical incenses

HOW TO USE

Burn kyphi before and during meditation and visualization and before sleep for past-world experiences, especially of ancient Egypt, where many old souls originated. • Use it to clear away any sense of paranormal malevolence, misfortune, anger, or sickness that seems to linger. • Use in more formal rituals, especially shared with those you feel you have known before in earlier lives, and in personal petitions to angels and deities for the help you most need.

Labdanum

from (*Cistus ladanifer*) and (*Cistus creticus*)

MAGICAL FORMS

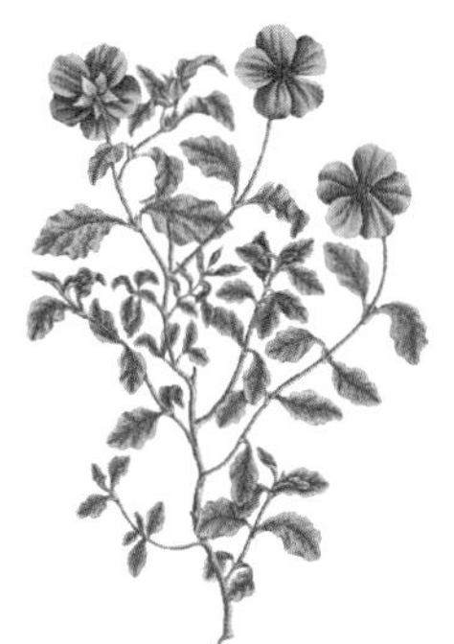

resin obtained from two shrubs in the rockrose species • *Cistus ladanifer* is also called western Mediterranean gum rockrose • *Cistus criticus*, Middle East/eastern Mediterranean hoary rockrose, is also called pink rockrose • produces a sticky, dark-brown resin, at one time combed from the beards and thighs of goats and the wool of sheep that had grazed on the herbs • the resin exudes from the glandular hairs of the leaves • offered to Aphrodite, the ancient Greek love goddess, in her temple on Cyprus • in modern times it is harvested with leather rakes or boiled from the leaves and twigs into a fragrant mass that becomes brittle as it ages, until heated • also found as dark, amber-green essential oil • especially when combined with oakmoss and patchouli in oil or incense, labdanum is an ethical substitute for ambergris that is produced from the endangered sperm whale and is largely banned • labdanum resin and oil are widely available online and it is an important ingredient in perfumes • magically use the resin and oil

PLANET AND ELEMENT

Sun • Fire

MAGICAL USES

found in antiquity in ancient Egypt and Canaan, a staple in many kyphi incense mixes • some consider it the biblical Balm of Gilead (see "Balsam Tree, Arabian," p. 48) • improves memory and concentration • preserves youthfulness

HOW TO USE

Burn labdanum as an aphrodisiac or dilute well and use as a love oil. • Diffuse the oil in the bedroom before sex magick and to restore passion to a relationship weighed down by everyday concerns. • Called the incense of the Black Sun, it can be used during partial and solar eclipses for rebirth and regeneration.

Labrador Tea

(*Rhododendron tomentosum*)

MAGICAL FORMS

also as *Rhododendron groenlandicum*, or bog Labrador, and *Rhododendron neo glandulosum*, or trapper's tea; previously called *Ledum glandulosum*, or western Labrador tea • all are wetland plants from the heather family with strongly aromatic leaves used to make a very weak, golden, aromatic herbal tea (see cautions, as if too strong or more than a cup a day it can cause cramps, paralysis, intoxication, and poisoning) • purchase from a reputable dealer and follow instructions for brewing if ingesting • also popular in cooking or for chewing raw among Indigenous people in the Arctic and subarctic, encompassing Alaska, Greenland, Canada, and the northern USA • magically use the essential oil, very well diluted, and safest of all, the nontoxic flower essence

PLANET AND ELEMENT

Venus • Earth

MAGICAL USES

used traditionally to smudge after a death, when a family member returns home after a long absence, and the first time a fisherperson goes to the sea to grant invisibility for the hunt • protection and blessing • dreams

HOW TO USE

Add the dried leaves to an incense mix of tree fragrances such as cedar and pine or add a drop or two of the essential oil to the mix to bless a new home before entering. • The same mixture is useful in removing illness or misfortune as well. • Drink a very weak tea before bed or consume the essence; some claim it will induce lucid dreaming.

CAUTION

Brew no more than a teaspoon of the dried tea or four to six fresh leaves for three to four minutes to avoid releasing toxins. • Though safe as a weak solution, and *only* as a weak solution, labrador tea is not to be consumed in pregnancy, by children and teens, or by older people who are frail. • For safety, seek advice from a health professional before consuming. • Labrador tea is toxic to animals.

Ladies' Tresses

(*Spiranthes* spp.)

MAGICAL FORMS

also called lady's tresses • small, wild orchids, growing near water, with spikes of tiny, white flowers spiraling up the stem like curly hair • bloom from late summer to early fall • produce a delicate fragrance of vanilla and jasmine • several varieties are found in the USA and Eurasia, including fragrant marsh lady's tresses (*Spiranthes odorata*) • can be cultivated in boggy areas of gardens • the source of the flower essence, hooded ladies' tresses or Irish ladies' tresses (*Spiranthes romanzoffiana*), was first described in the Aleutian Islands in Alaska in 1828 by N. Romanzoff, a Russian minister whose country ruled the area at the time • this species is also found in the northwest of the British Isles and Ireland and may have been there from before the last ice age • magically use the growing flower and the flower essence

PLANET AND ELEMENT

Moon • Water

MAGICAL USES

a fae flower • for love enchantments • as the flower essence, for recovering equilibrium after a trauma or injury, especially after attacks or assaults by known assailants or where an injury or accident has had life-changing effects, whether temporary or more permanent • for using setbacks to discover a new life purpose

HOW TO USE

Sit close to the flowers in moonlight, especially those growing near water, to have sight of the water spirits. • Make offerings of water crystals like fluorite or calcite in return for wishes. • Fill a love sachet with dried petals to be left near a would-be lover's door, or bring yourself into their thoughts by focusing on a picture of the flowers. • Use the essence added to a marigold- or rose-based cream, or give it to someone who has been the victim of a violent crime or witnessed a traumatic incident to overcome the effects of psychological or physical scarring.

Lady's Bedstraw

(*Galium verum*)

MAGICAL FORMS

also called yellow bedstraw • see "Cleavers" (p. 125), its close relative • releases the scent of honey when blooming and of mown hay when dried • if not in the wild or a large garden may need regular trimming back to avoid it taking over • magically use the whole, growing plant; leaves; flowers; stems; and yellow flowers

PLANET AND ELEMENT

Venus • Water

MAGICAL USES

attracts love • in dream pillows brings dreams or astral connection with a lover, known or unknown • entry into womanhood ceremonies • midsummer rituals to ask the fey to grant wishes by scattering the golden fresh or dried flowers from a hillside • to bring peaceful resolution to an unresolved conflict

HOW TO USE

Wear or carry in a sachet the fresh or dried flowers tied with red ribbon to call love. • Recite the fertility rune name *Geybo* (Gay-boe), which means *the gift*, nine times, followed each time by the name of Frigga, the Mother Goddess, after whom the plant was named as Frigga's grass, asking to conceive a babe. Then cast a sachet of the shredded plant into running water or burn on a ritual fire. • Originally put in mattresses of women about to go into labor, the leaves should be placed in a sealed jar to be released as the woman enters the hospital/birthing room, to create calm and a welcoming atmosphere.

CAUTION

Avoid while pregnant or breastfeeding, and be cautious if you are not familiar with the herb.

Laksa Leaf

(*Persicaria odorata*)

MAGICAL FORMS

also known as Vietnamese coriander • not related to true coriander (*Coriander sativum*) • used in southeastern Asian and northeastern Indian cooking • fast-spreading herb from the knotweed family, with aromatic, edible, lance-shaped purple or light-green leaves, often with burgundy, U-shaped markings • tastes lemony and peppery, becoming progressively spicier as it ages • grows worldwide, outdoors if warm and in pots indoors • Vietnamese coriander reached the USA and Europe with Vietnamese settlers in the mid-twentieth century • magically use the growing or dried herb and the leaves in magical cookery

PLANET AND ELEMENT

Mercury • Air

MAGICAL USES

to suppress libido if a love relationship would be unwise or destructive • increases psychic powers • use for obtaining recognition and rewards through artistry and creativity • use a bag of seeds to count yes or no for love, marriage, and fertility questions

HOW TO USE

Add the leaves or dried herb to cooking to ease tensions between those sharing the meal. • For overcoming heartbreak, stand in an open place when it is not windy and throw seeds over your left shoulder, making a repetitive chant, *So I leave heartbreak behind*. When they are all gone, say, *New love, new joy now shall I find*. Walk away, not looking backward. • Keep pots of Vietnamese coriander in your home studio or workspace while you are creating. • When you are ready to make your creation public, burn a few of the finely shredded leaves from one of the pots, in a success incense mix, based around frankincense, copal, or dragon's blood.

CAUTION

Avoid while pregnant or breastfeeding.

Lapacho Tree

(*Handroanthus impetiginosus*)

MAGICAL FORMS

also known as pau d'arco or pink trumpet tree • grows in the rainforests of Argentina, Paraguay (national tree), Brazil, and Mexico • called the divine tree, it predates the Incas • can be grown in pots • the inner lining of its bark can be made into a heal-all tea • magically use the whole, growing plant; tea (often combined with yerba mate and consumed ceremonially through a special metal straw from a gourd); dried bark; and herb

PLANET AND ELEMENT

Sun • Fire

MAGICAL USES

as a tea, it increases spiritual awareness • forges a connection with ancestors and spirit guides • aids in astral travel • drink tea before mediumship, ritual, and divination • used for anti-aging rituals and empowerments

HOW TO USE

Drink the tea or make an amulet bag of the dried bark hung inside your bedroom door to repel specters of the night, sexual demons, poltergeists, and evil presences that disturb your sleep. • Sprinkle the well-diluted tea, with its slight vanilla and nutty fragrance, in the corners of the bedroom and lightly anoint the window catches and doorknobs in the home with the tea for the same protective purpose. • Grow the potted plant or have a dish of the dried tea in your home or workspace to amplify good luck.

CAUTION

Lapacho may slow blood clotting.

Lapland Rosebay

(*Rhododendron lapponicum*)

MAGICAL FORMS

rare, low-growing, wild, dwarf rhododendron shrub • grows wild in the Arctic, the subarctic, and on alpine cliffs and in northeastern Canada around Hudson Bay • reaches northern New Hampshire • is found in Scandinavia, Lapland, and parts of Russia • cultivated, although not commonly, in the USA and the UK or Europe in gardens • blooms vivid pink-purple in June with leaves that are green all winter • magically use the growing plant in situ if you find it, or more easily and effectively, as flower essence

PLANETS AND ELEMENT

Venus/Saturn • Earth

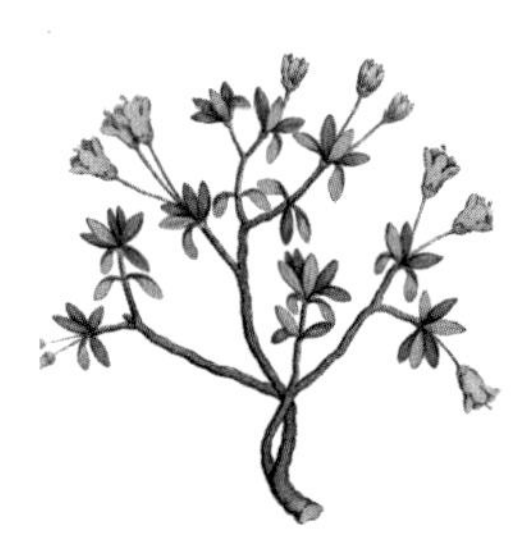

MAGICAL USES

as the flower essence and in meditation with the growing flower, brings clarity of purpose and freedom from circular and confused thinking if too dependent on the advice and opinions of others • breaks the habit of spending too much time with different clairvoyants or constantly seeking the latest spiritual expert or medical remedy • brings trust in the self and trusting the evidence of eyes and ears and personal intuition

HOW TO USE

Since it is so essential to insect life, especially in the Arctic regions when it blooms, use the essence in baths and humidifiers, and consumed diluted in water to discriminate between those who are genuinely knowledgeable and those who rely on ego and may be charging extortionately for seeming expertise. • Anoint your Third Eye with a drop of the essence to unblock your innate wisdom before divination if you are confused by reading too many books or attending too many classes. • Used in Lapland shamanic rituals, a drop under the pillow before sleep may induce prophetic dreams.

CAUTION

Avoid if pregnant.

Larch Tree

(*Larix* spp.)

MAGICAL FORMS

eastern larch, also called the American larch (*Larix laricina*), reaches forty to eighty feet and is native to most of North America • European larch (*Larix decidua*), a hundred feet high, is planted through the UK, Europe, Russia, Scandinavia, and North America • larches have soft, needlelike leaves that fall off in winter, turning yellow gold in the fall • first to sprout in the spring • an ancient tree, an eleven-thousand-year-old larch-wood idol was found in a peat bog in the Ural Mountains in Russia, the oldest known wooden sculpture in the world • in Siberia, the Siberian larch (*Larix sibirica*) is called Tuuru, the world tree connecting Earth to the polestar • magically use the whole, growing tree; needles; cones; and flower essence

PLANET AND ELEMENTS

Saturn • Air/Earth

MAGICAL USES

in Alpine folklore, the larch is home to tree maidens called the Blessed Ones, a name assigned to them by mortals wishing to incur their favor • wearing white and silver, the maidens dance around larches and sing mesmeric music • therefore, charms of dried bark or cones favor performers • use in meditation to connect with old worlds

HOW TO USE

Use the tree as a focus for shamanic rites or astral projection, as a ladder between the earth and heavens, and to overcome fears of the dark by gazing at the stars through its branches. • A couple of drops of the flower essence every morning or before you go out in the evening brings confidence and high self-esteem if others at home, work, or socially try to make you feel inadequate. • Tape a dried, golden leaf under your doormat to deter thieves.

CAUTION

Avoid if pregnant.

Lavandin

(*Lavandula* × *intermedia*)

MAGICAL FORMS

a hybrid, small shrub obtained from the mixing of the lavender plant (*Lavandula angustifolia*, see p. 252) with spike lavender, also known as aspic lavender (*Lavandula latifolia*) • sharper in fragrance and larger than true lavender with woody stems, gray-green resinous foliage, and spiked lilac-purple or violet-blue flowers, which bloom only once a year • though grown popularly in France and Bulgaria, lavandin will thrive in most places worldwide, including the UK and USA • magically use the fresh or dried plant, flowers, and flowerheads, as well as the essential oil

PLANET AND ELEMENT

Venus • Earth

MAGICAL USES

use fresh or dried flowers in love bouquets • use flowerheads in traditional lavender bags, potpourri, and sleep pillows • tougher emotionally than true lavender oil • for resisting emotional blackmail, subtle intimidation, and undermining • for revealing hidden love at the right time and maintaining love in difficult situations or against prejudice • its fragrance protects against all harm, earthly and paranormal, as well as from anger, violence, and accidents

HOW TO USE

Keep an empowered lavandin amulet bag, having added a drop or two of the oil to the dried flowerheads before sealing, to guard against the dangers of the road. Carry with luggage and documents before travel. • Hide lavandin bags close to precious artifacts and have one in your computer case to protect against theft and the hacking of electronic devices. • Grow lavandin in your garden or hang a dried bunch over your door to prevent anger within the home and external threats. • Diffuse or burn the oil to make telepathic communication with an absent lover if you cannot communicate openly. • Add a few strands of the dried plant to a smudge or smoke stick to cleanse the home if there are vulnerable, very old or sick people, children, or pets living there, and ventilate the home well.

CAUTION

Avoid if pregnant or breastfeeding.

Lavender, English

(*Lavandula augustifolia* 'Vera')

MAGICAL FORMS

has purple flowers and silver foliage, as does *Lavandula latifolia*, known as Portuguese lavender • flowering herb, in all shades of purple from pale to dark • magically use the whole plant, dried flowerheads, and oil

PLANET AND ELEMENT

Mercury • Air

MAGICAL USES

an all-purpose herb and flower for protection, especially of children and pets • for first love and rebuilding trust • happiness • heals abuse, especially among girls and young women • peace • past lives • increase of psychic powers through its fragrance • prevents cruelty • protection • purification, sleep, and beautiful dreams • to see ghosts, especially ancestral • use dried lavender heads for water scrying • particularly appropriate for the sixty-third wedding anniversary • any purple flowering lavender can be offered on the twenty-fourth anniversary

HOW TO USE

Use lavender to fill sleep pillows, which can bring beautiful and prophetic dreams and even enable you to see a twin soul, known or unknown, during sleep. • Keep bowls of dried lavender heads around the home to stop quarrels and rivalry. • Burn lavender as oil, in incense, or as part of a smudge stick to call reconciliation and acceptance within yourself of what cannot be changed. • Include the growing plants as part of a peace and domestic happiness garden. • Use lavender-scented furniture polish to fill the home with domestic contentment. • Use lavender for anointing the chakra psychic energy points to bring body, mind, and soul into alignment. • Wear the fragrance or oil or use in porous lavender bath bags to keep or drive away the evil eye and before a social occasion to attract new friends and romance.

Lavender, White

(*Lavandula angustifolia* 'Alba')

MAGICAL FORMS

there are other beautiful white kinds (about twelve in total) created by selective breeding, beginning, it is estimated, about four hundred years ago • white lavender has a sweet, powerful fragrance different from the purple lavenders • white lavender is far rarer than purple lavender but can be found in many parts of the world • many species bloom continuously from midsummer or before to the fall • ballerina lavender is especially noteworthy, as it is used as a charm by dancers, musicians, and artists: it's a specialty Spanish lavender with purple-pink spikes, topped by graceful white petals like ballerinas dancing in the wind • magically use the growing and cut plant, fresh or dried flowerheads, and as an infused oil

PLANET AND ELEMENT

Mercury • Air

MAGICAL USES

white lavender, mixed with other white flowering herbs in informal handfasting and commitment ceremonies, brings a sacred element if a formal ceremony is not wanted or possible • carry the dried, white flowerheads in a white sachet to inhale as a counterbalance to a fast, frantic world

HOW TO USE

Burn white lavender either on charcoal or as an incense stick to create an enclosed meditation or ritual space if your home is noisy or you lead a frantic lifestyle. • Keep a vase of white lavender on your altar or private space. • Also use the fresh-cut flowers to raise spiritual vibrations to connect with angels and guides and with the beloved deceased, to receive messages through automatic writing when you allow your hand to make the connection. • Use white lavender heads, especially celestial star, as part of an all-white herbal or floral potpourri in the home or in your workspace if family members are too brash and challenging, or work colleagues are inappropriate in what they say and do.

CAUTION

Lavendula angustifolia is toxic to dogs, cats, and horses. • Do not ingest the oil of any lavender. • Be cautious if you have low blood pressure, and use caution during pregnancy.

Ledum

(*Rhododendron groenlandicum*)

MAGICAL FORMS

formerly called *Ledum groenlandicum* • also known as bog Labrador tea or swamp tea • belonging to the heather family • an evergreen shrub that grows to about five feet in cold northern latitudes • its fragrant, white, cloudlike flowers appear in late spring to early summer • native from Greenland to Alaska within the tree line, as well as Russia and Scandinavia • cultivated in Canada, the northern USA, and northern Europe • known medicinally in Indigenous traditions for thousands of years • traditionally, the leaves, which have resinous, fragrant glands and silver hairs that turn red underneath, are made into a tea • also found as *Ledum palustre* or *Rhododendrum tomentosum* (called marsh Labrador tea or marsh rosemary), which is made into oil with similar properties and often sold as the dried herb, especially for making tea • magically use the essential oil (frequently sold as Greenland Moss), which is extracted from the leaves and flowers, and the growing plant

PLANET AND ELEMENT

Mercury • Air

MAGICAL USES

spiritual cleansing of people, places, and artifacts • revitalization after loss or stagnation • for leaving the past behind • lowers the temperature of potential anger, teen tantrums, and drama kings and queens at home or in the workplace

HOW TO USE

Sprinkle the tea infusion around objects you have bought if you are not certain of their origin or they are inherited from or given by potentially hostile relatives or neighbors. • Add a few drops of oil to a pump-action spray bottle filled with water or burn or diffuse the oil to lower a hyperactive atmosphere if family or colleagues are always dashing in and out. • Apply to an aroma bracelet or smell a drop or two on a tissue, cotton ball, or pillow, or massage diluted into the pulse points, to reduce unwise cravings for excess food, alcohol, nicotine, and recreational drugs.

CAUTION

Avoid if pregnant or breastfeeding.

Leek

(*Allium ampeloprasum* var. *porrum*)

MAGICAL FORMS

wild leeks, called ramps, are native to North America • the cultivated leek, a nutritious, bulbous vegetable with a leafy, green top and white, fleshy stalk • originating in the Middle East and eastern Mediterranean • originally recorded in ancient Egypt, Greece, and Rome, leeks may have traveled to Europe with the Crusaders in the Middle Ages and came from Europe to the USA with the early settlers • the stems grow through winter and are ready to harvest in spring before they flower • if unharvested and left to go to seed, leeks produce small purple and white flowers in large pompoms • the national vegetable of Wales since the sixth century, leeks are central to celebrations on St. David's Day, March 1 • magically use the empowered raw or cooked leeks, which are often steamed as a vegetable, stirred into casseroles, used dried in bouquet garnis, or as an ingredient in French vichyssoise soup

PLANETS AND ELEMENTS

Mars/Moon • Fire/Water

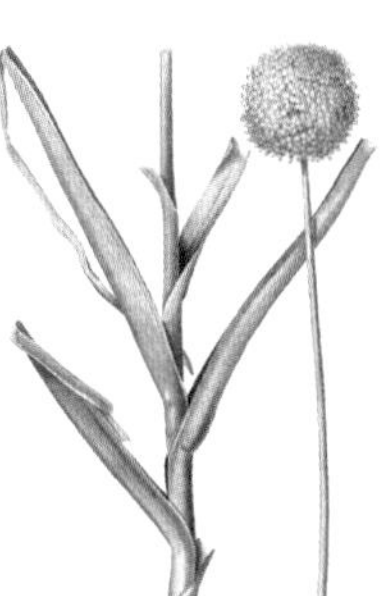

MAGICAL USES

to prepare for a physical or emotional challenge • to fight and win against seemingly impossible odds or corrupt organizations and officialdom • as a luck and prosperity bringer

HOW TO USE

Name what or whom you wish to lose from your life as you wash, peel, and chop leeks before cooking. • Bite through a cooked leek and bury the pieces at a crossroads to break hexes, curses, and jinxes. • Leeks are traditionally eaten before a battle to ensure victory. • Empower the leeks and add them to cooking if challenging family members are coming for a meal. • Because of their pungent smell, use leeks defensively to banish malicious spirits by hanging over doorways.

CAUTION

Poisonous to dogs and cats. • Avoid if on blood thinners because they are high in vitamin K.

Lemon

(*Citrus × limon*)

MAGICAL FORMS

flowering evergreen tree that produces aromatic, yellow fruit • like orange, a lemon tree can be a small container tree if space is limited • magically use the whole tree, blossoms, leaves, fruit, dried peel, juice, and oil

PLANET AND ELEMENT

Moon • Water

MAGICAL USES

grown together, orange and lemon trees represent the combined power of moon and sun into an energy greater than the separate plants • night and moon magick • the blossom or leaves for fertility rituals, especially for older people desiring a child • in Hindu lore, the lemon tree protects against the evil eye if planted close to the house • for safe travel, especially by sea • house moves • on the waning moon, to remove addictions, phobias, and bad influences; for new beginnings, good luck, and prosperity on the waxing moon

HOW TO USE

A planted lemon tree attracts prosperity, long life, and good fortune to the family. • Make a lemon pig by sticking pins in a lemon for legs, then roll the lemon in salt and burn it to take away misfortune. • Half a lemon pressed downward in salt until it dries out removes jealousy and spite. • Lemon juice added to a bottle of water and carried, but not consumed, absorbs negativity from others. • Use lemon juice mixed with water to physically cleanse amulets and artifacts belonging to others or gifts from someone ill-intentioned. • Lemon leaves in a sachet represent lasting love; replace when they lose their fragrance.

CAUTION

Phototoxic, so do not take the oil internally or go into sunlight for a few hours after using the oil.

Lemon, Amalfi Coast

variety of (*Citrus limon*)

MAGICAL FORMS

IGP (protected Geographical Indication) variety of lemon tree, twice the size of a normal lemon • sweet, tangy, and juicy with few seeds • strictly only trees grown along the twenty-mile strip between Vietri and Positano on the Italian Amalfi Coast can be called *Amalfi lemons*, however the species can grow in states and areas such as California and Florida with mild winters and hot summers • the tree blooms five times a year • the fruit is harvested between January and the end of October • perfume containing Amalfi citrus fragrance • magically visit the Amalfi Coast, a World Heritage site, on vacation to fill yourself with energy and happiness in the lemon groves or buy the fruit online

PLANET AND ELEMENT

Moon • Water

MAGICAL USES

for overcoming spite, sarcasm, and criticism with reason and positive words and actions • bringing happiness to gloomy people and situations • for spreading good luck, health, and light in the home, even on physically or emotionally dark days • removing lingering sickness or misfortune

HOW TO USE

Anoint your inner wrist points with any fragrance containing Citrus Amalfi to fill your heart with love and joy if you need to remain positive and cheerful rather than be dragged into others' pessimism. • Have a basket of the lemons in the kitchen or at family gatherings to share and spread happiness and goodwill. • Eat the fruit including the peel to absorb the energies of its native sunshine so the day ahead will be filled with laughter. • Shred the peel finely to add to a sunshine incense mix or potpourri, with chamomile flowers, yellow fragrant rose petals, sunflowers, marigolds, frankincense or copal (in incense), and orris root, adding blessings and specific wishes.

Lemon Balm Melissa

(*Melissa officinalis*)

MAGICAL FORMS

perennial herb known for its lemony scent • magically use the whole, growing plant; the aerial parts, fresh or dried; and the oil

PLANET AND ELEMENT

Venus • Water

MAGICAL USES

attracts love or a specific lover into your life • use for fertility, especially while undergoing IVF, artificial insemination, or otherwise conceiving through medical intervention • for letting go of emotional ties and healing wounds after betrayal • increasing all good things in life • promises long life and youthfulness • strengthens memory • attracts bees and butterflies to the garden and prevents bees from leaving and taking good luck with them • for full moon magick

HOW TO USE

Inhaling the fragrance from the leaves or plant, as well as anointing the Third Eye with the diluted oil or the oil in a diffuser, gives visions in meditation and aids spellcasting or divination. • Carry the fresh or dried herb in love sachets. • Drink the dried herb infused in wine before a social event to attract love, friendship, and popularity. • Add oil to water for an anti-negativity home spray. • Lemon balm melissa in the garden, or cut and displayed in a pot indoors, attracts health and abundance, and drives away all harm. • Burn as incense or smudge for prosperity. • For wish magick, hold the leaf, make a wish, leave it to dry, and then burn it.

CAUTION

Do not take the oil internally. • Excess or prolonged use can cause dizziness, high temperature, and stomach pains. • Dilute well or do a patch test before applying to skin.

Lemon Verbena

(*Aloysia citrodora*)

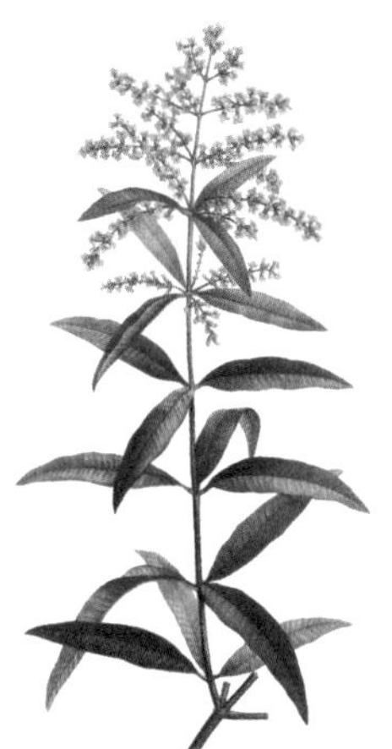

MAGICAL FORMS

flowering plant with a lemon scent • herb of the summer solstice • magically use the whole, growing plant; leaves; oil; and tea

PLANET AND ELEMENTS

Saturn • Moon/Air

MAGICAL USES

purification of bad atmospheres after love quarrels • protects against hexes or ill wishes in a love relationship by jealous relatives or rivals • breaks a streak of bad luck • maintains love and friendship through the years and life changes • increases family happiness • eases the pain of a relationship ending • gives confidence to succeed through perseverance • for use in magical cooking

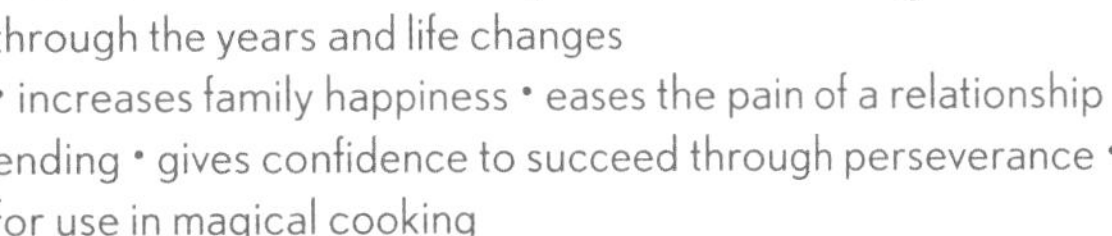

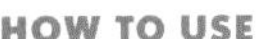

HOW TO USE

The oil can be added to purification baths before rituals. • Use as a floor wash or scatter the leaves and sweep them away to cleanse a ritual area. • Burn as incense or diffuse the oil to remove ill wishes and hexes and to break bad habits. • Grow in pots around the home to repel evil spirits. • Carry a sachet of the crushed leaves to increase radiance and charisma in love, self-love, and success. • Add to money spells to remove obstacles and make results come faster. • Lemon verbena increases the power of other spells. • Use lemon verbena as a meditation aid. • When placed under the pillow, it prevents nightmares. • Add to potpourri to silence complaints at home or work.

CAUTION

Do not use if pregnant or breastfeeding.

Lemongrass

(*Cymbopogon citratus*)

MAGICAL FORMS

plant known for its fragrant leaves • grows near the sea in Southeast Asia • magically use the grass or leaves and essential oil

PLANET AND ELEMENT

Mercury • Air

MAGICAL USES

repels spite • gives protection against jealousy, the evil eye, thieves, and attacks via social media • prevents online scams and keeps away bad neighbors • for smooth and efficient house moves of all kinds • swiftly removes what is redundant or stagnant in your life • attracts unexpected money or resources • also used to banish sad memories and past failures that hold back present and future achievements • increases passion

HOW TO USE

Move a lighted lemongrass incense stick counterclockwise in a spiral around a photograph or the written name of a human snake to take away their power to hurt you. Use the same motion, but clockwise, to give you confidence to face your enemy down. • Make a spray with a few drops of the oil mixed with geranium, orange, and lemon oil added to water for the workplace and home before a potentially confrontational meeting or a family gathering where there are inevitable rivalries. • Add a couple of drops of lemongrass oil before sealing a defensive mojo bag, bottle, or jar. • Burned as incense or in a diffuser, lemongrass brings prophetic dreams.

CAUTION

Dilute lemongrass well in olive or almond oil for anointing, as it is a skin irritant. • Avoid in pregnancy and if you suffer from glaucoma.

Lemon-Scented Tea Tree

(*Leptospermum petersonii*)

MAGICAL FORMS

fast-growing shrub, popular in and endemic to eastern Australia • intensely aromatic foliage • magically use as tea or essential oil, which is made from the leaves

PLANET AND ELEMENT

Moon • Water

MAGICAL USES

cleanses the home and workplace of gossip, spite, jealousy, and intergenerational or sibling rivalry at any age • empowers resistance to mind manipulation and emotional pressures from human parasites who visit or share the space

HOW TO USE

Use the tea, empowered by stirring counterclockwise while naming, as a silent chant, a person from whom you need protection or who is an emotional vampire, before you meet them. If you can get them to share the tea, so much the better. • Diffuse or burn the oil in the background if you know a relative or friend will visit or call to ask for a favor or loan they will never repay. • Use in an oil burner or diffuser when visiting a romance-oriented or financial website if you have doubts about its reliability. • Regularly scatter the tea as an infusion or add to a floor wash for doorsteps to deter not only physical cold callers, but telephone and computer intrusion, as well as time wasters if you work from home.

CAUTION

Avoid the plant during pregnancy and breastfeeding. • Dilute extremely well, especially for use on skin.

Lentil

(*Lens culinaris*)

MAGICAL FORMS

curved lens-shaped seeds, a legume related to the pea family • native to North America, the Mediterranean, the Near East, and western Asia • found in graves on the banks of the Euphrates dating from as early as 8000 BCE to nourish the deceased in the afterlife • cultivated in ancient Egypt and Rome • in modern times also grown in Canada and India • in the UK is grown in gardens and commercially, but not extensively • grows on bushy vines, one to two feet high • seeds can be red, yellow, brown, green, and orange • seeds grow in small pods after the white, pale-blue, and light-purple flowers have bloomed and closed • magically use the raw and cooked seeds

PLANET AND ELEMENT

Saturn • Earth

MAGICAL USES

use in magical cookery as part of harmonious, leisurely family meals if your family or partner usually grazes or rushes in and out • for defusing intergenerational conflicts and impatient family members • linking with the old Arabian world, lentils were a symbol of prosperity • old folktales recall numerous examples of lentil abundance, such as a magick lentil pot that was never empty and another of a man who shared his lentils with a genie in disguise and was given a bag of lentils that constantly renewed itself

HOW TO USE

Mix raw lentils of different colors in a dish, stirring clockwise seven times as you name the days of the week. For each day, ask for the happiness or resources you need. Put the lentils in a small gourd or sealable container and shake them seven times. Thereafter, shake whenever you lose faith in your wish being fulfilled. • Take a bag of lentils, scatter a few in the air outdoors, cast some in water, and add the rest to a meal shared with friends or family so that your resources will never run out.

Lesser Celandine

(*Ficaria verna*)

MAGICAL FORMS

a member of the buttercup family contains all the magical properties of greater celandine (*Chelidonium majus*), a member of the poppy family, but lesser celandine is safer to grow and handle • magically use the whole, growing plant; flowers; and leaves

PLANET AND ELEMENT

Sun • Fire

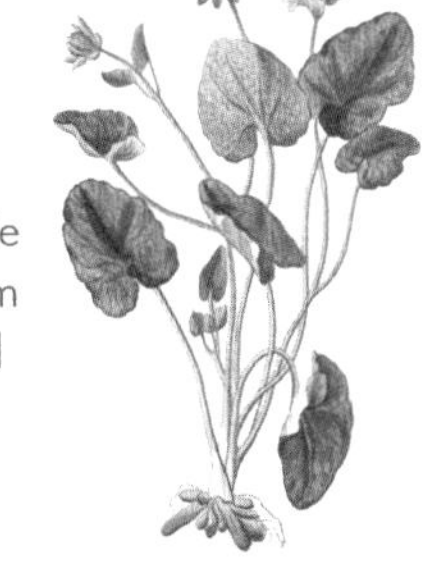

MAGICAL USES

happy vacations with good weather • flower of Imbolc, the first dawning of life after the winter • justice • a legend from Europe in the Middle Ages, associated with alchemy, tells that the swallow carried the flowering herb celandine in her beak, and two gems in her stomach, one a red ruby or garnet to bring wealth and the other a black jet or pearl to bring good fortune to those who found the stones on their doorstep with the plant • escaping emotional or psychic vampirism

HOW TO USE

Keep lesser celandine wrapped and taped to copies of official court papers or legal documents where there is dispute. • Give lesser celandine as a token of good fortune in a yellow purse with a small garnet and jet to bring luck or as a housewarming present. • Place the fresh or dried flowering plants in a vase on the altar for weather magick, to bring welcome change after loss, and for good vacations with the right weather conditions. • Use as a visionary plant for meditation, especially in sunlight.

CAUTION

Lesser celandine should not be used by anyone with chronic health issues, especially connected with the liver or tumors, or while pregnant or breastfeeding. • Though cooking the leaves is said to remove any toxicity, the plant is generally not recommended for consumption after it flowers (early spring). • It also can cause contact dermatitis with some people with sensitive skin so handle with care.

Lettuce

(*Lactuca sativa*)

MAGICAL FORMS

leafy vegetable cultivated and eaten raw or cooked • native to the Mediterranean and Siberia but grown almost worldwide • mainly green and red • generally harvested for culinary purposes, before it flowers yellow in late spring to early summer when it becomes too bitter to eat • prefers the cooler seasons • magically use the cut or whole, growing plant, or the leaves

PLANET AND ELEMENT

Moon • Water

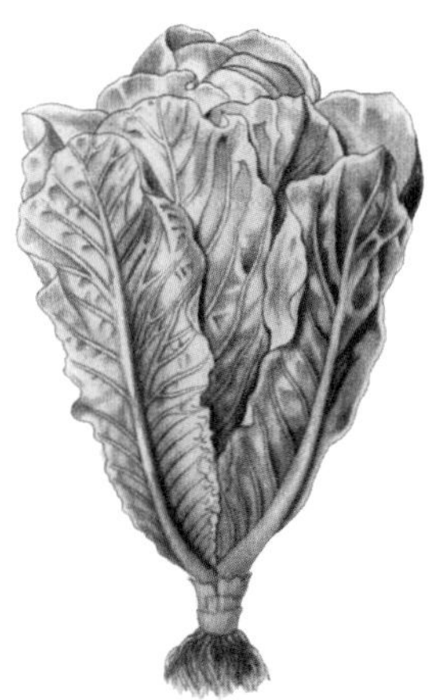

MAGICAL USES

deceptively powerful, the stronger and larger the leaves you eat, whether chopped or whole, the more you will gain advantage in a situation • mix and serve red and green leaves and different kinds of lettuce; for example, green romaine, iceberg (which can turn red), and red romaine when you need to blend two families after a remarriage or to bring acceptance of a new partner where there is opposition

HOW TO USE

Eat the leaves, preferably picked or purchased on a full-moon day or night, for a bonus or chance to make a one-off source of money. • Rub the leaves on your forehead before going to bed to bring sleep to insomniacs, prophetic dreams, and astral travel, especially if you are seeking the moon, stars, and starry realms. • Grown in the garden, even under glass, lettuce offers protection to the home against specters and fears of the night or restless spirits of the land.

Lewisia

(*Lewisia triphylla*)

MAGICAL FORMS

rare flower of the mountains of western USA, especially the Sierra Nevadas in California • appears for a few days in the high alpine regions on rocks when the snows melt • pink and white, iridescent, star-shaped blossoms with a very short stem • believed to be stars that have fallen from the heavens • magically use the flower essence, as it is hard to find as a flower

PLANET AND ELEMENT

Moon • Water

MAGICAL USES

for indigo children, star souls, and those on the autism spectrum to manifest their gifts in the world and for those gifts to be appreciated • for those whose spirituality is emerging but who find the experience unsettling or are discouraged from believing by others

HOW TO USE

For astral or mind journeying, anoint a drop of the essence in the middle of the hairline for the Crown energy center to visit star realms and talk with Star Guardians. • For pregnant women, use the essence in a gentle massage oil or lotion if it's hard to connect with the baby in the womb, especially if there have been problems with a previous pregnancy. • Place a drop beneath a dying person's pillow if they are ready to let go but afraid, as it will ease the passing.

Licorice

(*Glycyrrhiza glabra*)

MAGICAL FORMS

wild and cultivated, the deep root is used magically and for flavoring • the European form, *Helichrysum petiolare*, was naturalized in the USA, and the related *Glycyrrhiza lepidota* has a less intense flavor and is native to the USA • one of the most ancient healing remedies, used in ancient Egypt as a sweet drink by the pharaohs • placed in Egyptian tombs for the immortality of the soul and to ease the passage to the afterlife • magically use the root whole or chopped into small tube- or chip-shaped pieces

PLANETS AND ELEMENTS

Mercury/Venus • Air/Water

MAGICAL USES

used in herbal decoction teas to sweeten bitter tastes and ease difficult decisions • increases passion • promotes fidelity • to reduce addictions, especially smoking • for sexual potency • as an offering to love goddesses in love rituals

HOW TO USE

Share empowered candies (usually with anise added) with a lover or use the root in magical cookery to turn up the tempo of romance or friendship. • Carve the root into a wand to call an absent or hesitant lover in a spell. • Eat the root and absorb its power into your energy field to make yourself irresistible in your lover's mind, no matter how far away they may be. • Powder the herb and sprinkle it behind you as you walk a path your lover or desired lover would take to your front door or to a workplace you share, to imprint your essence in their footprints. • Burn the chips with pine resin as incense for honesty and fidelity in love if a partner is working away from home and you suspect their interest is straying.

CAUTION

Do not take in excess, especially if you have high blood pressure or are sensitive to estrogen. • Do not take during pregnancy.

Lightning-Struck Tree

MAGICAL FORMS

the most magical of all tree forms • ash, elm, oak, maple, poplar, and pine are among the most frequently struck, being the tallest and possessing a distinctive straight trunk • some trees are immediately at least partially destroyed, others as the effects are felt in the months ahead; some are able to heal • any lightning-affected tree becomes a source of transformation, its wood the most powerful protector against harm, as well as the luckiest • humankind's first introduction to fire, believed to be either gift or punishment from the deities

PLANET AND ELEMENT

Mars • Fire

MAGICAL USES

for change and transformation • making an interest or talent a second or major career seemingly overnight

HOW TO USE

Add the wood of a lightning-struck tree to any charm bag or amulet to greatly increase its power. • Carry the wood for transformation in any part of your life, especially for travel or sudden career change. • Make your lightning wood into a wand, whether a solid, uncharred piece or chippings or burned bark inside the wand for powerful fire rituals, to bring change, creative success, and any spell to more rapid manifestation. • If you witness a tree being struck or burning, you will receive sudden inspiration and illumination in the form of a message from the deities or an angel of fire and a matter that has been stagnant will burst into action in the weeks ahead. • Collect any ash and powder it, mixing it with cornstarch, talcum powder, or baking powder. • Scatter a little in front of your workplace or a desired lover's home to bring rapid actions in your favor.

CAUTION

Apart from fire hazards, if the tree sets others alight, be prepared for a psychological breakthrough or spiritual awakening that if embraced will bring new energies and an awareness that you are ready for a major step that others may not understand.

Lilac

(*Syringa vulgaris*)

MAGICAL FORMS

gorgeous flowering bush with distinctive purple and white flowers • magically use the fresh or dried flowers, leaves, bark, oil, and as a fragrance

PLANET AND ELEMENT

Venus • Water

MAGICAL USES

domestic happiness • family celebrations • connecting with old friends and past loves on social media • brings you the home you want • encourages and blesses permanent relationships • drives away unfriendly ghosts and all malevolence from the home and loved ones • calls home those estranged or far away • the flowers are not considered lucky in the home except on May Day or in unoccupied haunted houses

HOW TO USE

Lilac bushes and honeysuckle growing up external walls or set in corners are garden boundaries that keep domestic happiness within and repel all earthly and paranormal harm. • Use lilac water or fragrance to anoint door handles and window ledges after quarrels or sickness in the home. • Incorporate into empowered potpourri for family unity. • In dream pillows, incense, or in a diffuser, use lilac for manifesting guardian angel contact and for investigating past lives.

Lily

(*Lilium* spp.)

MAGICAL FORMS

perennial flowering plants that grow from bulbs • magically use the growing plant, flower, and oil

PLANETS AND ELEMENT

Venus/Moon • Water

MAGICAL USES

encourages spiritual powers • brings and preserves a happy marriage and permanent relationships • enhances beauty, radiance, and grace • used for fertility, mothers, and mothering spells • for purification rites • for solving mysteries and crimes • breaks vendettas from beyond the grave and generational curses • angel magick • sacred to the Mother Goddess and burned as incense in Goddess magic • especially linked with the ancient Egyptian goddess Isis • their use in ancient Egyptian rites dates back thousands of years • to bring peace if you are surrounded by noisy people • soothing if you are neurodivergent, including those with autism or ADHD

HOW TO USE

Each lily contains its own flower spirit; some believe it survives only as long as the flower and that the flower should not be picked, but kept in the garden or indoor pots. • Set white lilies in a front-facing window or plant them in the garden near the entrance to deter malevolent ghosts and ill-intentioned, deceased relatives who bring negativity. • A natural purifier, lily can be worn or carried until it fades to counteract negative influences in love and lessen the hold of addictions and obsessions. Bury or release faded petals into the air.

CAUTION

Some lilies are highly toxic if used medicinally, but are such an important magical and decorative flower it is worth taking extra care. • Canna lilies (*Cannaceae*) are generally regarded as safe and come in several varieties. • Easter lily (*Liliu longiflorum*), the related Tiger lily (*Lilium lancifolium*), Peruvian lily (*Alstroemeria aurea*), and Stargazer lily (*Lilium stargazer*) are considered less dangerous than many lilies, but are still very toxic for cats and small children. • Plant lilies in pots indoors or outdoors in a safe place.

Lily, Easter

(*Lilium longiflorum*)

MAGICAL FORMS

trumpet-shaped white flowers, grown in gardens, but mainly as potted plants sold commercially to guarantee their Easter blooming • around their Easter/springtime blooming, magically use the potted plant and afterward the dried petals and orange anthers (stamens inside the petals)

PLANETS AND ELEMENTS

Venus/Moon • Water/Air

MAGICAL USES

flower of the fifty-ninth wedding anniversary • if not in bloom, substitute the peace lily • symbolizing spring festivals, and especially Easter, whether celebrated as a family festival of spring or as the Christian resurrection • the Oregon-California border is called the *Easter lily capital of the world* as it is where 95 percent of Easter lilies are produced and shipped • the flower of Easter spring weddings • the flower for Easter funerals as a sign memories will live on and as a symbol in the spring of reconciliation and starting over • the flower for new mothers around Easter/springtime because the Easter lily is associated with motherhood, through its links with Archangel Gabriel who brought a sprig of white lilies to tell the Virgin Mary she would have a child

HOW TO USE

In the springtime/Easter, dome your hands over the plant without touching it to fill yourself with the energies and enthusiasm for new beginnings or a special new start you have been planning but hesitating. • Set your blooming Easter lily in the center of your altar or home and plant yellow crystal eggs, such as jasper, citrine, golden beryl, and rutilated quartz; lemon chrysoprase; and green aventurine in the soil, one for each member of the family or as wishes for your own future.

CAUTION

The Easter lily is toxic to humans and pets—especially cats—if ingested. • It may cause minor skin irritation.

Lily, Horse Tongue

(*Ruscus hypoglossum*)

MAGICAL FORMS

also known as spineless butcher's broom • there are six main *Ruscus* varieties of evergreen shrubs with thick, erect stems • *Ruscus hypoglossum* has tongue-shaped fronds, hence its name, and is less prickly than other *Ruscus* plants • grows indoors and in eastern North America as well as Europe • *Ruscus aculeatus*, the spikier and more hairy variety, though smaller leafed, is called the butcher's broom, and also now flourishes in the USA and Europe; magically, it has similar effects • both have flattened leaflike cladophylls, the *aculeatus* bearing clusters of flowers at the top of the stem and eventually red berries • the *hypoglossum* kind may only have a single flower and berry on each plant • magically use the cut or whole, growing plant; leaves, fresh or dried; stem, fresh or dried; berries; and root

PLANET AND ELEMENT

Venus • Earth

MAGICAL USES

horse tongue lily dates back to the ancient Greeks and was regarded as a secret ingredient in alchemy • either variety can be used, especially the chopped root, for rituals and charms to bring luck, fertility, and protection during childbirth • the butcher's broom variety is hung over a door to keep away malevolent spirits • *hypoglossum*, also known as mouse thorn, creates a low profile if you are seeking information that is being withheld from you, by increasing your clairaudient psychic hearing

HOW TO USE

Burn either kind of horse tongue lily in incense before divination to increase clairvoyance when using tarot, runes, or crystals. • Hide a tongue-shaped leaf in a brown amulet bag in your workspace to prevent gossip and spite and to bring harmony. • Push a dried leaf into any adjoining fence with an overly curious neighbor and replace it regularly, burning the old leaf as it crumbles. • Make a trail of berries leading away from your front door to deter unwelcome or hostile visitors, especially ones demanding money.

CAUTION

Do not ingest the raw plant.

Lily, Madonna

(*Lilium candidum*)

MAGICAL FORMS

also called St. Anthony's lily • originally from the Balkans and the Middle East, brought by explorers, traders, and settlers into parts of the USA, England, Europe, and beyond • one of the earliest cultivated flowers • it is called St. Anthony's flower because, when planted near statues and shrines to the saint, the flowers, it was said, would stay fresh and fragrant, continuing to blossom for months and even years • magically use the growing flower, fresh or dried flowerhead, petals, and leaves

PLANETS AND ELEMENTS

Mercury/Moon • Air/Water

MAGICAL USES

signifies purity • it is said that when the Virgin Mary picked a Madonna lily, which was then yellow, it instantly turned white • protects against sorcery, curses, and hexes • if Madonna lilies are picked when Venus and the Moon are in Taurus, they are considered powerful for love and fertility

HOW TO USE

Growing in your garden or as cut flowers near the center of the home, the flowers drive and keep malevolent ghosts away. • Carry flowers in a handfasting, commitment, or wedding bouquet as a symbol of spiritual, as well as earthly, love. • If you want to conceive a baby or add to an existing family as soon as possible after the ceremony, dry the flowers and leaves and then crumble them, placing the mix in a green bag. On a full-moon night, ask the Mother Goddess or Mother Mary to bless you with a child. Hang the bag on a thriving tree or bush near your home. If waiting before trying for a baby, keep the bag until you are ready and decorate the tree with white flowerheads, then hang the bag on it. • After a funeral, if you are allowed, plant Madonna lily bulbs around the grave. If not, leave growing bulbs in a pot near the gravesite and ask the kind divine mother of your own religion or spirituality to carry the loved one in their arms to rest and restoration.

CAUTION

Madonna lily is toxic to cats, but not to humans or other pets. • If you are pregnant or have a chronic condition, check with an expert before ingesting.

Lily, Mariposa

(*Calochortus* spp.)

MAGICAL FORMS

also called butterfly lily or globe tulip, though it is a lily • genus includes forty species of tulip-like plants, generally white, but can be other colors, including lilac or bluish • native to northwestern and western USA • several cultivated species include the sego lily (*Calochortus nuttallii*), the state flower of Utah, where its corms were used by early Mormons for food • the white mariposa lily (*Calochortus eurycarpus*) is found wild in meadows in northwestern USA • the purple sagebrush mariposa lily (*Calochortus macrocarpus*) is very common in arid regions of western USA • magically use the whole, growing plant; fresh or dried flowers; the cup-shaped fresh or dried white lily head; and the flower essence

PLANET AND ELEMENT

Venus • Earth

MAGICAL USES

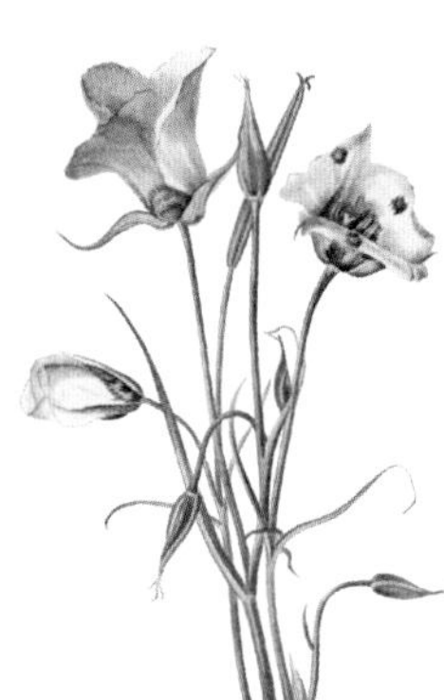

a sixty-second anniversary flower • send on Mother's Day if you are wishing to become closer to your mother • the essence is used in rebirthing ceremonies and for increasing self-love and freedom from the need to be mothered or to over-mother

HOW TO USE

Walk in a wildflower meadow (covering your legs to avoid possible skin irritation) as the flowerheads nod in the wind to free yourself from the need to seek approval from parenting role models. • Walk in the same meadow with your partner if you fear the responsibilities of parenthood, perhaps because of bad childhood experiences.

CAUTION

Avoid ingesting raw parts, especially the stems. • Check with an expert if you have pets, as opinion differs as to whether the lilies are poisonous to dogs and especially cats.

Lily, Martagon

(*Lilium martagon*)

MAGICAL FORMS

also known as turk's cap lily • wild, native to the mountain meadows of Switzerland and from Portugal east through Europe and Asia as far as Mongolia • cultivated, presently in many lands including North America, becoming up to six feet high, with dark green leaves and a tall stem • fragrant purple, white, pink, or dark-red, sometimes speckled, flowers • many flowers on the same stem • summer flowering from midsummer to early fall • magically use whole, growing plant; cut flowers; and flower essence

PLANETS AND ELEMENT

Venus/Moon • Water

MAGICAL USES

a national symbol in Turkey, named after sultans' turbans and regarded as a symbol of authority, perhaps back to the fourteenth century • because it lasts well as a cut flower, can be given in flower arrangements and bouquets as a token of appreciation, on anniversaries, birthdays, and for a central flower arrangement at weddings • as a flower essence, associated with overcoming fears of aggression in others • releases emotional blocks caused by childhood abuse or bullying • restores self-confidence and an ability to feel safe in the world

HOW TO USE

Grow these lilies or keep an arrangement in your home if you wish to attract opulence, luxury, and abundance to your life. • Use the essence in a humidifier, in baths, or sipped in water, or add a drop or two to food if you back away from confrontation or your children are naturally timid in the schoolyard. • A symbol adopted in art and literature, especially in the Near East, use the essence or meditate on the flowers to awaken creativity, especially if you shy away from vivid colors or dramatic scenes.

CAUTION

Martagon is fatal to cats if ingested. • Do not use if pregnant.

Lily of the Valley

(*Convallaria majalis*)

MAGICAL FORMS

flowering plant that spreads underground through networks of rhizomes • flowers appear as delicate, white or pink bells • magically use the whole, growing plant; fresh or dried root; and cut fresh or dried flowers

PLANET AND ELEMENTS

Venus • Water/Earth

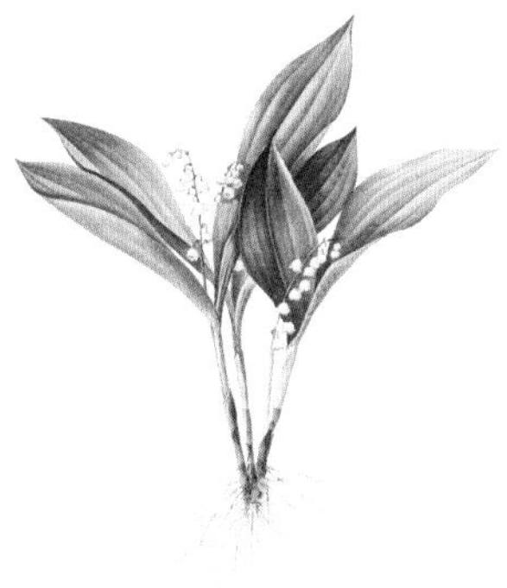

MAGICAL USES

brings luck and happiness in love, especially first love • return of happiness • improves memory and focus • for getting someone to listen to you • takes away regrets • lily of the valley, according to myth, appeared where drops of blood fell from St. Leonard after he was wounded slaying a dragon in the woods near Horsham in Sussex, UK • the flower is sometimes called Mary's Tears, to signify the tears that the Virgin Mary shed at the death of her son, which turned into lily of the valley as they hit the earth

HOW TO USE

Burn as incense, especially the dried bells or powdered root (handle with care), to clear energies before a ritual or if there has been a quarrel. • Also burn for the return of a lost love or to heal a fractured relationship, remarriage after divorce, or a major estrangement. • Plant lily of the valley to attract benign nature spirits into your garden and to repel any malicious spirits. • In Anglo-Saxon and Norse lore, lily of the valley was the flower of the goddess of spring, Eostre or Ostara. The first lily of the valley seen after winter heralded good fortune and wishes that would be granted.

CAUTION

Lily of the valley is toxic if ingested by humans and pets, especially the roots and berries, which are attractive to children.

Lily, Oriental

(*Lilium orientalis*)

MAGICAL FORMS

grows happily in temperate regions of North America, Asia, and Europe • in gardens, containers, or pots indoors • new kinds recently created as My Wedding flowers series, notably as a double lily • larger than Asiatic lilies, and there are no stamens in My Wedding lilies (stamens can be a problem, as they stain clothes) • magically use the whole, growing plant and fresh or dried flowers

PLANET AND ELEMENT

Venus • Water

MAGICAL USES

the Wedding series, mainly white with pink round edges and highly scented, is the ultimate bouquet flower for a wedding of twin souls and childhood sweethearts (two flowers or the double flower will make a distinctive bouquet) • the stargazer oriental lily is a great Mother's Day flower • the predecessor to the stargazer was the rubrum lily, preserved during World War II by a farmer in Japan, Hirotaka Ukida, and his son Masao • in 1949, Dr. Woodriff in California developed and named the hybrid stargazer, from the rubrum, so called because it faced the sky, blending East with West • like its name, it is linked with mystical experiences with stargazing and a portal for Star Souls

HOW TO USE

Meditate on fragrant oriental lilies to open your clairsentient psychic powers and experience visions of old worlds from the East and West, and other dimensions. • Gift yellow oriental lilies to your mother or grandmother at any time to express gratitude. • Keep a single crimson or pink oriental lily in your home to attract prosperity. • Buy three oriental lilies, one smaller than the others, to attract the blessings of a child. • The original rubrum forms are not sold commercially, so they can be preserved untainted.

CAUTION

Oriental lilies are toxic if ingested by small children and cats. • They should not be eaten by any pets or humans.

Lily, Peace

(*Spathiphyllum wallisii*)

MAGICAL FORMS

native to Asia and Central America, the peace lily grows outdoors in tropical and semitropical zones and indoors as a potted plant almost everywhere in the world • large, green, glossy, oval leaves and white spathe (large outer covering enclosing the tiny blooms growing in the center) • it may flower twice, in spring and again in the fall • magically use the growing indoor plant in every setting where harmony is needed

PLANET AND ELEMENT

Venus • Earth

MAGICAL USES

flower of the twenty-eighth and fifty-ninth wedding anniversaries to reflect any differences accepted or reconciled • also gifted for the birth of a new baby with wishes for a harmonious life ahead • sent to those who have lost someone, especially if the person was not able to say goodbye or died with unsaid words of love • with its message of peace and reconciliation, the plant forms a focus for rituals bringing peace to a community or between nations, such as International Day of Peace, or World Peace Day, on September 21 each year

HOW TO USE

A popular feng shui plant in the home or workplace, peace lily removes toxic atmospheres and rivalries along with its natural ability to physically remove pollutants from the air. • Set where chi life force can circulate and bring enthusiasm and a sense of well-being and cooperation if siblings are expressing rivalry for attention or in an overcompetitive workplace. • Offer an empowered plant as a sign of a truce if not agreement to a relative, friend, or colleague when there has been a major difference of opinion. • Place your peace lily in the center of a room if involved in mediation professionally or find yourself cast in the role of family, workplace, or social peacemaker.

CAUTION

Peace lily is toxic to people and pets if ingested and can irritate the skin.

Lily, Peruvian

(*Alstroemeria aurea*)

MAGICAL FORMS

also called the lily of the Incas, resembling a lily though not a true lily • originally grown in Peru, Chile, and Brazil but now beloved worldwide, particularly in warmer climes, such as California • brightly colored flowers reach for the sun • magically use the growing plant, indoors and out; cut flowers; and fresh and dried petals and leaves

PLANET AND ELEMENT

Sun • Fire

MAGICAL USES

a wedding flower in white and the kind called *Blushing Bride*, cream with brown speckles, treasured by childhood sweethearts • for loyal friendship, as a gift when a friend has stood by you in a crisis • itself a symbol of the ideal human with all the qualities desirable in or offered to a friend, lover, partner, family member, or work colleague • each of its six petals representing understanding, humor, patience, empathy, commitment, respect, while the twisted leaves represent unity • gifted to older relatives for a long and happy life

HOW TO USE

Send yellow and orange flowers representing health and vitality in a get-well-soon bouquet. • Send red flowers for romance, perhaps on Valentine's Day, to someone you would like to become more than a friend. • Send purple flowers to offer congratulations on a career success, promotion, or to say thank you for helping financially. • Grow mixed colors in your garden, a conservatory, or sheltered balcony to attract health, wealth, harmony, and unity to your home and all who live there or visit. • Take a sachet of dried leaves and flowers from a plant you grew in the months before you moved to hang on red ribbon inside your new front door to transfer the happiness and love of the family. • Set the actual plant near the front door to provide comfort if you are leaving the family home for the first time.

CAUTION

There is divided opinion as to whether the plant is mildly toxic to humans but not to pets, but the tubers of most kinds are generally considered edible.

Lily, Stargazer

(*Lilium orientalis* 'Stargazer')

MAGICAL FORMS

a hybrid oriental lily created in 1974 • fragrant flower that is a perfect star, blooming from the middle to the end of summer, dark pink or crimson, that fades toward the edge of the flowers, white to pale pink • in the center, large, yellow stamens release pollen • the whole flower can be yellow • so called because they gaze up to the stars not down like other lilies • each stem can produce up to ten blooms • magically cultivate in a pot or in the garden, or use as a cut flower arrangement

PLANETS AND ELEMENT

Venus/Moon • Water

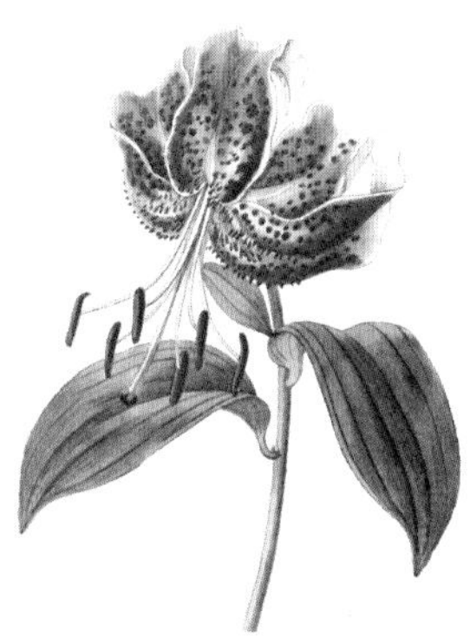

MAGICAL USES

for the fifty-fifth wedding anniversary, often considered the emerald anniversary, as a reflection of love growing deeper through the years • with the message from a partner, *You will always be precious to me as the years go by* • pink stargazers to wish prosperity on the couple and yellow for happiness, long life, and health

HOW TO USE

Give stargazers to anyone who is taking a starring role in any aspect of life or to send good luck before an interview, audition, or performance. • Stargazer lily is a symbol of rebirth and regeneration, when purchased as a cut flower, especially around Easter (often grown specially in hothouses) and other spiritual and religious festivals of rebirth. • Buy or plant for yourself after redundancy, job loss, or being or feeling abandoned as an act of faith. • Use your stargazer lily as a focus in meditation or as the subject of an empowerment with your hands close to the flowers, absorbing its power.

CAUTION

Stargazer lilies are considered less dangerous than many lilies but are still very toxic for cats and small children.

Lily, Tiger

(*Lilium lancifolium*)

MAGICAL FORMS

flowering plant • originally from Asia, tiger lily grows well in eastern North America and other lands • magically use the whole, growing plant indoors or out; fresh and dried flowers; essential oil; and flower essence

PLANET AND ELEMENT

Mars • Fire

MAGICAL USES

wealth • achievements • warding off evil spirits • in China, where it has been cultivated for two thousand years, a symbol of good fortune • in ancient Greece, represented motherhood and fertility • an icon of courage in Japan • promotes long life

HOW TO USE

Place the fierce, tiger-like, orange and black lily in a vase surrounded by golden tiger eye crystals in the center of the home or on your altar to ensure no unfriendly ghosts will hang around. • One growing in a pot in your workspace deters time wasters, gossips, and overcritical folk alike from intruding on your work time. • Make a mist spray with water and the flower essence in a room where a work meeting will take place to free the atmosphere from stagnant ideas and an inability of those participating to accept innovation and new practices. • Burn or diffuse the oil to encourage focused meditation and mindfulness. • Send a bouquet of tiger lilies with congratulations for a major success. • Keep the flowers in a new business to encourage prosperity. • Out of season, you can substitute a charm bag of dried flowers hung over the entrance or near your business computer to draw in clients and orders. • Grow tiger lilies in your garden with a clear quartz crystal buried in the center at the base to repel malicious spells and hostile land spirits if you live near where ley lines cross. • Bury purple amethyst and plant the tiger lilies on either side of the home entrance and exits if the negative energies flow through the house itself.

CAUTION

The tiger lily is extremely toxic to cats if ingested and can harm young children. • The jury is out as to their toxicity for adult humans and dogs, so do not ingest and avoid handling excessively. • Avoid if pregnant or while breastfeeding.

Lime

(*Citrus aurantifolia*)

MAGICAL FORMS

an evergreen shrub with glossy, fragrant leaves, sharp spines, and aromatic white flowers, followed by the round, green or yellow-green fruit about half the size of a lemon • originally from southern Asia, growing limes spread to North Africa and Egypt • during the thirteenth century, limes were carried by the Moors to southern Europe and from there to the coastal USA • limes were used on English ships in the eighteenth century and began to be adopted from 1809 by the US navy to prevent scurvy • magically use the fruit, the peel, and the essential oil, which is made from the fresh peel

PLANET AND ELEMENT

Moon • Water

MAGICAL USES

a fruit to protect against all harm, earthly and spirit • new beginnings, places, people, and original ideas • repels spite and jealousy, and hostile neighbors, family, and colleagues • for overcoming injustice and unfair or corrupt officialdom

HOW TO USE

To remove hexes, curses, and ill wishes—whether or not the source is known—pierce the skin of a lime fruit with rusty iron nails, pins, and needles, and then immerse it in salt. Place the salt and pierced fruit in a very deep hole in a strong, sealed box so it cannot harm burrowing animals. • Dry the lime peel and place it in an amulet bag to keep away jealousy, envy, and gossip if you must encounter an offender on a regular basis. Once a week, cast the peel in flowing water and replace. • Inhale the oil from a diffuser or burner, or alternatively carry lime oil in the form of a roller ball or a homemade small bottle of the diluted oil, to anoint pulse points and overcome food cravings, especially those with an emotional basis.

CAUTION

Use the oil very well diluted. • Lime is phototoxic, so avoid sunlight after use. • It is considered safe in pregnancy in moderation in the later trimesters. Check with your midwife or physician before use during pregnancy. • Some people are allergic to the lime peel.

Lingonberry

(*Vaccinium vitis-idaea*)

MAGICAL FORMS

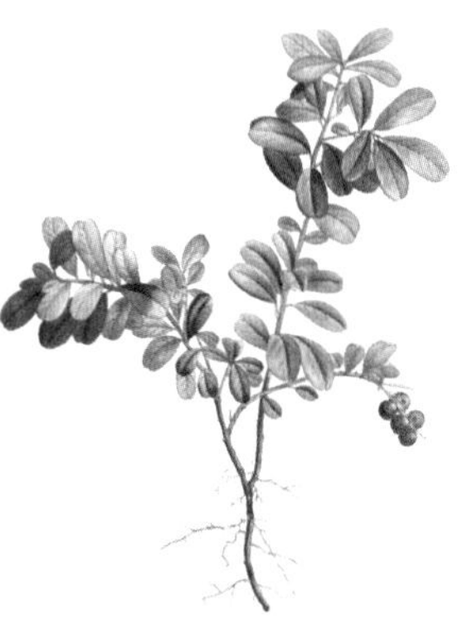

including American dwarf lingonberry (*Vaccinium vitis-idaea* subsp. *minus*) • part of the heather family • related to the blueberry and cranberry • growing wild and cultivated • the larger *majus* variety in the northern parts of the northern hemisphere, especially Iceland, Greenland, and northern Scandinavia • the dwarf form in the northern USA and Canada • small white or pink bell-shaped flowers between July and September produce the tart, round, dark-red fruit between August and October (sometimes as two harvests, the first from midsummer onward) • the fruit is nutritious, encouraging digestive health, weight loss, and heart health • magically use the berries or any cooked lingonberry product

PLANETS AND ELEMENT

Moon/Venus • Water

MAGICAL USES

in magical cookery lingonberries are empowered to give stamina, patience, and endurance to win despite difficult situations • use as jelly or jam, in desserts, cocktails, or in sauces, homemade or purchased • protect against paranormal harm • bring good luck • celebrate the passing of the seasons and life cycle

HOW TO USE

Associated with festivals of the sun such as midsummer or the fall equinox, whether growing, dried, or ready prepared, lingonberries transmit the pure solar life force and bring or restore hope, vitality, and enthusiasm. • Serve to enliven family meals with taciturn family members.

CAUTION

Lingonberries are too tart and bitter to be eaten raw. • Do not pick before ripe.

Lisianthus

(*Eustoma* spp.)

MAGICAL FORMS

including *Eustoma grandiflorum* • also called Prairie gentian and Texas bluebell • descended from wildflowers in the grassland of North America • magically use the whole, growing plant; cut flowers; and fresh and dried petals

PLANETS AND ELEMENTS

Sun/Jupiter • Fire/Air

MAGICAL USES

represents a lifelong bond between a couple who were friends for years before acknowledging love • red or apricot for Valentine's Day and anniversaries, and for courage to express your love if you face opposition • pink for romance, Mother's or Father's Day (especially for single parents), baby showers, and new mothers • purple for bereaved relatives or placed on a grave on the anniversary of a death to say love goes on forever • yellow for a *get well soon* or a *you make me happy* bouquet

HOW TO USE

If you want your best friend to become your lover, give them a bouquet of pink and red flowers with an invitation for a shared-interest event tucked in the flowers. • If love seems unattainable, bury twin rose quartz crystals beneath the growing roots of red lisianthus in the garden or a potted plant. Ask that as the plant grows, so will the attachment. • To attract twin soul love, take a double flower or two matching singles in white or cream, then tie them with cream or white ribbon and place them in a vase. With a lit white candle, burn a petal from each or the double flower, saying, *Find me my love forever, in fragrance and in flower, in fire and fragrance fulfill my desire*. Drop the singed petals in a bowl of soil. Bury the burned petals, still in the soil, near any growing plant, ideally lisianthus. When the flower(s) in the vase fade, drop a third of the petals into flowing water, cast a third into the air, and carry the rest in a sachet until twin love comes. • To overcome estrangement, set matching flowers in vases and each day move the vases closer together, saying, *Return love to me, estranged no more shall we be*.

CAUTION

Avoid using while pregnant.

Litsea

(*Litsea cubeba*)

MAGICAL FORMS

also called may chang • deciduous tropical tree often called the mountain pepper • fragrant leaves and flowers that are reminiscent of lemongrass • essential oil is made from the fruits that resemble large, dried, black peppers • grows in Southeast Asia and China, also in the Pacific Northwest of the USA and the southwest of the UK • magically use the essential oil • the oil has only been marketed since the 1950s, though the leaves, flowers, fruits, and roots have been used in traditional Chinese medicine for centuries

PLANET AND ELEMENT

Mercury • Air

MAGICAL USES

emotional well-being • clears a home or workspace of stagnation and negativity, earthly and paranormal • prevents overreaction by family members, friends, or colleagues • to help you say *no* to unreasonable demands without offending

HOW TO USE

Place a few drops of the oil in a roller bottle (available to buy empty online) or small stoppered bottle, adding, if you wish, a drop or two of peppermint oil, plus carrier oil, for anointing pulse points whenever you are weighed down by unenthusiastic or critical people or too much work. • Add the oil with a few drops of bergamot or lavender to a pump-action bottle of water to spray into dark corners if there is a spooky atmosphere in your entrance hall, and in your bedroom before sleep if you are troubled by paranormal nightmares or visitations by restless spirits. • Diffuse or burn the oil before a family celebration or workplace meeting when you know there will otherwise be a clash of temperaments or point scoring.

CAUTION

Though an edible plant, the oil is not established as safe in pregnancy, but is generally permitted while breastfeeding; seek professional advice. • Litsea is nontoxic and not a known irritant, but dilute before skin use.

Lobelia

(*Lobelia inflata*) or (*Lobelia erinus*)

MAGICAL FORMS

also called asthma weed because of its medicinal properties connected with the lungs • used medicinally by the Native North Americans and adopted by the late eighteenth-century eminent American herbalist Samuel Thomson • used by modern herbalists to clear mucus from the lungs, as well as to reduce smoking addiction • was used in smoking ceremonies where it was substituted for tobacco, hence it has also been called Indian tobacco • magically use the growing plant; fresh or dried flowers, especially in pale-blue form; powdered leaves; and bark

PLANETS AND ELEMENTS

Mercury/Saturn • Air/Earth

MAGICAL USES

to deter a lover from leaving or being unfaithful, subject to the constraints of free will • in an amulet to reduce hostility against you by ex-partners of your present love, spiteful neighbors, or jealous colleagues • enhances visions in meditation and increases psychic awareness, especially of the fey nature world

HOW TO USE

Keep the dried blue flowers or powdered leaves in a closed pot near the front door, and cast toward any approaching storms to avert damage. • Throw a handful out of the front door if you are expecting confrontational visitors. • Use in incense mixes to repel psychic attacks and unfriendly ghosts and to break hexes. • Growing the flowers outside the front door acts as a barrier against restless spirits of the land but encourages benign luck-bringing house spirits. • Make a wishing powder with crumbled, dried lobelia and cornstarch mixed with spices such as chile, then sprinkle it around your shoes at sunrise each morning so that your path will cross with a desired love who seems not to notice you.

CAUTION

The fresh plant is toxic to humans and pets. It should not be ingested and must be handled with care.

Locust Tree

(*Robinia pseudoacacia*) and (*Gleditsia triacanthos*)

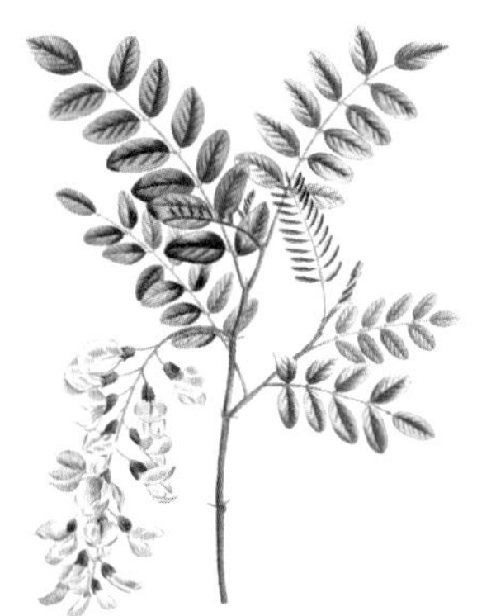

MAGICAL FORMS

flowering trees native to the eastern states of North America • two main kinds, most commonly black locust (*Robinia pseudoacacia*) and honey locust (*Gleditsia triacanthos*) • the black locust grows from Pennsylvania to Georgia but is naturalized over much of the USA • honey locust spans from New England to Texas with sweet-smelling flowers and sweet-tasting pods but fierce thorns • black locust also has dense clusters of flowers • called locust tree beginning in the 1630s because in some species the pods resemble a locust • magically use the fresh and dried flowers and leaves of either, as well as the honey locust thorns (with care!)

PLANETS AND ELEMENT

Sun/Mars • Fire

MAGICAL USES

black locust for developing potential, uncovering truth and secrets, and successful networking • as incense or on hearth or bonfires for all purification rituals • honey locust for both fertility and defensive magick

HOW TO USE

Use a black locust wand for protective and binding magick and for rituals requiring perseverance or where results are not immediate but will be long-lasting. • Use honey locust for fey magick, as well as for increasing charisma and creating good first impressions. • Use the thorns from the honey locust in defensive jars or bottles with the dried flowers and sweet red wine to protect against those who are vicious but masquerade as friends.

CAUTION

Honey locust should be ingested only with expert advice and moderately. • Black locust seeds, bark, and leaves are toxic.

London Plane Tree

(*Platanus × hispanica*)

MAGICAL FORMS

hybrid of the American sycamore (*Platanus occidentalis*, see "Sycamore Tree," p. 440) and the Oriental plane (*Platanus orientalis*) • London plane trees are arguably among the most famous and elegant city trees, planted extensively in the UK, especially in London, in parks and streets and in cities throughout the world • first planted in London in 1550, they became popular in cities because of the nineteenth-century worldwide urbanization • flourish in New York City, where more than 15 percent of all city trees are London planes • often seventy to a hundred feet tall and sixty to seventy feet wide with maple-like leaves • light brown bark peels to reveal creamy-olive, gray, green, or yellow wood inside • magically use the fresh and dried leaves, the fallen bark, and the whole tree, growing in a quiet spot in a park or botanical garden

PLANETS AND ELEMENTS

Sun/Moon • Fire/Water

MAGICAL USES

the shedding of the bark removes pollutants of city life and psychic and psychological toxicity • sacred in goddess rituals when the moon is full and god rituals at sunrise and noon • brings good fortune and protection from malevolent entities • for urban magick

HOW TO USE

Collect fallen bark and mix with a granular resin such as frankincense to remove sour emotional energies from your home or any poltergeist or restless spirit activity. • Sit beneath a plane tree in a quiet place so all you can see when you look up is the tree canopy. Inhale pure life force energies with this magical filter tree, exhaling all doubts, fears, and resentment until you feel free. • Circle a plane tree clockwise and counterclockwise at different moon phases and seasonal change points, especially midsummer and midwinter; while holding the tree, close your eyes and let it fill you with the changing powers of the time.

CAUTION

The tree is nontoxic to pets and humans. • Do not ingest raw parts, and be aware that leaves, flowers, and bark may cause skin irritation.

Loosestrife, Gooseneck

(*Lysimachia clethroides*)

MAGICAL FORMS

a wild flowering plant, named gooseneck because the flower spikes are long, arched, and slender • when growing together in colonies as is common, they resemble the white heads and necks of geese, especially when facing the same direction • native to China, Japan, and Indonesia • cultivated in most zones of the USA, in Russia, and in the UK and Europe • there are other kinds of loosestrife, especially purple • magically use the growing and cut flowers

PLANET AND ELEMENT

Jupiter • Air

MAGICAL USES

loosestrife, as its name implies, reduces anger and conflict, especially when meditating on the growing or cut flowers • considered to bring harmony and calm to families and communities • it was said that King Lysimachus, a Macedonian king, tamed a wild ox with the plant • it tamps down on gossip, spiteful comments, and rumor mongering

HOW TO USE

Plant gooseneck in the garden to deter troublesome neighbors from complaining or acting maliciously and to protect you from neighborhood cliques as a newcomer in a very established community. • Send a ready-to-plant small clump of gooseneck loosestrife or add it to a cut dried arrangement for a friend to mend a quarrel. • Ask your growing gooseneck what is being said about you behind your back and the answer will come as words or images in your mind.

Loosestrife, Purple

(*Lythrum salicaria*)

MAGICAL FORMS

lavender or occasionally magenta to red flowers in small clumps on long flower spikes forming a bell shape • the terminal flower spike can occupy the last foot or more of the plant • dozens of stems may rise from a single rootstock and the flowers on these can produce millions of tiny seeds • introduced from Europe and grows throughout most of the USA and Canada—except in far northern areas and parts of southeastern USA—as well as in Asia, Australia, South Africa, and New Zealand • classified as a noxious weed in some states in the USA • magically use the flowers on the stems, especially the tallest top flower, growing or cut and dried; fresh or dried flowers; leaves; and stems

PLANET AND ELEMENTS

Moon • Water/Earth

MAGICAL USES

for mending quarrels • bringing and keeping peace in the home, workplace, and any noisy or hyperactive environment • for quieting overly harsh earth energies beneath your home if grown in the garden or used as part of a charm bag (alternately, tape the dried plant beneath the doormat)

HOW TO USE

Loosestrife is considered most powerful when picked at midsummer. • Hide an amulet bag with the dried midsummer flowers in each corner of the house if you have a volatile family, or a single bag in your workspace facing where overly chatty or complaining people enter. • Set a bag containing dried leaves and the chopped stem or root in a stable or above an animal's sleeping place where they cannot reach it, to keep them calm. • Stash in the glove compartment of a car if you have a frustrating regular commute or have to drive demanding relatives.

CAUTION

Though traditionally used medicinally, loosestrife is poisonous if ingested by humans or animals.

Lotus

(*Nelumbo nicifera*)

MAGICAL FORMS

also called sacred Indian lotus and nelumbo lutea, the American lotus • grown within a water feature in your moon area in a deep bowl of soil or indoors with flowers, stems, and leaves above the surface • magically use the leaves, flowers, pods, stamens, seeds, and essential oil (expensive but beautiful)

PLANETS AND ELEMENTS

Moon/Sun • Water/Fire

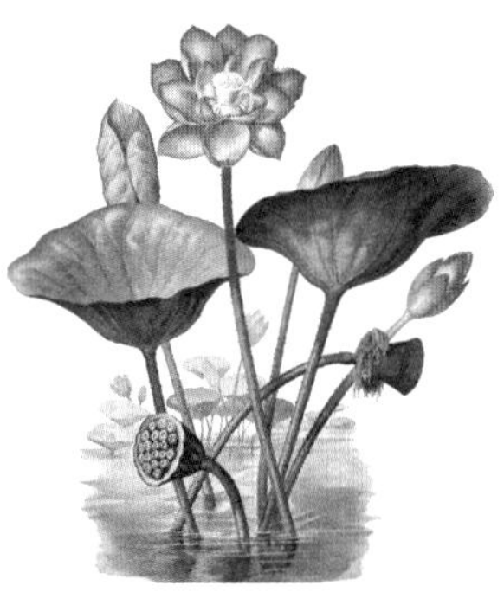

MAGICAL USES

to solve women's mysteries • for beauty, inner radiance, and sensuality • for secret love • fertility • an antidote to those who seek to control love by magick or emotional blackmail • good luck • giving those who are sick or despairing the will to live • a sacred symbol for peace and enlightenment in Hinduism and Buddhism and rebirth and regeneration in ancient Egypt and many cultures because the sacred lotus opens in the day, closes at night, and stays closed for three days

HOW TO USE

Plant a single white lotus to conceive a child. • Matching lotus flowers indicate a desire for twins; three lotus, triplets; or a lotus for each of the number of children you want. • Two lotus flowers side by side in water indicate the growth of twin-soul passion, and for rituals to bring the will to live to sick and sorrowing people. • Carry lotus seeds and pods in a sachet to break false enchantment in love. • Anoint white candles with lotus oil to connect with deceased relatives and your personal guides and deities.

CAUTION

Do not take or ingest lotus if pregnant or breastfeeding. • Avoid lotus if you are taking medication for diabetes, erectile dysfunction, high cholesterol, heart conditions, or certain psychological conditions (if in doubt check with an expert).

Lotus Root

(*Nelumbo nucifera*)

MAGICAL FORMS

originated in India, reaching Egypt, China, and Japan about two thousand years ago • tubular-shaped and often resembling a series of interconnecting chambers or holes, the edible root or stem from the lotus is featured in Chinese and Ayurvedic medicine and popularly in cooking • grows in muddy ponds and rivers • the root is sold in larger health stores and Asian markets as well as magick stores already sliced • magically use the root, especially, and also the seedheads, seeds (also called nuts), and leaves

PLANETS AND ELEMENT

Moon/Venus • Water

MAGICAL USES

brings new opportunities • blessings in whatever area they are sought • the ability to open any doors to career or business where advancement has been denied • enlightenment and regeneration after setbacks

HOW TO USE

Keep a dish of dried, chopped or powdered root in the kitchen to incubate wealth and health. • Lotus root is associated with Lakshmi, the Hindu goddess of Diwali and abundance who is depicted with lotus roots at her feet. • Burn the root or root powder in incense during Diwali, asking for the blessings of light. (The date of Diwali changes every year, but it falls in October or November, so double check the dates each year.) • Use the seed heads containing the seeds for fertility on the full moon. • Cast the seed heads or remove the seeds and cast them separately into flowing water the day after lovemaking to release the fertility. • Lotus root is also linked with Sarasvati, the Hindu goddess of music, creativity, and knowledge. • Keep the dried, sliced root in a charm bag, along with any books or scripts you are writing or have written or music you have composed. Take the bag along to any auditions concerning the performing arts or the media, or when selling your creative crafts.

CAUTION

People with diabetes should not ingest the root. • Not enough research about its safety in pregnancy or breastfeeding has been verified, so use medicinally only with expert advice.

Lovage

(*Levisticum officinale*)

MAGICAL FORMS

taken to the USA from Europe by the early New Englander settlers • the candied root was chewed in church to encourage alertness • magically use the whole, growing plant; flowers; fresh or dried roots (especially dug up on Good Friday, though roots are generally harvested in the fall); seeds; and oil, which is quite hard to obtain

PLANETS AND ELEMENTS

Venus/Sun • Earth/Fire

MAGICAL USES

popular in the gardens of Benedictine monasteries for medicinal and culinary purposes in the Middle Ages • since these monks built their monasteries along ley energy lines, lovage contains strong earth energies when grown that counteract any negative earth powers beneath land • used in magical cookery and medicinally in Greek and Roman times • resolving gender issues in relationships where there is uncertainty or opposition by outsiders

HOW TO USE

Add a lovage root decoction to your bath to experience its benefits (as listed above). • Alternatively, place dried, chopped lovage in a sachet in the bath with rose petals or float seven rosebuds in the water with your lovage sachet to attract love and romance. • It is especially potent on Valentine's Day morning and will help you find the right partner. • Hang the tied, dried plants upside down over an entrance or front-facing window to prevent negative spirits or ill-wishers disturbing your home. • When you are moving into a new home with a partner or carrying out renovations on your present home, tie a dried lovage root wrapped in a piece of paper with your names entwined, with red, green, and white thread. Place it either behind a fireplace, in a wall, or under a heavy piece of furniture that will not be moved for a lasting and happy relationship and, if wished, adding to the family.

CAUTION

Avoid in pregnancy or if you have reduced heart or kidney function. • Minimize exposure to the sun after use. • Do not use the root oil excessively.

Love-in-a-Mist

(*Nigella damascena*)

MAGICAL FORMS

a member of the buttercup family • each flower looks as if it is nestled within a mist of fern or threadlike foliage, giving the flower its name • though native to North Africa and southern Europe, the plant now grows in many parts of the world in gardens, containers, and hanging baskets • can reach almost two feet high • magically use the whole, growing plant; the delicate, shaggy, often-blue flower, fresh and dried; the seed pods still in the flowerheads after the flowers have died, dried; and the black, spicy seeds

PLANET AND ELEMENT

Venus • Water

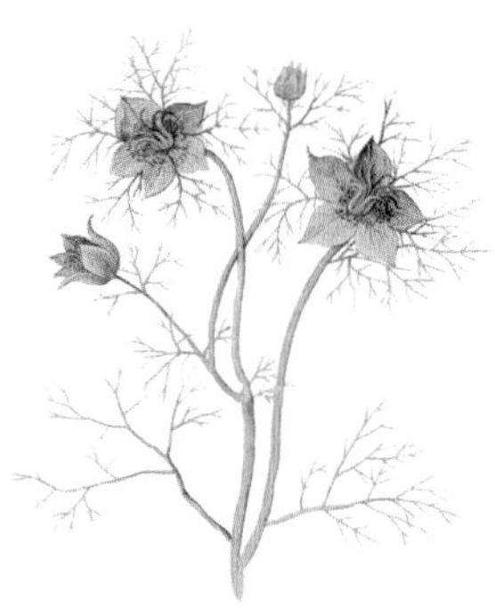

MAGICAL USES

the flower is associated with love and devotion • love-in-a-mist makes beautiful bouquets, fresh or dried, for any love connection • as a flower, because of its delicateness, give for the eighteenth wedding anniversary • giving the flower to a loved one for any occasion acts as a charm to hold a relationship safe from outside pressures

HOW TO USE

Love-in-a-mist is dedicated to St. Catherine of Alexandria, whose special day is November 25, when at her sacred wells she is entreated to bring good partners to those who ask her. • Take a blue flower to still water, surrounded by its mist, if possible on a misty day. Cast it into the water (best of all on St. Catherine's Day), asking for the right love. • When the flower dies and the seeds form within the seed pod on the flower, pop the pod. Keep the seeds in a clear glass jar in your home or workplace so that bonds of loyalty will grow.

CAUTION

The plant is considered slightly toxic and so should not be eaten. • The seeds are generally considered edible as a flavoring spice.

Lucky Hand Root

(*Orchis* spp.)

MAGICAL FORMS
also called salep root • several forms of orchids, popular in and beyond the Hoodoo tradition • a root resembling a hand and fingers, reaching out to grasp • magically use the root (unmistakable, though getting harder to obtain)

PLANETS AND ELEMENTS
Jupiter/Mercury/Venus • Air/Water

MAGICAL USES
gambling • speculation • good luck • employment • travel • help and opportunity when and where most needed in any area of life, using an open-hand root • substitute a closed-fist root in a red flannel bag if you know you face confrontation or are traveling to a hazardous place

HOW TO USE
Before gaming or placing a bet, carry the root in a charm bag with money herbs such as bay, basil, rosemary, or sage, plus any one of a small piece of gold, tiger eye crystal, or goldstone. • Traditionally, Psalm 23 is recited over the bag before sealing. • A small, whole lucky hand root (do not break or you will break the luck) added to a good-luck oil such as rose should be rubbed onto a lucky coin or gambling chip for cards, roulette, or lotto, or a silver horseshoe charm or St. Christopher charm for travel. • Burn a circle of five blue candles around your open-hand root, placed on a piece of paper that details a job you've applied for, your ideal job, or the name of a business you hope to start. Light a sandalwood incense stick from each of the candles in turn and write around and above the circle in incense stick smoke your future job title or business and your salary, and say, *So I reach out and so obtain, this night begins my life of gain*. Leave all to burn out and take the hand to the interview, exam, or loan application meeting in a blue bag.

CAUTION
As with any orchid, never ingest and keep away from children and pets.

Lungwort

(*Pulmonaria officinalis*)

MAGICAL FORMS
one of the earliest European wildflowers, now growing wild in North America and cultivated in informal gardens because of its beautiful flowers • magically use the whole, growing plant; leaves; fresh and dried flowers; and flower essence

PLANETS AND ELEMENTS
Venus/Mercury • Earth/Air

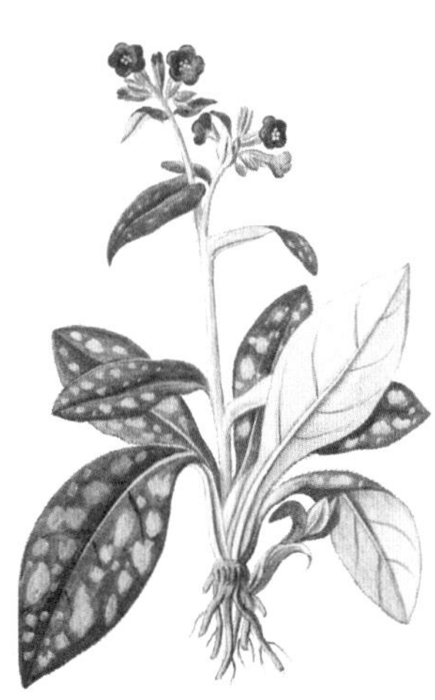

MAGICAL USES
in Germany, lungwort is called our lady's milkwort because of its green-and-white-spotted milky leaves, associated with the maternal milk of the Virgin Mary, which gives its leaves their protective qualities • a love herb meaning, in the language of flowers, *you are my whole life*, the first flowers presented as a token of devotion • for safe air travel and overcoming fear of flying

HOW TO USE
Because the flowers change from blue to pink or violet as they blossom and the flowers close at night and open in the morning, the dried flowers of the blossom are carried in amulet bags and burned in incense mixes to clear emotional blockages, solve situations going nowhere, and calm frustrations. • Because of traditional links with healing diseases of the lungs, scattering the chopped and dried plants where nothing grows breaks the stifling hold of an ex-partner or family member. • Empower the flower essence before taking it in the evening.

CAUTION
Lungwort is generally considered safe for adults, though not in pregnancy. • It is medicinally subject to restrictions in some countries but valued as a traditional magical herb.

Lupine

(*Lupinus* spp.)

MAGICAL FORMS

common varieties include sundial lupine or wild lupine (*Lupinus perennis*) and Texas lupine (*Lupinus texensis*), also called Texas bluebonnet • named after the wolf (lupus) because lupines often grew in barren places and were erroneously believed to steal nutrients from the soil, to the detriment of other plants, as the wolf killed livestock • in fact lupines increase soil nutrition by drawing nitrogen through their roots to fertilize the soil • native to North and South America and grows all over North America, in Eurasia, and the UK • the state flower of Texas is called bluebonnet because its blue flowers resembled the bonnets worn by early pioneer women • magically use the whole, growing plant; cut and dried flowers; and flower essence

PLANETS AND ELEMENTS

Sun/Jupiter • Earth/Air

MAGICAL USES

from ancient Egyptian and Roman times the pealike seeds within the pods were cooked for food • the flower was first said to grow in the USA when there was a famine • dried flowers in charm bags are used for protection and good fortune • like the wolf, lupine represents eagerness, health, and curiosity for life • use to see nature spirits or as a bridge between worlds

HOW TO USE

Use the cut flowers in the different quarters of your magick circle or altar. • Use pink in the north for memories of the departed and those removed from your life. • Yellow in the east is for travel, especially under uncertainty. • Red in the south is for courage and passion. • Blue in the west is for compassion. • White for Spirit in the center. • Use lupine to communicate with beloved ancestors by gazing into a glass bowl of water to which a little essence has been added. Close your eyes, *seeing* the sphere of light water in your mind. Open your eyes, blink, and in the water will appear momentarily an image of a loved one.

CAUTION

Seeds or pods should never be eaten raw, as they are toxic to humans and animals.

Lychee

(*Litchi chinensis*)

MAGICAL FORMS

red or pink oval-shaped small tropical fruit from the soapberry family • grown worldwide in subtropical regions, especially China and southeast Asia • increasingly popular in the USA in drinks, salads, and curries or raw as desserts • sweet, flowery flesh with leathery skin and a stone or seed that is removed before eating • magically use the whole and peeled fruit

PLANET AND ELEMENT

Mercury • Air

MAGICAL USES

for sweetening moods and tempers • the acquisition of beautiful artifacts • to strengthen quiet determination • for the granting of wishes • considered lucky in pairs, whether portrayed as such in pictures or naturally occurring on a tree • prints or paintings depicting a tree with a hundred fruits attracts profits and is often displayed in businesses

HOW TO USE

A bunch of raw lychees in their skins brings financial advantage. Subsequently, eating them raw or cooked sharpens the senses to become aware both of opportunity and concealed disadvantages. • Lychee is often combined with other fruits for success in examinations or a promotion, or with a date set on a newlywed couple's bed for fertility. • Keep it with a water chestnut to increase mental acuity and as a triplicate with a plum and finger lemon for the unity of yin and yang within the space where it is placed, whether the center of a room, the home, or office.

CAUTION

Lychee is generally regarded as safe if eaten in moderation, despite some unproven research in parts of Asia that suggests the fruit may be linked with brain inflammation.

Macadamia Nut

(*Macadamia integrifolia*)

MAGICAL FORMS

large evergreen tree, native to the rainforests of New South Wales and southeastern Queensland in Australia and a valued food for the Indigenous people • the tree is thirty to fifty feet high • white to pinkish flowers, blooms in winter and spring, followed by nuts that are creamy white inside a hard, smooth case • the toughest nut in the world to crack open • grows in the USA, first planted in Hawaii in 1837 • California produces the rough shell version (*Macadamia tetraphylla*) • magically use the unshelled and shelled nut

PLANETS AND ELEMENT

Mars/Sun • Fire

MAGICAL USES

youthfulness and improved memory in later years • positive body image • eaten shelled to give physical, psychological, and psychic protection • refusal to abandon principles

HOW TO USE

Collect the unshelled nuts (not always easy to find except from the tree) in a brown bag and add one every day to a ceramic lidded pot containing a coin with copper in it, such as a penny from the USA (or a two pence coin in the UK), or if you can obtain it, an old coin, like a fugio cent. Failing that, use a piece of copper jewelry. Shake the pot every day after closing it to keep money flowing into your life. When it is full, remove the copper, drop the nuts under trees, and refill the pot day by day.

CAUTION

Macadamia nuts are toxic for dogs if ingested.

Mace

from (*Myristica fragrans*)

MAGICAL FORMS

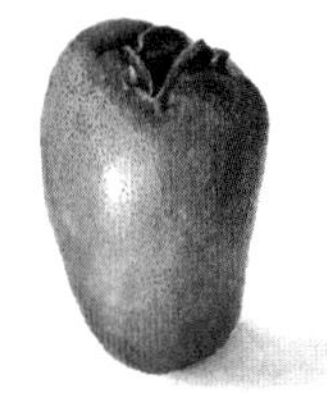

not to be confused with the protective spray of the same name, which is a chemical • the waxy, reddish seed covering that surrounds the nutmeg seed (see "Nutmeg," p. 308) • flattened and dried • the color changes to brown or orange • the remaining mace is smooth, hornlike, and brittle • usually used powdered in magical workings

PLANETS AND ELEMENT

Mercury/Jupiter • Air

MAGICAL USES

in incense blends, used to cleanse a ritual space or room and to increase psychic powers • improves memory, creativity, inspiration, and logic

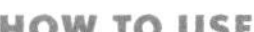

HOW TO USE

Mix with cardamom, clove, nutmeg, ginger, cinnamon, and coriander in a red prosperity bag. • Also use to attract good luck. • If you are being intimidated or subtly undermined at work or socially, add mace powder with crumbled dragon's blood incense and dried tarragon to a jar. Fill almost the entire jar with sprigs of fresh rosemary and red wine. Seal and shake the jar whenever you know you must meet the source of your fear. • For psychic visions and to gain answers to future directions, burn mace with bay leaves and myrrh resin as incense or cast with care on a bonfire or fire pit. In the smoke, you will see fleeting visions that will answer your question. • More delicate in flavor than nutmeg, mace can be used in magical cookery for strength and courage, and to focus your mind when matters are not clear or to encourage a lover or family member to speak the truth when you feel they are not giving you the complete answer.

CAUTION

Avoid using mace while pregnant.

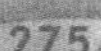

Magnolia

(*Magnolia* spp.)

MAGICAL FORMS

genus of flowering plants, including *Magnolia grandiflora*, *Magnolia virginiana*, and *Magnolia stellata* • growing as tree, it can be small • can also grow as a shrub or bush • magically use the aromatic bark, flower, oil, and seed pods

PLANET AND ELEMENT

Venus • Water

MAGICAL USES

enhances beauty, radiance, and sensuality • love of nature • altruistic love • promotes lasting fidelity and loyalty and the mending of estrangement after betrayal • romance, especially through social media • past-life recall from ancient times, for it is said magnolia predates even bees • reduces the power of addictions and obsessions, especially smoking • restores strength after a long illness

HOW TO USE

Place a sachet of the fresh or dried flowers under the mattress until they lose their fragrance to ensure a faithful partner. • On the side of a magnolia flower, use your finger to invisibly etch the name of the person you wish to marry or live with, then shred the flower and cast the petals on your doorstep just before they arrive. • Dried magnolia in a mojo bag or potpourri restores passion to a long-established relationship that has become routine. • Magnolia planted near the front of a house draws in happiness, and in the back preserves financial health. • Seven seed pods, each rubbed over its own Chinese divinatory coin, all placed in a sealed jar and shaken each full moon, bring prosperity and good financial luck.

CAUTION

Do not ingest the plant or use its oil during pregnancy.

Mahogany Tree

(*Swietenia macrophylla*)

MAGICAL FORMS

now rarely found as *Swietenia mahagani*, except as isolated forest trees • in the sixteenth century, mahogany was first brought to Europe by the Spanish • highly prized as a rich, red-brown, tropical and subtropical wood needing a dry climate • used for furniture in North America, the UK, and Europe • like many beautiful, magical trees, it is endangered through overforesting and there are now restrictions on the export or sale of new timber • mahogany is native to Central America, South America, India, and the West Indies and Florida Keys, where *Swietenia macrophylla* may be found growing in yards or in the wild • magically work with wood from specialty wood stores or adapt from pre-loved artifacts, unless you are lucky enough to see the fallen leaves and flowers from a living tree

PLANET AND ELEMENT

Jupiter • Air

MAGICAL USES

encourages musical gifts • as a wand for Earth and Fire balance • an altar made from a mahogany table or inlaid with mahogany (pre-owned) links powerfully with God and yang energies • a good balance for goddess/yin rituals

HOW TO USE

Pair two obsidian crystals with twin slivers of mahogany wood in a charm bag. • Keep in the bedroom or heart of the home for a mature, lasting, passionate relationship, often between star souls. • Use for a peaceful balance of power if one partner is more assertive. • Mahogany is also good for later-in-life relationships. • For blending different generations within the same home, buy a dried mahogany seed pod still on its stem (available online), one for each family member, and place in the center of the home.

CAUTION

Dust may irritate the skin and breathing if using the raw wood.

Mala Mujer

(*Cnidoscolus angustidens*)

MAGICAL FORMS

herb with white flowers blooming in late spring and summer • native to and growing in the Sonoran desert mountains of southeastern Arizona, northwestern Mexico, and southern Mexico • the name means *evil woman* in Spanish because its dark green leaves, which resemble maple leaves, are covered in white dots that form the base of stinging hairs • magically use the leaves, with the utmost caution, and the flower essence

PLANETS AND ELEMENTS

Moon/Mars • Water/Fire

MAGICAL USES

overcomes anger and irritability, expressed or repressed • counteracts effects of spite and negative reactions from and toward others • eases jealousy of a sibling at any age, especially if the remedy is combined with desert holly essence • for pets who resent a new baby or the arrival of other pets • hormonal swings of both sexes, particularly but not exclusively in adolescence • for PMS, postnatal blues, midlife crises in men and women, perimenopause, and menopause

HOW TO USE

With the greatest care, wearing gloves to handle, use the leaves, which are protective against spite and vicious gossiping, whether in the workplace, from neighbors, or in schoolyard cliques. • The herb can be used to protect teenagers and adults from trolling on social media. • To experience its effects, fill a dark-glass sealed bottle with the leaves (do not add liquid). When they wither, remove them safely and, if the issue is ongoing, refill the bottle. • Add a few drops of the essence to pet water or a child's or teen's bath or water bottle to create tolerance. Do the same for yourself if certain people automatically make you feel unsettled or resentful.

CAUTION

Contact with the leaves can cause severe dermatitis.

Mallow

(*Malva* spp.)

MAGICAL FORMS

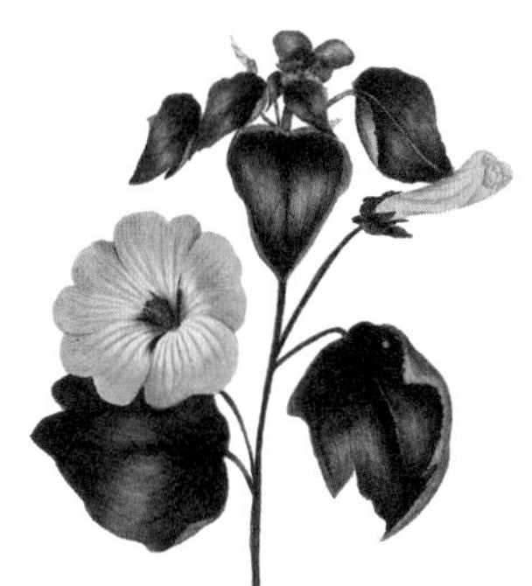

genus of flowering plants, including *Malva silvestris*, common or blue mallow, and rose mallow, *Malva trimestris* or *Lavatera trimestris* • related to hollyhocks • magically use the growing plant, cultivated or wild; fresh and dried flowers; leaves; and root

PLANETS AND ELEMENT

Venus/Moon • Water

MAGICAL USES

traditionally set in front of houses or worn as garlands on the morning of May 1 in celebrations for the fertility of land, people, and animals • love • protection • exorcism of fear and psychic attack • helps to overcome obsessions and love that can never come to being • water magick • used in anti-nightmare pillows

HOW TO USE

Set cut mallow plants in a vase at an out-facing window to call back an absent or estranged lover. • Steep mallow flowers in water as a protective floor wash. • Sprinkle the infusion from the edge of your property boundaries in a trail to your front door, calling the name of your lover or, if unknown, saying, *Come follow the path of love, you, whose love will be everlasting for me*. • Use as a magical ink, made on the Dark of the Moon for secret love messages, often smudged with the tears of the writer (a way of transmitting sorrow and regrets), for the color is not very resistant. • Burn as incense with rosemary and thyme to remove troublesome energies from restless spirits and to call the ancestors at Halloween.

Manchineel

(*Hippomane mancinella*)

MAGICAL FORMS

also called the little apple of death • poisonous apple tree, standing fifty feet high • called the most dangerous tree on earth as all its parts are highly toxic • found along coastal swamps from Florida throughout Central America and native to the Caribbean and South America • red bark, green leaves, green and yellow flowers, and apple-like fruit • the milky white sap that is present in every part of the tree causes blisters • the tree contains several toxins • the sap was used on the tip of poison arrows and is believed to have killed the Conquistador Juan Ponce de León in 1321 and used to contaminate the water supply of the invaders • a bite of the apple induces a burning sensation that could prove fatal • even standing beneath it in rain can cause severe burns • the tree's dried fruits were once used as a diuretic by Indigenous people • only the spiny-tailed black iguana can safely eat the fruit and leaves • not advisable to use magically (included here for informational purposes only)

PLANET AND ELEMENT

Saturn • Earth

MAGICAL USES

the fruit was traditionally used in baneful (harmful) magick for physically or psychically attacking or defending against foes, especially offering poison apples, mixed with other benign fruits • in modern positive magick, this destructive practice has died out and effects may rebound on the user

HOW TO USE

It was once valued for its exotic wood by Caribbean craftspeople to make artifacts and furniture. They first burned the tree at the base and left it to dry at a distance because the smoke is toxic. • If you were to buy any item made from the manchineel, it would certainly be a powerful, protective wood, but there are no guarantees that no toxicity remains.

CAUTION

With so many other tropical trees with healing properties available, this is probably best left untouched.

Mandarin/Tangerine

(*Citrus reticulata*) or sometimes (*Citrus tangerine*)

MAGICAL FORMS

although these fruits are not always the same, their botanical names and magical properties are interchangeable • small evergreens, both mandarin and tangerine trees have thorns • small, easily peeled fruit • fragrant blossoms • the tangerine is larger than the mandarin, rounder, and more yellow • the mandarin was brought to Europe from its native south China and Asia in 1805 and to the USA in 1845, where it was renamed the tangerine • tangerines grow in Texas, Florida, California, and Guinea • both tangerine and mandarin essential oils are extracted from the peel of the ripe fruit, though tangerine is used less in perfumes • magically use the blossom, fruit, and essential oil

PLANET AND ELEMENT

Sun • Fire

MAGICAL USES

well-being • makes anything seem possible • creative ventures • breaking safely through spiritual barriers in meditation • balances the body, mind, and spirit's psychic energy centers and aura field • the thorns in protective bottles will defend against spite from those who are physically vulnerable or very old • often used in a very diluted massage mix for older children if they are anxious

HOW TO USE

Take tangerines or mandarins, called the sharing fruits, to picnics and barbecues, and bring and share meals to promote friendship and goodwill. • Keep mandarins or tangerines in a bowl on your kitchen table to spread sunshine, happiness, health, and well-being. • Use the flowers at the wedding of someone getting married young or at the birth of a baby earlier in life. • Diffuse the oil with other citrus oils in the home or workplace to maintain optimism and protect against psychic and emotional vampires.

CAUTION

Mandarin and tangerine are generally considered safe in pregnancy in later trimesters, but check with an expert, as they are possibly phototoxic. • Dilute well if skin is sensitive.

Mandrake

(*Mandragora officinarum*)

MAGICAL FORMS

grown originally in the Mediterranean and Himalayas • a hallucinogenic plant of the nightshade family • with a short stem, basal leaves, a single bell-shaped flower with five petals, yellowish-green- to purple- and orange-colored poisonous berries • in the USA, the name mandrake may sometimes be applied to the mayapple, belonging to the barberry family • similarly, the so-called English mandrake (*Bryonia alba*) is not a true mandrake but is sometimes referred to as such • magically use the taproot, though expensive (is available in occult stores worldwide)

PLANET AND ELEMENT

Mercury • Air

MAGICAL USES

mandrake water (which should not be ingested as it is also poisonous) is used to sprinkle around the home and boundaries to protect against all malice, earthly and paranormal • once believed to hold the power of dark earth spirits, in the UK in medieval times, mandrake was said to grow on the graves of murderers • to be uprooted only by a black dog with a cord attached to the plant • its shrieks as it was uprooted were reputed to drive people mad

HOW TO USE

Once freed from the power of the dark spirits, mandrake became a charm for love, health, fertility, and wealth. • Use powdered in incense for purification ceremonies. • Because of the root's humanlike appearance, bind two roots together face to face with red twine to strengthen love, but never against the free will of the other person. • Where there is mandrake, no harm can ever enter, and so a root may be kept over a mantelpiece or on a shelf in the central room for good fortune and protection.

CAUTION

Do not ingest any part of mandrake and handle with care. • Avoid totally in pregnancy.

Mango

(*Mangifera indica*)

MAGICAL FORMS

large tree with a domed top • red drooping leaves when young, deep green and glossy when mature • clusters of flowers at the close of winter on the end of twigs with thousands of tiny blossoms in pink, yellow, brown, or white • the tree has been cultivated for more than four thousand years, mainly grown from India to Malaysia, and is found in Florida and Australia • suitable fresh or dried for making magical teas • magically use the whole, growing tree; fresh or dried blossoms; and fruit

PLANET AND ELEMENT

Venus • Water

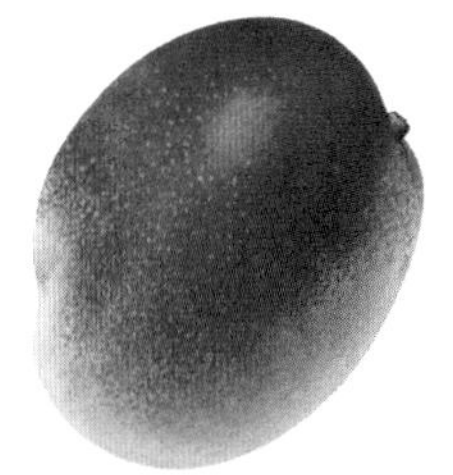

MAGICAL USES

family unity, spiritual growth • for strengthening friendships and increasing passion

HOW TO USE

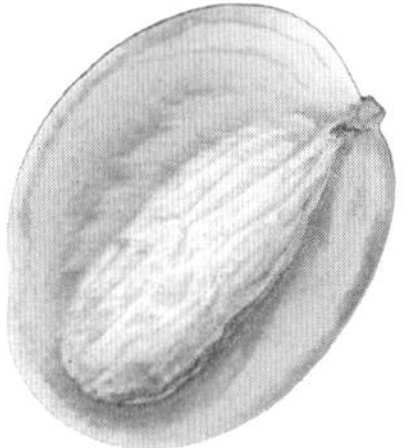

Sit beneath a tree as blossoms fall (you may find the tree in botanical gardens) or buy imported dried blossoms, catch or cast them in your hands, dry the fresh blossoms, and keep them in a charm bag to attract love when you go out socially, or hide the bag in the workplace if you desire the love of a work colleague. • The juice or pulp of the fruit acts as an aphrodisiac. • Write love or fertility petitions on the surface of the fruit, then cast into the ocean or running fresh water. • Mango is traditionally offered to Yemaya, goddess of the sweet waters, or Oshun, the Yoruban sea goddess. • Write the name of someone harming you or your loved ones on the skin of the fruit, remove the skin, and bury it. Bury the peeled fruit in a separate place.

Mangrove

(*Rhizophora* spp.)

MAGICAL FORMS

genus of trees in the mangrove family, including red mangrove (*Rhizophora mangle*) • though it is not classified as a true mangrove, the white mangrove (*Laguncularia racemosa*) is also notable here magically, as it has similar effects • other species are also commonly called "mangrove," such as the Australian milky mangrove (*Exoecaria agallocha*) and can also be used for the same or similar purposes • the mangrove tree grows along tropical and subtropical coastlines of more than a hundred countries, the white mangrove especially along the Atlantic coasts in the Americas from Bermuda and Florida to the Bahamas and in Western Africa • the red mangrove grows in coastal tropical USA and Africa • mangrove is the only tree with the ability to grow in salt water and has intertwining roots • can be planted as seedlings or small plants in a saltwater aquarium, vivarium, or tropical plant tank, or as a potted indoor plant • the USA has about eight hundred square miles of mangroves, mainly in southern Florida • magically use the whole, growing plant, or cuttings • dried mangrove leaves sold online for tea (especially the red) can be used if you cannot find growing mangroves

PLANET AND ELEMENT

Moon • Water

MAGICAL USES

to nurture self and others • increasing intuition • bringing inner strength, balance, and connection with the life force • raising confidence • banishing toxic people

HOW TO USE

Fill your magical aquarium, vivarium, or saltwater indoor garden with mini-mangrove as a focus for meditation and the visualization of subterranean worlds lost beneath the sea, as well as to restore your equilibrium. • Better still, take a vacation boat trip through mangrove swamps. • Use mangrove tea to sprinkle around your luggage for protection before a trip.

CAUTION

Do not ingest the leaves raw. • The sap of the Australian milky mangrove is highly poisonous and can cause skin irritation and temporary blindness if it comes in contact with the eyes.

Manuka

(*Leptospermum scoparium*)

MAGICAL FORMS

small shrub-like tree, found in Australia and New Zealand, the southernmost continental states of the USA, Hawaii, and the UK • magically use the leaves; blossoms, which only bloom for between two to six weeks a year; healing tea made from leaves, which is sometimes combined with green tea or manuka honey produced by bees from the nectar of the flowers; and essential oil

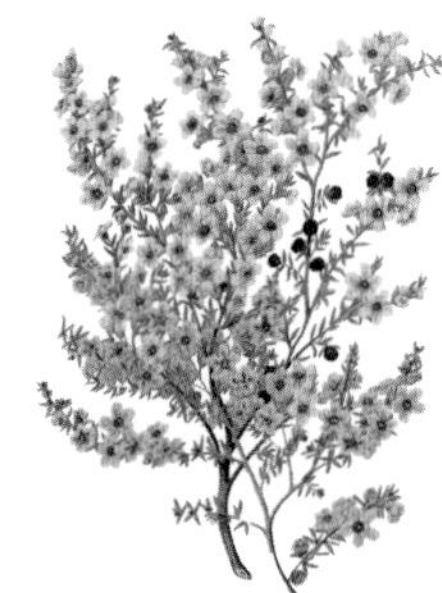

PLANET AND ELEMENT

Venus • Earth

MAGICAL USES

dried leaves and blossoms or a dish of the ultimate healing honey can be used in healing spells, as well as for empowering remedies for illnesses • for softening critical or discouraging attitudes in others • for generating family love and unity, combine bread and manuka honey for sit-down afternoons or high teas • for rituals for abundance and recovering from loss or setbacks, as the shrub or tree is one of the first to regenerate after fire or deforestation

HOW TO USE

Dilute a drop or two of the manuka oil in virgin olive oil for anointing candles for wealth, health, and healing spells. • Drink the tea (can be purchased as loose tea or teabags, as well as leaves that can be made into tea, online) before going for job interviews, bank loans, or any speculation, to activate natural entrepreneurial energies. • Feed children the honey, not only for health, but to give shy children confidence and to encourage those who are teased by peers or siblings to shine. • Buy the dried white blossoms online (though they may be hard to find as they are delicate) and add them to potpourri to bring prosperity to your home, business, or workplace, and to keep away illness and misfortune.

CAUTION

Avoid ingesting if you have blood sugar issues or diabetes requiring medication.

Maple Tree

(*Acer* spp.)

MAGICAL FORMS

genus including 125 species of trees • sugar maple (*Acer saccharum*) can be as tall as 150 feet • commonly cultivated through eastern and central North America • chief source of maple syrup in North America and Canada • red maple (*Acer rubrum*) is the most widespread in the eastern USA, with leaves that are green on top and silvery underneath in summer, then deep red in the fall • magically, leaves are best in fall when yellow, red, and orange may appear on the same leaf • magically use the whole, growing tree; wood; fresh or dried leaves; and syrup

PLANETS AND ELEMENTS

Venus/Jupiter • Water/Air

MAGICAL USES

use the empowered syrup in magical cookery for increasing money and domestic happiness (recommended for singles who would like a partner and family) • eat syrup to become more powerful, to enjoy a long life, and for a sense of well-being • use syrup as an offering in a small bowl for abundance rites, then share after the ritual • brings fertility, healthy children, and self-love, and increases personal radiance • helps children feel lovely or attractive if they are overlooked

HOW TO USE

Include a piece of wood in or above a front door when a house is built or renovated to keep all harm and danger away from the home, especially restless spirits on the land. • If you are on a family outing with a young baby, lift them up beneath a maple tree (or through its branches, if there is a cleft in the trunk) to ask the tree mother for a long, healthy life and good fortune for the infant. • If planning to gamble or speculate, put a spoon of syrup under your tongue before going out or making a bet, not only for good fortune but so that the fortune will bring happiness. • Choose maple wood furniture, so that love and financial security will grow and remain.

CAUTION

Red, sugar, and silver maple (*Acer saccharinum*) are not safe for horses, donkeys, alpacas, and llamas to consume.

Maple Tree, Japanese Red

(*Acer palmatum*)

MAGICAL FORMS

native to China, Japan, Korea, southeast Russia, and eastern Mongolia • can be grown in the USA and Europe, especially as the bonsai • called the "king of bonsai" since it can be grown indoors as well as outdoors • small, reddish-purple flowers in spring • leaves that change with the seasons from bright red in the spring through green in summer to deep red, orange, and yellow in the fall • in winter, sheds its leaves • as a full-grown outdoor tree, it can reach between four and thirty feet in height • magically use the whole growing tree, fresh or dried leaves, seeds, and helicopter-shaped seed pods

PLANET AND ELEMENT

Sun • Fire

MAGICAL USES

because the tree changes its leaf color with the seasons, it regulates the passing of the year and of the lifecycle in a harmonious way, especially as a bonsai centerpiece • offers enthusiasm in spring; fulfillment in summer; joy in the fall; and the ability to assess what can and should be carried forward, as well as patience and acceptance, in the winter • protects against accidents and misfortune to home and family

HOW TO USE

The bonsai, with its often five-lobed, human-palm-shaped leaves, should be placed on a divinatory table for accurate palmistry readings. • When the leaves fall, bury the pressed or dried red, orange, or yellow leaves from the bonsai, or a single large leaf from the ornamental tree, in a small bag in the soil to ensure money and resources flow in and remain until spring returns. • Eat some of the edible seeds in spring when they are young and green (you can buy them if necessary) for a harmonious but productive year ahead. • Scatter the seed pods, which are produced in September or October, to release what did not work out.

CAUTION

Though the seeds are edible to humans, the tree is not safe for horses, donkeys, alpacas, or llamas to consume.

Marigold

(*Tagetes* spp.)

MAGICAL FORMS

often found as French marigold (*Tagetes patula*) • originally from Mexico and Guatemala, but naturalized in many yellow and orange cultivars throughout Europe, the UK, and the USA • also as African marigold (*Tagetes erecta*), known as Aztec or American marigold, with large orange, yellow, and red blooms, sacred to the Aztecs as offerings to the sun gods • magically use the whole, growing or cut plant; seeds; and fresh or dried flowers

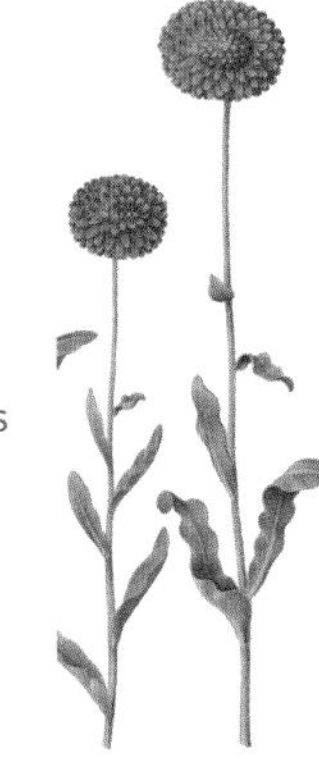

PLANET AND ELEMENT

Sun • Fire

MAGICAL USES

justice • love • spells to increase love and admiration, especially from an indifferent lover • to induce clairvoyant dreams • protection • success in legal matters and official accusations • increases psychic powers • for being positively noticed with admiration and respect • money

HOW TO USE

Hang garlands of fresh flowers at entrances to deter evil of all kinds. • Scatter the dried petals under the bed or in a sleep pillow to prevent nightmares and visitations from incubi, succubi, and sexual demons, as well as to bring prophetic dreams and reveal the identity of wrongdoers, especially thieves or those who secretly cause trouble at work. • A woman stepping over marigold plants without crushing them will understand the language of birds. • As an incense, marigold gives visions of nature spirits. • Use as part of a love bath sachet to increase radiance and attract the lover you most desire. • Each day, add a handful of dried petals to a jar; when full, scatter the contents to the winds to attract new sources of money.

CAUTION

Though used popularly medicinally, not enough is known about its safety in pregnancy and breastfeeding or its long-term side effects, so act with caution.

Marigold, Marsh

(*Caltha palustris*)

MAGICAL FORMS

also called Mary's gold since it was placed in medieval churches in honor of the Annunciation of the Virgin Mary • member of the buttercup family, blooming from late March or early April and May through June along ponds or marshes • at the end of the last ice age, the marsh marigold took advantage of retreating melting ice to take hold in boggy places in northern Asia, the UK, temperate Europe, and North America • magically use the whole, growing plant; fresh and dried flowers; heart-shaped leaves; and seeds

PLANET AND ELEMENT

Moon • Water

MAGICAL USES

in Celtic lands, marsh marigolds are called the yellow flower of Beltane, and on the morning of May 1 (May Morning) were strewn on doorsteps, made into garlands, pushed through letterboxes by children, and put in windows and over doorways with hawthorn, the original May blossoms that are only permitted indoors on May Day • a fertility flower during its bloom, especially around the May festival, traditionally the ultimate fertility celebration of the Celtic year

HOW TO USE

Because marsh marigolds are sacred to the Norse fertility and love goddess Freya, collect and dry their heart-shaped leaves at dawn on May Morning if you want to conceive a baby. Add dried flowers to sachets and keep beneath the mattress during lovemaking. Subsequently, put the sachet in full moonlight every month until conception. • In folklore, flowers are called kingcups because of their showy, gold, goblet-like flowers; so that money or prestige will come to you, pick five of the largest you can find and then cast them off a bridge over fast flowing water, followed by a small piece of gold. • Float the seeds on the surface of a glass bowl half filled with water, and the images formed will answer a love or money question.

CAUTION

The leaves and flowers are toxic to humans, pets, and livestock if ingested raw.

Marigold, Pot

(*Calendula officinalis*)

MAGICAL FORMS

scientific name comes from the Latin word for the first of the month because it can bloom every month, even in winter, though mainly from summer through to the first hard frost • for this reason, its flowers are ideal for magick • pot marigold has a large head with many tiny, yellow or orange flowers and aromatic leaves, forming a flower disk • flowers and leaves are edible • closes when it is going to rain • resulted from the hybridization of other marigolds • native to Canada and many states in the USA, though some claim its origin is the eastern Mediterranean • grows in Europe and the UK • magically use the fresh or dried flowers; oil made by infusing the flowers in olive or coconut oil; growing in a garden or as a potted plant; as a tea made from the flowers; in potpourri, with its herbal, earthy scent; and as incense

PLANET AND ELEMENT

Sun • Fire

MAGICAL USES

used in different cultures as an offering to the sun • wear or set the fresh or dried flowers in dishes at festivals for the sun • use in incense for success, health, and happiness rituals

HOW TO USE

Place as a sachet within your pillowcase to drive away nightmares and to call prophetic dreams. • Use the oil for anointing candles, ritual tools, and your Third Eye to open clairvoyant powers and protect against malevolent spirits. • Use potpourri with a little oil added to spread happiness, health, and sunshine through the home and workplace. • Send a wreath containing the flowers to a funeral or on the anniversary of a death because it was believed that the light from the flowers would illuminate the deceased person on their journey and in the afterlife.

CAUTION

Do not ingest any pot marigold product or tea during pregnancy or while breastfeeding. • Avoid if you are allergic to chrysanthemums, chamomile, daisies, or ragweed.

Marjoram

(*Origanum majorana*)

MAGICAL FORMS

also as sweet marjoram, *Majorana hortensis* • perennial herbs sensitive to the cold • magically use the dried and fresh plant; pink, white, and purple flowers; and oil

PLANET AND ELEMENT

Mercury • Air

MAGICAL USES

for luck in all joint ventures, financial or emotional • brings a sense of well-being that makes anything seem possible • drives away loneliness, alienation, and fear of separation or abandonment • encourages compromise • for increasing family loyalty and commitment in love or marriage • overcoming grief • protects against emotional and financial blackmail • for resolving divided loyalties • use dried or chopped, dried flowers for water scrying

HOW TO USE

Add marjoram to love charms to increase commitment when kept with a photo of the reluctant lover. • Use well-diluted oil or infusion for anointing the brow or Third Eye to increase clairvoyance. • Add to dream pillows for prophetic and past-life dreams and visions, and for banishing night terrors. • Gently inhale a little of the oil to remove doubt or despair. • Burn or add to a diffuser to empower wish magick. • Make and give magical potpourri that includes dried marjoram flowers to a grieving person. • Marjoram strengthens connection with others, especially friends and family, when added to food at communal meals. • It is protective when planted against a neighboring fence or in a pot against an indoor adjoining wall as it calms conflict and increases friendly vibes with difficult neighbors.

CAUTION

Use the oil in moderation, and avoid during pregnancy.

Marrow

(*Cucurbita pepo*)

MAGICAL FORMS

a summer squash • thick-skinned, often striped, cylindrical fruit • the swollen ovary of the yellow marrow flower • cooked and stuffed as a bland vegetable • the same species as the smaller zucchini (see p. 488) or courgette, which is an immature fruit that can be left on the vine to become a marrow • the marrow is believed to have been introduced from Mesoamerica by the Spanish Conquistadors, reaching Europe with them in the sixteenth century and the USA in the 1820s in its present form • magically use the whole, uncooked, large marrow or the cooked and stuffed version

PLANETS AND ELEMENT

Moon/Venus • Water

MAGICAL USES

for calling loved ones home • establishing friendships in new settings or workplaces • moderating angry or critical words in others

HOW TO USE

Add herbs and spices with the magical meanings you most need to the marrow before baking, empowering each herb while mixing it into the flesh. • Marrow flesh will act as an amplifier for wishes and needs. • Plant a few coins and money crystals like tiger eye and turquoise close to the growing immature zucchini fruits, then allow them to ripen into marrows; your financial good fortune will grow as they do. • A large, uncooked marrow in your vegetable rack attracts health, good luck, wealth, and happiness into the home, and, when cooked, transmits the same powers to the eaters.

CAUTION

Only eat a marrow cooked, and discard if bitter.

Marshmallow Root

(*Althaea officinalis*)

MAGICAL FORMS

a flowering herb grown ornamentally, as well as medicinally • originally from Europe and Africa, and naturalized in North America, especially in marshy areas near the coast • the sweet sap was once used in the production of marshmallow candy as far back as ancient Egypt • white to blush-pink flowers bloom from July to September • see also mallow (p. 277), a different plant though related • magically use the flowers, fresh or dried; the maple-like leaves; and the root (most commonly used in magick, especially decoction teas made from the chopped root or leaves)

PLANET AND ELEMENT

Venus • Water

MAGICAL USES

use the dried leaves and flowers on your altar or bedside table as an offering for fertility on the full moon, scattered outdoors at sunrise the next morning after lovemaking • soak the dried or fresh flowers in water and filter before anointing yourself before ritual • also use to bless artifacts and the corners of a sacred space

HOW TO USE

Use marshmallow, shared as tea or in magical cookery, as the entire plant is edible. • The leaked sap makes it sticky to handle but adds to the softening of even emotionally constipated folk. • Marshmallow will sweeten the tempers of guests, neighbors, and cantankerous family members. • Grow marshmallow in your garden or in a pot in your kitchen or the room where you relax (make sure to keep the potted plant moist) to spread abundance, health, and enthusiasm through your home if you have moody teenagers or an inert partner. It may inspire the latter to romance, especially if you feed them commercially prepared marshmallow candy.

CAUTION

Ingesting marshmallow may slow blood clotting. • Consult an expert before using during pregnancy.

Masterwort

(*Astrantia* spp.) and (*Peucedanum ostruthium*)

MAGICAL FORMS

great masterwort (plants in the genus *Astrantia*) and masterwort (*Peucedanum ostruthium*) are not scientifically related but have the same function magically • both are ideal in a wildlife garden but need to be cut right back after flowering to prevent excessive spread, as they can be considered invasive • magically use the growing plant, rhizomes, flowers, and leaves

PLANET AND ELEMENT

Mars • Fire

MAGICAL USES

magically, considered one of the most powerful defensive herbs • overcomes fears and intimidation • assists willpower • beloved by those involved in heavy physical work, as it gives strength and stamina • offers protection against evil, especially trolls, goblins, orcs, and malevolent nature beings • use in magical cookery for love, especially the leaves and flowers, which taste similar to lovage (see p. 272), or the roots and seeds, which can be pounded to make a strong pepper • *Astrantia* varieties are also called Hattie's pincushion because some kinds have a flower that resembles a pincushion • the identity of Hattie seems uncertain (readers, if you know, please write to me and I will update future editions)

HOW TO USE

Keep the cut herbs in a vase during a séance or mediumship session to call benign spirits and protect against malevolent ones. • Add the dried flowers to a red bag tied with red thread and hang it over the front door to repel all harm, curses, and ill intent from entering the home, as well as any negative spells being cast on your family. • Use a branch dipped in blessed salt water to asperge a ritual area if strong defensive spells are to be used or for mediumship if you are calling unfamiliar spirits. • To bring luck in love and a desired lover, mix with rose petal water and sprinkle a line from the front door to the bedroom.

CAUTION

Avoid exposure to sunlight after use as this may cause an allergic reaction to the skin.

Mastic Tree of Chios

(*Pistacia lentiscus* var. *Chia*)

MAGICAL FORMS

small evergreen tree found on the southern, more fertile part of the island of Chios, the fifth largest Greek island in the North Aegean Sea • produces sticky resin that is hard, brittle, transparent, and fragrant • tapped as semiliquid tears from the bark of the tree and placed onto specially spread white soil • it is left to harden for up to a month • magically use the resin and as essential oil

PLANETS AND ELEMENTS

Jupiter/Venus • Air/Water

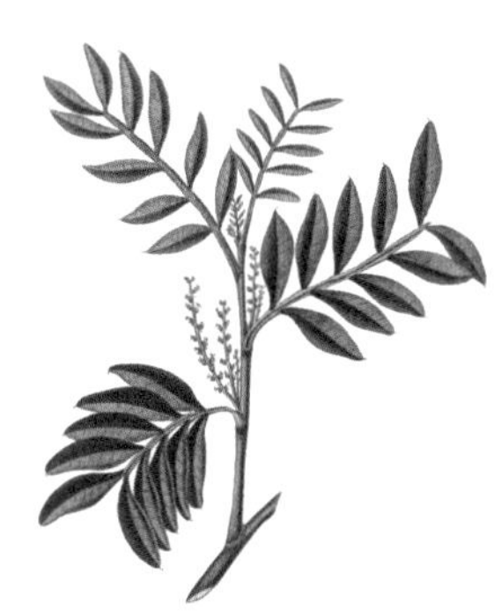

MAGICAL USES

the tree is said to weep tears for the local Saint Agios Isidoros, the patron saint of the mastic tree, martyred about 250 CE by the Romans, and the source of its association with relieving grief and suffering • used to raise magical power

HOW TO USE

Burn one part mastic gum, three parts frankincense, and one part sandalwood (see p. 399) to raise the power of formal rituals and to welcome the guardians who stand at the four directions of the circle. • Massage oil (diluted well in a coconut or almond carrier oil) on the skin or diffuse it in a vaporizer to connect with angels, guides, and higher beings, and to create a sacred space if life intrudes.

CAUTION

Dilute oil well before using topically.

Meadow-Rue

(*Thalictrum* spp.)

MAGICAL FORMS

genus including tall meadow rue (*Thalictrum polygamum*), common meadow rue (*Thalictrum occidentale*), and early meadow rue (*Thalictrum dioicum*) • a wildflower growing from rhizome roots, with lacy foliage • small yellow, lavender, white, or lilac flowers that can grow in pots as well as gardens • the *polygamum* and *dioicum* are native to eastern North America; the *occidentale* to the western USA and western Canada • meadow-rue also grows in the UK and parts of Europe • most meadow-rue has separate male and female flowers of different colors, the showier male flowers with numerous drooping, elongated stamens and the females with erect clusters of pistils resembling petals, containing the immature fruits or seeds • magically use the root and fresh or dried male and female flowers

PLANET AND ELEMENT

Venus • Earth

MAGICAL USES

not related to rue • dried female flowers represent the Earth element in goddess rituals • add mixed dried flowers to an amulet bag for goddess protection for all people moving away from home temporarily or permanently • all meadow-rue brings the thawing of coldness in relationships • any meadow-rue root also protects against malicious spirits and attracts love

HOW TO USE

Plant meadow-rue near your home so the cares of the day are filtered out. • Create a charm bag with pieces of the meadow-rue root you have grown to represent the number of children you hope to conceive with your partner. • Use mixed-gender dried flowers in a lucky charm bag to attract the right partner in an LGBTQ relationship.

CAUTION

Meadow-rue is toxic to dogs if ingested in large quantities.

Meadowsweet

(*Filipendula ulmaria*)

MAGICAL FORMS

though not categorized as the same plant, *Spiraea filipendula*, or dropwort, has the same effects magically • for both, magically use the whole, growing plant; flowering tops; leaves; and roots

PLANET AND ELEMENT

Jupiter • Air

MAGICAL USES

lasting love • reconciliation • diminishes rivalry in love and between warring factions in the family or workplace • domestic protection • happiness • psychic awareness about those who have wronged you or have malice in their hearts • recovery from abuse, especially sexual • sacred to the Druids

HOW TO USE

Use fresh or dried in love spells and sachets and for spells that manifest wishes. • Scatter on doorsteps and keep a pot indoors for peace in the home and to deter intruders. • If you have suffered a theft or been cheated, float meadowsweet leaves on water. If they sink, the thief is a man; if they float, a woman. Stir the water and blink, and you will learn the identity of the wrongdoer in images in the water or in your mind. • Burn as incense to call the right love or increase love and to remove negativity from the home after a quarrel. • Add it to baths for insight into problems with a relationship and to increase confidence in personal desirability.

CAUTION

Do not use meadowsweet if you are allergic to aspirin or are pregnant, breastfeeding, or using anticoagulants, as it can occasionally increase the risk of gastrointestinal bleeding.

Mesquite

from (*Prosopis* spp.)

MAGICAL FORMS

several plants in this genus are called by the common name "mesquite," including honey mesquite (*Prosopis glandulosa*), velvet mesquite (*Prosopis velutina*), and screwbean mesquite (*Prosopis pubescens*) • all present as a spiny tree with a crooked trunk • sacred to the Aztec sun god Huitzilopochtli, who was also god of war • grows in dry regions from California and the southwestern USA through Texas and Arizona to Central and Southern America, especially Mexico • the pods are ground into flour by Native North American and Mexican people and so mesquite is considered a tree of maternal blessings • magically use the growing tree; fragrant pods, which contain a brown seed in a sweet edible pulp; wood; thorns (with care); honey; tea made from the green or dried yellow twigs; pods (of velvet mesquite only); and incense

PLANETS AND ELEMENTS

Moon/Mars • Water/Fire

MAGICAL USES

creativity • purification rituals • fire magick • connects with spirits, the ancestors, and wise guides

HOW TO USE

Add mesquite to ritual fires on the full moon and on solstices and equinoxes, casting sticks of the wood (use care, as thorns grow at the base of the leaf stem) into the flames and naming petitions as the twigs burn. • Use the thorns in protective bottles, one for each threat. • Keep the thorns in a high place, immersed in bean wine made from mesquite. • Burn as incense or sit beneath the tree to induce astral travel. • Since mesquite thrives by extending its roots deep to find water, use a root, pointed twig, or a mesquite wand to locate buried treasure or what you have lost. The wood will vibrate close to the target. • Drink the tea if inspiration is not coming in creative ventures.

CAUTION

If pregnant, check with an expert before ingesting tea or flour products.

Mezereum

(*Daphne mezereum*)

MAGICAL FORMS

also known as the February daphne • a fragrant rounded shrub with tightly clustered purplish-pink, purplish-red, or light-purple flowers appearing as buds in twos and threes and flowering on the twigs before the leaves in the dark days of February • native to Europe, western Asia, and the UK • taken to the USA by the early colonists • naturalized in parts of the USA and Canada and sometimes considered invasive • known as a medicinal plant from the 1600s, and still used under expert supervision in homeopathy and traditional Chinese medicine • bright-red, fleshy, round, bird-dispersed berries • magically use the growing plant, flowers, and berries (all with great care)

PLANET AND ELEMENT

Venus • Earth

MAGICAL USES

heralds the coming of the early spring • sometimes used in baneful or harmful and defensive witchcraft in medieval Europe • in the modern world, grown with the utmost care in the garden as protection against those who would deceive or influence you or your family members through charm and sweet-talking • fae are often seen beneath the plant, but these may be tricksters

HOW TO USE

Its beauty, fragrance, and dangerous properties make its berries and dried flowers powerful in a tightly sealed, nonporous red amulet bag placed near a computer, tablet, or smartphone when on dating or friendship sites for protection against financial romance scams. Hold the closed bag if you are uncertain about a secretive lover or date having a double life, and the truth will come into your mind, or you will soon find evidence. • However, because of the toxic qualities of the plant, there may be a safer truth plant, such as honesty (see p. 220) or eyebright, to use against deceptive glamor.

CAUTION

Mezereum causes severe skin irritation (it was once used to create rosy cheeks) and should be handled with gloves. • The flowers, berries, bark, and twigs are very toxic so should not be ingested or applied topically.

Milkweed

(*Asclepius* spp.)

MAGICAL FORMS

genus including common milkweed (*Asclepius syriaca*), showy milkweed (*Asclepius speciosa*), rose milkweed (*Asclepias incarnata*), and swamp milkweed (*Asclepius incarnata*) • named after Asclepius, the Greek father of medicine who is reputed to have used milkweed extensively • host for monarch butterfly, also known as the wanderer, to lay eggs • magically use the leaves, dried and fresh flowers, and milklike sap

PLANETS AND ELEMENTS

Mercury/Moon • Air/Water

MAGICAL USES

for monarch butterfly magick, as they fly around or settle on the flowers • for wishes and rituals for freedom and taking the lead • in Air magick to shape-shift, and for astral travel • encourages the fae and friendly elves to the garden • fresh cut milkweed flowers (and the stems, sometimes seared to prevent wilting) in a workspace encourage inspiration and success in creative ventures

HOW TO USE

Use the fresh flowers to make a circle for midsummer fertility, abundance, and happiness rituals. • Release the fluff on the plant in fall rites for letting go of bad habits, sorrows, and what is no longer working as it flies in all directions. • Squeeze the sap (carefully, so you do not get any on your hands) into a hole in the ground before planting a tree to celebrate a new baby, asking the blessings of the earth, sun, and moon mothers to make the infant healthy, strong, brave, clever, and kind. Do the same for handfasting or anniversary tree planting, seeking good fortune, health, and wealth. • Rub a smooth stone on a wart, skin blemish, or wound that is slow to heal. Alternatively, hold the stone, naming a chronic illness afflicting you or a loved one, then dig a hole in soft earth and drop the stone into the hole, completely covering it with dried, crumbled milkweed leaves, and fill in the hole.

CAUTION

The milky sap in the leaves and stem is toxic to humans and animals, so the plant should be handled with care and not ingested.

Million Bells

(*Calibrachoa parviflora*)

MAGICAL FORMS

trailing plant with a blooming season from April to summer's end • native to southern North America • flowers resemble tiny petunias, but are hardier than their relatives, the petunia (see p. 346) • can be cultivated in warm zones throughout the continent, also in the UK and Europe • called million bells because of the numerous bell-like flowers in rainbow colors growing on each plant, some with patterns and double blooms • a magnet for butterflies and hummingbirds • ideal in hanging baskets and bowls, each individual flower is six to twelve inches tall with trailing stems • magically use a hanging basket or trailing container in bloom or the cut flower trails

PLANET AND ELEMENT

Sun • Fire

MAGICAL USES

long blooming though short-lived, the profusion of trailing flowers attracts rapid, major, short-term financial gain • for any plans that need to take root fast and bear tangible results for a few months rather than long-term • for networking that will open many doors • for intense romances and affairs without seeking or expecting commitment

HOW TO USE

If you need to make a good and fast-spreading impression, focus on a hanging basket or container, placed so you can easily reach the flowers. Touch different flowers, one after the other, speaking fast without conscious thought, naming one after the other the results you need or plans you wish to set in motion right now. Afterward, water the flowers and you will be filled with instant *go for it* power. • Cut a trailing stem with flowers attached and bind it around a folded paper on which you have written the amount of money you need fast. When the flowers fade, cut off the flowers and shred the stems, putting them both in a basket to tip off a bridge into fast-flowing water. Burn the paper.

CAUTION

Million bells is not toxic to humans but poisonous to pets, so it is best grown where they can't be reached.

Mimosa

(*Acacia dealbata*)

MAGICAL FORMS

this fragrant blossom tree, called the tree of happiness, can grow very tall • if you have a small garden or yard, you can grow a small one in a container or by pruning it; I had one for many years on my small, sheltered patio in the UK • magically use the growing tree, blossoms, and bark

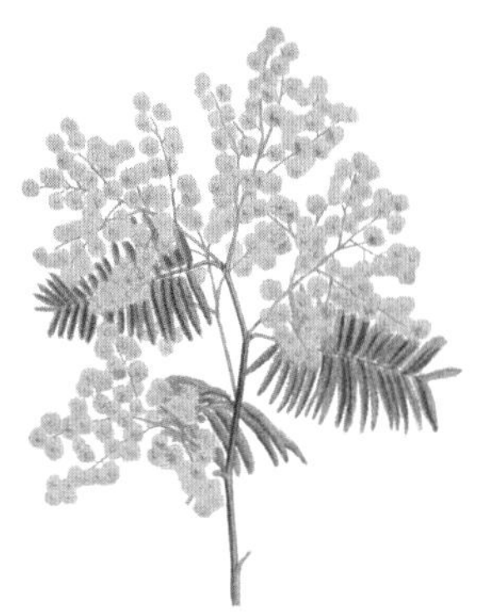

PLANETS AND ELEMENT

Moon/Saturn • Earth

MAGICAL USES

connects with angels • attracts a wealthy lover • brings love later in life • for overcoming grief for loved ones who have died or left forever • learning to love again • melts away hostility and opposition • sustains love in bad times • for keeping secrets and secret trysts • increasing charisma and personal radiance

HOW TO USE

To travel astrally in sleep to meet a known or unknown lover on the dream plane, put a sachet of blossoms under your pillow or in a sleep pillow. • Use for visiting past worlds in sleep and vivid past-life recall on waking. • Mimosa also prompts prophetic dreams and can be used to make dreams come true. • Called "the oil of tranquility" and "love without limits," mimosa oil is the ultimate oil for love and romance, and for sacred lovemaking when burned in scented candles, as incense, or diluted in massage. • As an infusion rubbed on the body, mimosa destroys hexes and curses while preventing future curses and ill wishes.

CAUTION

Avoid mimosa if pregnant or taking antibiotics, and do not take internally if pregnant. • Beware the houseplant *Mimosa pudica*, as it is toxic.

Mimulus

(*Mimulus* spp.)

MAGICAL FORMS

genus of flowering plants • yellow, orange, pink, purple, and red, with spotted or mottled throats and a musk fragrance • two of the redefined species are native to eastern North America and five more originated in Asia, Australia, and Africa • flourish in many countries, including the UK and Europe, in gardens and pots • related magically to the scarlet monkey flower (*Erythranthe guttata*), though they are not scientifically classified as part of the same genus • magically use the whole, growing plant; flower; and flower essence • can be used as part of the Bach Five-Flower Rescue Remedy (see p. 182)

PLANET AND ELEMENT

Sun • Fire

MAGICAL USES

named after the Latin word *mimos*, meaning mimic, linked with acting • because the flower resembles a grinning monkey, the flowers, cut or growing in the garden, strengthen anyone interested in the performing arts, especially the theater or comedy club • treats intolerance or phobias surrounding noise, crowds, heights, and enclosed spaces • calms pets who have been roughly handled or abused and horses that are easily startled • for courage, strength, and determination when part of the Rescue Remedy and also as a separate essence for removing fears of all kinds

HOW TO USE

Carry the dried petals, especially red, in a small, red bag or take the essence daily before you travel in elevators or to a crowded venue. • If using dried flower petals, scatter them in the open air after the last trial of the day. Reduce the amount of petals you carry and in time you will not need them. • Add to the water and food of pets from rescue centers and for horses who are afraid to enter a horse trailer.

CAUTION

Consult a physician before using while pregnant.

Mint, Apple

(*Mentha suaveolens*)

MAGICAL FORMS

see also "Pineapple Mint" (p. 292) • originally from North Africa, southern and western Europe, naturalized in central and northern Europe • found in temperate zones worldwide including the USA, where it grows wild from New England to Florida • perennial with light or bright green leaves, which, like the stems, are covered in fine hairs and called *woolly mint* • blossoms between the beginning and end of summer, small pinkish white or lavender flowers • with a peppermint and apple taste mixed, especially when the leaves are crushed or rubbed • flowers are bitter to taste • magically use the growing plant and fresh or dried chopped herb

PLANETS AND ELEMENTS

Mars/Venus • Fire/Water

MAGICAL USES

made into teas or jellies, eaten raw or as a potherb in magical cookery • for love and romance • as apple mint repels animal rodents, also deters human parasites and cheats

HOW TO USE

Grow apple mint in pots where you do tarot or other divinatory readings to open blocked psychic channels and give sudden insights. • Scatter chopped fresh or dried apple mint in ever-widening clockwise circles around yourself to call fertility, new energies, and new people into your life. Step across the circles and leave them to blow away. • Grow apple mint in your garden or kitchen pots to attract health and good fortune. • Place in your workspace to keep original ideas flowing and deter detractors who drain your enthusiasm.

CAUTION

Avoid with pregnancy and in excess quantities at any time. • Seek advice before ingesting if you are allergic to menthol or have asthma.

Mint, Chocolate

(*Mentha × piperita*)

MAGICAL FORMS

grow whole, dried aerial parts for teas and magical sachets • made by crossing orange mint (*Mentha × piperita citrata*) with ordinary peppermint (*Mentha piperita*) • some say it tastes like orange mint, but its fragrance is definitely chocolate and many detect this in the taste

PLANET AND ELEMENT

Venus • Water

MAGICAL USES

the minty-chocolate aroma flavor in magical teas and cookery can be empowered to lighten the mood for family occasions • encourages good humor • removes stagnation and obsession with routine • removes blocked anger and resentment • enhances enthusiasm for any task • an ideal diet substitute for the pleasure of chocolate without the calories

HOW TO USE

Plant in the garden to bring laughter and fun into family life and to overcome guilt when seeking pleasure and indulgence. • Use it for those who find it hard to spend on treats or outings. • Attracts benign nature spirits, who are drawn by its fragrance, and encourage a sense of well-being. • Plant it as another good addition to a well-being garden.• Being much softer than other mints in its energies, use it as a tea to encourage tolerance of the weakness and mistakes of others. • Place it in a charm bag kept with performance clothing or equipment to bring success to comedians and entertainers, especially children's entertainers, acrobats, jugglers, and cheerleaders. • Stuff a poppet or doll with the dried, chopped, or powdered plant, and keep it with a photo of (or, alternatively, send it to) someone who is depressed or has lost hope.

CAUTION

As with all mints, avoid excess consumption.

Mint, Eau De Cologne

(*Mentha × piperita citrata*)

MAGICAL FORMS

also known as orange or bergamot mint • a relative of peppermint (see p. 343) • citrus-fragranced, elliptical leaves on burgundy stems • originally from the Mediterranean and northern India • now nativized throughout the world • far more aromatic than other mints, with dense terminal spikes of tubular, mauve-pink flowers in late summer • can be grown in a pot • reputed to be used as an ingredient in the liqueur Chartreuse made by Carthusian monks • magically use the growing plant, the chopped and dried leaves, fresh or dried flowers, and essential oil

PLANET AND ELEMENT

Sun • Fire

MAGICAL USES

attracts success through creative ventures • gives confidence in both personal and professional communication • use in magical cookery and beverages for optimism and warm, loving vibes between partners and families

HOW TO USE

Burn or diffuse the oil if you have writer's block or another creative obstacle to your artistic or musical flow. • Grow orange mint in a pot for inspirational brainstorming sessions in your home business or workplace. • Combine dried orange mint with patchouli and add frankincense resin to create a money-drawing incense. Mix the two herbs in a money-attracting charm bag when you need to sell your own talents or a product to a reluctant market, or if you are offering an entirely new concept, to give you enhanced confidence and persuasive powers. • Carry the chopped, dried flowers and leaves mixed with golden glitter and a goldstone in a gold bag to take to auditions, interviews, competitions, reality shows, or performances when you are aiming for fame and fortune.

CAUTION

Dilute oil well before applying to skin and avoid sunlight immediately afterward. • Do not ingest the oil. • Consult your doctor before consuming orange mint while pregnant or breastfeeding, though drinking the tea and inhaling the scent is sometimes recommended to help with nausea.

Mint, Lemon

(*Monarda citriodora*)

MAGICAL FORMS

native to central and southern USA and northern Mexico • grows in parts of Europe and the UK • can be cultivated as an indoor potted plant almost anywhere • lavender, pink, or white flowers, generally blooming spring to midsummer • magically use the leaves and flowers, fresh and dried, and the whole, growing plant, especially in pots and cut in an herbal display

PLANET AND ELEMENT

Mercury • Air

MAGICAL USES

for concentration and focus • to avoid and clear misunderstandings • to draw psychic boundaries • breaks destructive habits, addictions, fears, compulsions, and phobias based in emotional trauma • for a quick infusion of logic if the emotional temperature is too high

HOW TO USE

Rub a picked leaf and inhale the scent, or slowly breathe in the scent of the growing plant, then breathe out. • Add the leaves to tea and the dried leaves and flowers to potpourri to create ongoing enthusiasm in the home and to minimize emotional outbursts. • Keep a potted plant in the workplace for clear thinking and concentration if there are a lot of distractions and gossip. • Carry the chopped, dried leaves in an amulet bag to stay alert if rest is not possible and to express yourself clearly and logically, as well as to avoid emotional manipulation and the effects of energy vampires. • Use mixed with lemongrass to ward off the evil eye and protect against spite.

CAUTION

Mint tea of any kind should not be consumed in excess and should be avoided in pregnancy and while breastfeeding.

Mint, Mexican

(*Plectranthus amboinicus*)

MAGICAL FORMS

herb with fuzzy, velvety ornamental leaves with a pungent oregano taste and fragrance, though it is not oregano • also called Cuban oregano • trumpetlike pink flowers • originating in southern and eastern West Africa, Middle Eastern traders brought the herb to the Middle East and India • thereafter it came through Europe and via European settlers to the Americas • used as a spice, Mexican mint can be grown in tropical and subtropical regions worldwide • it can be grown as a potted plant indoors or, if grown outdoors, can be brought indoors in the fall in temperate regions • used in Ayurveda and medicinally as a diuretic, for IBS, for removing toxins from the body, and for relieving arthritic pain, colds, and coughs • magically use the growing plant or the growing or dried herb

PLANETS AND ELEMENTS

Mars/Venus • Fire/Water

MAGICAL USES

acquired the name Cuban oregano because it is added to Cuban jerk-inspired dishes • the dried leaves, empowered as herbal tea, reduce stress and anxiety • share with those who are potentially confrontational and will not listen • because of its oregano-like pungency, it combines the protective powers of true oregano with the active energies of mint (to whose family it belongs) • since it stores water within its evergreen leaves, a few leaves can be floated in water for the Water element in a magick circle and/or the potted plant in the Fire quadrant element in defensive magick

HOW TO USE

Grow in a pot placed in your workspace or near the entrance to your business to repel timewasters and pettiness and attract profitable encounters. • Add the chopped herb to celebration meals to raise the fun tempo and spontaneity, especially if those present are naturally inhibited or the event is one you are attending strictly out of duty.

CAUTION

The bristly leaves and stems may cause skin allergies, so handle with care.

Mint, Pineapple

(*Mentha suaveolens* 'Variegata')

MAGICAL FORMS

cream and green fragrant variegated leaves • hybrid of apple mint (see p. 290) • like the parent plant apple mint, which is native to southwestern Europe and the Mediterranean, pineapple mint is now naturalized in North America and Australia, growing wild and in gardens in many parts of the world and in containers or pots almost anywhere • magically use the cut or whole, growing herb, fresh or dried, and tea made from the herb

PLANETS AND ELEMENTS

Mars/Venus • Fire/Water

MAGICAL USES

for cleansing homes and sacred spaces • removing negative entities • connects with the spiritual world • magical cookery • sweeter than many mints, so encourages kindness and tactful words when offered as a tea

HOW TO USE

Because it spreads rapidly via horizontal underground roots and will revert to its parent, pure green apple mint, if unchecked, pineapple mint, with its slight fragrance of pineapple, can be used potted to encourage networking in business and also to resist undue parental influence at any age. • In potpourri, grown in the garden, or as an indoor kitchen herb, pineapple mint deters not only rats, mice, and insects but also all who would invade or disturb the peace with their petty irritations by creating a psychic exclusion zone around you and your home or workspace. • Sprinkle a little of the tea on doorsteps and wash it away out of the door with a cascade of clear, hot water to prevent complaining neighbors or interfering relatives from overstaying their welcome; this also cleanses the home of illness, financial worries, or misfortune.

CAUTION

Though pineapple mint has many medicinal and culinary benefits, as with all mints, avoid ingesting it in pregnancy and if breastfeeding. • It can interfere with blood pressure and diabetes medicines.

Molasses

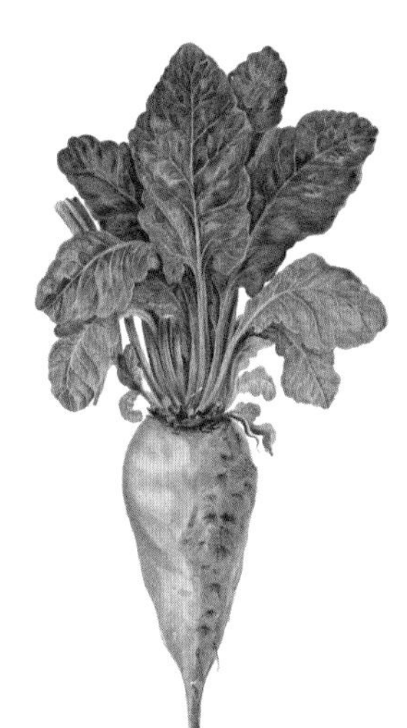

MAGICAL FORMS

molasses, or treacle, is a thick, sweet, dark syrup • a byproduct made from juice extracted from sugar cane or sugar beet • used as a sweetener • was more popular than sugar in the USA and the UK until the 1880s • contains vitamins and minerals, including iron, magnesium, and calcium • magically use the syrup in magical cookery

PLANET AND ELEMENT

Venus • Earth

MAGICAL USES

use in magical cookery • in love magick to attract a new lover or enchant an existing hesitant one • given to children on waffles and pancakes instead of maple syrup to protect them in the day ahead from recess conflicts • for safe journeys

HOW TO USE

Keep a sealed clear jar of molasses on a shelf in the kitchen to attract health, wealth, and good fortune to the home. • Hide another small dark glass jar almost filled with molasses in which you have added symbols of what you most desire: coins for prosperity, an old key for a new home, dried rose petals for love, a tiny clay baby in a cradle for fertility. Each week, hold your jar and shake it gently, repeating its purpose nine times before re-hiding it. You can add more than one symbol for different needs.

Money Tree

(*Pachira aquatica*)

MAGICAL FORMS

grown indoors, usually as a bonsai plant with braided stem • can grow outdoors in warm climes • magically use the whole, growing plant and leaves

PLANET AND ELEMENT

Saturn • Earth

MAGICAL USES

brings prosperity and good luck in feng shui • encourages chi or positive life force to flow freely through the home or workplace • health and happiness

HOW TO USE

Twisting the stems to make braids and adding red ribbons creates and maintains financial success and positive energies. • To draw in money, set the tree near the front door in homes and workplaces, the financial section of a workplace, or in the southeast wealth corner of the home. • Set a second plant in the east of the home for ongoing good health and to clear stagnant energies. • Five-leaf plants attract money; six, exceptional good luck; and seven, major financial success. • Give money trees as a housewarming gift or the first item to be placed in a new home to ensure money flows in and not out and that the home will be a haven of peace.

CAUTION

Though the plant is not toxic for humans, cats, or dogs, the nuts are considered by some sources to be dangerous to eat. • Cats who eat an excess of leaves may get an upset stomach.

Monkey Puzzle Tree

(*Araucaria araucana*)

MAGICAL FORMS

evergreen with often horizontal branches the shape of long monkey tails, covered in spirals of sharp, triangular leaves • cones on tips in older trees • trunk resembling elephant skin • a 200-million-year-old species native to Argentina and Chile, first introduced to the UK at the end of the eighteenth century • now endangered • grows in the USA along the coastal zone from Virginia to the Atlantic, west through Texas and up the Pacific coast to Washington • can eventually grow to eighty feet • traditionally planted near graveyards in the UK to keep away evil spirits • sold in specialty stores, and may be grown initially in a container • often seen in arboretums and botanical gardens • magically use the living tree, dried leaves, cones, seeds, and white wood from specialty craft stores (or occasionally pre-loved artifacts)

PLANET AND ELEMENT

Mars • Fire

MAGICAL USES

to encourage problem-solving and ingenious solutions • for adaptability and versatility and getting out of difficult situations • it is said to be unlucky to speak while passing near or under the tree or your plans will be disrupted by the mischievous spirits within

HOW TO USE

Sit beneath this ancient tree to receive visions not only of your own past lives, but of times when the dinosaurs lived. • Collect the rounded, spiny female cones that contain up to two hundred seeds. • Fill a charm bag with them when you need to brainstorm or talk your way out of a potentially difficult situation. • Carry a small piece of wood or make a monkey puzzle tree wand by obtaining the wood from a wood craft outlet. • This is the ultimate magick wand for manifesting positive outcomes to any situation and to draw unexpected help, resources, and rescue.

CAUTION

Avoid ingesting the leaves or any part of the tree if uncooked. • Avoid while pregnant.

Monkshood

(*Aconitum napellus*)

MAGICAL FORMS

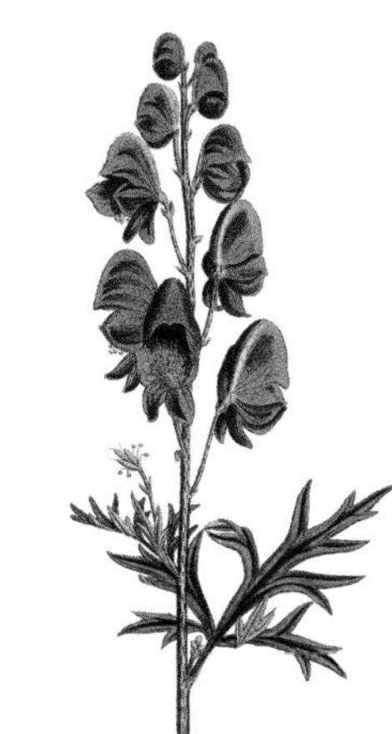

also called aconite or wolfsbane • dark-lobed leaves • violet or blue delphinium flowers on spikes • from the buttercup family • can reach five feet tall • native to North America, as well as central and southern Europe • introduced to Australia and New Zealand, where it is considered invasive • magically use only the dried or fresh herb with extreme caution, as it is poisonous

PLANET AND ELEMENT

Saturn • Earth

MAGICAL USES

named monkshood because of the shape of the flower • traditionally used in arrow tip poisons • said to kill werewolves • in myth, aconite was used by the sorceress Medea to poison Theseus after he defeated the Amazonian women • especially in medieval times, there are many accounts of using the herb for getting rid of unwanted rivals and foes • applied only in very strong defensive magick if at all

HOW TO USE

The only recommended uses by more extreme practitioners in modern magick are to carry it in a strong, sealed bag for protection in a life and death situation and to use it as an amulet for extreme sports and stuntpeople. • Note that this plant is best left alone, as there are many more benign defensive herbs that can be empowered for critical situations.

CAUTION

All parts of the plant are highly toxic and the roots and seeds of the raw plant are especially hazardous. • Although it is still used in Chinese and Ayurvedic medicine and homeopathy, it is subject to restrictions in a number of countries, including the USA, and is prescription-only in the UK.

Monstera

(*Monstera deliciosa*)

MAGICAL FORMS

also called the Swiss cheese plant, one of a variety of monstera plants, including the rarer closely related *Monstera albo borsigiana*, with large splashes of white on the split leaves • houseplant • native to the South American rainforests; in the wild is a vine that grows up trees and can reach sixty-six feet high • even indoors, monstera plants can reach six to seven feet high and eight feet wide, so they are ideal in conservatories or garden rooms to create the feel of being in an exotic jungle • magically use the whole, growing plant and cut leaves

PLANET AND ELEMENT

Sun • Fire

MAGICAL USES

long life • respect • honoring wise and older people, as well as ancestors • the patterned leaf holes admit the power of the sun as good luck • for a healthy life and prosperity • for grandparents and great-grandparents, to wish them a long, healthy life • given to beloved family members on the eve of the Chinese New Year • a natural filter in both the home and workplace, monstera eliminates toxins from the atmosphere—both physical and as lingering resentment and fixed viewpoints

HOW TO USE

In feng shui, the plant, when placed in the center of a room or workspace, filters the life force. • The patterned leaf holes transmit the gentle but not overwhelming power of the sun, bringing a healthy lifestyle and energy without hyperactivity. • Monstera calls wealth and good luck to flow in and not directly out again. • Empower the plant with enthusiasm, calm, and optimism when you encounter discouragement, hyperactive or overly driven people or situations, or if you have yourself become a workaholic with diminishing returns.

CAUTION

Monstera is toxic to humans and pets: do not ingest.

Moonflower

(*Ipomoea alba*)

MAGICAL FORMS

night flower growing on a vine • a night-blooming form of morning glory • large, heart-shaped leaves • slightly prickly stems • iridescent, trumpetlike flowers that unfurl as sun goes down or on cloudy days and stay open all night, exuding beautiful fragrance and closing at dawn • though best in tropical USA, moonflower grows happily in more temperate zones • magically use the whole, growing plant; leaves; fresh or dried vine; and fresh or dried flowers

PLANET AND ELEMENT

Moon • Water

MAGICAL USES

for all moon magick, especially full moon rituals, in particular the full moon nearest to midsummer, when the flowers begin to bloom • night magick • women's rites of passage • clairsentience, by inhaling the growing fragrance to open psychic awareness • protective magick against paranormal and human attack by night • moth magick for overcoming hidden fears

HOW TO USE

Set a moonflower (cut it while open) on the altar for the goddess, with a sunflower head for the god. • Burn the dried leaves and flowers in incense with myrrh moon resin for Drawing Down the Moon ceremonies. • Use moonflower petals, scattered in an outdoor space to create a magick circle, for crescent moon rites for love and romance. • Chop and powder the vine, adding with fresh, heart-shaped leaves and two fresh moonflowers to a jar to call back a lover from your past or one from whom you are estranged, or if your current lover seems indifferent. Shake the sealed jar before sleep, keeping it next to your bed. When the leaves and flowers fade, tip the mix into flowing water saying, *Flow free, come back to me, in love and unity, willingly.*

CAUTION

Moonflower is mildly toxic to adults, and care should be taken around pets and children; it should not be ingested in remedies in large quantities. • The seeds are hallucinogenic. • Beware of *Datura*, which is poisonous and may be sold as moonflower, but it has an unpleasant smell and opens in the daytime.

Moonwort

(Botrychium lunaria)

MAGICAL FORMS

also called common moonwort, and in ancient times, Unshoo-the-horse • tiny but powerful fern with crescent-moon-shaped paired leaves and fronds resembling keys • much grows below ground • a circumpolar herb found in Scotland, Wales, and north and west England, as well as in North America, Eurasia, and Australia • worth seeking out as one of the most magical and mysterious alchemical herbs from times past • magically use the fresh or dried plant

PLANET AND ELEMENT

Moon • Water

MAGICAL USES

linked with love rituals associated with the moon phases • also for secret love • a money herb traditionally believed to turn base metals to silver, the metal of the moon • according to the seventeenth-century herbalist Nicholas Culpepper, moonwort was potent for undoing locks and less usefully was known for pulling shoes from the horses who passed over it • helpful to the fey

HOW TO USE

Use in spells for romance and attracting love on the waxing moon. • When used on the full moon, moonwort brings passion and fertility, and on the wane, it can be useful in ending destructive relationships and codependency. • Traditionally, it is placed in safes where cash or jewelry is kept to ensure their security. • In alchemy, it is called the white celestial herb and used in transformational and manifestation rituals. • Use in rites for overcoming obstacles and opposition to love, especially on the full moon, by placing moonwort in the keyhole of a closed box with what is forbidden written inside, then opening the box and throwing away the actual key. • Conversely, lock a box with moonwort inside and throw away the key to keep a lover's identity safe or to protect secret information.

CAUTION

Consult an expert before using if you are pregnant or taking medication.

Moringa Tree

(Moringa oleifera)

MAGICAL FORMS

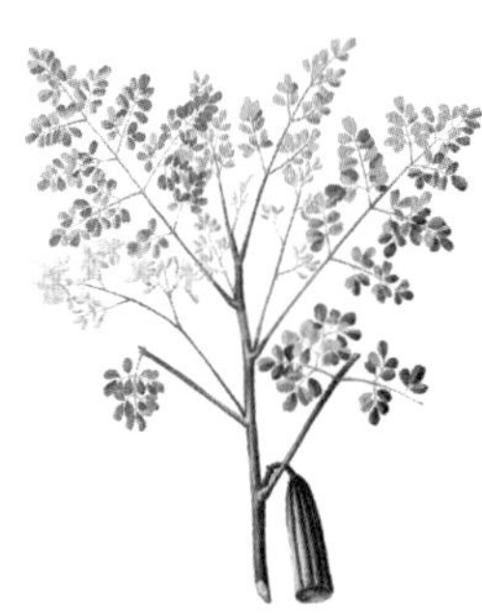

native to the Indian subcontinent and dry desert landscapes in the Middle East • grows in Florida and other tropical regions, where its fragrant white flowers blossom through the year • magically use the flowers, leaves, powdered leaves made into a tea to absorb its healing powers (often with turmeric or ginger), and seed oil

PLANET AND ELEMENT

Sun • Fire

MAGICAL USES

seed oil was found in the tomb of Maiherpri, an ancient Egyptian noble in the Valley of the Kings dating to the fourteenth century BCE • oil was also prized in ancient Greece and Rome cosmetically and medicinally • for anti-aging, abundance, and healing rituals and spells • also called the Miracle Tree or Tree of Life because of the numerous health-bringing and culinary properties of its flowers, stems, seeds, fruit, and leaves

HOW TO USE

An aphrodisiac, the tea should be shared with a lover to inflame passion and before sex magick. • Anoint a red candle with seed oil before lovemaking if you seek to conceive (note that adding oil makes candles more flammable). • Use the dried, chopped herb in incense for fire and sun rituals, or cast on bonfires to generate power and courage, especially on sun festivals such as midsummer and at noon when the sun is shining.

CAUTION

The roots and bark (the latter questionably) are toxic. • While it is generally considered safe to ingest leaf tea in pregnancy, check with your maternity team for sure. • Do not ingest the seed oil.

Morning Glory

(*Ipomoea purpurea*)

MAGICAL FORMS

originating in Mexico and other parts of Central and South America • naturalized throughout much of the USA and eastern Canada • brightly colored, trumpet-shaped flowers on a climbing plant, the flowers tightly curled, unfolding to their full glory as the sun comes up • the flowers last only one day • magically use the growing vine, pieces of entwining vine, the flowers, and the seed pods (with care)

PLANETS AND ELEMENTS

Mercury/Moon • Air/Water

MAGICAL USES

the day-blooming version of the night-blossoming moonflower, a good pairing for magick when sun and moon are both in the sky • the unfolding flowers can be used in dawn rituals to infuse a surge of the life force, promising new beginnings if yesterday did not work out; to overcome inertia and pessimism; and to protect against the false illusions of others • a number of Native North American people and later Spanish and European settlers used morning glory to induce psychic visions • for binding spells using the vine • create a circle with the flowers on the vine to mark the boundary between the magical and everyday world and to ensure any intruders are magically tangled • use a thick vine stalk as a dowsing tool to find what is lost

HOW TO USE

Meditate on the growing plant to get priorities right if others are throwing you off course, as well as to develop mindfulness and to ascend to higher levels of awareness especially by focusing on the blue or purple flowers as a celestial stairway on the ascending vine. • Since morning glory will spread over anything horizontally as well as vertically, make a wheel of good fortune using an old wagon wheel. • Train morning glory to trail all over it and set the wheel outside the dwelling to protect the property.

CAUTION

The seeds, which are hallucinogenic, are toxic to people and pets, especially when ingested, and are illegal in the USA and many other countries.

Moss, Irish

(*Sagina subulata*)

MAGICAL FORMS

an emerald-green mosslike plant, forming a thick, dense mat with short, thin, creeping stems, covered by short leaves • sometimes used in place of a lawn in gardens • tiny, white, star-shaped fragrant flowers cover the tufts from late spring until midsummer • found in temperate regions in central and western Europe, Ireland, Wales, Scotland, and other Celtic lands, as well as those where Celtic ancestors settled • can be grown in gardens in the USA • magically use the mossy plant in situ or the flowering plant, fresh or dried

PLANETS AND ELEMENTS

Saturn/Moon • Earth/Water

MAGICAL USES

planted to mark out a sacred area for outdoor rituals to absorb the energies of the Earth Father or Mother • as an infusion of the dried flowering plant, sprinkled around the home or home business to banish debt and fears of financial loss • made into a moss baby on a wicker frame for fertility

HOW TO USE

Fill poppet dolls with dried Irish moss for money or luck. Tie the poppet to a tree with a moss agate crystal inside to speed up financial matters in a business you cannot get off the ground or funds that seem slow coming. • Mix the dried flowers and leaves in incense with chamomile and scatter the ashes outward along a garden path or outside the front door to keep opportunities flowing in the long-term. • Roll a green unlit candle in dried, shredded greenery, then light the candle on Fridays as it grows dark, sending love to absent friends or relatives. This also deters ill-wishers and any who drain resources, financial or emotional, from intruding on your life and family.

Moss, Spanish

(*Tillandsia usneoides*)

MAGICAL FORMS

hanging, branching, rootless air plant, not actually moss, that grows on trees, shrubs, or any supporting surface without being parasitic, using the host for support • long, cascading stems of up to twenty to twenty-five feet, with silver-green foliage • native to tropical and subtropical USA, especially the Southeast, and some parts of Central and South America • also grows as a houseplant, especially in bathrooms, attached to a frame or under glass in cooler climates • magically use the whole, growing plant and the cut, stringy strands

PLANETS AND ELEMENT

Mercury/Jupiter • Air

MAGICAL USES

protection in the home • for increasing financial assets • reducing codependency • knot magick • obtaining financial, physical, or emotional support

HOW TO USE

Add cut, chopped moss to a money incense to increase your assets and savings, passing a green dollar note or a gold-colored coin through the smoke and keeping it afterward in a purse, wallet, or business cash register. • Grow the climbing moss close to or on the outside of the house, or indoors in a warm place, to bring protection and avoid division, disunity, and dissension with a partner or family, and to attract good fortune. • Fill a poppet doll with the dried moss, chamomile, and rose petals for healing sorrow after loss or betrayal and to call back love (using twin dolls positioned face to face).

CAUTION

Check with a physician or midwife before using Spanish moss if you are pregnant.

Moss, Square Goose Neck

(*Rhytidiadelphus squarrosus*)

MAGICAL FORMS

species of moss known as springy turf moss in the UK and square goose neck moss in the USA • grows extensively throughout Eurasia • common in lawns and in the wild • may be pale green with a starry appearance when seen from above • leaves grow up to six inches tall, bent back on the red stem at ninety degrees • magically use the moss in situ or cut and dried, and the flower essence

PLANET AND ELEMENT

Saturn • Earth

MAGICAL USES

as a flower essence, releases self-imposed and familial restrictions about freedom, and lack of spontaneity • for those who as children feared the dark and may still do so as adults, as well as children indoctrinated when young in a religion or community that warned of the dangers of sin and even of thought • a particularly lucky form of moss that adds to the power of any spell

HOW TO USE

Fill a featureless poppet doll or sachet with the dried moss and dried basil or sage for money. • Stuff twin poppet dolls with moss and dried rose petals for lasting love. • For healing, fill a poppet or sachet with moss and dried lavender. • Grow the moss on your lawn and press hard on the plant with your feet, pointing your fingers downward to give yourself a sense of stability if you are restless or situations have made you feel insecure. • Give the essence to children who are afraid of the dark.

CAUTION

Though used in some traditional medicines, it is not generally ingested. • Be careful using if the plant has been treated with herbicide.

Motherwort

(*Leonurus cardiaca*)

MAGICAL FORMS

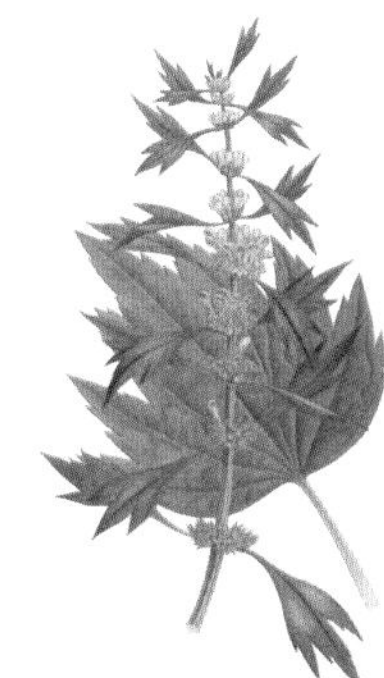

also known as lion's tail • native to central Asia, now naturalized throughout much of Europe and North America • cultivated in gardens and growing wild • magically use all aerial parts, the growing plant, the pink clusters of flowers, fresh and dried palm-shaped leaves, and dried leaves as a tea

PLANETS AND ELEMENTS

Moon/Sun • Water/Fire

MAGICAL USES

for power animal connections • rituals for male potency • women's magick, especially rites of passage • protects against misfortune • cleanses people, places, and situations • strengthens purpose if you have lost sight of your life path • for moon rituals

HOW TO USE

Drink the tea to invoke the courage of a lion to stand against injustice and intimidation. • Use the dried, chopped herbs as the Earth element in protective rituals conducted by mothers for their offspring of any age who may be threatened or cannot find their purpose, and afterward keep with their photographs. • If you are a parent, grow the herb in your garden so your children and their families will hold you in their heart. • Also grow in the garden, in pots indoors, or hang dried motherwort in a red bag over the front door to keep away all malicious psychic and psychological attacks and ill wishes. • Add another over the back door if you have one, to keep happiness and love within.

CAUTION

Avoid ingesting during pregnancy and if trying to conceive or taking blood-thinning medication.

Mountain Mahogany

(*Cercocarpus* spp.)

MAGICAL FORMS

genus containing several species of flowering plants, including *Cercocarpus montanu* (alder-leaf mountain mahogany) and *ledifolius* (curl-leaf mountain mahogany) • a small, wild shrub or tree with grayish-brown bark, yellowish-white flowers, and egg-shaped leaves • from the rose family • native to northern Mexico and the western USA in dry canyons and rocky outcrops in northwest Oregon, on the lower foothills of the Rockies, and the Great Plains • was a Native American remedy for earache, stomachache, and sores • may only become three and a half feet high as grazed by wildlife or up to thirty feet if undisturbed • can be cultivated as a hedge plant • environmentally valuable, as it fixes nitrogen levels in the soil and prevents erosion • magically use the growing tree, wood, or essence

PLANETS AND ELEMENTS

Jupiter/Mars • Air/Fire

MAGICAL USES

as the flower essence, used to overcome suddenly expressed anger, sometimes masked as chronic irritability, due to inner fears and frustration of not moving forward naturally, often alternating with false complacency • for learning to recognize and flow with both opportunity and challenge

HOW TO USE

Cast small pieces or bark scrapings into water to remove fears or frustration. Since the wood is so dense, it will not float on water. • As it is brittle and burns intensely, use the wood on ceremonial or celebration fires to welcome the changing energies of a new season or life stage. • Planted in the garden, the tree is believed to protect the home against storms and fire. • Use the essence if you are out of rhythm with your natural stages of progression or for children who are either easily frustrated or overconfident about life's natural challenges.

Mugwort

(*Artemisia* spp.)

MAGICAL FORMS

also called the traveler's herb • plants from the genus *Artemisia* (see "Wormwood," p. 479, and "Davana," p. 154) • can grow tall, so if in a wildlife garden, keep it cut back or as hedging • magically use the growing plant, especially the leaves and stems, and the flowers

PLANET AND ELEMENT

Saturn • Earth

MAGICAL USES

drives away evil spirits, disease, and earthly harm • for enhancing visionary powers • the ultimate herb for walking between worlds and shape-shifting • increases fertility • protective on journeys of all kinds, especially from attack and predators, human and otherwise

HOW TO USE

Wash magical mirrors with a mugwort leaf infusion before and after scrying. • Fresh leaves can be placed beneath a crystal ball to aid visions (replace as the plant dries out). • Make the leaves and stems plus bay leaves into smudge sticks to cleanse a ritual area and magical tools, and to clear the home of negative influences, both earthly and paranormal. Smudge your home before going away to create a barrier against all intrusion in your absence. • Burn as incense with sandalwood chips and fennel before meditation. • Water darkened with mugwort is used for scrying, illuminated by candles; its aroma also increases psychic and prophetic powers. • Use as part of a dream pillow with lavender and dried rose petals for predictive dreams, astral travel, and lucid dreaming. • Traditionally, the plant is added to Midsummer Eve fires and the ashes scattered on the garden for year-round fertility and protection in the way most desired.

CAUTION

Avoid mugwort if pregnant or allergic to celery, carrot, ragweed, or caraway.

Muhuhu

(*Brachylaena hutchinsii*)

MAGICAL FORMS

also called the silver oak tree • grown in Kenya, Tanzania, Uganda, Angola, and the African coast • the essential oil is made from the aromatic golden-brown heartwood and bark • produces a wood that is similar to sandalwood • the tree is rare and endangered • magically use the essential oil and artifacts made from the wood, such as a statue or prayer beads • artifacts should be obtained only from an ethical seller who can trace their environmental history

PLANETS AND ELEMENTS

Jupiter/Saturn • Air/Earth

MAGICAL USES

for compromise and peaceful interactions • panic and stress relief • takes the heat out of confrontations at home and in the workplace • for successful negotiations • quiet rest and pleasant dreams

HOW TO USE

If you find it hard to "switch off" and focus during meditation, or if you are perpetually anxious, diffuse the oil or put a little oil diluted on your wrists or aroma bracelet. • Hold a muhuhu artifact between your hands—this could be as small as a wooden pen, a handful of beads, a prayer necklace, or a small polished offcut from a specialty wood store—then close your eyes to let go of expectations. • Burn the oil as a background fragrance if your home is constantly hyperactive and loud. • Relax in the fragrance before bed so you can switch off from the world, especially if you frequently bring work home.

CAUTION

If pregnant or lactating, consult a physician or midwife before using the oil, as not enough is known about effects on mother and baby. • Do not ingest. • Dilute before using on the skin.

Mulberry Tree

(*Morus* spp.)

MAGICAL FORMS

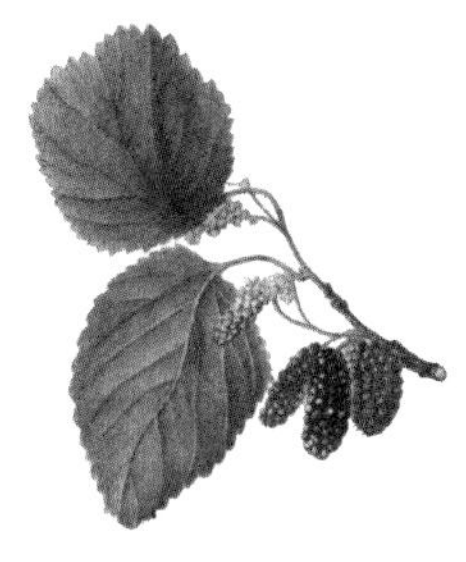

genus of flowering plants, including American mulberry or Beautyberry (*Callicarpa americana*), black mulberry (*Morus nigra*), and white or common mulberry (*Morus alba*) • the children's nursery rhyme, "Here We Go Round the Mulberry Bush," refers to the mulberry tree in Wakefield Prison in Northern England that in Victorian times female prisoners circled for exercise • magically use the growing tree, wood, and berries

PLANET AND ELEMENT

Mercury • Air

MAGICAL USES

protective against all kinds of malevolence • an anti-lightning tree • the white mulberry supports silkworms, and so mulberry chippings or dried leaves can be part of an incense mix to encourage the accumulation of wealth • in Chinese legend, the mulberry tree is the sacred World Tree, up which the three-legged sun bird climbs each day to bring in the morning • the tree serves as the link between heaven and earth, so is central in new beginnings and dawn outdoor rituals

HOW TO USE

Add the dried berries to success, money, and creativity charm bags. • As a magic wand, mulberry can be used for spontaneous rituals where words and form evolve naturally and with inspiration, without preparation. Use the point of the wand like a pendulum to vibrate over the correct choice out of a number of written options. • Protect babies in a nursery by hanging a white silk amulet bag filled with the dried fruit and leaves in a safe place in the nursery. This also signifies the child will never lack resources during their life. • Sit beneath the tree at dawn for successful astral travel.

CAUTION

The milky white sap from the fresh leaves, as well as the unripe berries, are toxic to humans.

Mullein

(*Verbascum* spp.)

MAGICAL FORMS

genus of flowering plants with over 450 species • magically use the growing plants; fresh, dried, and powdered leaves; and fresh and dried flowers

PLANET AND ELEMENTS

Saturn • Earth/Fire

MAGICAL USES

sometimes called lady's candles, because in early times its stem was dried, tipped into tallow, and lit on festivals linked with the Virgin Mary • also known as hags' candles, the hairy stems and leaves substituted as wicks in oil lamps to illuminate magical rituals and offer protection within the light • large, dried flower stalks were soaked in tallow and lit on Halloween to keep away restless spirits • for courage • protective against hostility, accidents, psychic attacks, and natural hazards, especially while camping or backpacking in the wilderness • mullein was traditionally carried by hunters and travelers to guard against injury from wild animals

HOW TO USE

Cast on ritual fires to call Fire elementals. • Added to a dream pillow, mullein prevents nightmares, incubi, and succubi. • Mullein is hung over doors and windows in lands including India to banish evil, spirits, poltergeists, negative enchantment, and all entering the home with evil intent. • Carry a tiny, dried sprig to an overcompetitive workplace. • Powdered mullein leaves were substituted in spells created in the past that demanded graveyard dust.

CAUTION

Mullein is not to be used during pregnancy. • The fine hairs covering the plant should be removed, as they can be an irritant.

CAUTION

Avoid if pregnant.

Mushroom

(*Agaricus* spp.)

MAGICAL FORMS

genus of over four hundred mushrooms, including the white button mushroom (*Agaricus bisporus*) • fungus with a cap, the spore-bearing fleshy part, and gills (the thin, papery part beneath the mushroom) • growing wild, cultivated, and in pots • reproduces constantly • magically use the growing mushroom • for *bisporus* and any other edible variety, use raw and cooked

PLANET AND ELEMENT

Saturn • Earth

MAGICAL USES

avoiding illusion and those who would deceive • for contact with nature spirits, especially on May Eve, Midsummer, and Halloween • fertility

HOW TO USE

Fairy rings are circles of mushrooms (beware the archetypal red with white spots that are probably poisonous toadstools, *Amanita muscaria*) growing in grassy places from Europe to North America to Australia and the Far East, especially in the morning after rain. These are natural circles within which it is said the fey hold their revels. • A fairy ring that appears in your garden or a field nearby brings blessings. Never enter the ring; but if you find one on full moon night, run around the outside three times clockwise, then three times counterclockwise, followed by three times clockwise to catch glimpses of the fey. Leave a coin or crystal outside the circle in return for a wish for good fortune. • As you stir mushrooms into cooking, ask to see through illusion, and you will gain sudden insight of those in your friendship or work circle who are less than reliable, however friendly they appear.

CAUTION

If picking wild mushrooms, great care is needed because of toxicity.

Muskflower

including (*Malva moschata*)

MAGICAL FORMS

common name for several varieties of plants whose musk scent is used in perfumes and essential oils instead of the banned animal source • notably the pink or yellow musk mallow from tropical Asia, Europe, including the UK, introduced to the USA by settlers, with a musky fragrance that produces a heavy, sweet musk oil from its seeds • also the more subtly fragranced yellow muskflower or musk monkeyflower (*Erythranthe moschata*), found in western North America and parts of eastern North America, naturalized in parts of Europe, the UK, and Finland • however, the *Erythranthe moschata*, grown in the UK, and cultivars of the plant are scentless • sticky monkeyflower, or orange bush monkeyflower (*Mimulus aurantiacus*), also has a strong musk fragrance • magically use the flowers, incense, and essential oil, or in musk-based fragrances (choose organic products that are not synthetic)

PLANET AND ELEMENT

Sun • Fire

MAGICAL USES

is used to create one of the most spiritual, mystical incenses from ancient times, still used in formal rituals and as offerings • the essential oil, made from the seed of the musk mallow or from another muskflower, can be used for love-attracting spells and for twin soul love and sex magick

HOW TO USE

Anoint the throat energy center with the diluted seed oil or one of the Egyptian musk oils that do not contain alcohol before divination and automatic writing for prophetic words. • Anoint the brow energy center for clairvoyant visions and the center of the hairline for the crown energy center for astrally traveling in meditation to ancient worlds, sacred temples, and your own past lives. • Meditate among fragrant muskflowers to move from the everyday world to a state of merging with the flower energies.

CAUTION

Always dilute musk essential oil well, and some experts say to avoid sunlight immediately after use. • For determining the safety of a particular muskflower species, check with a physician, and avoid in pregnancy if uncertain.

Mustard

including (*Sinapis alba*)

MAGICAL FORMS

Sinapis alba is also called white or yellow mustard • also black mustard (*Brassica nigra*) or brown or Indian mustard (*Brassica juncea*), which is of Himalayan origin • magically use the seeds, dried powder, dried yellow mustard flowers, or as a condiment

PLANETS AND ELEMENT

Mars/Sun • Fire

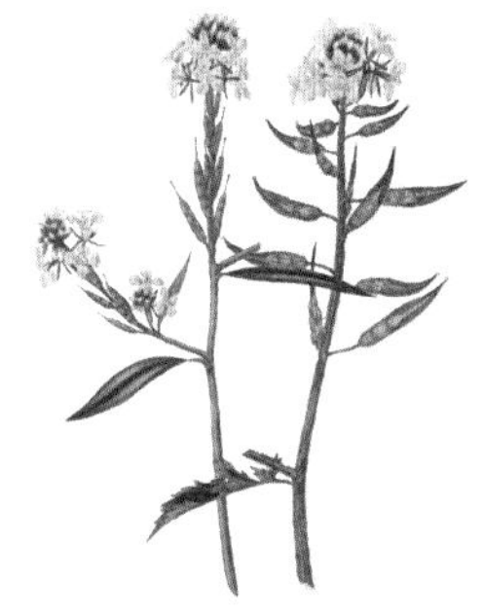

MAGICAL USES

for fertility • protection • courage to stand up to bullies • overcoming seemingly impossible odds to scale great heights even from small beginnings, given faith in oneself • the mustard seed is likened in the New Testament to the Kingdom of Heaven; from the smallest beginnings, it grew into a mighty tree in which birds could shelter • black, brown, or white mustard can be grown in the garden and the seed pods split to release the seeds in the fall, which should be dried separately rather than in a heap; however, both kinds of spice can easily be bought

HOW TO USE

Add to a red charm bag with ginger, chile, allspice, and cinnamon for a swift, urgent infusion of money. • Chew black or brown seeds to aid in astral travel, according to an old Hindu tradition. • Mustard seeds buried under the doorstep or taped under a doormat repel supernatural evil and negative earth energies attempting to enter the home. • Fill half an eggshell with mustard seeds and on the day or evening of the full moon, float the eggshell on flowing water before lovemaking to conceive a child. • Scatter seeds or flowers across a pathway a desired lover will walk along.

CAUTION

Consuming excess black mustard seeds can damage the throat. • People with thyroid problems should avoid the raw seeds. • Mustard oil is not allowed in the USA. • Care is advised in pregnancy.

Myrrh

(*Commiphora myrrha*)

MAGICAL FORMS

primarily used as thick, yellow gum resin extracted from a desert thorny tree • resin is a core and very ancient ingredient in incense, the kind burned on a charcoal block • essential oil is extracted from the resin • myrrh incense is rarely used alone • myrrh trees are native to the fabulous and fabled Land of Punt, described by the ancient Egyptians, probably a region in northeastern Africa in modern Somalia from where the ancient Egyptians obtained their myrrh • myrrh is found today still in Somalia, Ethiopia, Saudi Arabia, India, Iran, and Thailand • magically use as resin, incense, and essential oil

PLANETS AND ELEMENTS

Saturn/Moon • Earth/Water

MAGICAL USES

like frankincense, and often paired with it, myrrh is one of the main ceremonial incenses, burned in the ancient Egyptian temple of Ra the Sun god at noon • used to begin again after difficulty or loss • use in post-redundancy and retirement spells, for all who would wish to or already work in alternative therapies • healing rituals • for meditation, visualization, and enhanced psychic awareness, especially of past lives • for prayers against prejudice and war • for blessings, especially on homes and on wedding, engagement, or eternity rings and pearls

HOW TO USE

Myrrh increases the power of any other incense and rite because its thick, aromatic smoke heightens spiritual awareness. • Use to mark out sacred space for formal magick and dedicating ritual artifacts. • Myrrh incense rituals are integral to crone or wisewomen ceremonies and also for wise men to assume their magical and spiritual authority. • Once used for funeral rites, a single drop of myrrh can be added to olive oil to anoint a white candle before lighting it to ease the passing of a beloved friend or family member in the last stages of life. • Mix myrrh oil with benzoin and sandalwood in an aroma lamp or diffuser after a stressful day.

CAUTION

Do not use while pregnant. • Do not take the essential oil internally.

Myrtle

including (*Myrtus communis*)

MAGICAL FORMS

the common name "myrtle" generally refers to *Myrtus communis*, the common myrtle, but also encompasses several other species in the *Myrtus* genus and beyond • magically use the leaves, fresh or dried blossoms, fruit, or berries, as incense, and as essential oil made from flowers

PLANET AND ELEMENT

Venus • Water

MAGICAL USES

for lasting love and stable relationships • dried myrtle flowers carried in charm bags keep love alive; hang from a plant on full moon night to call a child into your life if you are trying to conceive • berries from common myrtle can be eaten as an aphrodisiac when ripe, or used in magical love cookery • essence made from the giant honey myrtle (*Melaleuca armillaris*) brings clarity and freedom from undesirable influences

HOW TO USE

For visions of your true love if you have not yet met, or to call them back if they have left your life, light myrtle incense sticks in front of a mirror in total darkness at midnight, then stand to the side so you are not reflected and look through the smoke: you will see your true love (who may not be whom you expected to meet!). • Add a small flowering branch as the center of a love altar. • Grind the dried flowers and leaves into a powder and sprinkle it near your desired lover's home or workplace to bring ailing love back to life or to make yourself noticed if they seem unaware of your presence. • Burn myrtle, lemon, and thyme oils in an aroma lamp or diffuser while your partner is away so that they will have thoughts only of you and resist temptation to stray.

CAUTION

Do not take the oil internally or use undiluted on skin. • Avoid the oil in pregnancy, while breastfeeding, or if you suffer from epilepsy. • Common myrtle may be slightly toxic to pets if ingested. • Chilean myrtle (*Luma apiculata*) is not toxic to pets.

Nag Champa

(*Plumeria pudica*)

MAGICAL FORMS

incredibly fragrant white flowers with yellow centers and leaves like cobra hoods growing on this shrub • related to frangipani • native to warm, temperate, subtropical and tropical regions, including Mexico, Central America, and Polynesia • grows also in warmer parts of North America and other warm areas • the most fragrant varieties found in Southeast Asia, especially India • can be grown in a pot indoors almost anywhere, up to two feet high • used to make incense by combining with the sweet-scented, golden flower from the large Indian evergreen tree *Magnolia champaca*, as well as sandalwood (see p. 399) (and in some blends, camphor, honey, ghee, patchouli, and other secret ingredients) • magically use in incense as sticks, powder, cones, or ropes, and as essential oil

PLANETS AND ELEMENTS

Sun/Venus • Fire/Water

MAGICAL USES

brings peace from fear and insomnia • exceptionally powerful against all earthly malevolence and hostile or restless spirits • as incense, sacred for formal and informal rituals • to calm minds always racing ahead, and to make the home a place of calm

HOW TO USE

Burn the incense or diffuse the oil to create a sacred space for personal or group meditation, yoga, Reiki, or any energy transference work. • Use before divination and mediumship to open psychic powers and call the protective wise guardians. • Nag champa stimulates sexual desire if burned in the bedroom, diffused as background, or used during erotic massage diluted in jojoba and almond carrier oil.

CAUTION

Keep away from cats. • Ventilate rooms well if using indoors.

Narcissus

(*Narcissus* spp.)

MAGICAL FORMS

there are more than fifty varieties of narcissus • daffodils and jonquils belong to the *Narcissus* genus, but while all daffodils are narcissus, all narcissus are not daffodils • named after Narcissus, who, in one version of the ancient Greek myth, fell in love with his own beauty and stared at his reflection in a pool until he faded away • in this place, the first narcissus flower grew • the paperwhite narcissus (*Narcissus papyraceus*) is especially magical • more delicate in energies than the more upfront daffodil • magically use the whole, growing plant and cut fresh or dried flowers

PLANET AND ELEMENTS

Jupiter • Air/Water

MAGICAL USES

often found growing in areas that were once burial grounds, so is considered a flower that opens the gates to the afterlife and therefore is used for contacting the ancestors • heals eating disorders and obsession with excessive cosmetic surgery • for maiden magick and rites for entering into womanhood

HOW TO USE

To release sorrows from the past, put a white narcissus in a vase of water, then hold your hands around the vase and visualize passing all you wish to leave behind into the water. When you are ready, shred the flower and cast the petals to the four directions, then skyward and downward. • Hold a clear crystal pendulum or point over a narcissus as it grows and allow it to draw healing from the plant. When you feel that the pendulum is filled with life force, pass it around your body and energy field, pausing over areas of pain or tension. When you feel healed, thank the flower. • Keep dried flowers in a green sachet with six small peridot or olivine crystals to bring prosperity when speculating.

CAUTION

Narcissus is regarded as toxic to humans and pets, so handle with care. • Avoid totally during pregnancy and breastfeeding.

Nasturtium

(*Tropaeolum majus*)

MAGICAL FORMS

flowering plant beloved by Benjamin Franklin, who grew it in his garden • magically use the whole, growing plant in a garden or pot; fresh or dried cut flowers or petals; tea or infusion; flower essence; and essential oil

PLANET AND ELEMENT

Jupiter • Air

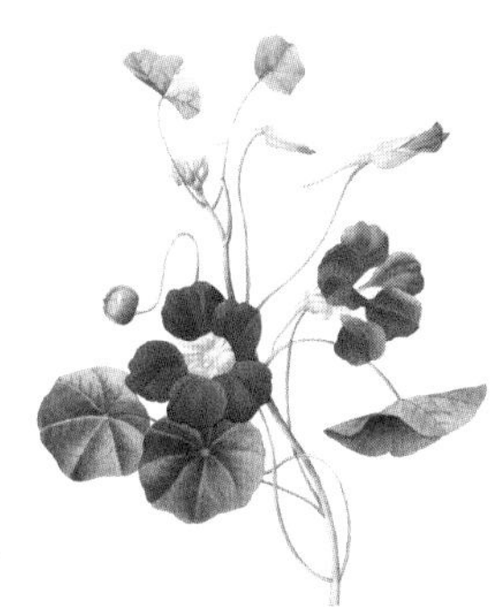

MAGICAL USES

creativity • independence, creating your own reality, not conforming to the status quo • freedom through releasing fear • overcoming prejudice • for matters concerning fathers, especially domineering ones • magical cookery • flower psychometry

HOW TO USE

Since its leaves resemble shields, inhale the fragrance of the flower or use the flower essence to follow your own path and resist intimidation from father or authority figures. • Carry the dried petals when you know you will face opposition and narrow-mindedness to your ideas or lifestyle. Afterward, release the petals to the wind to blow away any lingering effects. • Diffuse or burn essential oil if you lack inspiration in your creativity. • Take a potted nasturtium as a gift if you go home for Father's Day and your father tends to override your opinions. • Blend the well-diluted oil into lotions and creams if you have been told you are a failure or unattractive to restore your self-belief and speak up for yourself. • Use the tea or infusion sprinkled on the threshold and boundary walls to deter critical, biased neighbors.

CAUTION

Avoid if pregnant, as well as if you have kidney disease or stomach ulcers. • Oil and flowers can be a skin irritant for some people, particularly if used excessively or if not diluted well.

Neem Tree

(*Azadirachta indica*)

MAGICAL FORMS

also called the margosa tree • belongs to the mahogany family • grows on the Indian subcontinent and parts of Southeast Asia • also in the southern USA and can be grown in pots elsewhere in the world as houseplants, kept indoors in winter • magically use the whole, growing tree; leaves; and oil made from the fruit and seeds (use as a carrier rather than the pure oil)

PLANETS AND ELEMENT

Sun/Mars • Fire

MAGICAL USES

often called Earth's wish-fulfilling tree, the tree is planted near homes and hospitals because it is said to bring blessings and purify the atmosphere • to ward off evil spirits, the leaves are hung over doors to protect the home • dedicated to Kali, who is sometimes portrayed with a neem leaf • linked also with Sarasvati, Hindu goddess of wisdom, medicine, healing, divine knowledge, poetry, speech, and learning

HOW TO USE

Use the carrier oil or diluted oil for massage to bring calm and stillness to the unfocused mind. • Anoint the throat energy center at the base of the throat and Third Eye in the center of the brow for releasing creative blocks and before public speaking or performing, and the palm energy centers or inner wrist points before healing self or others. • To naturally beautify skin and hair, add a little carrier oil to shampoo or bath and, as you massage it in, picture the radiance spreading through your aura energy field for a special date or occasion where you wish to shine. • Keep your potted neem near the front door to repel all harm and filter disharmonious energies as family returns from the day.

CAUTION

If the neem oil is pure, dilute it with coconut, jojoba, or olive carrier oil (one ounce of carrier to twelve drops of pure neem) to avoid skin irritation. • Neem should not be ingested or used by those with autoimmune diseases, MS, lupus, rheumatoid arthritis, or nut allergies, or in pregnancy.

Nepalese Paper Plant

(*Daphne bholua*)

MAGICAL FORMS

winter flowering, very fragrant shrub or semishrub with yellow, pink, or white flowers and a sweet citrus scent, followed by purple berries • grows in the foothills and mountains of the Himalayas • cultivars are grown in the USA, the UK, and Europe, including Jacqueline Postill, which blooms in January and so is a herald of the New Year, with white, pink, and purple flowers and slender, smooth, brown to gray woody bark • Lokta paper has been handmade from the inner bark for thousands of years • magically use the growing plant, cut and dried flowers, and paper

PLANETS AND ELEMENTS

Moon/Jupiter • Water/Air

MAGICAL USES

paper from the plant is prized for paintings, calligraphy, and origami, and was historically used for religious and government documents • monks would embark on long journeys to obtain the paper for their sacred books • use the paper for writing magical petitions, automatic writing, and psychic artistry, and the fragrant flowers as dried flower decorations in your sacred place or altar

HOW TO USE

Recall loved ones who have passed by displaying photographs alongside a vase of the fresh or dried flowers or a bowl of potpourri in which the flowers have been added as a centerpiece on a table in your home. • Set a vase of the flowers or a bowl of potpourri and an inspiring statue, especially if Himalayan, near the door as an indwelling place for your house guardian. • Use the paper with a nonporous pen to allow your guardian angel or spirit guide to dictate messages or answer questions spontaneously via your hand and make these into a leather-bound volume.

CAUTION

The plant is toxic if ingested. • It can irritate the skin, so wear gloves when handling the plant.

Nettle

(*Urtica dioica*)

MAGICAL FORMS

used since Anglo-Saxon times in food and folk medicine • if you're growing it yourself, keep well maintained and cut back frequently, as it spreads • magically use the whole, growing plant or fresh or dried flowers, often chopped for rituals

PLANET AND ELEMENT

Mars • Fire

MAGICAL USES

a very defensive and cleansing plant traditionally grown to repel strong attack or danger or to be added to healing bags • said to encourage elves • protects the home against storms and attracts money • use in magical cookery to deter spite and jealousy and induce passion

HOW TO USE

Fill a poppet or doll with chopped fresh or dried nettles and it will act as a guardian for the home, banishing negative atmospheres, unfriendly people, and ghosts, and will return curses to their sender. • A nettle patch close to a boundary fence forms a natural magical barrier. • Freshly cut nettles, placed in a sealed jar beneath the bed, are believed to drive away any sickness and misfortune. • Burn on a bonfire if you fear you are under psychic attack.

CAUTION

Handle with care to avoid stinging yourself, and grow where small children will not be hurt.

Niaouli Tree

(*Melaleuca quinquenervia*)

MAGICAL FORMS

evergreen tree or shrub with spiky, pale-yellow, cream, red, or green flowers • native to Australia, Papua New Guinea, and the French Pacific Islands • related to the tea tree (see p. 444) and cajeput tree (see p. 94), but with a gentler, sweeter fragrance • the trees were introduced into the USA in 1900, where they became regarded as exotic but invasive, and are also found in Europe, especially France • the oil is obtained from the young leaves and twigs and is increasingly valued worldwide in aromatherapy • there are three different kinds of the essential oil from different trees of which *Melaleuca quinquenervia* and *viridiflora* are the most common, but all have similar properties • magically use the essential oil

PLANET AND ELEMENT

Moon • Water

MAGICAL USES

overcomes psychic and psychological attack, earthly and paranormal • for self-healing rituals and cleansing the aura

HOW TO USE

Diffuse or spray a few drops of the oil diluted in a water pump bottle to cleanse artifacts, rooms, and spaces for rituals. • In the morning and after the day, massage the oil mixed with sweet almond carrier oil counterclockwise into the center of your hairline, the center of your brow, your throat, and your two inner wrist points for your heart energy center, saying at each point, *May only goodness and light enter here*. This protects you from and removes all mind attacks or psychic clutter during the day and while you sleep.

CAUTION

Niaouli tree is not to be used during pregnancy, while breastfeeding, or if suffering from epilepsy, low blood pressure, or asthma.

Norfolk Island Pine

(*Araucaria heterophylla*)

MAGICAL FORMS

not actually a pine, but a relative of the monkey puzzle tree (see p. 294) • native to the South Pacific Norfolk Island, an external territory of Australia • slow growing to a towering two hundred feet outdoors in subtropical areas of the USA, such as southern California and southern Florida • can be grown indoors in a pot in more temperate climes to three feet or more (if a mini Christmas tree is rooted, it can be kept as a potted plant), even as a bonsai tree • found also on the Isles of Scilly, south of England, and in some UK arboretums • magically use the growing tree, outdoors or potted; soft bright-green needlelike leaves, which can be added to charm bags; and cones containing edible seeds

PLANET AND ELEMENT

Jupiter • Air

MAGICAL USES

Brings assurance that you and your family will never go without the necessities of life • friendship • hospitality • official symbol of Norfolk Island, shown on the flag, symbolizing harmony and unity • for winter solstice celebrations

HOW TO USE

Display cut branches as a Christmas wreath, or decorate a potted plant in the hall at Yuletide. • Adorn with small, gold ornaments and red ribbons to attract the true spirit of Christmas. • Sit close to the growing tree or use your potted plant or Christmas tree for meditation to connect with the natural world or, if you know where one grows, as the center of a magical ritual circle with small potted plants or four growing trees to mark out the magick directions of the circle. • Connect through the Norfolk Island pine in any form psychically through visualization with Zuphlas, angel of the forests, or the Norfolk Island pine indwelling spirit, who offers insight through your inner voice of unthought-of ways of increasing prosperity.

CAUTION

The Norfolk Island pine is mildly toxic to pets but not to humans, though some may experience some skin irritation from the needles.

Nutmeg

(*Myristica fragrans*)

MAGICAL FORMS

tree native to the Moluccan islands of Indonesia • cultivated in tropical zones, including those in the south of North America (see "Mace," p. 275, the waxy, reddish seed covering surrounding the nutmeg seed) • part of the spice trade as early as sixteenth century BCE • magically use the whole nutmeg with the mace coating removed, powdered or freshly ground as a culinary or magical spice, and the essential oil

PLANETS AND ELEMENTS

Saturn/Jupiter • Earth/Fire

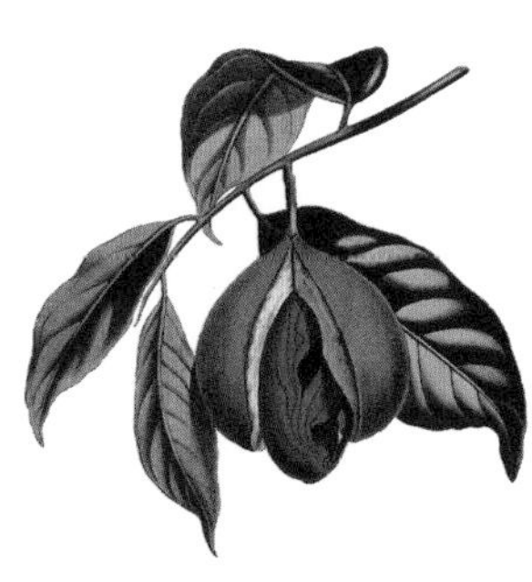

MAGICAL USES

seeds are carried as good luck charms, worn often as a necklace with star anise • powdered in an incense mix for prosperity • freshly ground in magical cookery, in small quantities only, often mixed with cinnamon, ginger, and cloves for fidelity if a partner is frequently absent or flirtatious • also for abundance and well-being to all sharing the empowered food

HOW TO USE

Make a good luck bag for gambling and games of chance with three whole nutmegs and a silver dollar. • Shake the bag three times before gaming or a lottery is drawn. • To increase clairvoyant powers, light a candle that you have rolled in a little powdered nutmeg before reading the cards or conducting a séance. • Diffuse or burn the oil sparingly in a room with ylang-ylang, jasmine, and clary sage as an aphrodisiac before lovemaking.

CAUTION

Oil should never be ingested and must be well diluted. • Do not eat the whole nuts or eat or inhale excess quantities of the spice in any form, as it is very toxic and hallucinogenic. • Do not use large amounts of the spice or oil while pregnant.

Oak Tree

(*Quercus* spp.)

MAGICAL FORMS

genus of trees including *Quercus robur*, the English or brown oak; *Quercus alba*, the white oak; and *Quercus rubra*, the red oak • called the father tree • a tree associated with the father gods of ancient Greece and Rome, Zeus and Jupiter • magically use the growing tree, wood, bark, twigs, fresh or dried leaves, and acorns

PLANET AND ELEMENT

Sun • Fire

MAGICAL USES

many oaks are up to a thousand years old, representing magical and earthly power, wisdom, expertise, and the ability to control the elements; in modern times interpreted as mastery over the self • drives away harm, fear, and impotence (actual and psychic), replacing with strength and courage • used ceremonially for purification and to create an enclosed circle for nature rituals • sitting against an oak at twilight offers a doorway to the otherworlds and prophetic insights following the ancient Greek and druidic tradition of the oak as an oracular tree • acorns symbolize fertility and new beginnings

HOW TO USE

Oak is traditionally burned on hearth or bonfires or as dried oak leaves or bark chippings in incense to remove illness from an individual or the home and to protect the home from further illness. • Oak wands and staffs are symbols of authority and power, and used in protective rituals for charitable and altruistic ventures as well as bids for leadership and increased authority, recognition of expertise, and resulting advanced financial status. • Two oak twigs bound with red thread, forming an equal armed cross, should be placed indoors facing an entrance to drive away all threats, earthly and paranormal, and to attract good fortune. • Plant an acorn once the moon is no longer visible, but before the crescent reappears, to germinate growing money in the months ahead.

CAUTION

The white oak's leaves and acorns are particularly toxic when immature and should not be ingested raw. • Bark can cause skin allergies.

Oak Tree, Arizona White

(*Quercus arizonica*)

MAGICAL FORMS

long-living, slow-growing tree whose small thick evergreen leaves, normally lasting a year, fall in spring and are immediately replaced by new ones • the most common white oak in Arizona, New Mexico, and Texas, extending south to Mexico, growing wild on sandy hillsides and rocky canyons, • its dark brown acorns are enclosed in a half cup with pointed top scales • does not thrive in the UK • magically use the bark, acorns, and flower essence (obtainable worldwide)

PLANET AND ELEMENT

Jupiter • Air

MAGICAL USES

essence counteracts depression and lethargy • fears of aging and limitations old age might bring • for adolescents who avoid responsibility, encouraging facing challenges such as learning to drive

HOW TO USE

Crumble fallen bark or buy shredded bark online to add to incense to cleanse yourself of inertia or the fear of facing up to a challenge that will bring advantage. • Bury the acorns on the new moon, when it can no longer be seen in the sky after the end of the waning cycle, to accept your current fear and on the crescent moon, two days later, to press ahead regardless. • If fears return, take the flower essence either in water or as drops under your tongue four times a day to help you keep going. You will gradually realize that, like the hardy tree, you also are filled with strength.

CAUTION

Pregnant women should avoid taking any form of white oak bark supplement medication.

Oakmoss

(*Evernia prunastri*)

MAGICAL FORMS

a lichen growing on oak trees and other deciduous trees and conifers • until recently highly prized for perfume until banned by the International Fragrance Association because it was considered a skin irritant • used in ancient Egypt in embalming mummies • also called tree moss, found in forests all over the northern hemisphere including the USA • hard to cultivate and sometimes to buy • magically use the whole plant as greenish-white or olive-green dried moss, or the oil

PLANETS AND ELEMENTS

Mars/Jupiter • Fire/Earth

MAGICAL USES

protection from storms and from natural disasters or malevolent strangers entering the home • connection with nature and nature essences, tree magick, and divination • in crone or wisewomen ceremonies • for slow but continuing financial growth

HOW TO USE

Create a money and good fortune charm bag by including a tiny piece of dried oakmoss in a red bag with a cent coin; the next day, add a slightly larger piece of oakmoss with an additional five-cent piece. On day three, include an even larger piece of oakmoss and a ten-cent piece. Keep the sealed bag where you do your accounts at home or in a cash register or near a credit card machine at work. • Make a figure out of the moss and set as a guardian outside your front door to protect against restless and malicious spirits on the land, as well as earthly intruders. Bury a green jasper or tree agate beneath it to attract the blessings of the spirits of nature. Replace the figure when it crumbles. • Mix dried oakmoss with neroli, lavender, patchouli, and cypress in incense or an oil diffuser to call a mentor or backer to further your career.

CAUTION

Oakmoss comes with many contraindications, so avoid if you have allergies to any moss or lichen. • Do not use if pregnant, breastfeeding, or suffering from epilepsy, or if you have broken skin. • Inhaling the oil or incense may irritate mucus membranes.

Oat

(*Avena sativa*)

MAGICAL FORMS

grass with small spikes containing seeds • once used to stuff mattresses, to relieve rheumatism, and as cereal eaten to speed recovery from illness • eaten mainly as oat bran or flour • magically use the whole, growing plant; seeds, raw or dried and chopped as the grain; dried stem with grain; and rolled oats in magical cookery

PLANETS AND ELEMENT

Venus/Saturn • Earth

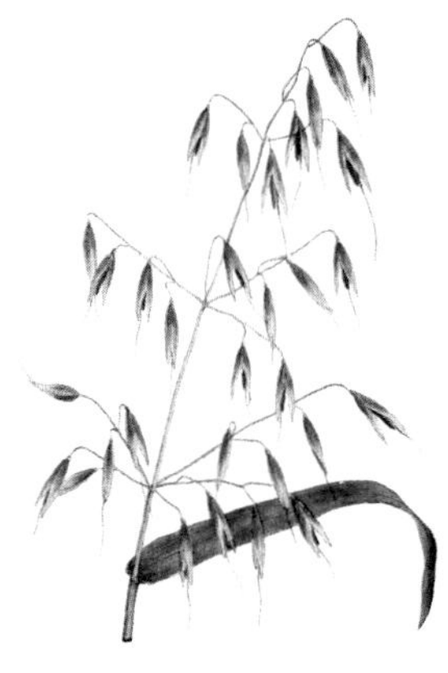

MAGICAL USES

for money, security, stability, and restoring the balance in any situation • for Lammas and other first harvest celebrations • fertility, family happiness

HOW TO USE

Sprinkle the grain on the earth at harvest time for future prosperity and as a tribute to the Earth Mother. • Gain the right employment and increase sources of income, such as with a raise, by using in magical cookery, stirring oatmeal or oat flour while chanting empowerments and then eating the empowered cooked oatmeal or oatcakes while visualizing what you are after. • Add the growing or dried grain, still on its stem, to a wedding bouquet as a symbol of fertility and abundance in the years ahead. • After the wedding, keep the dried bouquet grain hanging in the kitchen or make into a grain knot to keep the kitchen safe from accidents and to bless food that is prepared and served there with health and happiness. • Add oatstraw—the dried, chopped plant—to fertility- and money-attracting sachets and bottles. • The seeds, mixed with those of other grain seeds in a prosperity jar, should be sealed and shaken every day for a lunar month, from full moon to full moon, then scattered with the contents over a wide area of open, uncultivated land to symbolically, and maybe actually, grow.

Ocotea Tree

(*Ocotea quixos*)

MAGICAL FORMS

a large evergreen tree, native to the wilderness of the Amazon basin, on the west side of the Andes • oil is distilled from the leaves • oil has a softer, sweeter, less intense fragrance than cinnamon, which it resembles • magically use the oil and *ishpingo*, the spice made from the flowers, used since Incan times and often sold as dried flower powder mixed with the bark as tea

PLANET AND ELEMENT

Sun • Fire

MAGICAL USES

for self-confidence and personal well-being • improves body image and self-esteem • used in rituals and meditation to connect with higher nature beings and spiritual realms

HOW TO USE

Used by Indigenous people in purification ceremonies, the oil forms a powerful cleansing and protective barrier when diluted in massage. • Burn the oil, diffuse, wear as a lava aroma bracelet, or use in a roller massager for pulse points and as a personal portable diffuser to top up the psychic shield during the day or evening whenever needed. • Ishpingo spice is used as a tea to give confidence and restore self-esteem and good fortune, and as an offering that brings sight of higher nature spirits. • Ocotea can be bought online or from specialty food or herb stores. • Traditionally, ocotea is offered to the ancestors on the Day of the Dead, November 1, in ritual foods and drinks. • Sprinkle the tea infusion in a circle to protect precious artifacts or magical tools set within.

CAUTION

Avoid the oil and spice in pregnancy and if breastfeeding. • Dilute the oil very well before topical use, as it can irritate the skin.

Okra

(*Abelmoschus esculentus*)

MAGICAL FORMS

a flowering plant five to six feet tall • the green edible pods, of which there may be up to thirty on a plant during a season from midsummer to fall, are technically a fruit, but are commonly known as a vegetable • also found as red, purple, orange, and burgundy • first grown in Egypt in the twelfth century BCE • arrived in the USA three centuries ago • now grown in tropical, semitropical, and warm temperate regions of the western as well as eastern hemisphere, also in pots or in greenhouses • the elongated pods, two to three inches long and covered with fine hairs, are added to soups and stews in many countries, including the Creole cuisine of Louisiana • magically use the whole, growing plant and the fruit in cooking

PLANETS AND ELEMENT

Mars/Sun • Fire

MAGICAL USES

the seeds were used for making coffee during the blockades of the Civil War, so represent adaptability • okra increases yang energies when sudden action or assertiveness is needed • served in a communal meal to cast protection on all present from outside threats and internal divisions

HOW TO USE

Grow okra in rainbow colors, setting them on your altar or in your kitchen (for only a short time, as they go mushy) to attract abundance. • Crush okra into a bowl of water, stir well to release the sticky internal liquid, and then throw the mix out of the front door to remove curses, hexes, jinxes, or ill wishes. • Lemon juice, if added to okra, will act as an aphrodisiac. • If you sense unfriendly ghosts in the home, dry and scrape out the inside of a pod, making a lid at the top. • Wash and dry okra seeds, then add them to the dried pod to create a mini rattle.

CAUTION

Okra interferes with diabetic medicine and anticoagulants and may increase arthritic pain and occasionally causes allergies.

Oleander

(*Nerium oleander*)

MAGICAL FORMS

an evergreen shrub, originally from Africa and the Mediterranean, now grown in the USA and the UK and where the temperature does not drop below zero • flowers in summer are large, open, single or double clusters in red, peach, white, and pink, with upright stems and silvery-green leaves • can grow in pots in conservatories • a problematic plant as it is very beautiful but so lethal it may not be worth the risks • magically use the plant and flowers, fresh or dried, with extreme caution, or consider using the flower essence in lieu of actual plant matter due to the plant's toxicity

PLANET AND ELEMENT

Saturn • Earth

MAGICAL USES

for wise caution, especially with money • in the language of flowers, oleander means *Beware those who are draining you of money with flattering words* • probably too risky to send to others, but good to keep the flowers for yourself if you are gullible and fall for people's hard luck stories and "too good to be true" offers, as a reminder that what may seem appealing may also be dangerous

HOW TO USE

The red flowers are used in defensive magick to deter restless ghosts or poltergeists from remaining in the home. • A pot of the flowers set in the center of the house will drive them away. • The red flowerhead dried somewhere out of harm's way can be hung high near the entrance in a sealed, thick red bag as an amulet against spite and jealousy entering, traditionally over the doorway to keep out venomous creatures. • However, even the oil must be handled with great care—it is not recommended for aromatherapy or topical use—and there are safer psychic defense solutions in this book.

CAUTION

All parts are poisonous and should not be ingested. • Foliage may be a severe irritant. • Wash hands after handling the flowers or preferably wear gloves, and keep oleander well away from children, pets, and unsuspecting adults.

Olive Tree

(*Olea europaea*)

MAGICAL FORMS

can be found as small trees, often potted and so suitable in a small garden, yard, or balcony if space is limited • magically use the whole, growing tree; blossoms; leaves; and fruit; or as a carrier oil (virgin oil is generally used in magick)

PLANET AND ELEMENT

Sun • Fire

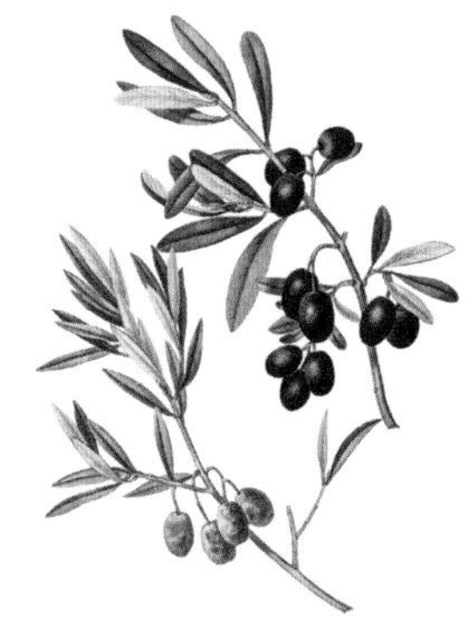

MAGICAL USES

for fertility and potency • wealth (especially green olives) • protection (black olives) • love (red Cerignola olives) • health • protection against storms and the evil eye • promotes peace (personal, family, community, workplace, global) • for divination using olive oil on water • aligned with the Fire element • for forgiveness rituals, especially of our own mistakes • in magical cookery and food (both the fruit and the oil)

HOW TO USE

Use to anoint candles and the Third Eye for protection, opening psychic powers and to attract all that is positive. • Eat an olive daily for a week, or whatever time period you desire, for a financial boost, burying the stone or pit and asking for the urgent finances you need by the end of that time period. • Make a circle of olive oil on water, or trace a pointed crystal on the surface of a pool of olive oil until the shape disappears, to remove the evil eye from loved ones, yourself, or property. • Use in spells for prosperous partnerships in love or business. • Olive blossom, when worn by brides, brings fertility and peace within the marriage.

CAUTION

Olive leaf extracts can cause dull headaches, a sore throat, body pain, and other side effects. • Avoid olive leaf if you have diabetes or low blood pressure.

Olive Tree, Wild

(*Olea oleaster*)

MAGICAL FORMS

including *Olea europaea* subsp. *cuspidate* and *Olea europaea* var. *sylvestris* • the wild olive tree is often overlooked in favor of its cultivated cousin, which was developed from the wild olive eight thousand years ago • growing still in forests of the Mediterranean; Africa, where in some regions it is a protected species; North and South America; China; and increasingly in gardens throughout the world, often in a large container, as an ornamental shrub or tree • magically work with the living tree (try a botanical garden or arboretum if you cannot find one locally); the dried, dark leaves with silver undersides; its lightly scented sprays of tiny, white flowers, fresh or dried; and small, thin, fleshy fruits, purple or yellowish-green, resembling olives, but not edible raw

PLANETS AND ELEMENTS

Jupiter/Moon • Air/Water

MAGICAL USES

brings different qualities than the peace-loving, cultivated olive • in Greek mythology, the club wielded by Hercules against the Nemean lion that was destroying the land was made from the wood of a wild olive tree • represents courage, strength, and resistance against seemingly impossible odds • during the Olympics in ancient Greece, a sacred wild olive tree stood near the temple of Zeus, patron of the games, so the wild olive is symbol of achievement

HOW TO USE

Make a small circlet on wire or raffia of the dried leaves and flowers and hang it in your workspace or home office, empowering it for achieving a dearly desired goal that will bring fulfillment or altruistic, rather than monetary, gain. • Wild olive leaf fossils have been found in Pliocene deposits in Mongardino in Italy dating up to five million years ago. • Wild olives can be used for past-life visions and sights of ancient worlds. • If you cannot obtain a wild olive, use a digital image as a screen saver or lock screen or look at a physical printout of a photo of the tree as a focus for empowerments if others treat you as second rate, to help you value your own unique nature and independence, without the approval of others.

Onion

(*Allium cepa*)

MAGICAL FORMS

common or bulb onion • an herbaceous vegetable from the amaryllis family with an edible underground bulb • the most popular kind of onion now cultivated worldwide in temperate regions • originally from southwest Asia • one or more leafless stalks growing between two and a half and six feet high, producing a spherical cluster of greenish-white flowers at the end of the season • onions came to the UK with the Romans, and the bulb onion was first recorded in the USA in 1629 • Indigenous North Americans also used a strong-tasting wild onion, *Allium canadense*, in cooking • protection of the home, like garlic hung on strings in the kitchen, is a custom attributed to the settlers in the USA • magically use the uncooked onion bulb

PLANET AND ELEMENT

Mars • Fire

MAGICAL USES

attracts good luck, money, and health • if buried, takes away illness or misfortune

HOW TO USE

To overcome sickness, obsessions, fears, and addictions, etch the name of the affliction on the outer onion skin and bury this outer skin before cooking the remaining onion. • Alternatively, bury half a cut onion after rubbing the inside of the onion on an afflicted body part or growth. • Stick black-headed pins in an onion and set it on an indoor out-facing window ledge to guard against malevolent spirits or sharp-tongued visitors. • Peel away layers of an onion, for each layer naming a wrong done to you or by you, unfair treatment, or accusations, your words mingled with the tears caused by the onion. Dispose of whatever is left, as well as the peelings, by burning or burying rather than discarding in garbage to avoid the scattering and loss of resources.

CAUTION

Onions are not toxic to humans but are to dogs and cats. • The volatile, sulfur-rich oil that gives the onion its pungency causes irritation when peeling and can irritate sensitive eyes.

Onion, Hooker's

(*Allium acuminatum*)

MAGICAL FORMS

also known as tapertip onion • a flowering plant, Hooker's onion produces bright-magenta-colored flowers on narrow stems in late spring and early summer • there may be as many as forty flowers on a stalk • strong onion smell and taste from all parts of the plant • attracts hummingbirds, bees, and butterflies • native to North America, east of the coastal ranges, in open rocky places, through Oregon, Washington, northern California, and British Columbia • can be cultivated in other parts of the USA, the UK, Europe, and southern Asia (where it is valued in cooking) • magically use the crushed and chopped plant and the flower essence, which has no odor

PLANET AND ELEMENT

Mars • Fire

MAGICAL USES

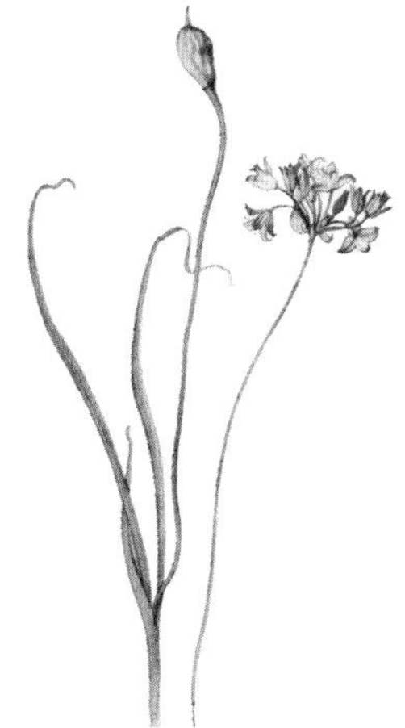

for discovering spontaneity and fun • awakens creativity and the inner child • breaks down stereotypes of parent/child interactions at any age, especially if these are very formal • helps in relating with people outside their societally assigned roles, especially in a small community, and in learning to be friends with the real person • like other pungent plants, it can be grown in the garden or made into a protective amulet to banish negativity, misfortune, and illness

HOW TO USE

Make an amulet of the crushed, dried plant and tip it away, replacing it with golden flower petals before travel if you find it hard to leave work behind on vacations. • For those undergoing rebirthing, take before preliminary sessions, or use in massage or baths to awaken or reawaken the inner child.

CAUTION

The bulbs, leaves, and bulblets are edible, but should only be eaten in small quantities.

Oppopanax Resin

MAGICAL FORMS

from the scented myrrh (*Commiphora erythraea*) tree native to Somalia and Ethiopia • called sweet myrrh as a cousin of the more astringent myrrh resin • honey and balsamic fragrance • extracted from the tree by breaking the bark and tapping or by snapping twigs • the brown or dark-red gum seeps out and solidifies • magically use as resin and essential oil

PLANET AND ELEMENT

Moon • Water

MAGICAL USES

used as incense since biblical times and in Roman temples as offerings • still burned for making petitions to higher powers • spiritually uplifting • for protection against psychic attack and emotional vampires • for revealing secrets • for meditation if focus is difficult

HOW TO USE

Burn as incense if thought forms or low-level spirits seek to take over during or after amateur seances or spirit board sessions. • Diffuse the oil or light the incense to make connection with ancestors and receive messages through smoke images or in your mind. • Anoint your brow energy center with a drop of well-diluted oil in a carrier oil such as almond, or on a candle before lighting if you need protection from those playing mind games or attempting to manipulate you through guilt.

CAUTION

The oil may cause sensitivity if the user is exposed to sunlight in the hours afterward. • Do not ingest the oil, and dilute well before applying topically.

Orange, Bergamot

(*Citrus bergamia*)

MAGICAL FORMS

cultivated plant with orange or red flowers and citrus fruits • with similar properties to and a lemony scent like wild bergamot (see p. 473), though a different plant • if a climate is tropical or subtropical, can be grown in a prosperity garden, or otherwise, often most successfully, in a pot that in more temperate climes can be brought or kept indoors to avoid frost • magically use the whole, growing plant; fresh or dried flowers; flower water; leaves; fruits; oil; and fragrance

PLANETS AND ELEMENT

Mercury/Venus • Water

MAGICAL USES

for successful property deals, encourages returns on investment and attracts both fast and substantial, longer-lasting money • reduces addictions, fears, and the hold of destructive relationships • brings new love • increases persuasiveness

HOW TO USE

Anoint your home and Third Eye chakra with flower water (beware sensitivity near eyes) to bring fresh energies and to reveal hidden truths. • Bergamot is an ingredient in many commercial perfumes, which can be enchanted as a signature fragrance to increase charisma and radiance. • Burn or diffuse the oil for communication with angels. • Bergamot leaves and dried blossoms should be kept with money to increase wealth.

CAUTION

Citrus oil users should avoid direct sunlight immediately after applying it to skin. • Avoid oil during pregnancy, and always dilute well at other times, as any citrus oil can be irritating to the skin.

Orange, Bitter

(*Citrus × aurantium*)

MAGICAL FORMS

evergreen tree, growing to thirty feet • leathery dark leaves • delicate white flowers and bitter orange fruit • native to tropical Asia • now grown throughout the tropics and subtropical Mediterranean coasts, especially Spain and through the southern USA • a blossom given by the Roman sky god, Jupiter, to his bride, Juno, on their marriage • magically use the whole, growing tree in the wild or cultivated; leaves; flowers; or flower water • most popularly used as neroli essential oil, which is made from the flowers (see "Orange Tree," p. 317; "Orange Blossom," p. 316; and "Petitgrain," p. 345)

PLANET AND ELEMENT

Jupiter • Fire

MAGICAL USES

a gentler substitute for orange oil • for all commitment ceremonies and rituals for fidelity • for abundance • a natural enhancer of confidence and self-esteem • for restoring happiness, good fortune, and trust after betrayal

HOW TO USE

Use in an aroma lamp or diffuser at home to create calm and lessen mood swings and panic attacks. • Rub a drop or two of neroli oil diluted in a carrier oil into a white candle before lighting if a proposal or plans for living together are imminent but your intended is slow in popping the question. • Anoint a yellow candle with diluted neroli oil and burn it the night before an audition or the launch of a creative venture. • Add fresh orange blossoms or a dried sprig (or the two mingled) to a bridal or handfasting bouquet for love that will last through good times and bad. • Bless magical tools, amulets, and charms with a drop or two of neroli oil. • Add neroli flower water to sacred baths before love rituals or lovemaking to bring a spiritual dimension, or wear as a perfume for the same results.

CAUTION

Dilute well as massage oil. • Do not ingest the oil or go out in the sun after using the oil. • Avoid bitter orange during the first trimester of pregnancy and seek advice after that.

Orange Blossom

from (*Citrus × sinensis*)

MAGICAL FORMS

flowers growing on orange tree, which have their own unique magical properties (see "Orange Tree," p. 317, and "Orange, Bitter," p. 315) • kept in Chinese homes and shops to welcome good fortune • magically use the cut, fresh, and dried blossoms; essential oil; flower essence; honey; and flower water

PLANET AND ELEMENT

Venus • Water

MAGICAL USES

according to myth, the Roman father god, Jupiter, gave his bride, Juno, orange blossom on their wedding day • associated strongly with weddings, commitment ceremonies, and handfastings, and sometimes handed down in carefully preserved form from mother to daughter as something old to be carried to a wedding to bring luck and a lasting happy marriage • fertility, since the fruit and blossom may appear on the tree at the same time • happiness in the home, prosperity, and abundance • health

HOW TO USE

Add fresh or dried blossoms, or a few drops of the oil, to a bath sachet to enhance radiance. • Give a massage with the well-diluted oil before lovemaking. • Inhale the oil in a diffuser or burner or as cut blossoms to calm the mind, especially prior to hypnotherapy, massage, counseling, or past-life work. • Use the water distilled from orange blossom flowers in love potions and mist oil, well diluted in water, around the home before a lover arrives. • Make a blossom love tea or use in magical cooking as an aphrodisiac. • Eat or cook with honey made from bee hives set in blossoming orchards, which increases fertility and attracts abundance to the home.

CAUTION

Orange blossom is edible to humans, but the blossoms are not generally consumed raw. • They can be toxic to pets. • Do not ingest the oil or use it undiluted. • It is mildly phototoxic, so beware going into sunlight directly after using the oil. • If pregnant, check with an expert before using the oil.

Orange Hawkweed

(*Pilosella aurantiaca*)

MAGICAL FORMS

a small lawn weed with a flat-topped circle of orange petals with russet red underneath, resembling a paintbrush • also called fox-and-cubs • similar in size to dandelion (see p. 153), to which it is related • flowers bloom from May to September • brought to the UK from its native Europe, especially alpine regions in Europe in the seventeenth century, and introduced as an ornamental plant in the USA around 1818, perhaps from contaminated lawn seed • found in Australia, where it is considered invasive • the ancient Greeks believed the milky sap of hawkweed gave hawks their acute eyesight • according to research conducted in 2009, all orange hawkweeds in the USA come from the same original flower • magically use the dried flower and flower essence

PLANET AND ELEMENT

Mercury • Air

MAGICAL USES

use the plant and essence for adults to productively express their creativity if they have a constant rush of ideas but can never settle or channel them in viable ways • for artists and writers overwhelmed by deadlines or exhibition or commission dates that freeze them into inaction • the essence helps children express creativity and imagination and channels disruptive, unfocused, and overactive energies into worthwhile interests and projects • calms ADHD

HOW TO USE

Anoint your Third Eye with the flower essence to increase clairvoyance and also for astral travel and remote or distant psychic viewing. • Use the dried flowerheads in a sachet as a fertility symbol, especially if you want many children. • Plant orange hawkweed in the garden or let it grow on the lawn so you can see it from wherever you paint, create, or write, to inspire you to shape and finish your creations. • Make a hawkweed design for your website or company logo.

CAUTION

The plant is nontoxic, but the sap can cause skin allergies and blisters.

Orange Tree

(*Citrus sinesis*)

MAGICAL FORMS

magically, the properties of the *Citrus aurantium* (bitter orange) are similar (see p. 315) • species of orange that contains several varieties of fruiting trees, including Valencia and navel oranges • can be found as miniatures in containers or pots grown in sheltered places, even in cooler climes • magically use the whole tree, leaves, fruit, blossoms, seeds, and oil made from the fruit and peel

PLANET AND ELEMENT

Sun • Fire

MAGICAL USES

prosperity • health • enhanced libido • fertility • wedded happiness • attracting love • good fortune

HOW TO USE

The planted tree brings fertility. • Hang a petition for a child to Mother Earth on the tree or plant on the night of the full moon, using a luggage label and string. Replace the petition monthly until conception. • Grate peel from an orange and add to potpourri as a luck and prosperity bringer. • Dried peel, burned with benzoin and lavender as incense, will call your soulmate. • Add peel and seeds to a sachet and place under your pillow to dream of your future marriage or commitment.

CAUTION

Avoid going into the sun after using orange, or indeed any citrus oil, as most will irritate the skin and have a phototoxic effect. • Do not take the oil internally. • Some experts advise avoiding orange oil in the first trimester of pregnancy.

Orchid

(*Orchidaceae* spp.)

MAGICAL FORMS

family of flowering plants encompassing approximately 28 thousand species • some orchids, such as *Calanthe striata*, are remarkably hardy outdoors • magically use the whole plant, fresh flowers, oil, and flower essence

PLANETS AND ELEMENT

Moon/Venus • Water

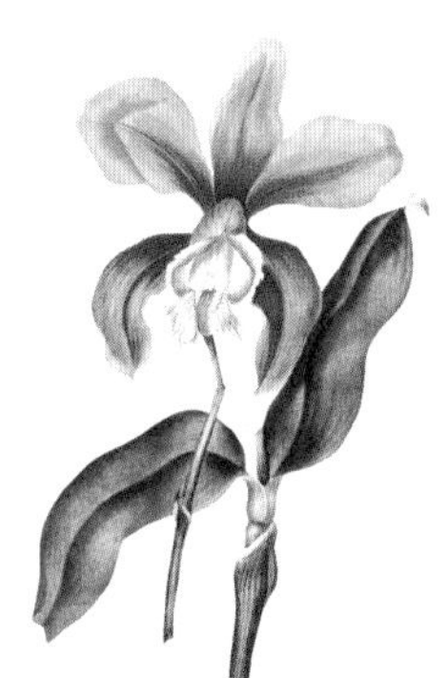

MAGICAL USES

increases visions and prophetic powers • fertility • for overcoming love rivals • striving for perfection • in spells for love, charisma, and sexual allure • also for success through recognition of achievements

HOW TO USE

Use the flower essence mixed with rose water sprinkled around your aura to enhance radiance. • Add a few drops of the oil in bath water as an aphrodisiac for reviving romance in a relationship or before a first date. • Add small quantities of the flower essence to wine, rose petal tea, or champagne as a love potion. • Keep the potted or cut flowers on your altar to manifest your unique qualities. • Plant scented orchids in sheltered places or keep indoors in your home or office for harmony—some claim to increase work production and to soften critical words. • Grow orchids to maximize the flow of positive chi.

Orchid, Bee

(*Ophrys apifera*)

MAGICAL FORMS

also known as bee flower • grows in a garden or a pot • distinguished by its brown velvety lip with yellow markings, like a female bee • magically use the petals, fresh or dried

PLANET AND ELEMENT

Mars • Fire

MAGICAL USES

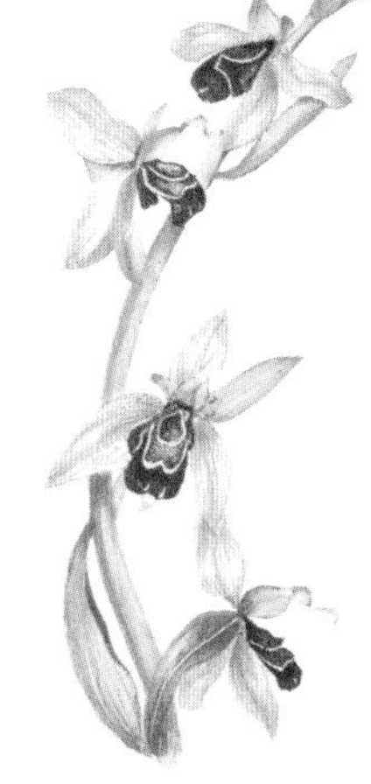

though not popular in the US or the UK, bee orchids are well worth tracking down from a specialty garden supplier • they are such wondrous plants that mimic the female bee in order to attract the male bee (though in fact they are mainly self-pollinators) • bee orchids are ideal for stealth magick where you cannot reveal your true self or purpose because of prejudice, whether in a social or work situation • the flower of actors and actresses, impersonators, drag artists, comedians, ventriloquists, and those who work undercover to solve crime or protect the vulnerable • for Goddess magick • send as a gift for putting right misunderstandings

HOW TO USE

Focus on your bee orchid in meditation (best in informal gardens or specialty potting material), and see yourself creating whatever favorable impression you need, whether at an interview, attending an audition, or assuming a more confident persona if others put you down. • When the petals fade or fall off, dry them and carry them in a protective amulet bag for whenever you need to conceal your true feelings or beliefs. • Use this only on special occasions and crises as, when you sense their power is waning, you will need to set them free and replace them. • Increasingly, it is used to offer determination to LGBTQ individuals facing community prejudice.

Orchid, Butterfly

(*Psychopsis papilio*)

MAGICAL FORMS

five known species, with bright orange and yellow flowers • though native to northern South America, Central America, and Trinidad, butterfly orchids are quite rare in gardens elsewhere, but can be grown in most areas in pots indoors • worth searching for, as they are magically the most exotic of all magical orchids • magically use mainly the potted plant in situ, which flowers through the year, and the flowers when they fall off, fresh or dried

PLANET AND ELEMENTS

Venus • Earth/Air

MAGICAL USES

a seventeenth anniversary flower, given in a pot, as a reminder of every precious day spent together and perhaps a ticket to a local butterfly conservancy • hold the pot or, if lucky enough to obtain a butterfly orchid for the garden, focus on the growing flower to connect with a beloved deceased relative on a special anniversary or when you suddenly think strongly of them • departed souls are often believed to manifest as butterflies • set the orchid in the center of the altar or spellcasting table as focus for a transformation or renewal ritual

HOW TO USE

Meditate on your butterfly orchid for astral flight, especially to shape-shift in your mind into the form of a butterfly in the colors of your plant. • When your flower falls off, dry it and mix with lavender heads and rose petals plus a small rainbow quartz in a white bag, and keep the bag until you see a rainbow in the sky. Then attach the bag to a flowering bush or tree, knowing that your plant will flower again and asking for the regeneration or rebirth you most need (worth waiting for the right conditions). • If you do need an urgent revival of happiness, love, or good fortune, bury the rainbow quartz in the soil of your plant, and as you hold the pot, ask Iris the angel of the rainbow or Psyche the ancient Greek butterfly goddess and symbol of the soul to restore joy and love in a new way.

CAUTION

The butterfly orchid is toxic if ingested. • It may occasionally cause some skin irritation.

Orchid, Green Bog

(*Platanthera huronensis*)

MAGICAL FORMS

native to Alaska, widespread throughout boggy areas in the Rockies and in the eastern half of the USA, in western Europe, Scotland, and scattered areas of northern England and Wales • one of the smallest wild orchids, fragrant at night • can be cultivated in boggy areas of a garden • green flowers, of which there may be up to seventy-five on a single plant • magically work with the growing wild orchid or flower essence (note that some common essences are derived from similar species, such as *Platanthera obtusata* or *Platanthera aquilonis*)

PLANET AND ELEMENT

Moon • Water

MAGICAL USES

removes fears of all kinds that manifest as an inability to connect with others or to become emotionally and physically intimate • for city or apartment pets that have become detached from nature, add to pet water or food

HOW TO USE

Add the essence to cut-flower water or the soil around a growing plant, especially any orchid, to become aware of and connect with natural cycles in urban settings. • Spritz the essence in water or add a few drops to a humidifier for teens and children who are obsessed with video games or their smartphones and do not communicate with others or spend time outdoors. • If you can find the growing flowers or create your own bog garden, merge with what the early Medieval mystic Hildegard von Bingen called "the greening principle" to fill yourself with the life force and the ability to flow with the natural cycles of the seasons. • Cast small green crystals into the boggy area around the flowers to let go of old hurts and pains that have caused you to cut yourself off from others so you can reach out once more.

Orchid, Lady's Slipper

(*Cypripedioideae* subfamily within *Orchidaceae*)

MAGICAL FORMS

the yellow version of this small exotic flower (*Cypripedium calceolus*), the Greek name of which means "the foot of Aphrodite" • lady's slipper is also known as the fairy slipper • belonging to the orchid subfamily, has a pouch that gives the flower its name • presently subject to preservation efforts, as some species are threatened or endangered • the state flower of Minnesota • magically use the growing plant and petals

PLANETS AND ELEMENTS

Saturn/Venus • Earth/Water

MAGICAL USES

to find love at first sight • guards against hexes and curses • the pink kind is often called the moccasin flower (*Cypridedium acaule*) because it was said to have grown for the first time in the spring after an Ojibwe maiden made a perilous journey through the snow to obtain medicine for her sick people • she lost her moccasin and left a trail of blood in the snow; therefore it represents happiness and love after suffering, as well as altruism • as its name suggests, it attracts the fae and benign household spirits to the garden, especially in its yellow or pink shades • its purple form brings wealth and the white new or first love

HOW TO USE

Give the lady's slipper in a pot as a special love gift, as well as after a loss or at anniversaries and birthdays to express lasting devotion through good times and bad. • The orchid is a perfect addition to a newlywed couple's first home, as it brings lasting happiness, especially if the couple has experienced difficulties being together. • Use the dried, pink, mildly fragrant petals in a sleep pillow with lavender or rose petals for calm sleep and peaceful dreams. • Carry the petals of a lady's slipper in a sachet and keep with printouts of your tickets and other documents before traveling if you are uncertain about a journey or vacation, especially if you are traveling in the wilderness or where there are many diseases or conflict.

CAUTION

As the stem can be covered with hairs, handle carefully to avoid contact dermatitis if your skin is sensitive.

Orchid, Laelia

(*Laelia* spp.)

MAGICAL FORMS

the best-known kinds are the fragrant *Laelia rubescens* and *Laelia anceps* • usually white, pink, or pale lavender • grows wild in Mexico and Brazil and in tropical regions of the USA on the bark of trees, especially oaks, and sometimes rocks • blooms naturally in fall and winter • can grow in extreme temperatures • magically buy as cultivated cut flowers, or grow in pots or on tree bark

PLANETS AND ELEMENT

Moon/Venus • Water

MAGICAL USES

a fourteenth wedding anniversary flower that communicates the message *I will love no other but you* • symbol of dedication, purity, and lasting fidelity in love • according to the American Orchid Society, Laelia was the name of one of the Vestal Virgins in Rome who guarded the sacred flame of Vesta, mentioned by Tacitus in 62 CE

HOW TO USE

Because the Vestal Virgins dedicated their lives for thirty years to the goddess Vesta, Laelia orchids also represent single-minded devotion if a couple cannot be together and have sacrificed their love because of prior commitments and will wait many years if necessary until free to love openly. • Light a white candle near a potted white Laelia orchid of any kind if you have decided to remain celibate before marriage because of a spiritual or religious calling. • If you have decided to postpone serious relationships while pursuing an all-consuming course of action, or you devote your life to care for a chronically sick adult or child, breathe in the light and fragrance of the Laelia orchid when you find your promise too hard to keep.

Orchid, Sparrow's-Egg Lady's-Slipper

(*Cypripedium passerinum*)

MAGICAL FORMS

a multistemmed flower, growing up to twenty inches • found farther north in North America than any other slipper species, just south of the Arctic and subarctic regions of Canada and Alaska, and south to northern Montana • known as sparrow's egg because of the white, oval shape of the flower with purple spots • the plants are rare and protected but can be grown in gardens with care • magically use the whole, growing plant in situ or as flower essence

PLANETS AND ELEMENTS

Saturn/Venus • Earth/Water

MAGICAL USES

to repair insecure body/soul connection, where life is either experienced only practically and materially or as dreams and illusion that may be at odds with reality • for overcoming shock and trauma after a problematic birth, whether for mother, child, or both • for gentle healing of deep-seated wounds from years before or even from a past life

HOW TO USE

Begin with a drop of the essence on each sole of your feet to move forward from the past. • Add a drop behind each knee to overcome grief, trauma, and regrets. • Place a single drop on the sacral chakra around the navel to restore a desire for living, and to mend any birth traumas or postnatal depression. • Add a drop on the inner side of each wrist to heal the heart of pain, and in the middle of the hairline to connect or reconnect body and spirit and to remove any past karma causing fears or restrictions in the present life.

CAUTION

Parts of the plant are considered poisonous to ingest, but no sufficient research has been done to affirm or deny safety, so it is best avoided in pregnancy. • Handling the plant may cause a skin allergy.

Orchid, Vanilla

(*Vanilla planifolia*)

MAGICAL FORMS

fermented climbing orchid on vine • cultivated in the USA in Florida, Puerto Rico, and Hawaii • the bean is the fruit of the orchid plant, which grows as a long, brown seed pod containing hundreds of tiny black seeds • magically use the pure extract, essential oil, powder, and whole bean

PLANET AND ELEMENTS

Venus • Water/Earth

MAGICAL USES

passion • fidelity • marriage vows and renewal of vows • for a good self-image • health and harmony • preserving youthfulness • sexual and personal vitality and increasing radiance

HOW TO USE

Add a bean or the extract to magical cookery, especially in a cake also containing rose petals and angelica to increase romance and charisma when your lover calls. • Add vanilla powder or a few drops of the essence or oil to potpourri in a mint and sage mix in your work or study space to improve focus and concentration, and aid in memorizing important facts. • Keep dried vanilla powder and dried yarrow leaves or flowers in a small, natural fabric bag or purse over your bed for seven years for a faithful and joyous marriage (or replace when it loses its fragrance).

Oregano

(*Origanum vulgare*)

MAGICAL FORMS

sometimes called wild marjoram, although this name also refers to a cross between sweet marjoram (*Origanum majorana*) and wild marjoram (*O. vulgare*) • magically use the whole, growing plant; flowers; leaves; and both essential and extracted oil

PLANETS AND ELEMENT

Jupiter/Mercury/Venus • Air

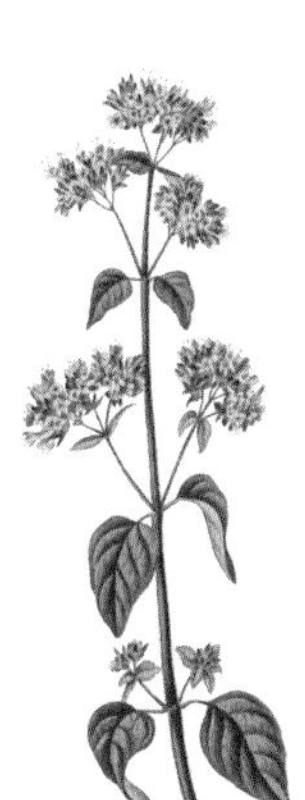

MAGICAL USES

protects against interference in your business, home affairs, and love life • use in magical cookery • in healing spells • a ceremonial plant for bereavement and mourning • for prophetic dreams • for safe travel • for justice

HOW TO USE

Burn sprigs of the oregano plant for a private memory of someone you cannot mourn openly or who found passing hard. • Place sprigs or a pot of oregano on or near a grave once the funeral flowers have faded. • Inhale the oil or crushed leaves to let go of past loves, especially if you must still see your ex. • Burn the oil before a court case or official inquiry. • Plant in the garden to protect home and pets or in a pot in the kitchen to bring lasting peace, security, and wealth, and to prevent kitchen accidents and quarrels at home. • Make a travel charm bag, adding a citrine, dried bay leaves, and oregano, and keep with travel documents to avoid last-minute panics. Make it the last thing you place in your hall before going on vacation to speed your journey and keep your home safe while you are away.

CAUTION

Do not take the essential oil internally, and be sure to dilute it well for skin use. • Avoid oregano if you are allergic to mint, and do not use while pregnant.

Oregano, Greek

(*Origanum creticum*) or (*Origanum vulgare* subs. *hirtum*)

MAGICAL FORMS

compact, woody, bushy plant with very aromatic dark-green leaves and spikes of small white, pink, or light-purple flowers in clusters • blooming from midsummer to fall • the plant is six to eight inches tall • oregano in its many forms is one of the most powerful magical herbs • Greek oregano is native to Greece, Turkey, and the Aegean, where it grows wild • can be cultivated in the UK and USA and in gardens in most temperate regions in the northern hemisphere • keep as a potted plant or in an indoor herb garden • magically use the dried spicy herb, whether purchased in a store or dried and chopped from your own leaves; fresh or dried flowers; or the whole plant in situ

PLANETS AND ELEMENT

Jupiter/Mercury • Air

MAGICAL USES

for all empowerments for family matters • often added to pizza and pasta for dealing calmly and firmly with teenage sulks and rebellion • for healing relationship rifts • resolving matters where plain speaking and tough love are needed

HOW TO USE

Because Greek oregano is stronger than ordinary oregano in flavor, it will bring extra power to spells and empowerments. • With its Greek origins, it has strong connections with Aphrodite, the ancient Greek love goddess. • Woven into a bridal headdress, Greek oregano in flower or the dried flowers ensure the marriage will be strong and faithful. • A few grains of the dried and chopped herb sprinkled into the flame of a lighted red candle will deter a love rival and love temptation. • Burn only for a minute as the flame sparkles. • Extinguish (do not blow out) the candle and dispose of it in a paper bag in which you have tipped more Greek oregano. • Throw the bag in a garbage bin near the rival's home if possible (it will not harm, just protect your love).

CAUTION

Avoid in pregnancy as all oregano is a uterine stimulant.

Orris Root

from (*Iris* spp.)

MAGICAL FORMS

the fresh or dried root of the Iris plant, often *Iris × germanica* or *Iris × florentina* (see "Iris," p. 231) • fragrance similar to violets • orris root essential oil has been treasured as a perfume since ancient Greek times, so it is very rare and expensive • the oil is sometimes sold in the modern world diluted with olive or jojoba oil that is good for diffusing • magically use as whole fresh or dried root, essential oil, and fragrance

PLANETS AND ELEMENTS

Mercury/Moon • Air/Water

MAGICAL USES

powdered or whole dried orris root is used in rituals and charm bags for female leadership, authority, and breaking through glass ceilings • as a potpourri fixative, especially valued if the mix is empowered to fix domestic or workplace situations that stand between you and happiness • positive change • prosperity

HOW TO USE

Orris root aids focus and concentration for intellectual as well as spiritual purposes if combined with celery seeds and added to incense or a charm bag. • Use before a date to give yourself extra charisma. • Dilute essential oil well to massage your inner wrist points. • Carry the root in an orange bag with dried lavender heads and rose petals and a few drops of the oil added before closing the bag, so that the right person's eyes will fix upon you and remain on you. • Diffuse the oil for confidence and authority in the room in which you will be gathering if you are coming out sexually to a family you know will not approve. • Use a well-shaped and well-trimmed root inverted as a pendulum to answer love questions and choices. • Suspend a dried orris root with dried sage as high as possible inside your home so air circulates to protect the premises and family against physical, psychological, and psychic malevolence, and harm is turned back upon the sender.

CAUTION

Though orris root has traditionally been used medicinally, it may not be safe to ingest the fresh juice or root. • The root may cause allergic reaction for those with sensitive skin. • As a precaution, avoid in pregnancy.

Osmanthus

(*Osmanthus* spp.)

MAGICAL FORMS

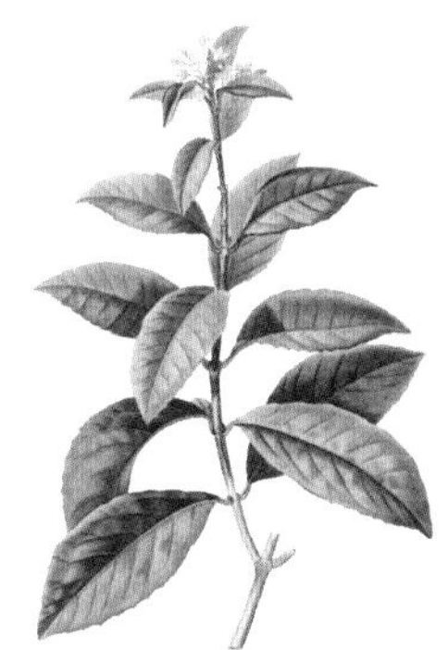

flowering evergreen shrub or small tree whose name comes from the Greek for *fragrant flower* • with small, tubular, white, yellow, or orange intensely fragrant flowers, appearing in later summer and fall • blue-black ovoid berries are native to Japan, China, Thailand, Cambodia, and the Himalayas • now, especially as *Osmanthus fragrans*, grown in North America, Europe, and other warm, temperate regions • can be potted • magically use the whole, growing plant; fresh or dried flowers or flowerheads; and essential oil made from the flower

PLANET AND ELEMENT

Mercury • Air

MAGICAL USES

cleansing • fertility • twin soul love • fidelity • making a permanent love commitment • the flowers added to wedding bouquets • protection against rivals and opposition to a relationship • peace • magical cookery • essential oil for spiritual heightening and overcoming setbacks • in China, a bride offers the flowers to her new family

HOW TO USE

Grown in a garden, cut or potted osmanthus draw good fortune into the home. • Give the flowers to a rival to disarm their intentions. • Osmanthus essential oil (from *Osmanthus fragrans*) can be burned, diffused, or added to a ritual bath. Can also be diluted for massaging the center of the brow or the Third Eye psychic energy center, or to lift meditation, yoga, and energy transference to heightened spiritual awareness.

CAUTION

Consult a physician or midwife when using the oil if pregnant, as the jury is out on safety. • Dilute the oil very well if applied to the skin.

Pale Pitcher Plant

(*Sarracenia alata*)

MAGICAL FORMS

also known as yellow trumpets • a carnivorous plant with modified green or purple leaves, forming pitchers producing nectar and a pleasing scent • insects attracted to the pitchers lose grip on the pitcher's waxy surface and drown in the fluid at the base • the pale-yellow flower nods forward behind the pitchers and blooms slightly ahead of the pitchers, allowing for safe pollination • blooms in the second half of the spring • the plant is six inches to four feet tall • grows in Texas, Louisiana, Mississippi, and Alabama, and is becoming endemic in the southeastern regions of the USA • also grows in the UK and parts of Europe • can be produced in large pots indoors in many places • magically work with the growing plant, outdoors and in

PLANET AND ELEMENT

Mars • Fire

MAGICAL USES

for removing what is destructive in your life, including bad habits, addictions, and obsessions • for avoiding fatal attractions, unwise influences, romance scams on- and offline, and making risky investments or gaming

HOW TO USE

Work with an indoor plant, tangling thick, red thread to represent temptation and destructive impulses, or people you know are bad for you, around the pot. Cut the pot free and burn the thread. • Alternatively, tie the thread around the stem of one of the outdoor plants. Cut that carefully and bury it beneath the plant. If hoping to kick an addiction, afterward bury a small symbol of the temptation, for example a crushed cigarette, a drop or two of alcohol, or a gambling chip.

Palm

(*Arecaceae* spp.)

MAGICAL FORMS

a large family of plants commonly known as palms • grown either indoors as potted plants, such as the nontoxic parlor palm (*Chamaedorea elegans*), or outdoors in warm climates, such as the smaller dwarf date palmetto (*Phoenix roebelenii*), the even smaller minor palmetto that is suitable for limited outdoor areas or containers indoors (*Sabal minor*), or if you have room, the full-sized date palm (*Phoenix dactylifera* or *roebelenii*) • magically use the whole tree, leaves, fronds, fruit, and small berries of the palmettos, or as a carrier oil

PLANET AND ELEMENT

Sun • Fire

MAGICAL USES

brings immense good fortune • prosperity • fertility and potency • abundance • health • protection against harm, earthly and paranormal • potted palms powerfully transmit the life force throughout the home • for scrying with oils

HOW TO USE

In feng shui, indoor plants such as parlor palms draw good fortune, divert poison arrows, and prevent excessively fast chi from rushing through the home. • Palms purify any emotional toxicity. • Use palm oil to anoint white candles for fall and midwinter rituals to bring prosperity. • Palm fronds, woven into crosses and placed in olive or palm oil bottles, make the oil sacred. The crosses are then either burned and the ashes rubbed on the forehead for purification or added to cleansing incense mixes. • The pits of the fruit or the berries are carried in a small charm bag to increase potency and fertility or placed beneath the mattress when trying to conceive a child (see "Date Palm," p. 154).

CAUTION

While many palms are not toxic, always check the species and beware some also have spikes. • Sago palm (*Cycas revoluta*), for example, is highly toxic.

Palmarosa

(*Cymbopogon martinii*)

MAGICAL FORMS

sweet with grassy leaves that have a roselike fragrance • the oil comes from the fresh or dried grass and is popular in perfumes • native to India and Pakistan, also now growing in Africa, Brazil, the Comoro Islands off the southeast coast of Africa, and Indonesia • magically use the essential oil

PLANETS AND ELEMENTS

Mercury/Venus • Air/Earth

MAGICAL USES

dispels jealousy and unkindness in self and others • assists concentration, especially in later years (diffuse while learning new facts or techniques) • creates a sense of security in uncertain situations

HOW TO USE

Prepare a party or celebration room with dishes of potpourri infused with the oil on every table. You may end up with a budding romance or two by the end of the evening. • If you are anxious with unfamiliar people, crowds, or new situations, subtly inhale a drop of the oil or use your roller massager or aroma bracelet to restore your equilibrium and draw people to you who are natural kindred spirits. • If uncertain whether a person you are due to meet is safe with your heart or money, float a few drops of the oil on the surface of a small bowl of water. Mix the water with the index finger of your writing hand, then close your eyes as you stir and you will see with your inner eye an image of what you need to know about the person and their reliability.

CAUTION

Avoid in pregnancy and when breastfeeding. • Dilute well if you have sensitive skin.

Palo Santo

(*Bursera graveolens*)

MAGICAL FORMS

related to frankincense and myrrh • from South and Central America, especially Peru • milder and sweeter than sage • magically use the dried wooden sticks or essential oil

PLANETS AND ELEMENTS

Mars/Jupiter • Fire/Air

MAGICAL USES

traditionally used by shamans from Inca times for healing, to remove bad luck, unhelpful thought patterns, and malevolent spirits, still offered today to any respectful user • removes stress and agitation • energy cleanser and balancer in the home, aura, and business (subject to fire regulations, or draw a plan of the workplace and smudge that) to clear discord, disharmony, minor ills, and sick-building-syndrome energy • replaces it with a sense of well-being and compassion toward even rivals

HOW TO USE

Ignite the tip of the piece of wood, holding it at a forty-five-degree angle in the flame, and allow it to flare briefly, then blow it out. Set the smoking stick either in the center of your home in a fire resistant bowl or carry it in a heatproof dish from room to room to lift the vibrations. • Each morning, use the oil, diluted well with a carrier such as coconut or jojoba oil, to anoint the center of the forehead above the eyes, the brow chakra energy center (Third Eye). Avoiding eyes, nose, and mouth, also anoint the throat energy center at the base of the throat and the two inner wrist points for the heart, at each chakra or energy center, sealing the entrance to your spirit from all that is not from the light. • Mix the oil with frankincense, lavender, or bergamot in a diffuser to remove any lingering negative vibes in the home after difficult visitors or quarrels and to infuse the air with loving vibes. • Burn shavings of the wood as incense before meditation, mediumship, or healing rituals, and to connect with the higher realms of angels, saints, and guides.

CAUTION

This sacred wood should be treated with respect. • Check oils and wood to ensure they are genuine and come from ethically produced sources and not prematurely cut trees. • If using topically, do a patch test and always dilute well.

Palo Verde Tree

(*Parkinsonia aculeata*)

MAGICAL FORMS

Spanish for *green stick*, referring to the trunk, also called Jerusalem thorn • magically similar to the yellow or foothill palo verde (*Cercidium microphyllum*), found mainly on rocky slopes, and the blue palo verde (*Cercidium floridum*) with a blue-green trunk, which grows near water sources • foothill palo verde can live up to four hundred years • spiny desert shrub or tree, native to the southwestern USA and northern Mexico, introduced into Spain, Africa, and Australia • in Spain, Africa, and Hawaii it is regarded as invasive • colorful, fragrant, yellow flowers with orange patches • the desert museum palo verde tree is thornless, hybridized at the Arizona Sonora Desert Museum in Tucson • leaves and roots are used medicinally in infusions and the beans are traditionally eaten cooked, raw, or in flour by Indigenous people • magically use the growing tree, flowers, fresh or dried leaflets, upright reddish thorns separated from the branches or cut and left on small branches, and seeds

PLANET AND ELEMENT

Mars • Fire

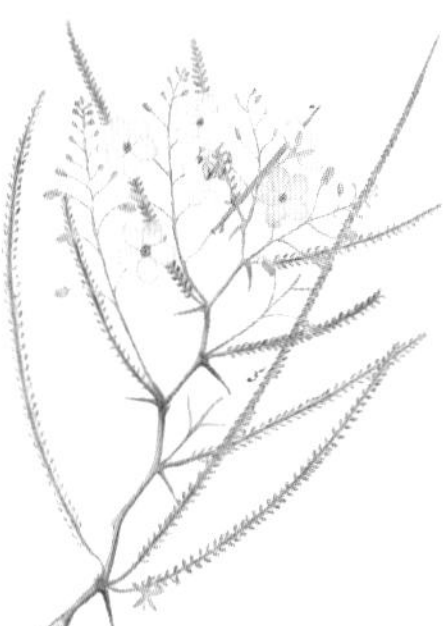

MAGICAL USES

attracts abundance, happiness, and fertility • protects against and removes negative energies • defensive against all earthly and paranormal ill wishes and intrusion • aligns body, mind, and spirit

HOW TO USE

To create a sacred space around yourself, meditate close to a thornless tree for harmony and the removal of obstacles and unhelpful people, and near the thorned kind (with care) for fierce defense if you or loved ones are being threatened by spirits or human intimidation. • Use the dried leaflets to sprinkle around artifacts, to form a ritual circle, or scatter on the front and back doorstep and sweep outward to remove misfortune or illness, or if there have been curses or ill wishes set against the house or family.

Palo Verde Tree, Foothill

(*Parkinsonia microphylla*)

MAGICAL FORMS

also called little-leaved palo verde or yellow palo verde • the toughest and most resilient of the spiny desert palo verde shrubs and trees • found wild in hot and arid areas of Arizona, eastern California, and Mexico • the smallest of the species, needing less water than its sister the blue palo verde, so it can grow in desert upland areas • like other palo verde, if there is a drought, it will shed its leaves and branches but revive when water returns • magical tea can be made with the dried flowers or the seeds • can be ground into flour • widely obtainable as a flower essence (see "Palo Verde Tree," p. 325) • magically use the growing tree with yellow trunk, yellow green leaves, and yellow blossoms

PLANET AND ELEMENT

Mars • Fire

MAGICAL USES

the growing tree, seeds, and flowers share the energy to overcome harsh judgments of self and others and the too-high demands of perfectionism • the flower essence, which is also sometimes sold combined with buffalo gourd essence for extra strength, assists in conserving energies in crisis or unpromising situations until the time is right to try again

HOW TO USE

Take the flower essence regularly to accept imperfections in yourself and others and accept that the present may not be the right time to squander energies in an unpromising situation. • Add a few drops to a bath or a chamomile-based massage oil to prevent overthinking or overreaction and to create an inner stillness. • Visit the plant in the wild or a botanical garden to see the flowers in bloom. • Breathe yellow into your aura energy field and find peace and joy in the moment. • Alternately, to receive these energies, meditate on a large printout of the blossoming trees.

Pampas Grass

(*Cortaderia selloana*)

MAGICAL FORMS

feathery white plumes • grows up to ten feet high, blooming in summer and fall • silver, pink, and purple flowers • dwarf pampas grass (*Cortaderia selloana pumila*) with ivory or yellow plumes only grows to about five feet so can be developed in containers • though native to South America, pampas is very hardy, flourishing naturally not only in warmer parts of North America, where it was introduced by the Spanish conquistadors, as well as Australia and New Zealand, but also in cooler climes such as the UK • magically use the whole plant, growing or cut and dried to fit in a tall floor-standing vase; the dried flowerheads for good luck; freshly cut pampas for special occasions; and the sharp leaves as defense—a magical practitioner's store in one plant!

PLANETS AND ELEMENTS

Saturn/Jupiter • Earth/Air

MAGICAL USES

for meditations and in spells where it is important to maintain dignity and determination for what is of worth • indoors, its feathery plumes continually filter out stagnation, misfortune, quarrels, and ill health • cut fresh pampas to fit bouquets, for celebratory arches, and for Thanksgiving or Yule arrangements

HOW TO USE

Carefully hang part of a stem with dried leaves high over the outer door to keep away spite, envy, critical words, and unkind actions. • Plant pampas grass, full size or dwarf, in the corners of your property outside as guardians of your boundaries. Keep the small pots indoors in the corners of your home. • Meditate on growing pampas, if necessary in a botanical garden, as a focus for astral projection and ancient ceremonies from its pre-Columbian past. • In the 1970s, pampas grass in the front garden was taken as a sign that the residents were sexually liberal. Harness this fun aspect as an aphrodisiac in existing relationships and put a few cut plumes in a red bag under the mattress before lovemaking.

CAUTION

Beware of sharp leaves.

Pandan

(*Pandanus amaryllifolius*)

MAGICAL FORMS

tropical shrub similar in appearance to the palm with fragrant leaves • there are over six hundred species in the genus *Pandanus* that all have similar effects magically, including *Pandanus odoratissimus*, sometimes called the fragrant screw-pine • native to Indonesia, grows in the Philippines and Southeast Asia and in those parts of the USA and beyond where there is a consistently warm climate • generally edible • female trees have fragrant flowers • males in many species bear red-orange pinecone-like fruits • magically use the fruit and fresh or dried leaves as tea

PLANET AND ELEMENT

Sun • Fire

MAGICAL USES

protection • reliability in others • brings stability of emotions • use leaves in magical cookery • use whole, dried leaves (pandan leaves can be bought fresh, frozen, or dried from many Asian grocery stores or online) to wrap magical tools when not in use, tied loosely with red thread

HOW TO USE

Etch what you most desire on the inside of a dried whole leaf with a sharp awl or thin-bladed knife. • Secure a crystal or coin inside, and offer the parcel to the ocean or a fast-flowing river. • Share with friends as a tea or a cold drink to reinforce friendship, some given first to the earth along with a handful of dried flowers if available, to ask Earth Mother blessings. • Leave the pinecone-like fruit in a cairn (a pile resting one on top of the other in a pyramid shape) in a high place to attract the blessings of the wind spirits.

CAUTION

Avoid if you have kidney problems.

Pansy

(*Viola × wittrockiana*)

MAGICAL FORMS

species of flowering plant within the *Viola* family • magically use the fresh flowers and dried petals

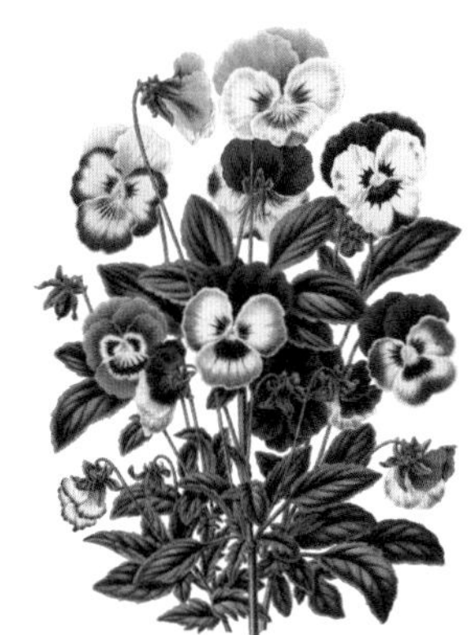

PLANETS AND ELEMENTS

Saturn/Venus • Earth/Water

MAGICAL USES

for rain magick • healing • connecting two lovers, family members, or friends telepathically • bringing thoughts of the home and garden if someone is far away • happy stepfamilies • friends and lovers from the past returning • in the language of flowers, pansies signify nostalgia • in Shakespeare's *A Midsummer Night's Dream,* the mischievous Puck, on the orders of the fae king Oberon, pressed wild pansy juice or heartsease into the fae queen Titania's eyes while sleeping so she would fall in love with the first person she saw on awakening, signifying illusion

HOW TO USE

Young lovers used pansies to represent secret love, in bouquets tied with pink or green ribbons. They would plant it in the shape of a heart. If the flowers flourished, love would be true and lasting. • A sailor's wife or mother would traditionally bury sand or shells beneath pansies to keep her in his thoughts and so he would return safely; in modern times any sailor's partner left at home can do this. • Pansies are found in many rainbow colors: red invokes passion, purple calls back lost love, and pink planted in a garden brings romance and faithful love.

CAUTION

Do not ingest in pregnancy, as pansies can bring on labor.

Pápalo

(*Porophyllum ruderale*)

MAGICAL FORMS

ancient herb, native to Mexico, Central America, and the southwestern USA • can be grown in warmer climes or indoors in pots • the leaves are especially popular in Mexican cooking, and taste like a mix of cilantro, lemon, arugula, and parsley • best harvested at the end of summer when the herb is about six inches tall and leaves can be taken as needed, as more will grow • magically use the fresh, dried, or frozen leaves, available in specialty cookery stores, farmers' markets, or online

PLANET AND ELEMENTS

Mercury • Air/Fire

MAGICAL USES

the Mayans and Aztecs used pápalo for medicinal, magical, and culinary purposes • believed from Aztec times to increase spiritual awareness and bring connection with the deities • will cut through earthly clutter for clear psychic and mental vision

HOW TO USE

Take a few leaves from the top of the plant or defrost frozen leaves (dried are good magically but not so flavorful). • Shred and add them to cooking or use them whole as garnish, asking as you stir for blessings on your home and family. • Display a pot of the sprigs on your meditation or divinatory table to make connection with angels, spirits, guides, ancestors, or your personal deities. • Scatter a few leaves outdoors on a windy day to clear confusion and see through those who would deceive or deliberately create misunderstandings.

CAUTION

Pápalo is an allergen for some; use caution before ingesting if pregnant.

Papaya

(*Carica papaya*)

MAGICAL FORMS

growing tree can reach twenty-six feet • yellow flowers • native to southern Mexico, northern South America, and Florida, papaya can now be grown in any tropical regions, including Arizona, southern California, Hawaii, and Texas, and the fruit can be obtained worldwide • magically use the fresh or dried flowers, branches with fresh or dried leaves, wood, tropical fruit, and flower remedy

PLANET AND ELEMENT

Sun • Fire

MAGICAL USES

for abundance • fertility • absorbing the power of the sun • transformation and renewal • rituals to bring positive energies and good fortune • dried or powdered leaves in incense mixes to attract money, increase the tempo of love, and enhance self-image • opens the path to angelic communication (often called the fruit of the angels)

HOW TO USE

Hang twigs in an equal-armed cross tied with red twine just outside and over the door to keep earthly and spirit malevolence away. • Keep a small fallen branch as a prayer tree on which to hang wishes and petitions in the form of white cloth strips with the petition written visibly or invisibly on each. • Scoop out the seeds, share some of the fruit with a lover, bury the rest, and cast the seeds into water at precisely sunrise (verify the time) before lovemaking to conceive a child. • Carry a piece of dried skin from fruit you have eaten plus five gold-colored coins in a gold bag for an inflow of wealth.

CAUTION

Skin and seeds are toxic and should not be ingested.

Papyrus

(*Cyperus papyrus*)

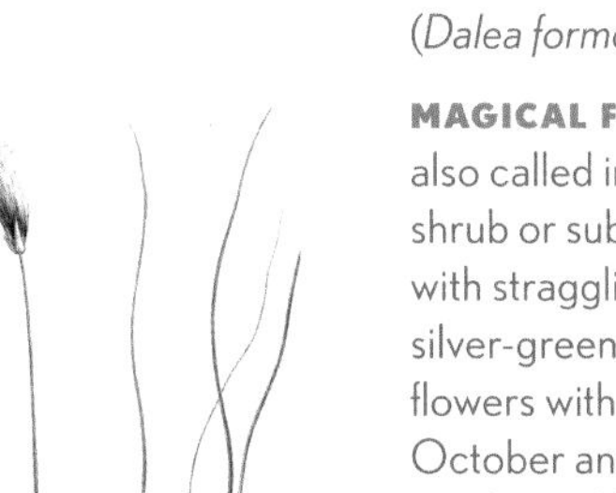

MAGICAL FORMS

also called papyrus sedge or Nile grass • tall (thirteen to sixteen feet high), stately, green sedge growing wild, cultivated in water gardens and containers (as dwarf papyrus plant *Cyperus haspan*) • found in wetter parts of Africa, Madagascar, and the Mediterranean countries; the Indian subcontinent; the Caribbean; and southern parts of North America • magically use as pure fragrant oil without alcohol, as essential oil, as sacred paper for magical petitions, and as a reed pen

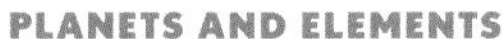

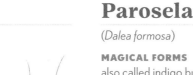

PLANETS AND ELEMENTS

Venus/Mercury • Water/Air

MAGICAL USES

traditionally placed in boats to ward off the Egyptian crocodile god Sobek, cut and woven into knots as an amulet for safe sea voyages and to repel those who are false • the dried flowers or diffused oil recall ancient worlds • for drawing talismans or images of Egyptian deities set on the altar in Egyptian-inspired rites with a reed pen and red or black ink • papyrus wrapped around a printout of a book you are writing or even your tablet brings inspiration

HOW TO USE

Use oil to anoint your Third Eye or brow energy center clockwise to open your psychic channels and counterclockwise to keep out all harm. • Anoint your throat energy center at the base of your throat for clear communication and to speak the truth with kindness. • Draw the ankh (♀), the sign of Isis and Osiris, the Egyptian divine couple, in red ink on a square of papyrus. Keep the drawing in a clear glass bottle for attracting your twin soul or preserving existing love.

Parosela

(*Dalea formosa*)

MAGICAL FORMS

also called indigo bush or feather plume • a many-branched shrub or subshrub that can grow between three and six feet, with straggling woody, gray-brown stems and small, feathery, silver-green leaves • bright purple-and-pink, pea-shaped flowers with yellow throats, blooming March or April to October and after the monsoons • found in southern and southwest USA, including Colorado, Arizona, New Mexico, Oklahoma, Texas, and northern and northeastern Mexico • magically use the plant in situ, dried foliage, and flowers (which are ideal for rituals and spell bags)

PLANET AND ELEMENT

Sun • Fire

MAGICAL USES

worn by Native Americans to attract a successful hunt • more generally used to seek and find whatever is needed • use the feathery, silver leaves as the Air symbol in an Air spell

HOW TO USE

Scatter a circle of dried flowers or leaves (alone or mixed with knotted devil's shoestring or goldenseal, see p. 202) for good luck around lottery tickets or before sending a talent show application. • Carry a charm bag of the crushed, dried flowers or foliage if you have a physically demanding job or need extra strength when you cannot easily rest. • Shred the dried or fresh leaves in a windy place to call back what you have lost or has been stolen.

CAUTION

Use with care and avoid if pregnant.

Parrot's Beak

(*Pedicularis racemosa*)

MAGICAL FORMS
a unique flower with petals resembling a parrot's beak • native to coniferous forests in western North America, in the Rocky Mountains from southern Canada to New Mexico, in the Cascade Mountains from British Columbia to California, and in the mountainous regions of Arizona • white to cream, yellow, or pink flowers that bloom in summer, growing profusely at the base of spruce trees • magically use the plant, cut and sifted dried herb stem, flower, and leaf, or as tea and incense

PLANET AND ELEMENT
Moon • Water

MAGICAL USES
brings calm and ability to connect with other dimensions • anti-addiction • prevents repeating mistakes

HOW TO USE
Burn in incense or drink the dried herb mix as a tea before meditation or divination to increase your psychic awareness, especially clairaudience. Do the same to hear and repeat messages from ancestors on the Other Side—your own relatives and those of others. It's also an excellent tool for learning mediumship. • Add the herb to an amulet bag to touch when cravings and anxiety attacks kick in. • Carry in a charm bag if you are speaking on behalf of a company or need to accurately deliver information you have recently learned to an audience.

CAUTION
Parrot's beak is not recommended if trying to conceive, in pregnancy, while breastfeeding, or if taking regular medication for a chronic condition. • It may also pick up toxins from nearby plants through its roots.

Parsley

(*Petroselinum crispum*)

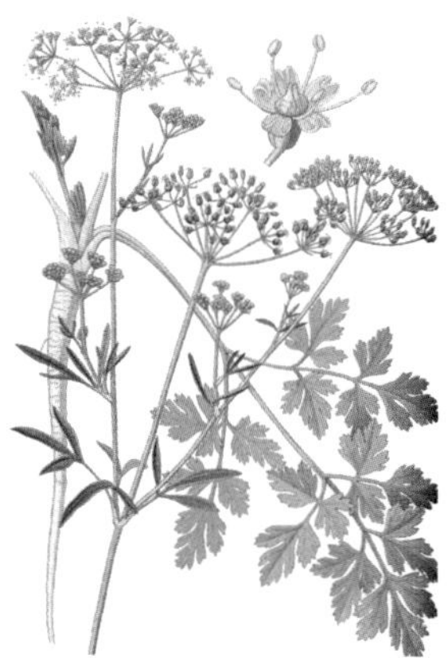

MAGICAL FORMS
species of flowering herb • magically use the fresh or dried herb, root, as tea, and in magical cookery generally

PLANETS AND ELEMENTS
Mercury/Mars • Air/Fire

MAGICAL USES
anti-debt • anti-intimidation, whether official, personal, or in the workplace • one of four divinatory herbs with sage, rosemary, and thyme • banishing • promotes fertility • for learning new technology • increases libido • passion • physical, emotional, and psychic protection • protection of pets and wild habitats • for purification • removes bad luck • rights inequalities • for water scrying

HOW TO USE
Roll a candle in the herb and use in candle magick to draw passion or money. • Add to a charm bag. • Grow the plant to create a defensive garden. • Use in dragon rituals (with tarragon). • Add parsley to infusions, teas, and decoctions from roots to pour away misfortune or bad influences. • Mix with magical salt to draw money and luck after loss. • Use with magnets or meteorites to call back money or love.

CAUTION
Avoid larger medicinal quantities during pregnancy. • Beware if picking from the wild, as it resembles poison hemlock.

Parsnip

(*Pastinaca sativa*)

MAGICAL FORMS

Edible, aromatic, thick, root vegetable with creamy-yellow, knobbly skin and white flesh, related to the carrot (see p. 104) • native to Europe and Asia and, until potatoes were introduced from Virginia in 1586, parsnips were the staple food for less wealthy people in the UK and Europe • in the Middle Ages, parsnips were eaten in their present cultivated form, but the Romans consumed wild parsnips, from which the cultivated parsnip was developed • harvested mid-fall to January • introduced into the USA, Quebec, and Ontario by British colonists • magically use the root

PLANET AND ELEMENT

Mars • Fire

MAGICAL USES

anti-debt • the parsnip in Christmas meals and other family winter celebrations brings good luck and lasting prosperity on both sides of the Atlantic • at Christmas, parsnips promise incoming wealth through the year ahead, a good harvest (in the urban world, sufficient financial resources to meet demand and also to save money), and to drive evil spirits away

HOW TO USE

Because it is considered an aphrodisiac, physically as well as psychically, and a symbol of virility, a couple wanting a baby and/or a more passionate sex life should eat a meal to which empowered parsnip has been added; having been left the previous night in full moonlight. • Make a floor wash with hot water and shredded root. Stir well, strain, and pour the liquid into a conventional floor wash for uncarpeted areas of the home and the doorsteps, ending at the front of the house. Afterward, bury the shredded, discarded parsnip near the front door (if possible) with a small gold item like an earring to avoid unexpected household expenses, house and vehicle repairs, and drains on family finances through extra demands.

CAUTION

Parsnip leaves can cause serious skin irritation, and some are allergic to ingesting the vegetable.

Parsnip, Cow

(*Heracleum maximum*)

MAGICAL FORMS

wild flowering plant and flower essence, related to the carrot • originally from Europe, naturalized throughout the USA and Canada except far northern areas and in the Deep South • cow parsnip can grow up to ten feet high and its leaves one and a half feet to two feet across with umbrella-like clusters of creamy white blooms from February to September • magically use the flower essence (easiest and safest) or grow the plant in a wildflower garden away from children

PLANET AND ELEMENT

Mercury • Air

MAGICAL USES

the blooming flower and the flower essence bring strength, courage, and determination in times of change, for example, moving house, children changing schools, going to college or leaving home, taking a new job, or new members joining the family • for quietening anxiety in those who take total responsibility for the happiness and well-being of others • myth links the name of the plant with the Greek hero Hercules, who ate the plant to give him the strength to complete tasks far from home

HOW TO USE

Focus on the sea of growing blossoming flowers at twilight and call a distant ancestor or a living family member if you are feeling homesick or rootless. • Picture a pathway through the flowers to the place you call home. • Spritz the essence (diluted in water) around a new home, around children's new uniforms, or around your own or a partner's work equipment to create confidence in a new environment or in one where you or they seem to not fit in. • Add the essence to pets' water to stop them trying to find their way back to the old home.

CAUTION

The sap can cause serious irritation and burns because its toxins interact with UV rays causing photosynthesis in sunlight. • The seeds are very toxic, and even the inner young shoots should be ingested only on expert advice. • Care must be taken if picking in the wild as its larger relative, giant hogweed, causes serious burns on contact. • Poison hemlock is also quite similar.

Passionflower

(*Passiflora incarnata*)

MAGICAL FORMS

may also be shrub or dwarf • associated with Christ's crucifixion, as there are ten petals for the apostles who were at the crucifixion, five stamens for the five wounds, the blade-like leaves for the sword that pierced Christ's side, styles for the three nails, white for purity, and purple for heaven • magically use the climbing vine, aerial parts, flowers, and essential oil

PLANETS AND ELEMENTS

Mars/Venus • Fire/Earth

MAGICAL USES

for finding or reuniting with your twin soul under difficulty • love affairs with consequences • in mojo bags in times of hardship • reduces arguments and keeps all harm from the home • attracts new friends and increases bonds with existing ones • passionflowers help to acknowledge and express strong feelings positively and to be open to love and life • soothes anxiety, panic attacks, and phobias • used in flower psychometry

HOW TO USE

Grow around or near the door to bring peace into the home if there are many quarrels. • Carry the leaves or roots in a red bag with a hummingbird or exotic small bird charm to bring new love or revive passion. • Fill dream pillows with dried flowers for peaceful dreams and to meet a lover on the astral plane while asleep. • Use flower petals in incense on the fall equinox to manifest abundance and sufficient resources through the winter. • Burn the dried petals to bring understanding when others are being difficult or obstructing your plans. • For five nights, add the oil to a floor wash or a magical bath (or place the flowers in a bath sachet) to open the way to finding or increasing love. • Inhale the fragrance of the oil in a diffuser, use well-diluted as part of a massage, or use in an oil burner to induce calm, a sense of well-being, and for some, euphoria.

CAUTION

Passionflower can cause drowsiness and dizziness when inhaled, so beware if taking blood pressure medicine, sedatives, or sleeping tablets. • Avoid in pregnancy. • Do not ingest the oil.

Passionfruit

(*Passiflora edulis*)

MAGICAL FORMS

flowering vine that produces the widely consumed fruit • white flowers are followed by oval, yellow (*Passiflora edulis* f. *flavicarpa*) or purple (*Passiflora edulis* f. *edulis*) fruit • originating from Amazonian Brazil, but since the nineteenth century increasingly cultivated in tropical and subtropical areas worldwide • the purple fruit is especially popular in the USA, cultivated in Florida and Hawaii and wild in Hawaii • may be grown in containers in hothouses and conservatories in more temperate climes • magically use the seeds and the fruit

PLANET AND ELEMENT

Venus • Water

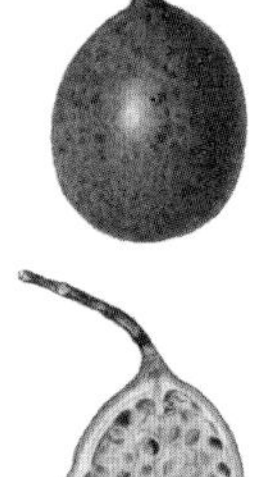

MAGICAL USES

for finding love at first sight • for dreams of your lover or the person you will meet who will inflame your heart • passion for a creative interest or performing art that overrides all other priorities • dedication to spirituality or a particular religious faith

HOW TO USE

Traditionally, plant one seed for each child you would like or for the health of existing children, ideally close to a passionfruit or passionflower vine. • For a love and fidelity charm, melt beeswax from a burned candle, then shape it into a heart and drop the dried seeds into the melted wax, the seeds forming the initials of you and a loved one or desired love. • Wrap in silk when cool and keep until it crumbles. • The fruit can be halved and the fleshy mesocarp scooped out from either side and mixed in a bowl to share as a sign of the mingling of love, particularly for a couple who has previously been married when two existing families are moving in together.

CAUTION

Use with caution if you have a latex allergy.

Patchouli

(*Pogostemon cablin*)

MAGICAL FORMS

aromatic flowering plant often cultivated for its fragrant oil • grows indoors or outdoors in warmer climates • magically use the whole, growing plant; young shoots and roots; fresh and dried leaves; oil; and fragrance

PLANET AND ELEMENT

Saturn • Earth

MAGICAL USES

for attracting money and money-making opportunities • brings stability for business ventures and property matters • sex magick • environmental and personal protection and healing • Earth mysteries and magick • connecting with Earth spirits and elementals • reconciliation • balance and peace • substitute for graveyard dust in traditional spells

HOW TO USE

Use in prosperity spells with green candles. • Make into a money charm bag by adding the dried herb to purses and wallets. • Use as incense to stop a lover from straying. • Use the dried herb as the Earth element in rituals instead of salt. • Carry the dried herb in a fertility bag with a carnelian crystal and dried rose petals empowered on the full moon. • Keep a root in a small bag under the mattress to enhance lovemaking and fertility if anxiety has slowed conception and spontaneity. • As an aphrodisiac, the infusion can be added to water when washing bed sheets. • Empower the diluted oil or commercial perfume scented with patchouli to stir a lover to passion. • Burn as clairvoyance- and divination-enhancing incense.

CAUTION

Do not use the oil internally.

Peach

(*Prunus persica*)

MAGICAL FORMS

flowering tree, probably native to China • peaches were introduced to the USA in the 1500s by Spanish monks living around St. Augustine, Florida • flowers are normally white, pink, or red • magically use the growing tree, leaves, fruit with stone or pit, and as essential oil

PLANET AND ELEMENT

Venus • Water

MAGICAL USES

make love charms with the blossoms • share the fruit with a lover for increased sensuality if lovemaking has become routine, and for fertility • use oil mixed with water in a bedroom spray, in a diffuser, or diluted for a massage as part of sacred sex • for making wishes, sit in a peach orchard, picking a peach for each wish • gift peach blossom to a bride or new parents, and a basket of peaches for older relatives, representing a wish for long life and health

HOW TO USE

The fruit, when eaten alone before you meet a lover, is an aphrodisiac and increases radiance. Say, *This fruit I eat, does taste so sweet, and so as one our hearts shall meet*. Bury the stone so that love may grow, indoors in a pot of soil if in a cooler location. • The same ritual is also effective on the full moon if you want a baby. • Hang branches with fruit outside houses or business premises, or place in a vase indoors to drive away malice and restless spirits. • Crush the stone and powder it to create circles around a lighted red male and female entwined candle if a partner is going away, reciting, *Think only for me, be only for me, return faithfully*. Scoop up the peach powder and keep it in a closed box until they come home.

CAUTION

Do not ingest the oil, and be sure to dilute it before applying it to your skin.

Peanut

(*Arachis hypogaea*)

MAGICAL FORMS

pods that develop in the soil • each pod consists of the shell and inner kernel • often called groundnuts because they grow underground, not on trees • more closely related to chickpeas and lentils than nuts • peanuts grow in a bush, with red, orange, or yellow flowers resembling butterflies • the modern peanut is a hybrid of two wild species that were first grown in Bolivia more than 7,500 years ago • cultivated in thirteen states, including Alabama, Florida, North and South Carolina, and Texas, and in other warm lands such as in Asia, especially China, and in India, Africa, Australia, and South America • magically use the nuts, either in the shell or without it

PLANETS AND ELEMENTS

Saturn/Jupiter • Earth/Fire

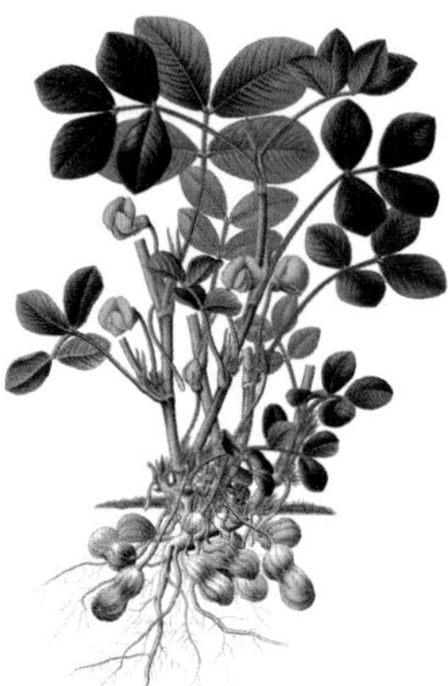

MAGICAL USES

represent financial growth from small beginnings or over a period of time • encourage sociability and networking at gatherings

HOW TO USE

Carry a small green bag of unshelled peanuts when you are speculating, applying for financial assistance, or performing monetary transactions. If the outcome is uncertain afterward, shell the peanuts and discard the shells, keeping the nuts or eating them. • Empower dishes of peanuts before a gathering of friends and family, having prechecked for nut allergies, for a happy noncontroversial gathering. • Keep the shelled nuts by your computer, smartphone, or tablet and eat one before each networking transaction or request for business.

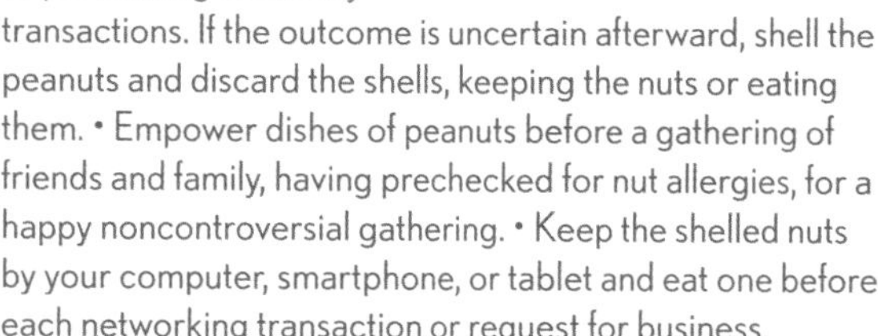

CAUTION

Be extra aware of nut allergies in others whom you do not know well, especially with unfamiliar products that may contain peanut extracts. • The shells are not edible.

Pear

(*Pyrus* spp.)

MAGICAL FORMS

genus of fruit trees • white blossoms, sweet fruit • the tree was introduced to Europe and Britain around 995 CE • fruit of the flowering ornamental pear (*Pyrus calleryana*) is too small and sour to eat, but the tree brings profuse spring blossoms and beautiful fall leaves—purple, red, yellow, or orange depending upon the species • cultivated in western Asia from 2000 BCE • now more than three thousand cultivars of pears worldwide • magically use the dried and fresh blossom, fruit, wood, and seeds

PLANET AND ELEMENTS

Venus • Earth/Water

MAGICAL USES

called a gift from the gods by the ancient Greek poet Homer • sacred tree of Hera, Greek goddess of marriage, fertility, and women, and once the supreme mother goddess in pre-Hellenic Greece • the Chinese believed it was a symbol of immortality • for rituals for new life, health, girls' and women's needs, fertility • to ask for and welcome a baby girl (use an apple for a boy)

HOW TO USE

Growing a pear tree, even a miniature one, is believed to bring good fortune and blessings from the higher spirits. • Use a pear wood wand for fertility rituals, goddess mysteries, and women's rites of passage. • Share a pear with a lover before lovemaking. • Save the seeds and stalk to bury beneath a thriving tree, so that love and passion will continue to grow.

CAUTION

Avoid eating the seeds or core, as these are toxic to humans and pets.

Pear, Nashi

(*Pyrus pyrifolia*)

MAGICAL FORMS

also called Asian pear • a fruit from eastern Asia, especially China, Japan, and Korea • round like an apple with a thin, golden or yellow skin • the tree can grow fifteen to thirty feet high with glossy, green leaves that turn bright red, orange, or yellow in the fall • white flowers in the spring • popular as an ornamental • grows in the UK, Europe, and the USA • first seen in Queens, New York, around 1820 and planted extensively by Chinese miners along the Sierra Nevada during the nineteenth century • magically use the fresh or dried blossoms, fruit, as an ingredient in fragrances, and in perfume oil mixed often with lily, lily of the valley, sweet pea, or other sweet fragrances

PLANET AND ELEMENT

Venus • Water

MAGICAL USES

the apple shape of this pear is a fertility symbol, combining the traditional meaning of an apple for a boy and pear for a girl, for a couple who are equally welcoming of a healthy baby of either sex • share two pears for an addition to a family if you only have one and want two or more children • reputedly ideal for conception of twins

HOW TO USE

Collect the blossoms, drying or preserving them until the first fruits appear, then releasing them outdoors for the fulfillment of an earlier wish if slow to materialize or for the next stage. • Choose a fragrance containing nashi pear or a nashi oil mix. • Add a few drops of the fragrance or oil to a spritzer bottle of water (shake well) and spray around the home if illness is lingering or money is not flowing as quickly or as plentifully as hoped. • Alternatively, add a few drops to fruity or floral potpourri, so that good fortune will enter the home.

CAUTION

Consume in moderation if you are diabetic because of its sweetness.

Pearly Everlasting Flower

(*Anaphalis margaritacea*)

MAGICAL FORMS

as wildflowers and in gardens or containers • growing in many areas of the northern and western USA and Canada • also can be found in India, Asia, and parts of Europe and the UK • silvery foliage and long-blooming, small, white flowers on tightly formed buds with yellow centers, resembling strings or clusters of pearls • magically use the plant, growing wild or cultivated in a nature garden (beware of it spreading too fast); as cut flowers in bouquets, fresh or dried; and as arrangements and clusters of the fresh or dried pearly flowers or bracts

PLANET AND ELEMENT

Moon • Water

MAGICAL USES

Given in bouquets for the sixty-ninth wedding anniversary, fresh or dried • to express romantic love at any time • on the birthdays of much older people to wish them a long and healthy life • for all craft ventures using flowers and foliage in potpourri, with its slight balsamy fragrance • as an altar centerpiece or decorating a ritual circle, outdoor space, or room for moon ceremonies

HOW TO USE

Weave a wreath on a wicker circle using dried flowers, silver foliage, and silver thread, then hang on a bedroom wall to protect against paranormal nighttime threats. This is especially effective for younger women who may suffer from poltergeist activity or sexual demons. • Place a circle of the small fresh flowers around a photo of a beloved, recently deceased relative or a memento of them. Replace the flowers as soon as they begin to fade (or use dried ones if out of season, replaced weekly) to sense their loving presence if you have not been able to make contact.

CAUTION

The flowers may cause skin irritation to those with sensitive skin. • If this is the case, use gloves or wash hands immediately after handling.

Pea, Black-Eyed

(*Vigna unguiculata*)

MAGICAL FORMS

a variety of legume related to green beans, its light- to medium-green pods resembling green bean pods • a cowpea cultivar • grows as a flowering bush or climbing plant • the round inner seed or pea is white to buff color with an identifying black spot where it joins the pod • native to West Africa but now grows in many parts of the world • magically use the shelled peas

PLANET AND ELEMENT

Mercury • Air

MAGICAL USES

increases clairvoyant vision • protects against the evil eye and spite • nine peas and nine coins mixed in a sealed jar in a warm place such as the kitchen ensure sufficient material resources • if they sprout, plant them

HOW TO USE

Black-eyed peas are eaten in celebrations in different parts of the world to incubate wealth, health, fertility, and good fortune; they are also symbols of prosperity. At New Year celebrations in the southern USA, especially North Carolina, at least one bowl of black-eyed peas can be found, served alongside cornbread or rice. The dish is called Hoppin' John when ham hock is added. • Black-eyed peas are eaten at midwinter in Brazil at the Festas Juninas, the celebration of the birth of St. John the Baptist on June 24; midsummer in the northern hemisphere. • A black-eyed-pea-centered feast can be adopted for any seasonal celebration or major family change point. • Draw an eye shape invisibly with the index finger over the black center of a pea, and carry the pea in a small bag to protect against jealousy and rivalry in the workplace or socially.

Pea, Green

(*Pisum sativum*)

MAGICAL FORMS

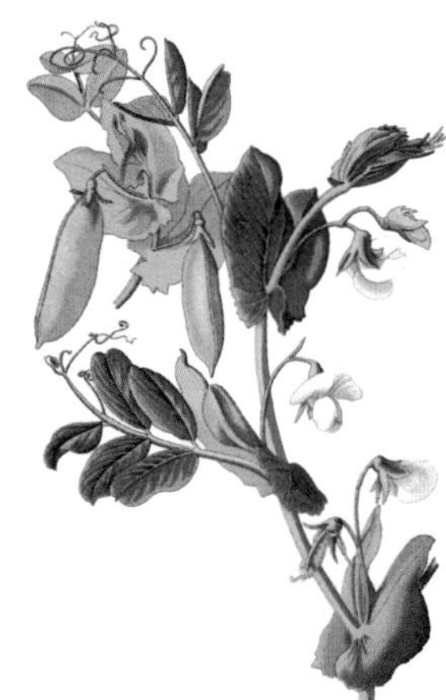

flowering green plant that grows against a pole or trellis and can reach up to four to six feet high • developing pods containing seeds (peas) • three main varieties: garden, snow (*Pisum sativum* var. *macrocarpon*), and snap peas (*Pisum sativum macrocarpon* ser. cv.) • can be eaten raw or cooked • snow and snap peas have edible pods • one of the oldest cultivated crops, found wild in the Mediterranean and from late Neolithic times in the Middle East • green peas are most cultivated in India, China, the USA, Canada, Russia, and the UK, but are found worldwide • in the USA, especially in the northern plains and the northwest • originally reached the USA with the colonists • magically use the seeds in the pod and shelled

PLANET AND ELEMENT

Mercury • Air

MAGICAL USES

shell peas for business and money-spinning opportunities • seven peas found in a pod means unexpected money is coming • if there are nine peas in a pod, it promises luck in love or new love if alone

HOW TO USE

Eat raw peas to enhance charisma and the ability to attract who and what you want into your sphere. • A dish of empowered cooked peas represents, as they are eaten, the resolution of small worries and calls small benefits and favors. • The last spoonful is especially lucky for small wins.

CAUTION

Do not eat in excess, especially if taking blood thinners.

Pea, Rosary

(*Abrus precatorius*)

MAGICAL FORMS

also called jequirity bean • a climbing plant that can reach thirteen feet, twining around trees, shrubs, and hedges with pink flowers, becoming seed pods containing scarlet or occasionally white, green, or black seeds • usually red or orange with a black eye • highly poisonous • the plant grows in India, Asia, the Caribbean, northern Australia, and Africa • used for landscaping in the southeastern USA, but considered invasive, growing wild in hotter parts of the USA • called rosary or paternoster peas because the hard, colorful seeds were and still are used for rosaries • Lord Krishna is pictured with a rosary (mala or japamala) of the seeds • magically use the seeds

PLANET AND ELEMENT

Mars • Fire

MAGICAL USES

the seeds have been used for centuries in India to weigh precious gems including the Koh-i-Noor diamond and gold and therefore magically represent wealth fraught with dangers

HOW TO USE

In Trinidad, the seeds are worn as protective bracelets or anklets to ward off malicious spirits and the evil eye (blue turquoise is safer). • Seeds may be attached to wooden tourist items or made into jewelry bought overseas or imported from the Caribbean, Africa, or India. • If you keep the seeds at all (they are said to be less toxic if they have been boiled before the making, but since the seed is water-impenetrable this may not be foolproof), preserve the jewelry or wooden item in a locked box set in a high place away from children or pets. • Draw an eye over the box in incense stick smoke to protect the home and family from jealousy.

CAUTION

Rosary peas are highly poisonous seeds containing the poison abrin, for which there is no known antidote. • The plant is prohibited in Canada. • If you have any of the seeds, keep them well away from children, unwary adults, and pets.

Pea, Split

(*Pisum sativum*)

MAGICAL FORMS

an agricultural preparation of *Pisum sativum* • split peas are dried, yellow or green peas that are allowed to split naturally into two sections or are split mechanically or by hand • magically use the dried peas

PLANET AND ELEMENT

Mercury • Air

MAGICAL USES

peas in a sealed container act as a shamanic rattle for trance work or astral travel • yellow split peas bring fame and fortune • the old nursery rhyme "Pease Pudding Hot" (made from yellow split peas) was first recorded in 1760 and may be a covert protest by the poor who were forced to eat "pease" pudding at every meal

HOW TO USE

Add green split peas to a green love bag and shake it night and morning at an open window (upstairs if possible) calling your twin soul to find or return to you if estranged. • Mix empowered dried split peas into a soup or stew you are cooking. Eat it on a Wednesday, Mercury's day, to give yourself or a loved one the confidence to raise their profile if there is stiff competition for advancement or to increase your or their recognition and tangible approval.

Pea, Sweet

(*Lathyrus odoratus*)

MAGICAL FORMS

climbing plant with strongly scented flowers • magically use the whole, growing plant and flowers

PLANET AND ELEMENT

Venus • Water

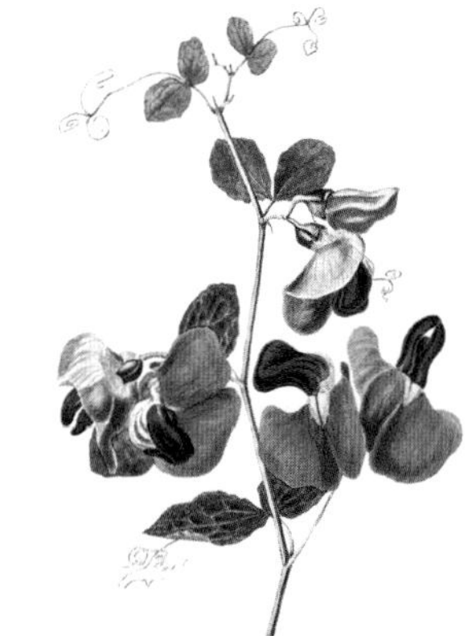

MAGICAL USES

for developing love, friendship, and amicable encounters with strangers who may become friends • purity in love • truth, especially in love, and ability to know if your lover speaks the truth on- and offline • partings • passion fulfilled • develops clairsentience, especially with other fragrant flowers • for quiet courage and strength to outface intimidation

HOW TO USE

Wear or carry sweet pea flower blossoms in a sachet or offer the flowers as a bouquet to attract good friendships and strengthen the bond in existing ones. • A vase of sweet peas in a room encourages the truth to be told over lying to gain money; it also encourages loyalty as well as love, especially when you are doubting a particular person. • Kept in a mojo or amulet bag over the front door, the dried blossoms and seeds will protect children in the home and ensure worries and the burdens of the day are left at the front door by adults and children alike. • Attach the dried flower in a small, sealed bag to a dreamcatcher in the bedroom to keep away sleep disturbances and phantoms of the night. Replace when the fragrance disappears. • Inhaling the scent from the growing or cut flowers attracts abundance and luxury into your life.

CAUTION

Do not ingest, as the flowers and seeds are toxic if consumed. • Be careful around pets and small children.

Pecan Tree

(*Carya illinoinensis*)

MAGICAL FORMS

belonging to the walnut family • native to the southeastern USA, where the tree is cultivated in orchards and grows wild in forests and near rivers, such as along the Mississippi • also in Spain, Australia, and South Africa • growing tree nuts with a tough brown shell (from a mature dried fruit) • bright-green leaflets • compound leaves containing up to seventeen small leaves in approximately symmetrical pairs with an extra small leaf at the end, turning rich yellow in the fall • the only major nut tree indigenous to North America, traded by the Native North Americans and taken to Spain and beyond by early explorers • magically use the leaflets or leaves and nuts

PLANET AND ELEMENT

Mercury • Air

MAGICAL USES

keep unshelled nuts in a bowl in the center of the altar for wealth rituals for enhanced career • eat the nuts and hide the shells in your workplace or business for financial stability • for a happy inheritance, unexpected but deserved family monetary gift, maturity of a financial bond, a new opportunity in retirement or redundancy based on previous hard work and interests, and successful small investments that bear fruit within a year • keep the dried yellow fall leaves in a money charm bag

HOW TO USE

When the moon is waxing, take seven pecan nuts, shelling and eating one every day, naming what you most need in terms of wealth or abundance. Name the day you begin the ritual; for example, on a Monday say, *Monday and every day I ask abundance comes my way*. On day two, continue shelling and eating, and say, *Monday, Tuesday, and every day. . . .* Continue eating, shelling, and speaking until on day seven you name all seven days and eat the final nut. Bury an eighth unshelled nut on day eight, and say, *Let abundance unfold.* • At Thanksgiving, let each person present touch the center of their piece of pie before eating, and give thanks for the year (even if not brilliant), also naming blessings for the next twelve months.

Pennyroyal

(*Mentha pulegium*)

MAGICAL FORMS

a smaller version of the mint family, also called lurk in the ditch because it springs up easily wherever it lands • pennyroyal grows wild and in natural gardens • brought to North America by European colonists and adopted medicinally among the Native North Americans • beautiful, purple flowers bloom in the last half of the summer • magically use the growing plant; dried, chopped aerial parts; fresh or dried leaves; and fresh or dried flowers

PLANET AND ELEMENT

Mars • Fire

MAGICAL USES

a mystical herb to aid those who walk astrally between worlds; the ancient Greeks used the herb when initiating novices into secret rites of the Eleusinian rebirth ceremonies in honor of the Earth mother Demeter • pennyroyal is burned as incense in a room before divination or a pot of growing pennyroyal is kept on the table during divination or mediumship • it is burned also in incense to break curses and hexes or scattered along doorsteps of home and business • the dried herb is carried in a sachet on sea journeys to prevent motion sickness and misfortune and to relieve tiredness on any travel

HOW TO USE

If you or a loved one are anxious or fear a panic attack before a meeting, exam, or interview, fill a green poppet doll with pennyroyal. Before sealing, add a written statement of the fear and then sew it up, saying, *I leave all fear behind*. Leave the poppet at home. • Tie an eye charm to pennyroyal growing in the garden or add the charm to a sachet containing pennyroyal flowers or the dried herb, and draw a blue eye on the bag. Hang it hidden as far from your entrance as you can within your boundaries.

CAUTION

Pennyroyal oil should not be used in pregnancy or if trying for a baby; nor should the plant be inhaled. • Pennyroyal oil has been removed from commercial sale in many locations because of its many contraindications, and there is dispute about the safety of ingesting the plant or using it directly on skin.

Pennyroyal, Mountain

(*Monardella odoratissima*)

MAGICAL FORMS

a fragrant herb, member of the mint family • also known as coyote mint • reaches up to two feet tall wild in scrublands and forest edges throughout western North America from northern Idaho to eastern Washington and south to New Mexico, Arizona, and California • will also grow in gardens, especially rock gardens in the USA, in the UK, and Europe, where it is valued in the wild for conservation purposes • its puffball-shaped blooms in white, pale pink, or purplish blue (often tangled) attract pollinators • magically use the growing plant, edible fresh and dried flowers, aromatic leaves with silvery fine hairs and stems, and flower essence

PLANET AND ELEMENT

Mercury • Air

MAGICAL USES

the herb and flower essence clear confused thoughts and cut through indecision • can help in attuning to unseen forces by increasing clairvoyant powers • protects against and removes psychic as well as emotional parasites, especially when used with garlic, rue, and aspen essences

HOW TO USE

Make a spritz by combining the essence and water to spray where there are spooky atmospheres in the home or workplace, or in the bedrooms of children who are afraid of ghosts. • Make a drink by infusing the fresh or dried flowerheads and leaves in cold water, straining away the plant after a few minutes, and consuming when extra energies and focus are needed. • Sit close to the plants with half-closed eyes for connection with Earth and Air spirits.

CAUTION

Medical advice should be taken before ingesting in pregnancy or while breastfeeding.

Peony

(*Paeonia officinalis*)

MAGICAL FORMS

beautiful flowering plant known as the king of the flowers in ancient China and Japan • magically use the whole plant, flowers, roots, buds, and seeds

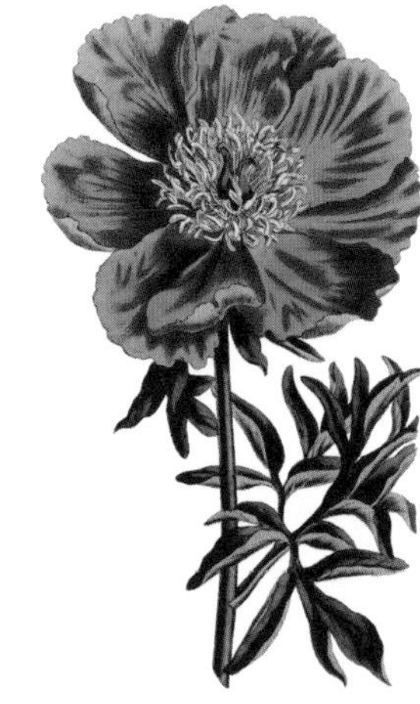

PLANET AND ELEMENT

Sun • Fire

MAGICAL USES

for good luck, especially when in bloom • prosperity • authority and leadership • honorable deeds and words • protection

HOW TO USE

Plant peonies in the garden or keep potted or cut fresh flowers indoors to attract good fortune and happiness and to protect against all harm and storms. • Burning the root in incense brings blessings on the home and loved ones, guarding against threatening spirits or sexual demons such as succubi and incubi. • Carved seeds or roots worn as a necklace or hung in an inaccessible place in children's rooms keep away mischievous fey and changelings. • Peony blossoms in water or peony flower essence, when sprinkled around a room, remove negative feelings from the space after a quarrel or sickness.

CAUTION

Consult with your doctor before using while pregnant or breastfeeding. • Peonies can slow blood clotting. • They should not be taken with contraceptive pills containing estrogen.

Pepper, Bell

(*Capsicum annuum*)

MAGICAL FORMS

also called capsicum in the UK • flowering member of the nightshade family, though not poisonous • countless varieties, from spicy to mild • native to the Americas but cultivated all around the world • ripening on the plant as green, then yellow, orange, becoming progressively sweeter and finally red • indigenous to the original people of Mexico between six thousand and seven thousand years ago • Christopher Columbus took the seeds to Europe • magically use peppers, fresh or dried (often in magical cookery)

PLANET AND ELEMENT

Mars • Fire

MAGICAL USES

use dried slices of the green capsicum or indeed any pepper to add determination and power to amulet bags against bullying or being shouted down • see also capers (p. 101) and chili powder (p. 121)

HOW TO USE

In magical cookery, use sliced bell peppers to spice up a relationship sexually, adding each color in turn, as you stir to increase passion while maintaining the sweetness and romance. • A basket of the different colored bell peppers in the center of your kitchen will stimulate an unenthusiastic partner or family while preserving good-natured relationships. • Use bell peppers to encourage positive interactions with visiting relatives and neighbors while discouraging them outstaying their welcome.

CAUTION

The foliage is toxic to humans. • Eat in moderate quantities, and keep raw peppers away from your eyes and children. • Avoid if you are taking aspirin or other anticoagulants or diabetic medications.

Pepper, Black

(*Piper nigrum*)

MAGICAL FORMS

dried mature fruits of the flowering vine • native to southern India and Indonesia for two thousand years • often grown as an annual plant in the southernmost USA and other warm locations around the world • reaches ten to thirty feet • magically use the peppercorns, whole or powdered, and the essential oil

PLANET AND ELEMENT

Mars • Fire

MAGICAL USES

black pepper spice was so valued in ancient Rome it was traded as currency • in the fifteenth century, the Portuguese explorer Vasco de Gama discovered black pepper in India and made it part of the spice trade where it was called black gold • the oil brings protection against anger, threats, and fear of violence, relieving inertia, and fears of tackling new pursuits or taking center stage in any area of life

HOW TO USE

Burn or diffuse the essential oil when unwise cravings strike. • Carry whole peppercorns for protection in an amulet bag, especially against the evil eye. • Add a few peppercorns every day to a charm bag to accelerate the accumulation of money and to attract money. When the bag is full, stir the peppercorns into cooking. • Powdered peppercorns mixed with salt and placed on doorsteps weekly are swept away (outward) to remove misfortune and keep danger away.

CAUTION

Do not ingest the oil, and dilute it very well, as it can be an irritant. • Avoid the oil during pregnancy.

Pepper, Cayenne

(*Capsicum annuum* var. *acuminatum*)

MAGICAL FORMS

long, thin, bright red pepper • grows on the cayenne shrub and is cultivated in tropical climates around the world and in parts of the USA • most usually ground into a spice • magically use the whole pepper and the spice

PLANET AND ELEMENT

Mars • Fire

MAGICAL USES

popular in Creole and Cajun cooking • for increasing passion • adding fire to a spell if the need is urgent • defense against curses, hexes, and ill-wishing • first cultivated between 5000 BCE and 3500 BCE in South America and transported to Europe by Christopher Columbus

HOW TO USE

Use the ground pepper as the ultimate doorstep guardian, sometimes mixed with coarse salt, sprinkled to keep away intruders and ill-wishing, and swept outdoors with a broom kept for that purpose. • Dry whole peppers and string them across your kitchen ceiling to protect against accidents and fires, burying them when you replace them. • Add chopped or whole peppers to spicy dishes (you can remove them if you wish after cooking), or use the spice to restore life to an ailing relationship or project for which you have lost enthusiasm but know is worth preserving.

CAUTION

Keep away from eyes. • Avoid if you take aspirin, blood thinners, or ACE medications to lower blood pressure. • Do not ingest if breastfeeding.

Pepper, Jalapeño

(*Capsicum annuum* var. *jalapeño*)

MAGICAL FORMS

bushy plant that bears one of the most popular capsicum peppers in cookery • jalapeño pepper plant grows between two and three feet high and each pepper plant produces between twenty and twenty-five peppers per season • white flowers are followed by hanging green fruit that ripens into bright-red, medium-hot chile peppers • originally from Mexico, they grow well in southern New Mexico and western Texas • the plant can be grown indoors anywhere or in very warm but not overly hot climates • magically use the jalapeño peppers fresh, dried, or powdered

PLANET AND ELEMENT

Mars • Fire

MAGICAL USES

for silencing unfair criticism, gossip, and untrue accusations • to face challenges head-on and overcome them • because the pepper is dedicated to the warrior god Mars and the Yoruba deity Shango, who commands thunder, lightning, and justice, use in defensive magick (but the latter figure should not be invoked unless you are very experienced in magick and are working with pure intent to right a matter of severe injustice) • it is safer to seek help in defense from the archangels Mars, Camael, Samael, or Azrael • as with all pepper or fire plants, never use for revenge or when angry

HOW TO USE

Cook the peppers in a meal to share with a lover or intended lover to increase passion. • Use for sex magick between committed partners. • Grow the peppers indoors if you have hostile neighbors, live in a potentially dangerous area, or are facing threats against your home and family. • Slit a ripe red pepper open and slip a piece of paper naming the outcome or compensation you need in a court case inside. When the pepper dries or if the case is heard before that, bury both pepper and paper beneath a healing plant such as lavender or chamomile.

Pepper, Pink

(*Schinus molle*)

MAGICAL FORMS

from the ripe dried fruit of the Peruvian pepper shrub or tree; it's native to Peru and Brazil but grows worldwide, including Arizona, California, Texas, Alabama, Louisiana, Florida, and Hawaii • also commercially available under the same common name but derived from the Brazilian pepper tree (*Schinus terebinthifolius*) • both have similar magical effects • sweet and spicy • member of the cashew family, not actually a pepper • not as intense as black pepper • magically use the ground or whole peppercorns and essential oil

PLANET AND ELEMENT

Mars • Fire

MAGICAL USES

for restoring life and vitality • promotes self-love • for goddess rituals for men and women • to attract the right friends • protects against those who are spiteful or jealous but are vulnerable

HOW TO USE

Use the oil, well diluted, in a massage or burn in a diffuser if you lack confidence because of unkind words spoken many years before that still haunt you. • Mix pink and black peppercorns in a sealed amulet bag. Shake it nine times every morning if you are naturally reluctant to defend yourself, but need to speak out at work to avoid being overlooked or shouted down. Keep the mix with a photo of children or pets if they are being bullied, making sure they cannot open it. • Tape a few pink peppercorns beneath the doormat if your children are expressing sibling rivalry or are competing for your attention.

CAUTION

Before using the oil, consult a physician or midwife if pregnant or breastfeeding. • Dilute it very well. • Avoid pink pepper if you have a nut allergy, high blood pressure, or heart conditions.

Pepper, Szechuan

MAGICAL FORMS

a spice made from the dried, papery fruit husks of several species of the prickly ash—shrubs or small trees with multiple trunks that grow in the Chinese form (*Zanthoxylum simulans*), twenty-three feet high • mild, citrusy, and numbs the mouth when eaten • one of the Chinese five-spice mix, the others being star anise, cassia (Chinese cinnamon), fennel, and cloves • magically use as infused oil, peppercorns, and ground spice

PLANET AND ELEMENT

Mars • Fire

MAGICAL USES

for galvanizing self and others when urgent action is needed • protects against threats and intimidation, inducing the buildup of passion

HOW TO USE

Eat the spice in a meal before divination to bypass its numbing effect, for logical words and responses, and for direct connection with messages from the spirit world. • Keep peppercorns in an amulet bag along with one of the true peppers, such as powdered chili or black peppercorns, to prevent unwise temptations to passion if your natural caution is overridden. Once temptation has passed, tip away the contents. • Szechuan pepper is also useful to deter sexual predators who use their status or power to intimidate you sexually. • Add to a love meal if you and/or your partner are anxious and so inhibited or too eager to enjoy a gradual buildup to prolonged lovemaking.

CAUTION

Avoid eating in large quantities as effects of long-term usage have not been fully researched. • Avoid totally in pregnancy and while breastfeeding.

Peppermint

(*Mentha × piperita*)

MAGICAL FORMS

herb frequently used in cooking • magically use the whole, growing plant; leaves for teas; and essential oil

PLANETS AND ELEMENTS

Mars/Mercury • Fire/Air

MAGICAL USES

money spells • travel and protection during journeys of all kinds • love and passion • attracting good fortune • healing spells • banishing magick and exorcism • increases instinctive awareness of good versus bad investments and scams • attracts money through overseas or online business

HOW TO USE

Keeping a dried mint leaf in your purse ensures that money will come in. • Carrying dried leaves in the glove compartment of a vehicle protects against accidents and aggressive drivers. • Peppermint tea or cocktails will attract a lover, especially if offered to the desired lover. • To increase psychic powers, fill an herb jar with peppermint, cinnamon, cloves, fennel, and sage (see p. 395); shake; and then inhale before mediumship or divination. • Add mint infusions to floor wash to clear and cleanse the home of sickness and misfortune.

CAUTION

Peppermint is not suitable for children, and no form should be used in excess by adults or for more than eight weeks at a time. • Peppermint tea can occasionally cause mouth sores and allergic reactions (the latter is true also for the oil, which should always be well diluted). • Peppermint should be avoided in pregnancy and lactation. • It can interfere with blood pressure and diabetes medications.

Perilla

(*Perilla frutescens*)

MAGICAL FORMS

including *Perilla frutescens* var. *crispa*, called shiso in Japan • called perilla or deulkkae in Korea • an aromatic herb belonging to the mint family • native to the mountains of China, Japan, India, and Vietnam • a sacred plant in Japan • made popular internationally with the advent of sushi and sashimi • red, purple, or bright green, with ruffled leaves • used to separate items of sushi or the food in a traditional Japanese bento box • food is wrapped in leaves to keep it fresh, or leaves are eaten as a snack wrapped around food • can be grown in pots indoors or gardens in warm to hot climates • magically use the fresh leaves, which you may find in Asian groceries, imported dried and ground, or frozen in sesame oil, and the essential oil, which is steam distilled from the leaves with an aromatic mix of citrus, mint, basil, and cinnamon

PLANETS AND ELEMENTS

Mars/Venus • Water/Earth

MAGICAL USES

red or purple for passion and the preservation of love through the ages • green, called *oba*, for releasing the inner self • spiritual growth • expressing spontaneous spiritual connection with the land

HOW TO USE

Add dried, ground shiso to an incense mix to cleanse the house of restless spirits or poltergeists, or after a run of lingering sickness or misfortune. • Add shiso essential oil to a diffuser or aroma lamp to bring harmony to the home. • Step away from a potential confrontation at work by inhaling the fragrance of the oil on a tissue or from the bottle.

CAUTION

Some people may be allergic to the leaves, particularly if sensitive to mint. • Dilute the oil well and consult an expert before using if pregnant.

Periwinkle

(*Vinca* spp.)

MAGICAL FORMS

flowering plant known since Roman times for its medicinal and ornamental uses • often called the sorcerer's violet, as it was a staple of medieval witchcraft • magically use the growing plant and fresh and dried flowers

PLANET AND ELEMENT

Venus • Water

MAGICAL USES

for first love and uncertainty in new love • recalling memories and lost love returning • as incense in goddess rituals, also to call abundance • a sign of immortality and rebirth • offers protection in affairs or romances where there is opposition • use in binding magick because its vines naturally stick together

HOW TO USE

Hang a garland of periwinkles over an entrance to protect against evil spirits. • Grind periwinkle into a powder and keep in a sealed sachet under the mattress to bring or rekindle passion into a relationship. • Give periwinkles growing in a hanging basket if you suspect the recipient may be extra sensitive to toxicity. • On the Feast of St. Matthias, February 24, in a modern version of an old love ritual, fill a small bowl with water and float nine periwinkle flowers on it. Float nine daisies in a second bowl, and leave the third bowl filled only with water. Blindfolded, twirl around nine times clockwise, nine times counterclockwise, and then nine times clockwise again. If you touch the periwinkle bowl, a new love will come to you within the year; the daisy bowl predicts you will connect with an old love; and if you touch the third, you should let go of a love who will not return. • Meditate on the growing plant or cut flowers to retrieve memories both from earlier in this life and from past lives. • Set periwinkles close to whatever or whomever is precious, such as a photo of your family or of a vacation location to which you wish to return.

CAUTION

Periwinkle is toxic to pets, especially cats, and to humans if the plant is ingested raw. • Do not use periwinkle if you are pregnant or breastfeeding. • Avoid the tea if you have liver or kidney problems or low blood pressure.

Persimmon

(*Diospyros* spp.)

MAGICAL FORMS

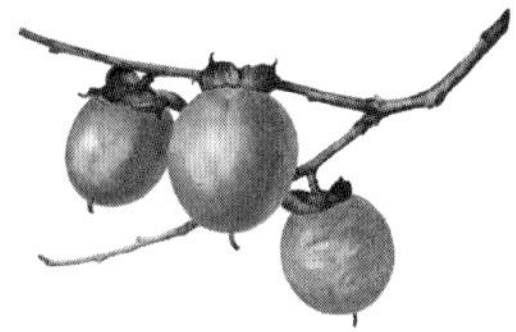

genus of fruiting tree • the fruit grows from the fall through December • pale yellow to deep orange with a jellylike texture • the sweet fuyu variety of *Diospyros kaki* possesses a honey-like flavor • the *kaki* tree flourishes in California and the Gulf states • the smaller American persimmon (*Diospyros virginiana*) is found from the Gulf states to central Pennsylvania and Virginia to central Illinois • leaves turn yellow and orange to bright red in the fall • magically use the fruit, leaf powder collected from the growing *kaki* tree, and the leaves

PLANET AND ELEMENT

Venus • Water

MAGICAL USES

for gender issues • bringing the right partner to LGBTQ couples and overcoming prejudice • in earlier times a young woman might have to disguise herself as a boy for safety if she was traveling alone • this herb or fruit psychically and psychologically helped maintain her new identity • a persimmon brings good fortune and prosperity through one's own efforts • the first fruit picked from the *virginiana* tree in the Ozark Mountains was traditionally cut open to divine the weather • if spoon-shaped inside, a hard winter lay ahead; if fork-shaped, mild; if knife-shaped, it heralded icy winds

HOW TO USE

Seal the dried, powdered leaves or, if you can obtain them, the brightly colored dried fall leaves, in a charm bag to help older people, especially those who want to acknowledge and live by their true inner sexuality but also wish to explore their unique gifts and maybe totally change their lifestyle.

CAUTION

Do not eat unripe persimmon—the Hachiya kind in particular is very bitter before it ripens.

Petitgrain

MAGICAL FORMS

essential oil from the bitter orange tree (*Citrus* × *aurantium* var. *amara*) (see "Orange, Bitter," p. 315) • this is a particular blend of essential oil made from the leaves and stems of the tree combined with neroli essential oil, which is made from its blossoms • petitgrain is stronger and more pungent • native to southern China and northwest India, the finest-quality petitgrain, obtainable worldwide, is distilled in France • also a major ingredient in eau de cologne and in orange leaf and flower water absolute, a byproduct of the manufacture of neroli oil

PLANETS AND ELEMENTS

Sun/Venus • Fire/Water

MAGICAL USES

banishes unwelcome energies, entities, fears, and threats • for meditation if concentration eludes • removes anger and anxiety from home or tensions lingering during the evening after workplace conflict

HOW TO USE

Dilute a drop or two of petitgrain oil in virgin olive oil and anoint an unlit red candle, having previously scratched on the candle with a thin knife or a fingernail the name of what or whom is causing fear or intimidation. Let the candle burn away, and with it, the negative influences. • Add petitgrain with a drop or two of chamomile, lavender, and ylang-ylang to evening bath water or on a shower cloth for quiet sleep and peaceful dreams if the day has ended in anger or reproach or you suffer from nightmares.

CAUTION

Consult a doctor or midwife before use if you are pregnant, particularly in the later trimesters of pregnancy or if breastfeeding.

Petunia

(*Petunia* spp.)

MAGICAL FORMS

genus of approximately twenty species of flowering plants • part of the *Datura* family, and so related to tomatoes, tobacco, and potatoes • magically use the whole, growing plant; fresh or dried flowers and petals; and flower essence

PLANET AND ELEMENT

Venus • Earth

MAGICAL USES

for vacations • inspires creativity • for environmental concerns, settling into committed relationships • overcoming despair, debts, or fear • bringing calm • flower psychometry

HOW TO USE

If you have a bad quarrel, send petunias as peacemakers and to defuse anger. • Keep a pot near the center of the home if a recent committed relationship has settling-in clashes. • Grow petunias in the garden if you have hormonal teenagers or temperamental relatives and to keep away aggressive debt collectors and unfriendly officials. • If you desire a vacation or have one planned, scatter fresh petunia petals over a map of your planned destination. Afterward, tip the flowers outdoors to fly free. • Do the same with a map or large photograph of an area of beauty that's being threatened by pollution or developers. • Add petunia flower essence to your bath or take a drop or two under your tongue if you have been unfairly treated but know you must respond calmly. • Keep petunias in pots in your creative space and inhale the fragrance when you experience a creative block.

Phlox

(*Phlox* spp.)

MAGICAL FORMS

found in traditional gardens in the USA and as wild plant • the Native North American pink full moon around April is named after the pink phlox flowering in eastern North America at this time • its name means *flame* and especially the red variety is called the flame flower because it resembles a lighted torch • it is said phlox was created when a young Choctaw boy, helped by his animal companions, tried to save his people in a battle from a wall of flame and the Great Spirit turned the fire into red phlox • magically use the whole plant, fresh and dried flower petals, and sprigs of the plant

PLANETS AND ELEMENTS

Moon/Venus • Earth/Fire

MAGICAL USES

unity among partners, family, friends, organizations, covens, and colleagues • use if contemplating marriage or major love commitment or planning a proposal • flower psychometry

HOW TO USE

Phlox can be given as a bouquet when a person proposes marriage or lasting commitment, especially white or pink. • Plant outside a first home set up with a partner as a reminder of love if life gets fraught. • Use dried purple phlox petals in dream pillows or a sachet beneath the pillow for beautiful dreams, especially of love. • Tie two sprigs of fresh phlox with seven red twine knots and place on an altar with red candles to ritually bind a newlywed couple in lasting unity. • Sometimes the sprigs are attached to the handfasting cord as part of the ceremony and kept by the couple over the marital bed until the flowers die. • White petals can be used to create a magick circle for ceremonies to ensure unity of purpose.

Pine Tree

(*Pinus* spp.)

MAGICAL FORMS

genus including approximately 187 species of pine trees • magically use the whole, growing tree; dried needles; cones; nuts; resin; and oil

PLANET AND ELEMENT

Mars • Fire

MAGICAL USES

protects against tricksters, emotional vampires, liars, and psychic attacks • purifies homes and ritual areas • associated with birth, baby blessings, and new beginnings • for healing • ending destructive relationships • fertility • money • an herb of the winter solstice, although its powers to overcome negativity are strongest when its needles and cones are gathered at midsummer

HOW TO USE

Pass pine cones through pine needle or pine resin incense smoke to bring blessings to the home, cleansing away what is no longer wanted or needed and returning ill wishes to the sender. • Add the dried needles and nuts with a small gold item to an orange bag or cloth and hide within the branches of a Yule tree to attract prosperity and good fortune through the winter and to give thanks for what has been received. • Burn dried needles mixed with equal parts of juniper and cedar on a hearth fire or bonfire, or mix the oils in a diffuser to purify the home in winter, especially on New Year's Eve. • Traditionally, pitch was added when sealing a new boat to keep it safe from the dangers of the sea. A modern equivalent is taping nine pine nuts in the glove compartment of a vehicle, under the saddle of a bicycle, or beneath the sails of a boat to keep travelers safe. • For fertility, collect a pine nut on a white cloth each day from the end of a menstrual cycle to ovulation, or traditionally from the crescent moon until the full moon, to aid conception. The next morning, keep the cloth tied with the nuts inside a drawer, to be replaced with new nuts on the new cycle until conception.

CAUTION

Some pine needles, such as Ponderosa, are toxic, so do not ingest without consulting a doctor.

Pine Tree, Pinyon

(*Pinus edulis*)

MAGICAL FORMS

pine tree native to the southwestern USA and northern Mexico • the resin or sap is taken from the bark of the tree, but also is present in the branches and needles • this sap or resin is sometimes referred to as colophony and is also called rosin • magically use resin as incense or mix with non-resinous ingredients to create rich, aromatic smoke

PLANET AND ELEMENT

Mars • Fire

MAGICAL USES

resin is sacred to Native North American healing and purifying ceremonies • use for fertility, both creativity and for welcoming a baby into the world • protection • returns hostility to sender • for increased influx of money • for cleansing homes psychically

HOW TO USE

Burn the resin to clear a sacred space before a ritual, meditation, or divination, especially if you are working in a less-than-ideal environment. • Waft the incense smoke with a fan or feather around your aura energy field to increase clairvoyant powers and create boundaries with the everyday world. • Spiral the incense over a healing crystal or a sachet of healing herbs you are sending or giving to a sick or troubled person as you speak blessings.

Pineapple

(*Ananas comusus*)

MAGICAL FORMS

bush with sturdy stem and tough, waxy, spiny lancet-shaped leaves that grow into a rosette • juicy reddish-yellow fruit, growing close to the ground and only producing one pineapple, after which it dies • native to South America for thousands of years • introduced to Europe by Christopher Columbus in 1493 and Spanish explorers reintroduced them to the USA in 1521 (they had been found wild in Hawaii long before that) • cultivated in tropical areas and can be grown in warmer climates or in pots indoors in more temperate lands • magically use the plant in situ, fruit, and juice

PLANETS AND ELEMENTS

Sun/Venus • Fire/Water

MAGICAL USES

for striving for a luxury lifestyle • the juice, when consumed on its own, acts as a deterrent from pursuing unwise sexual attractions or being pursued • however, with rose petals and honey added, pineapple juice will attract the right love • the whole fruit set in a meditation place or on your altar aids connection with other dimensions and opens clairvoyant and clairsentient powers • magical cookery

HOW TO USE

After preparing the fruit, dry the skin and chop or finely grind it, carrying a scoop or two in a money sachet to obtain the resources for a major purchase. • Pineapple fruit baked into a cake and shared endows good fortune and creates a bond among all who eat it. • Scoop out the pineapple flesh and share it with a partner on full moon night to conceive a child, or eat alone if you are trying for a baby as a single parent. Fill the skin with white flowerheads, sesame or pumpkin seeds, and uncooked rice—symbols of fertility. Float the filled skin on the silver pathway the moon makes across the sea or down a moonlit river, and afterward make love or baby plans.

Pineapple Weed

(*Matricaria discoidea*)

MAGICAL FORMS

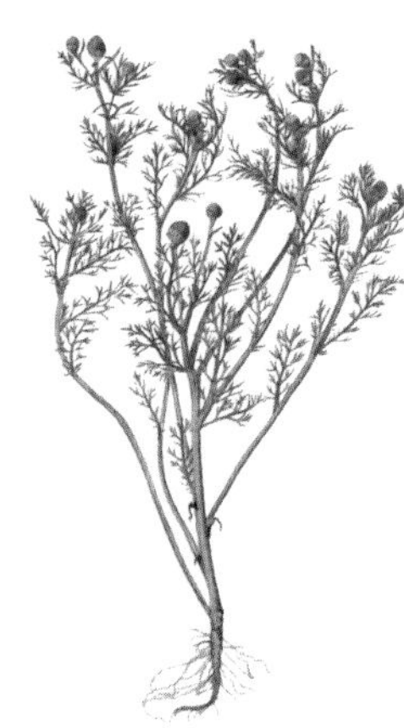

feathery leaves with a pineapple scent, and yellow flowerheads that look like small pineapples, blooming May to November • a wildflower that can grow up to sixteen inches but often remains low growing • resembles a small chamomile plant without leaves • pineapple weed may have traveled from northeast Asia to the USA on the feet of prehistoric dogs via the land bridge across the Bering Strait • grows on farmland and along tracks throughout the USA • in 1869, having been introduced to Kew Gardens in London, it escaped, and by the twentieth century it spread across the country via car tires • magically use the dried flowers, growing plant, and flower essence

PLANET AND ELEMENT

Mercury • Air

MAGICAL USES

for positive parent/child interactions at any age, especially with mothers where these were severed by absence in childhood or traumatic early life issues • strengthening connections with nature if you are a city person • for environmental warriors to make effective peaceful protests

HOW TO USE

Use the leaves and flowers in love and fidelity charm bags, hung over the bed and replaced when they lose their fragrance. • Anoint your inner wrist points with a drop of the essence if you are going to see your birth mother for the first time or if you have become estranged from your mother because she cannot show affection, to insulate yourself from potential hurt.

CAUTION

Avoid pineapple weed if you are allergic to daisies.

Pink Plates

(*Mesophyllum lichenoides*)

MAGICAL FORMS

a red marine algae, brittle and calcified with concentric bands • pink to purple with white around the edges • found in tidal pools or on rocks depending on the location • in the UK as far north as the Orkney Isles, further south in the Atlantic, the Mediterranean, the Aegean Sea, Algeria, and Turkey • may grow overlapping in a heap or attached to other plants, but are not parasitic • magically use the seaweed in situ or dried and as essence

PLANET AND ELEMENT

Moon • Water

MAGICAL USES

as the essence, for patience before or in the early stages of a new beginning or relationship • for being ready to embrace necessary change harmoniously without forcing it • for thinking before acting • moving out of the comfort zone

HOW TO USE

Cast the seaweed, or a bottle of water collected from the ocean with four drops of the essence added, back into the sea, saying, *I return what is yours, send what I ask for back to me*, asking for the safe return of a lost opportunity, a lost love, or a precious item that has been mislaid or stolen. • Pink seaweed represents the acquisition of money within a joint business or financial venture you are undertaking with a partner. • Add a little of the dried seaweed or another red or pink seaweed with four drops of the essence into a glass jar, then half fill with brandy to cover the seaweed. Seal and keep from New Year to the next New Year.

CAUTION

There is not yet sufficient scientific evidence to safely ingest pink plates seaweed or use it medicinally.

Pipsissewa

(*Chimaphila umbellata*)

MAGICAL FORMS

also called prince's pine or spotted wintergreen • low-growing, erect, evergreen, wildflower plant with several stems • shiny, wedge-shaped leaves • native throughout the cool temperate zones of North America from Canada to Mexico, Europe, and Asia, with pink and white flowers in June • pleasant flavor and taste, used in root beer, candy, and tea • quite difficult to cultivate • magically use the crushed leaves, whole aerial plant, and shredded and hulled wild herb (available online and perfect for ritual purposes)

PLANET AND ELEMENT

Saturn • Earth

MAGICAL USES

attracts good spirits and your own spirit guides • a money magnet, for rituals for life transitions, especially if you can meditate on the growing plants in the wild to take you first to past worlds, then to the future you can make and the steps you should take to get there

HOW TO USE

Before mediumship or divination, burn the shredded herb with dried sage, sandalwood, and cedar chips on a bonfire, mixing in myrrh resin if using incense on charcoal, to seek the advice of the wise spirits and keep out those spirits who would do harm. • Add the dried, shredded leaves to a dollar bill in a charm bag, including a gambling chip or three small, green aventurine crystals if you plan speculation or if you are entering a competition, and keep the bag with you as you take a chance.

CAUTION

Pipsissewa can interfere with absorption of prescription medicines. • Avoid while pregnant, breastfeeding, or if you have an iron deficiency. • It may cause skin irritation.

Pistachio Nut

(*Pistacia vera*)

MAGICAL FORMS

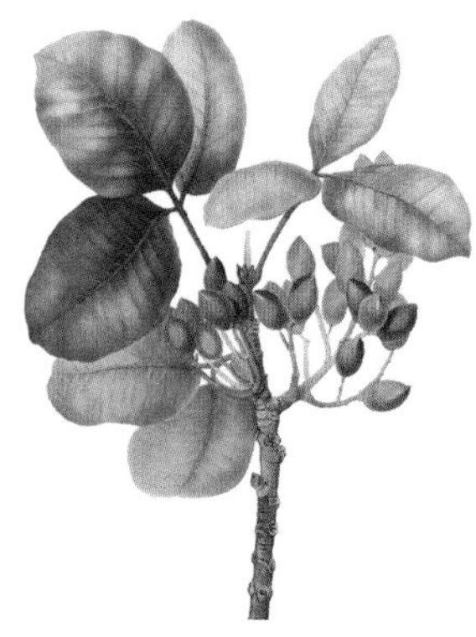

the pistachio tree has taproots as long as the tree is tall, up to thirty feet • produces pistachio nuts that are seeds rather than fruits • encased in a hard nonedible shell, the nuts may burst through when ripe • green when raw and light brown when roasted • native to Asia and Iran, where they are still grown in large quantities and in California and parts of New Mexico and Arizona • harvested in October • magically use the nuts, shelled and unshelled

PLANETS AND ELEMENT

Mars/Sun • Fire

MAGICAL USES

to attract generosity in those who hold back from sharing • to herald in a new phase that will bear results in the months ahead • when dyed red, the nuts are used for love-attracting spells and for protection against unwise love temptations and love cheats

HOW TO USE

Eat to break the hold of a love enchantment and mind manipulation, discarding the shells before meeting or communicating with a person when you know your willpower is overridden. • Shell the nuts and share them with those who find it hard to part with their money, affection, or praise. • Eat the nuts and decorate the empty, creamy-yellow shells with bright colors (sometimes you can prise the nut out and leave the two halves still joined, which is extra lucky). Name each one for a wish, desire, or need for the six months ahead. Varnish and keep them in a sealed glass jar as a reminder of those dreams that can be fulfilled.

Plai

(*Zingiber cassumunar*)

MAGICAL FORMS

the plant, which is eight to twelve inches tall, is native to India, Indonesia, and Thailand • essential oil is produced from the rhizomes (roots) and is central to Thai massage • a relative of ginger and galangal, the rhizome is used medicinally and in traditional Thai cookery • magically work with the essential oil and the rhizome, usually sold powdered from Asian specialty stores and online from herbalists

PLANET AND ELEMENT

Mars • Fire

MAGICAL USES

protects against psychic attacks and mind manipulation • for peaceful but lively social occasions • enables workaholics to switch off

HOW TO USE

Carry the powdered root or, if you can get one, a whole root in a small bag to guard against people playing mind games or twisting your words, or if adversaries are trying to convince you that you are wrong and you are doubting yourself. Add a single drop or two of the oil before sealing the bag. • Use the diluted oil in self-massage or a few drops in your bath or on an infused cloth in the shower in the evening. • Pay extra attention to the back of your neck, the base of your spine, your inner wrist pulse points, the soles of your feet, and your knees to seal your energies against lingering external pressures and demands of the day and so that no psychic or psychological harm will befall you as you sleep. • Use anywhere you have regular pain, as that may indicate a weak spot in your aura energy field.

Plantain Tree, Broadleaf

(*Plantago major*)

MAGICAL FORMS

often called a lawn weed, this is arguably an herb since it has both medicinal and edible properties and was used extensively in healing and folk magick • an example of how disregarded plants can possess magical powers • found in Europe, Asia, and eastern North America • magically use the whole, growing or dry plant; the chopped or powdered oval leaves set in a rosette near the ground; the tall, thin spikes develop into tiny club-shaped flowers; or as a flower essence

PLANET AND ELEMENT

Saturn • Earth

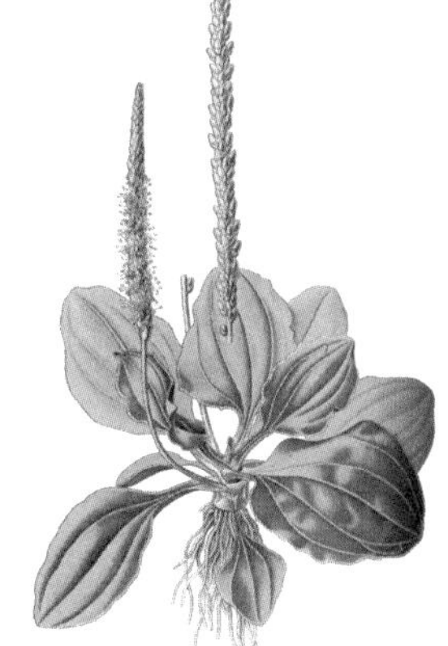

MAGICAL USES

because broadleaf plantain will grow on barren land, in spells it represents stamina and perseverance • alternatively, a tiny piece stuck to the inside of shoes signifies overcoming weariness • as a flower essence, removes anger due to bitterness and resentment from the past

HOW TO USE

Hang the dried, chopped herb or dried flowers in a tiny sachet on the rearview mirror of a vehicle or in a glove compartment to increase alertness while driving. • The dried, powdered herb, burned regularly in an incense with a courage resin like dragon's blood, allows your influence to spread and is useful if you long to be recognized for your abilities. • Scatter the seeds on barren land, calling as you turn in all directions what you need to plant in your life and whom to attract. • Bury some to represent what or whom you no longer want to dominate your life or denigrate you.

CAUTION

Do not take while pregnant or breastfeeding.

Plantain Tree, Cooking

(*Musa × paradisiaca*)

MAGICAL FORMS

the scientific name encompasses both edible plantains and bananas (see p. 50) • the cooking plantain tree is grown in tropical climates • native to Southeast Asia, especially Malaysia and Indonesia, it may be found outdoors in a few areas of California, notably Sacramento, San Diego, and San Juan Capistrano, as well as in Florida • can be grown in pots, for example as the Puerto Rican dwarf plantain • plantain fruits, which are green, yellow, or brown, are longer and firmer than bananas with less sugar and thicker skin, and are cooked as vegetables rather than eaten raw • the fuchsia-colored tree flowers bloom around midsummer, then in late summer to early fall and mid-fall, becoming the hanging fruit four to eight months after flowering • much loved by Alexander the Great, who in 327 BCE imported plantain fruit from India to Europe • magically work with the fruit and peel in all its forms

PLANET AND ELEMENT

Moon • Water

MAGICAL USES

like the banana, plantains are associated with male power and virility • the fruit brings healing and protection, increases stamina, and repels spite and human snakes, malicious people, and restless spirits

HOW TO USE

Tie a piece of the dried peel with red ribbon over the door at home or your business to keep away all malevolence, ill-speaking, and ill wishes, and to attract harmony and good fortune. When it withers, replace it, as it has lost its power. • While cooking your plantain, making plantain bread, or eating commercially prepared plantain chips, make wishes for abundance, health, wealth, and fertility in the ways most needed. • Do not throw away the peeled skin in the garbage, but recycle it as compost or burn in an outside fire to avoid throwing away happiness and luck.

Plum

(*Prunus* spp.)

MAGICAL FORMS

commercially produced plums grow on a medium-size pruned tree • the wild plum is a naturally small tree or shrub • both producing red, purple, green, or orange-yellow, smooth, round or oval fruit, each containing a single stone • cultivated plums are larger and sweeter • the cultivated plum is grown in most temperate zones • wild plums are native to North America, originally growing extensively across northeastern and southeastern USA and southeastern Canada and the Midwest • in modern times the USA is an important producer of cultivated plums • during the nineteenth century wild plums became widely cultivated in backyards in the USA and during the railroad era wild plums dramatically declined, though fifteen species still exist in the USA • wild plums are increasingly found in gardens once more • magically use the fresh and dried blossom and fruit

PLANET AND ELEMENT

Venus • Water

MAGICAL USES

the five petals of the Chinese plum blossom, a structure found in some other plum blossoms, represents in China the five blessings: old age, wealth, health, love of virtue, and an easy natural death • the blossom is an important symbol at Chinese New Year • plum blossoms and fruit signify in Western traditions sensuality and heightened libido, riches, radiance, fertility (especially in all-female relationships), attracting or maintaining love, and healing

HOW TO USE

Place a bowl with plums in it at the center of the home for protection against intrusion by spirits. • Eat three plums and carry the washed and dried stones in a charm bag to bring novelty and exciting change into your life. • Bury an overripe plum to mark the end of a relationship—especially sexual, without commitment—or life phase, trusting new happiness will in time regrow.

CAUTION

Plums should only be eaten ripe or dried as prunes. • The stone is toxic and should not be ingested.

Plumeria Tree

(*Plumeria* spp.)

MAGICAL FORMS

also called the frangipani • small, rounded tree of the dogbane family • also found as shrubs and woody climbers • native to Central America and Mexico, naturalized elsewhere in subtropical and tropical zones including southern North America • can be grown as house or conservatory plants in temperate areas of the USA, Europe, and Great Britain • traditionally used as a scented oil in Pacific Islands such as Hawaii • a tree sacred to Buddhism and Hinduism outside temples in the Far East, the flowers are made as offerings to the deities • magically use the fragrant frangipani flower (popular as necklaces in Cambodia for protection and to attract love), scented oil, potted plant, and living tree

PLANET AND ELEMENTS

Venus • Water/Earth

MAGICAL USES

for love spells, sensuality, and enhancing sexual magnetism • friendship, romance, and preserving love far away • for a long life, loyalty, protection against emotional vampires

HOW TO USE

Anoint a white candle with the scented oil (just a drop diluted in olive oil) before lighting to call an absent love home. Blow out the flame and send the love to where your lover is. Relight every night for a few minutes until it is burned through. • Use flowers for weddings and births, or place a small plumeria or potted frangipani on the grave of a female relative so its fragrance rekindles fond memories. • They are best given in a pot rather than cut flowers so the love will grow.

CAUTION

Do not use while pregnant or breastfeeding. • Do not ingest any parts of the raw plant. • Dilute the oil well before putting on the skin. • The plumeria trunk and branches and flower stems secrete a milky sap that is highly toxic.

Poinsettia

(*Euphorbia pulcherrima*)

MAGICAL FORMS

scientific name means "most beautiful" • native to southwest Mexico and Guatemala • bracts (holding the small flowers) are most popularly scarlet, though there are a hundred varieties and different colors • the poinsettia was used by the Aztecs and Mayans ritually and medicinally for centuries and adopted by Franciscan missionaries in Mexico to adorn their elaborate nativity altar • poinsettia was brought to the USA and Canada, eventually spreading worldwide, by the amateur botanist and United States ambassador to Mexico, Joel Roberts Poinsett, in 1828 • magically use the whole, growing plant and fresh or dried flowers

PLANET AND ELEMENTS

Sun • Fire/Earth

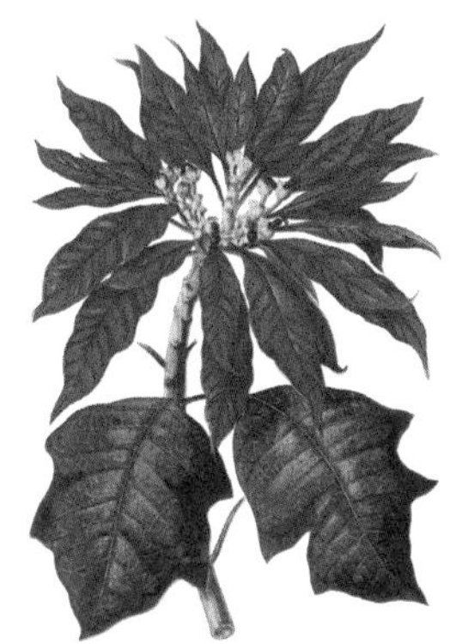

MAGICAL USES

signifies the return of light at the darkest time of the year or when life seems without hope • poinsettia is a magical centerpiece for the home, a joy bringer, a family unifier if money is short around Christmas, and a gift of love for all mothers

HOW TO USE

In Yuletide celebrations, place the poinsettia in the center of the altar or family table to represent the birthing of Jesus, or the sun king or maiden in the earlier goddess tradition that many still celebrate. • On Christmas Eve or the midwinter solstice (the shortest day of the year), take a large, red bract and make a wish for what you most desire to come into or return to your life. Take a second bract and wish for someone or a place in need. Wrap both in tissue paper between the pages of a Bible or sacred book. On New Year's Eve before midnight, burn the leaves and give thanks for blessings received or still to be granted.

CAUTION

Poinsettia is mildly toxic to household pets.

Poison Hemlock

(*Conium maculatum*)

MAGICAL FORMS

poison hemlock is a flowering plant growing to eight feet with red, speckled stems; small, clustered, white flowers; and seeds with beaded ridges • native to Europe, China, and northern Africa, and naturalized in the USA • Socrates ended his life in 399 BCE by drinking poison hemlock, having lectured his students on the immortality of the soul • used as a form of capital punishment among the high born of ancient Greece • not recommended for magical use (the below is for informational purposes only!)

PLANET AND ELEMENT

Saturn • Earth

MAGICAL USES

added to flying medicines for out-of-body experiences in medieval times • even in small quantities, hemlock is highly dangerous and some practitioners lost their lives • in ritual magick, its juice was rubbed into magical knives and tools in the tradition of King Solomon to purify them and give them potency • hyssop (see p. 228) infusion is just as good and lacks risks

HOW TO USE

Hemlock is known as a baneful herb, which means it has been used to harm others physically or magically or in fierce defense in days when justice was only for the rich. • In the modern world there are many alternative, safe magical defensive herbs. • Some practitioners keep the chopped plant in a dark jar on a high shelf to be held and directed to repel danger or protection of the vulnerable, but the risks of having it around the home are, in my view, too great to merit this—even if handled with extreme caution.

CAUTION

Poison hemlock is a fast-acting poison to humans and livestock through ingestion, inhalation, and touching any part of the plant.

Poison Ivy

(*Toxicodendron radicans*)

MAGICAL FORMS

as ground cover, vine, or shrub, poison ivy differs botanically and in appearance from common nontoxic ivy (see p. 232) • identified by three shiny leaflets on a stem and white berries • common ivy retains its leaves all year but poison ivy turns red in the fall and its leaves drop off • grows wild and in gardens in all states in the USA, especially the east, as well as in parts of China • magically use (without touching!) the whole, growing plant and fresh or dried leaves, handled with care

PLANET AND ELEMENT

Moon • Water

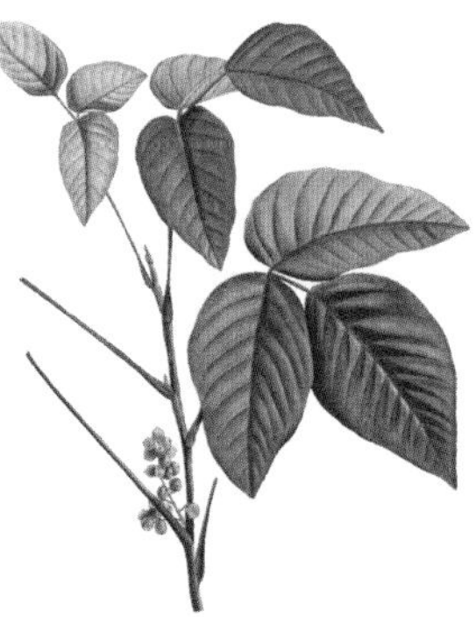

MAGICAL USES

for establishing personal and domestic boundaries • driving away temptation to behave unwisely in love if the desired lover is not free or is destructive but exciting • for defensive magick if an attack is particularly vicious, whether psychic or actual

HOW TO USE

Dried leaves were traditionally added to fierce defense bottles. • In dire circumstances, though common, non-poisonous ivy is effective for most protective bottles. • Chopped poison ivy handled with gloves can be added to thorns and a strong vinegar in a dark sealed bottle to establish boundaries. Store high off the ground in a safe place. • Poison ivy growing naturally up a tree in a place in the garden safe from children, unwary strangers, or pets acts as a psychic barrier if you live on land with disturbed energies where sorrow or a tragedy has occurred in the house, land, or nearby, or you have a poltergeist predator spirit.

CAUTION

Touching the plant causes dermatitis and severe skin inflammation, up to forty-eight hours after handling. • The effects may last for three weeks.

Poison Oak

(*Toxicodendron diversilobum*) and (*Toxicodendron pubescens*)

MAGICAL FORMS

the Pacific or western poison oak (*diversilobum*) is a low-growing shrub or woody climbing vine • found throughout western North America, especially coastal regions from British Columbia to Mexico with usually round, shiny, three-leaflet leaves, turning red in the fall • the Atlantic or eastern poison oak (*pubescens*) is not a creeper, but a shrub about three feet tall with three lobed, hairy leaflets • native to the southeastern USA with orange-red leaves in the fall • neither is an oak (*Quercus*) • magically use the dried leaves or twigs collected with gloves, checking that there is no exposed flesh around ankles, and more safely as flower essence

PLANET AND ELEMENT

Jupiter • Air

MAGICAL USES

the essence reduces fears of all kinds, especially of physical touch or intimacy that may be linked to sexual trauma or abuse in childhood • use when finding physical contact hard, even with children • for those who are overprotective of personal boundaries

HOW TO USE

Add a few drops of the essence to massage oil if working with a partner if one or both of you has sexual inhibitions. • Alternatively, anoint your inner wrist points to open your heart to receive and give physical love. • The poison oak plant is like its close relative poison ivy, another baneful herb used for fierce defense. • Take three equal-length twigs with leaves cut, and tie them together with red cord, using gloves. Wrap in a tightly tied, biodegradable bag and bury deep beneath the poison bush or tree to remove hexes, curses, and ill wishes, or to banish the memory of abuse.

CAUTION

Tree leaves, branches, and bark contain urushiol oil, which causes a severe skin rash if the leaves are touched. • Avoid burning the wood because of toxic smoke inhalation. • It may be safer and as effective to use another, less-toxic, banishing magick plant unless matters are dire.

Poison Sumac

(*Toxicodendron vernix*)

MAGICAL FORMS

a woody shrub or small tree, with a distinct trunk, branches, and twigs, growing in the eastern USA, Texas, and Canada • related to poison ivy but even more toxic • thrives in wet areas • identifiable by clusters of white or light-green berries hanging down and glossy leaves with a reddish tinge • between seven and thirteen leaflets attached to each stem by a reddish stalk • magically use the whole, growing plant or cut leaves with the utmost caution, if at all, and do not allow any exposed skin to make contact

PLANETS AND ELEMENTS

Mars/Saturn • Fire/Earth

MAGICAL USES

for banishing what or who is destructive in your life • for defensive magick when a crisis is acute or a vulnerable person is under threat, although generally other strong banishing herbs such as peppermint (see p. 343) or juniper (see p. 241) are safer to use

HOW TO USE

Place a paper leaflet stem or an image cut from a printout in a sealed bag, then add salt. Cut the leaflet and three small, dark-colored cords in half, put the cords in a bag before sealing, and throw away the bag in a trash can somewhere away from your home to once and for all remove a generational curse, or when you feel you are being ill-wished or jinxed.

CAUTION

The pollen, oil, and resin cause a painful rash. • The tree can be fatal if parts are ingested. • It would be best to leave poison sumac alone or work from photographs of the tree that with ingenuity you can adapt to all kinds of banishing spells.

Poke Root

(*Phytolacca americana*)

MAGICAL FORMS

a flowering, tall shrub with pinkish-red stems and purple-black berries • native to southwestern and eastern regions of the USA • grows in other parts of the country, and in Europe, Asia, and South America, as does the related common poke root (*Phytolacca decandra*) • magically use the root, most usually sold as shredded, dried poke root that can be purchased online • probably more wieldy than the actual root, as the average taproot is over a foot long and four inches thick

PLANET AND ELEMENT

Mars • Fire

MAGICAL USES

for breaking curses and hexes during the dark of the moon • courage • use the berries for magick ink to write petitions or archangel messages on thick, white paper

HOW TO USE

Deeply bury a root mix in sealed wildlife- and pet-proof containers near your property boundaries to deter hostile neighbors and vandals. • To remove any ill wishes, curses, hexes, jinxes, or a sense of paranormal restlessness, create an infusion of the root to sprinkle on doorsteps. Using clear, hot water, wash away and then discard any remaining infusion down outside drains. • To discover the culprit when someone has stolen something precious or deliberately sabotaged an effort, use the crushed berries as an ink. Pour a little ink into a bowl of clear, cold water, half closing your eyes. In the swirls, you will either see a face or hear a name before the water turns black. Take calm action without making accusations.

CAUTION

Poke root is poisonous, so handle with care, using gloves. • Keep the plant away from children and pets. • Berries are the most poisonous. • Avoid totally if you are pregnant or nursing.

Polyanthus

(*Primula × polyantha*) or (*Primula variabilis*)

MAGICAL FORMS

a natural hybrid created in the 1670s and often called the false oxslip, through the combination of the cowslip (*Primula veris*) and common primrose (*Primula vulgaris*) • much underrated magically and botanically, polyanthus is a long-stalked version of primula with brilliantly colored, showier flowers, including red, yellow, blue, and purple with basal rosettes • most precious magically as the smaller gold or silver lace polyanthus, golden-eyed with deep-burgundy petals and gold or silver margins around the petals • magically use the whole, growing plant; cut flowers (with care, as they can be delicate); and fresh or dried flowerheads

PLANETS AND ELEMENTS

Venus/Sun • Earth/Fire

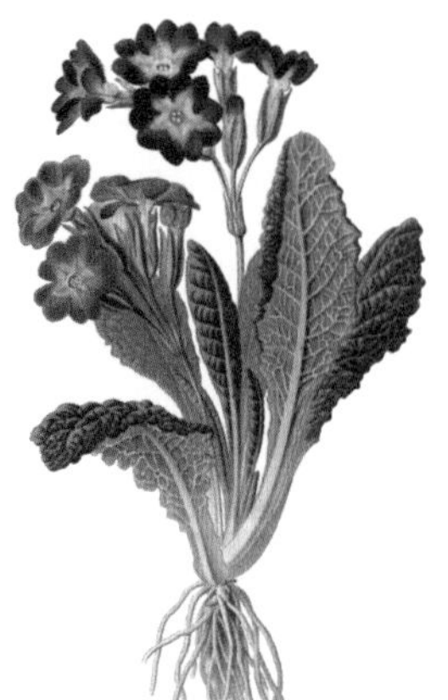

MAGICAL USES

use the gold and silver varieties for all forms of money magick, to obtain beautiful objects, to bring beauty out of ugliness and to bring happiness out of sadness

HOW TO USE

Add a silver and a gold flowerhead with a piece of silver and a piece of gold (such as an earring or thin ring) to a silver or gold charm bag. Pass the sealed bag through the smoke of a frankincense or sandalwood incense stick, both wealth bringers. • Set different-colored, taller polyanthus in a vase, inverting your cupped palms, fingers together, a few centimeters above the flowers. Allow the color energies to pass through your fingertips into your aura energy center. When you feel the power filling your aura, shake your fingers over your head and around your heart to fill your energy system with radiance, charisma, and beauty. • Tape a few dried petals of polyanthus in a tiny bag to the back of valuable antiques or beautiful artifacts in your home to prevent breakages or theft.

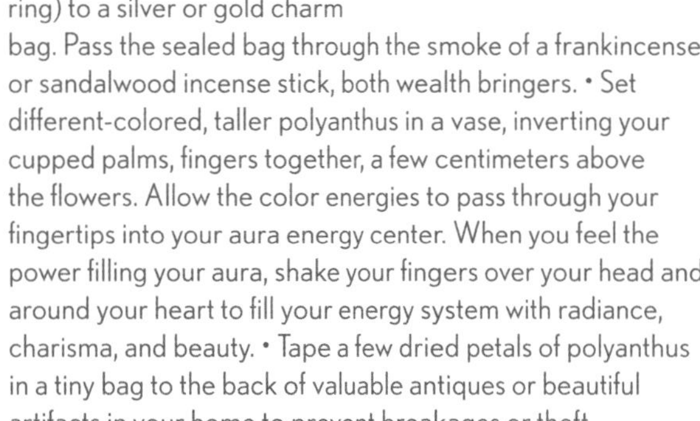

Pomander

MAGICAL FORMS

a plant-based decoration made from a large citrus fruit, especially oranges, grapefruit, or the even larger pomelo (see p. 358) plus cloves and chosen spices (typically allspice, cinnamon, and nutmeg) • the combination of fragrances is more powerful than the individual, separate ingredients • a pomander represents a treasure house of health, wealth, love, and good fortune • magically use pomander to work alone or with a loved one or family members, preferably with a fresh citrus fruit you have been given as a gift

PLANET AND ELEMENT

Sun • Fire

MAGICAL USES

dating from medieval times when a sailor might bring an orange home from an exotic voyage as a love token, pomanders were created to call an absent lover home, for domestic health and happiness, family celebrations, a first home together or alone, or more prosaically to fragrance the house • each of the spices chosen represents a different quality: allspice for prosperity; cloves, fidelity; cinnamon, passion and fertility; nutmeg, good fortune; coriander for business or workplace success; and orris for unity • the citrus fruit represents health and abundance

HOW TO USE

To create a pomander, pierce the skin of the fruit all over with a barbecue fork, kitchen skewer, or knitting needle, not cutting through to the flesh. Test a hole for size; they should be no less than a quarter of an inch apart or the pomander may break up. Place dried cloves with sharpened ends in the holes and roll the pomander in a bowl or plate of mixed allspice, cinnamon, and nutmeg, plus any other spices whose magick you need, not just those suggested above, speaking wishes or blessings aloud for each spice as you roll to empower your pomander. Additionally, you can create a chant as you press in the cloves. Shake off any residual powder and leave to dry in a warm but not hot, dry place. Criss-cross red ribbons and hang the pomander from a hook on the ceiling in your kitchen or the center of your home so air can circulate.

Pomegranate Fruit

(*Punica granatum*)

MAGICAL FORMS

this entry is specific to the fruit of the pomegranate, which has strong magical associations apart from the tree • ruby flesh, filled with seeds inside and an amber-gold skin • said to have been the original fruit of temptation in the Garden of Eden, pomegranates are associated with the maiden Greek goddess Persephone, who ate pomegranate seeds when she was abducted by the underworld god Hades, and so for part of the year returned to Hades, her grieving mother Demeter bringing winter • magically use the fruit

PLANET AND ELEMENT

Moon • Water

MAGICAL USES

for overcoming lack of nurturing as a child and breaking the pattern with one's own children • also for creativity • pomegranate fruits attract unexpected wealth or a source of income previously dismissed • fertility because of the number of seeds

HOW TO USE

Keep the seeds of the fruit after preparation and ask a yes–no, go–stay, act–wait, or speak–be silent question using the seeds to count. • The juice can be used as a magical ink for writing petitions and used instead of blood in ancient spells with equal effect, more ethically. • Add the crushed skin to money incenses and as an aphrodisiac when tea is made from the seeds or dried flowers, or purchased commercially, or the juice is shared before lovemaking.

CAUTION

Pomegranate may interact with ACE inhibitors, drugs for high blood pressure, or blood thinners.

Pomegranate Tree

(*Punica granatum*)

MAGICAL FORMS

the fruit-bearing pomegranate tree is native to southern Europe and southern Asia, but grows in warmer parts of the USA and even the UK in a hardy form • produces deep-red, funnel-shaped flowers in late spring/early summer and early fall, and fruit if pollinated five to seven months later • generally deciduous but can be evergreen in warm climates • the bonsai form originated in Japan and is now grown worldwide indoors, and represents all the powers of its full-size big sister • flowering in most regions but bearing fruit mainly in Japan and Mediterranean-type climates • magically use the growing tree, whether full-size or as a bonsai tree if the full size does not grow in your region; flowers; or flower essence

PLANET AND ELEMENT

Moon • Water

MAGICAL USES

the full-size pomegranate tree represents good fortune, prosperity, and connection with the ancestors, and heralds the birth of future generations • the pomegranate bonsai signifies charisma and fertility when in leaf • once it loses some or all of its leaves in fall and winter, it encourages the need to allow life and nature to take its course until the leaves return • as a flower essence, represents maternal and mothering issues, especially combining parenthood or motherhood with career

HOW TO USE

Since the tree signifies in Greek myth the rebirth of Dionysus, the god of wine and ecstasy, use the dried red flowers in a charm bag for the regeneration of abandoned creative projects, the restoration of fortune, and happiness, prosperity, and fertility when hope has been lost. • Make the bonsai the center of a miniature indoor garden (outdoors in summer if a warm climate), and use while meditating when the tree is in leaf to allow creative solutions to achieve desired results. • When partially or totally leafless, use the bonsai for patience and allowing the natural flow of events to replace anxiety and seemingly fruitless efforts.

Pomelo Tree

(*Citrus maxima*)

MAGICAL FORMS
tree native to Malaysia, Thailand, and South China, growing wild on river banks in Fiji • the largest citrus fruit and sweeter than grapefruit • an ancestor of the grapefruit • often pear-shaped with pale rind and greenish-yellow flesh • the tree came to the USA in 1902 • magically use the fruit, essential oil made from the peel, and the oil, which can sometimes be found in perfumes

PLANET AND ELEMENT
Moon • Water

MAGICAL USES
traditionally, displaying the fruit brings joy to any occasion and celebration, especially Chinese New Year, when it is a symbol of ongoing good luck throughout the year • the fruit also brings abundance, confidence, and a sense of well-being when kept in the home, especially when decorated with ribbons and bells • the oil and fragrance soften bad news and critical words • promotes tolerance of difficult people and situations and opens new possibilities and approaches

HOW TO USE
Anoint the center of the throat and the brow with the empowered diluted oil or a fragrance in which the oil is used to inspire creativity if you run out of original ideas or have artistic or writer's block. • Pierce the skin of the fruit all over with cloves and roll it in allspice, cinnamon, and nutmeg, naming any prejudice or attempts to stifle your true self or hold you back through unfair bias. Display it in a wire fruit dish in the center of your kitchen so air can circulate, and turn the fruit over every day, adding more spice until eventually the fruit decays (see "Pomander," p. 356). Bury it in soil where nothing grows so the prejudice or obstacles will not return.

CAUTION
Do not use the oil while trying to conceive or while pregnant or breastfeeding. • Also avoid oil and fruit if suffering from kidney or liver problems.

Poplar Tree

(*Populus* spp.)

MAGICAL FORMS
genus of plants with twenty-five to thirty species • grows through western North America from Alaska to California • white European poplar (*Populus alba*) is a broader tree with pale gray or white bark and distinctively woolly undersides of leaves • magically use the whole, growing tree in situ; buds, which are golden, fragrant, and sticky on the black cottonwood; catkins (flowers containing pollen); balsam-fragranced leaves of the black cottonwood; and fruit, with hundreds of seeds released as fluffy cotton on the wind (see "Aspens," which are closely related, p. 38)

PLANET AND ELEMENT
Moon • Water

MAGICAL USES
white poplar is sacred to the ancient Greek hero Hercules and garlands were worn to signify victory over great odds • as distinctly different catkins appear on the separate male and female trees in many species of poplars, the male and female catkins can be used for twin soul rituals and sacred sex (this works just as well in same-sex or gender-fluid relationships as the coming together of animus or anima)

HOW TO USE
Crush buds or dried leaves in an incense mix for employment, money, and increased business. • Inhale the balsam fragrance from fresh leaves or sit beneath any poplar tree for astral travel. • The taller, slender kinds of poplars such as the black cottonwood or the Lombardy poplar (*Populus nigra* 'Italica') are associated with otherworlds as world trees. Ascend them shamanically to higher realms when the full moon is shining through the branches as you gaze upward.

CAUTION
The sap can cause skin irritation. • Do not ingest the raw plant or its parts.

Poplar Tree, Balsam

(*Populus balsamifera*)

MAGICAL FORMS

also known as the balsam poplar • including *Populus balsamifera* subsp. *trichocarpa*, known as America western poplar/black cottonwood • the buds are gummy, releasing a balsam-like fragrance and red balsam-smelling resin was used medicinally for centuries by Native North Americans • the female trees release clouds of cottony tufts containing seeds in the early summer • native to North America, transcontinental from Alaska to Nova Scotia, though may grow in northern Minnesota, Michigan, and parts of the Rockies • magically use the flower essence, the cotton-like tufts, and the inner bark as tea

PLANET AND ELEMENT

Jupiter • Air

MAGICAL USES

as flower essence, awakens all the senses • overcomes sexual difficulties and suppressed libido, often caused by earlier sexual trauma, abuse, or rejection • restores harmony with natural and astrological cycles • as a tea, overcomes inhibitions in revealing the true self unbound by others' rules • the dried, unopened buds, inner bark, and balsam-fragranced resin were used by Native North American people for respiratory illnesses and skin conditions

HOW TO USE

Release the cotton-like seeds, collected in a bag, in high spaces to bring renewed connection with the spiritual self and especially the spirits of the Air and Mountain wherever you live in the world. • The floating seeds can be used for wishes. • Add a few drops of the essence to an erotic massage oil if sex has become limited to certain times and places.

CAUTION

Do not ingest during pregnancy or breastfeeding, and avoid if allergic to aspirin and bee stings or if taking blood thinners. • The flower essence does not absorb any of the plant's chemical properties, but use other balsam poplar products in moderation and with advice.

Poppy

(*Papaveroideae* spp.)

MAGICAL FORMS

a wide variety of flowers growing within the *Papaveroideae* family • the opiate found in the milky sap within the pod of this plant is illegal in the USA, though it is still tolerated as an ornamental • magically use the whole plant, dried petals, pods, seeds, and seed oil (note that the opiate is not contained within the seeds or the seed oil)

PLANET AND ELEMENT

Moon • Water

MAGICAL USES

psychic visions and divination • peace • increasing imaginative and creative gifts • quiet sleep • remembering ancestors • fertility • lowering physical and psychological profile in times of danger or potential confrontation • reversing bad luck • taking away grief and mental anguish

HOW TO USE

To create a fertility charm, fill a sachet with seeds, to be set on a window ledge on the full moon or outdoors if possible (keep hidden for the rest of the month). • A dried seed pod in which the seeds are replaced by a written question, set by the bed, brings the answer in a dream or immediately upon waking. • Attract prosperity by placing the pod or seeds in a sachet with a small piece of gold such as an earring, then hang on a tree; the growing flowers have the same effect. • Enchant a lover with a bath sachet filled with petals.• Sprinkling seeds or growing poppies around your property confuses and drives away malevolent spirits.

Poppy, California

(*Eschscholzia californica*)

MAGICAL FORMS

not a poppy as such, but shares their ancestry • native to the southwestern USA, including Oregon, Arizona, Nevada, and New Mexico, and to Mexico, including Baja California • magically use the whole, growing plant; cut flowers (short life unless dried); flowerheads, fresh and dried; leaves, fresh and dried; and seeds

PLANETS AND ELEMENTS

Sun/Mercury • Fire/Air

MAGICAL USES

mainly golden orange though can be red or yellow, called the *cup of sunlight* or *California sunshine,* and the state flower of California since 1903, with its own day on April 6 each year • for wealth, success, and as the first plant to regrow after fires • for rituals and talismans for regeneration and recovery after loss or illness • in folk magick, used to gain attraction

HOW TO USE

Since California poppies are associated with the Californian gold rush, use the golden orange flowers for accumulating money and discovering new sources of income. Each day add a handful of seeds to a wealth jar, then close the lid and shake the jar, saying, *Incubate to accumulate, more and more each day, for growing wealth lies that way.* Incubate the jar in sunlight or near a source of heat, and when the jar is full, shake out the seeds in the open air in bright sunlight, leaving just a few in the jar. With these, start a new collection in the same jar, continuing the cycle so you will never be short of money. • Also for protective nighttime rituals to slow personal overactive energies and restless spirits, as the golden poppy closes its flowers every night. • Use the dried crumbled herb with dried valerian and lavender in an incense mix with myrrh resin for shedding the cares of the day, removing any paranormal disturbances or darkness from the home, and bringing quiet sleep.

CAUTION

Avoid eating the fresh flowers or leaves.

Poppy, Mexican

(*Argemone mexicana*)

MAGICAL FORMS

Mexican poppy is a common name for several plants • magically, the *Argemone ochroleuca*, or pale Mexican prickly poppy, has similar effects • both are hardy, small, flowering, thistlelike poppies with sharp, spiny stems, white-veined leaves, and large, yellow flowers with delicate petals • indigenous to Texas, southern and western USA, parts of Mexico, the West Indies, and Central America • introduced into Australia in 1845, where it is regarded as a troublesome weed • buy the chopped and crushed aerial parts online (handle with care) for magical use, or use the seeds and the growing plant • can also be used as a flower remedy

PLANET AND ELEMENT

Moon • Water

MAGICAL USES

the growing yellow Mexican poppy represents wealth, gain, optimism, and joy • because the Mexican poppy is toxic, it signifies advantages involving risk and danger • one version of a Mexican folktale recalls a woman turned into a yellow poppy by a malevolent magick woman, whose husband searched the fields until he found her • because of the poppies' sleep-inducing properties he kept falling asleep but he persisted and she was restored, making this a poppy of not giving up, especially in terms of lost love

HOW TO USE

Pour a few seeds mixed in beer down an indoor water source—an old West African remedy for impotency if conception is hard and your partner is having problems making love. • Fiercely defensive, chopped stems with spines still attached, well wrapped in a workplace drawer, should be used if you are facing gossip, malice, or misrepresentation.

CAUTION

All parts of the plant are toxic, so only take the remedy in a professionally prepared form and dosage. • Avoid handling the poppy (except with gloves), and never ingest the picked plant. • Poppy should not be used excessively, nor by pregnant or lactating women or those with diarrhea, IBS, or colitis.

Potato

(*Solanum tuberosum*)

MAGICAL FORMS

a root vegetable grown for its tubers, the swollen end of the underground stems • often produces white, purple, and yellow flowers with yellow stamens and berries with seeds • a single plant will produce up to five or even ten smaller potatoes • the more potatoes on the single plant, the more prosperity and good luck • cultivated by the Incas in South America • now grown worldwide as a food staple • also grown in containers or bags • magically use the raw or cooked potato, or as the very popular potato chip

PLANETS AND ELEMENT

Moon/Saturn • Earth

MAGICAL USES

for building up opportunity step by step • perseverance • long-term security • buying and selling property to obtain a good deal • share empowered potato chips to encourage love commitment • for a reliable longer-term investment • if your potato has eyes, the more eyes in the same potato, the more opportunities will appear to you

HOW TO USE

Peel a raw potato during the waning moon to lose an addiction, fear, or phobia; discard the peel in the garbage; then cook the potato and eat it or add it to a meal for friends and family. • If growing potatoes, leave one potato at harvest in the ground as an offering to the land spirits, so that lasting prosperity will follow. • An early form of poppet or magick doll was made from a human-shaped potato with eyes. The root or potato poppet was named for a person in need of healing or blessings and planted when it withered or the positive results were obtained.

CAUTION

All parts of the potato plant except the tubers are highly toxic, including seeds, fruit, and flowers, so keep children and pets away.

Potato, Sweet

(*Ipomoea batatas*)

MAGICAL FORMS

large, sweet-tasting, underground, tuberous root • these are root rather than stem tubers; in this way, sweet potatoes are different from yams (see p. 480) • native to tropical and subtropical USA • becoming popular to grow and cook in more temperate zones worldwide as an alternative to ordinary potato • generally orange flesh, though there are white-, brown-, yellow-, and purple-fleshed varieties • edible, young, green shoots and leaves • magically use the raw and cooked sweet potato

PLANETS AND ELEMENTS

Saturn/Moon • Earth/Water

MAGICAL USES

for connecting with your roots, ancestors, and family at gatherings • sweetens friendship and kinship bonds that may have become distant • sweet potato is much more concerned with harmony in relationships than the more money-oriented and practical potato • serve both together for a good balance in your home life

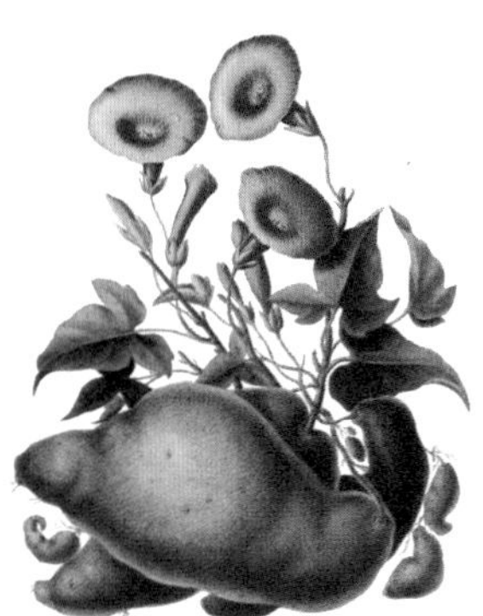

HOW TO USE

Empower before cooking as part of Thanksgiving and other family celebrations to encourage gratitude and family unity among taciturn or hard-to-please partners or relatives. • Serve in a meal to welcome new friends and catch up with old ones with whom you may have lost touch. • Eat after meditation, divination, or mediumship to restore the everyday world if you are feeling disoriented.

CAUTION

Avoid sweet potatoes that are turning green, as they contain a toxin.

Potentilla

(*Potentilla* spp.)

MAGICAL FORMS

genus containing over five hundred species of flowering plants, sometimes called cinquefoils • as *Potentilla sterilis*, or barren strawberry, presents as a small, delicate, woodland wildflower with five heart-shaped, white flowers enclosing yellow stamens, surrounded by five star-shaped leaves • appearing as early as February in warmer areas, as one of the earliest spring flowers • called the barren strawberry because unlike its cousin, the wild strawberry, it does not produce edible fruit • can be cultivated in gardens common throughout mainland Europe, the UK, North America (it is known as strawberry cinquefoil in Newfoundland), and many areas of the northern hemisphere including Asia • magically use the growing and dried flower and flower essence

PLANETS AND ELEMENT

Moon/Venus • Water

MAGICAL USES

use as a flower and flower essence for teens who have body-image problems or are teased about their appearance or a physical or intellectual disability • for adults who constantly self-sabotage through lack of self-belief and who consider themselves unworthy of happiness or success

HOW TO USE

Anoint the navel and the solar plexus area with a drop of the essence mixed with a lavender or rose massage oil or sip the essence in water if you are going to a social event or at work when you will be in the limelight, to speak and act with confidence and authority, or if you cannot avoid the company of those who criticize your appearance or weight. • Keep the dried flowers in a charm bag when going to choose new clothes so you trust your own judgment. • Look for the flowers if you know where they grow after they have stopped blooming in your area and grass or plants are obscuring them as a reminder that you do not need to be admired by others to be of worth.

CAUTION

Use with caution if pregnant.

Praline

MAGICAL FORMS

a smooth, sweet candy confection made according to various recipes, from almonds, pecans, or hazelnuts • pecan praline candy, popular in the south of the USA, especially Louisiana, is created with pecans, brown sugar, butter, and cream • praline is originally from France, where it is made with almonds and caramelized sugar • Ursuline nuns brought them to New Orleans from France in the 1700s and they became an early street food • there are many excellent recipes online • magically use purchased pralines or your own favorite homemade form, or use in a fragrance (often found as a base note in perfume)

PLANETS AND ELEMENT

Mars/Sun • Fire

MAGICAL USES

a praline is an alchemical magick mix for bringing fun, laughter, sweet words, and harmonious gatherings, whether homemade or purchased • as a perfume ingredient, a natural money magnet, making doors open and previously closed opportunities become possible

HOW TO USE

Make pralines as part of a group activity for binding together new members of the family, especially stepchildren, as you collectively stir in goodwill. The baking part of the process seals in the sweetness. • Wear a praline fragrance if your workplace is confrontational or you have sarcastic, gossipy, or overcritical colleagues. • Take a batch to the workplace or to a community event if there will be a meeting or discussion where compromise is needed and one or two people will try to shout others down.

Prickly Ash

(*Zanthoxylum americanum*)

MAGICAL FORMS

also called the common or northern prickly ash • the *Zanthoxylum clava-herculis*, the southern prickly ash, is similar • neither is an ash (see p. 36), but the northernmost New World tree belonging to the citrus family • small, aromatic tree indigenous to North America • highly regarded by Native North Americans medicinally and called the toothache tree for its apparent ability to relieve teeth and gum problems • magically use the whole, growing tree; fresh or chopped dried bark; berries; and, with care, its yellow or dark-brown branches, which have prickles

PLANET AND ELEMENT

Mars • Fire

MAGICAL USES

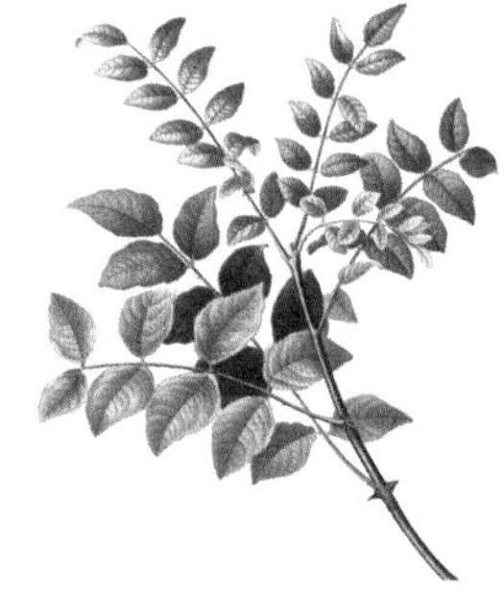

the fruits are used in love potions and to increase libido • the bark, sealed in an amulet bag, is used for safe travel • a fiery herb that will add energy and increase the power of other herbs and flowers in spells and charm bags • carry out shamanic initiation rites in a circle around a prickly ash to absorb its fire into the new shaman

HOW TO USE

Using string, hang tags with the names of yourself and any family members and the address of your home or business that has been cursed, jinxed, or hexed, on the branches of a prickly ash. The protective prickles break the connection by forming a boundary through which ill wishes can no longer pass. • Crumble and powder the bark and rub it on the mouths on printouts of images of those in your life who are constantly malicious. Shake off any excess powder outdoors and fold the images into small squares and put them in a closed box.

CAUTION

If ingested or even touched, prickly ash can cause a severe allergic reaction. • Avoid ingesting decoctions and prickly ash medicine if pregnant or if taking anticoagulants.

Prickly Custard Apple

(*Annona squamosa*)

MAGICAL FORMS

also the cherimoya (*Annona cherimola*) • pale-green or creamy-yellow cone-, round-, or heart-shaped fruit that can grow up to ten inches • leathery skin and creamy, sweet flesh, made up of small individual fruits fused together to resemble one large fruit, with dragon scales • ancient and originally grown in the Andes Mountains • cultivated in tropical and subtropical zones and now imported around the world • sweet banana- or pineapple-like taste, with soft flesh that is spooned out like custard • the fruit can be harvested four to five months after flowering • in the USA, they are found in South Carolina and southern California • magically use the whole, dragon-like fruit and the scooped-out flesh (being careful to remove the seeds and skin) as an addition in magical cookery

PLANET AND ELEMENT

Mars • Fire

MAGICAL USES

for increasing romance and passion in a routine relationship or with a reticent partner • for unity and the creation or restoration of loyalty in any family or community group

HOW TO USE

Use for dragon magick with a gold-colored model dragon in rituals to call wealth or opportunities hidden from your life. Afterward, eat the fruit flesh. • Add to smoothies, salads, fruit salad, and any recipe instead of apples, or top pancakes for family meals or for your partner if there is a conflict of loyalties and to include any new partners or children who are resisting joining the family circle.

CAUTION

The skin and seeds contain toxins that may damage the nervous system. • Avoid custard apple if you suffer from Parkinson's disease or another nervous system condition.

Prickly Pear Oil

(*Opuntia ficus-indica*)

MAGICAL FORMS

seed oil from the prickly pear fruit of the cactus of the same name, grown in parts of the Americas, Australia, the Caribbean, the Mediterranean, and the Middle East • the oil is sold in health food stores and online as 100 percent pure prickly pear oil, with the cold pressed or virgin kind being of higher quality • magically use as a carrier oil mixed with essential oils or alone

PLANET AND ELEMENT

Mars • Fire

MAGICAL USES

called the oil of overcoming challenges, brings resilience to overcome unexpected setbacks and seemingly immovable obstacles • absorbed physically to prevent aging and the effects of the sun, prickly pear cactus oil can be empowered before use to enhance radiance and give confidence if you worry about your body image

HOW TO USE

Before lovemaking, anoint or massage the womb with the undiluted oil, asking that you may be fruitful (you can also use the essence, see "Cactus, Prickly Pear," p. 92). • Rub the pure oil clockwise into the skin or a little in your hair to strengthen your aura energy field before going out socially or if you cannot avoid supercritical people. • Massage counterclockwise on your Third Eye in the center of your brow to keep ill wishes away, on the center of your throat to protect you from unkind words, and on your inner wrists to guard your heart from those who would manipulate you.

CAUTION

Though considered a nonirritant for most skin types, do a patch test if you have very sensitive skin. • Proportionately, add no more than five drops of essential oil such as lavender or geranium to a teaspoon of the carrier oil (often one or two drops is sufficient for delicate skin).

Primrose

(*Primula vulgaris*)

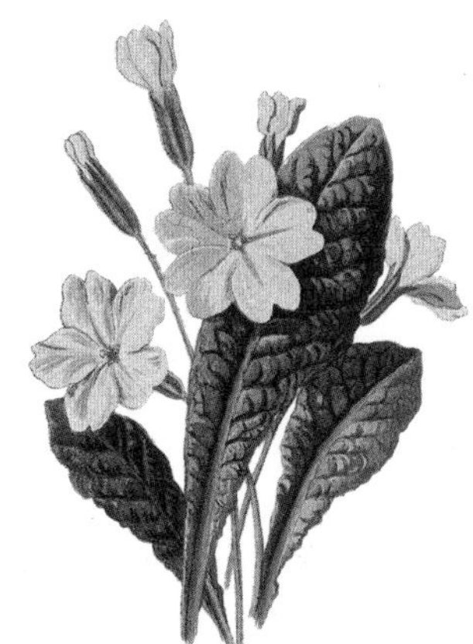

MAGICAL FORMS

flowering perennial • magically use the fresh, growing, and dried flowers and the yellow and white leaves

PLANET AND ELEMENTS

Venus • Fire/Water

MAGICAL USES

protection against adversity • uniting a family if children or teens feel alienated • attracts and brings awareness of nature essences • sacred to the Mother goddess, the Celtic Druids, and Freya, the Norse goddess of beauty and magick, primroses are said to grant invisibility and so are used magically for creating a low profile in times of conflict or threat • a flower of the spring equinox

HOW TO USE

Five newly picked primroses, growing around a tree close to water or near an ancient standing stone, offer an entry to the land of the fae, especially when placed on an ancient sacred stone. • Though not considered lucky indoors, a bunch on the doorstep will bring the blessings of the fairy folk into the home and call telepathically the person or people you would most like to visit. • In the language of flowers, primroses represent young love and send the message *I cannot live without you.*

CAUTION

Toxic to dogs, cats, horses, and those using blood-thinning medication or with allergies to acetaminophen. • Do not use while pregnant. • While yellow or white *Primula vulgaris* is edible, some colored primroses are not so safe and may be poisonous.

Primrose, Dune

(*Oenothera deltoides*)

MAGICAL FORMS

flowering plant member of the evening primrose family, blooming January through May • opening in early evening and closing midmorning • grows on desert sand dunes or beach fringes • native to southwestern USA and northern Mexico, especially the Mojave, Sonoran, and Great Basin Deserts • saucer-shaped white blooms with yellow stamens, growing in a rosette near the base of the plant • the flowers become pink as they mature • beloved of butterflies • magically use the flower essence, unless you can find the growing plant in situ

PLANET AND ELEMENT

Moon • Earth

MAGICAL USES

resolves issues with your mother or with mothering • aids grief and conflicting emotions if your mother has passed on, you were abandoned young, or a birth mother refuses contact • to overcome trauma giving birth and afterward • for children who are fostered or adopted who may suffer feelings of rejection • for night or moon magick

HOW TO USE

Meditate on the growing flowers (can occasionally be bought from a garden center to grow in sandy soil) to connect with the soul of the Divine Mother to mother yourself. • Alternatively, bury in the sand with desert rose crystals, creating a bird cage formation when the stems die and curl upward and inward, to let go of maternal rejection pain. • As an offering, every week, use a diluted essence to anoint the heart area of a nonporous statue of mother goddesses such as the Paleolithic Venus, religious icons from any faith, abstract figures representing pregnancy, or your own inner wrists to ease the pain of mothering or motherhood issues. • Add the essence to a rose oil or lotion whenever you feel unloved and massage your knees where rejection energies collect.

CAUTION

Check with an expert, especially if pregnant or taking regular medication, and read the precautions of its sister, evening primrose. • Dune primrose is nontoxic for animals.

Primrose, Evening

(*Oenothera biennis*)

MAGICAL FORMS

opens in the evening like many other forms of the plant • *Oenothera lamarckiana*, the common evening primrose, opens in later afternoon from May to July • evening primrose is native to North and South America and Canada and was used therapeutically by Native North Americans • also grows in Europe and Asia • magically use the whole, growing plant; yellow flowers, fresh and dried; and oil made from the seeds

PLANET AND ELEMENT

Moon • Water

MAGICAL USES

overcoming jealousy • regeneration, healing, and restoration • moon spells • finding what is lost • self-love and esteem • magical cookery

HOW TO USE

Add to a moon garden to attract the fey, but ask their permission to pick it—even when grown in your garden. • Place the flowers in the center of the altar for goddess rituals in all her phases, especially connected with the changing cycles of the woman's life: the girl entering puberty; celebrating the new mother; and wisewoman ceremonies, linked with crescent, full, and waning moon. • To open your psychic powers and seek opportunities in career, money, and love, anoint candles and your Third Eye with the oil diluted in a little grape-seed oil, as the oil is quite thick and sticky. • Once used in hunting rites, the dried open flowers can be taken in a yellow sachet when going to an employment agency or a job interview, or when asking for a loan (place by your computer if applying online). • Add the flower tea to a bath to enhance beauty and in the weeks before you plan to conceive a child to call the infant into your aura.

CAUTION

Avoid if you live with epilepsy, are pregnant or trying to conceive, or are taking anticoagulants or schizophrenia medication.

Primrose, Scottish

(*Primula scotica*)

MAGICAL FORMS

small, delicate, dark-purple flowers with yellow centers and five heart-shaped petals • bloom twice: from May to June and again from July to August • found only in northern Scotland, usually near the coast in the Orkney Isles, Caithness (also growing inland), and Sutherland • visit the flower on a vacation, especially if you are of Celtic descent, though they are rare and are protected by law • magically use the flower essence

PLANET AND ELEMENT

Venus • Earth

MAGICAL USES

Scottish primrose is a survivor against seemingly impossible odds because of its harsh environment, so as a flower or essence it brings inner peace • connects with natural biorhythms, including lunar and seasonal cycles • restores equilibrium during and after times of crisis and conflict • the growing plant is associated with the fey

HOW TO USE

Meditate near the growing flowers if you can visit them, or try to grow some in your garden—the seeds are occasionally sold from a few Scottish nurseries. • Alternatively, print an image of the flowers or make it a screen saver or lock screen on any device to connect with the natural flow of life if you are fighting against circumstance. • Sip the essence, put it under your tongue, or mix a drop or two of the essence with a peace-bringing essential oil such as chamomile or a gentle carrier oil like virgin olive oil and add a few drops of the blend to your bath to allow all anxiety to flow from you.

Protea

(*Protea* spp.)

MAGICAL FORMS

goblet-shaped flowers • bloom in clusters, especially as cut flowers • also called sugarbush or honeybush because of sweet nectar • native to Australia and South Africa but growing naturally in warmer parts of the USA and worldwide under glass • a very ancient flower named after Proteus, the sea lord of ancient Greece, who could change his form as he wished • magically use the fresh or dried cut flowers and the seeds

PLANETS AND ELEMENT

Mars/Sun • Fire

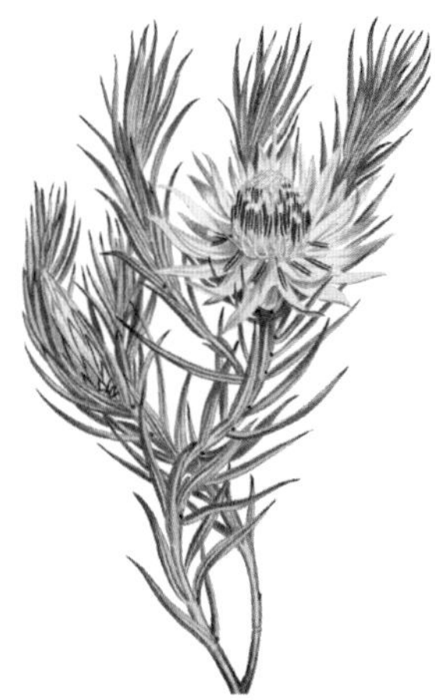

MAGICAL USES

in celebratory Thanksgiving and Yule holiday wreaths as a late fall or winter flower • pink, cream, and white proteas have strong connections with weddings, for example *Protea serruria*, a creamy cultivar called 'Blushing Bride' • another wedding variety is linked to bridesmaids, 'Pretty in Pink' • use also in vibrant colors for tropical, beach, or exotic weddings, especially as king protea (*Protea cynaroides*), which resembles a crown with red and yellow flowers

HOW TO USE

The flower in all its forms is symbolically gifted or used ritually for new life after loss or hardship; regeneration, especially after business reversal or a serious illness or operation; or a housewarming for a newly divorced friend or family member. • Since it retains its shape and color well when dried, keep as an altar flower for longer-term, slower-manifesting spells. • Use in meditation for shape-shifting, astral travel, and past-life journeying, as well as for transformation rites.

CAUTION

Flowers, seeds, and leaves are toxic to humans and pets if ingested.

Psyllium

(*Plantago ovata*)

MAGICAL FORMS

psyllium, or Indian wheat, is a small, bushy plant that grows between twelve and eighteen inches high • cultivated worldwide mainly for its medicinal purposes, especially as a source of plant dietary fiber • native to central Asia, especially India and Iran • the plant lives for only 130 days • edible seeds and husks—the outer part of the seeds are used medicinally and the husks in soups and smoothies • seeds are pink or brown, boat- or ear-shaped, within capsules on the plant after flowering • important in Ayurvedic medicine • magically use the whole seeds and the husks (crushed or as a powder)

PLANET AND ELEMENT

Saturn • Earth

MAGICAL USES

to remove emotional, psychological, and psychic blockages from your life • for lessening excessive cravings, whether for food, excitement, alcohol, gambling, or cigarettes • banishing an unwise liaison or influence or helping you refrain from returning to the same relationship that holds you back

HOW TO USE

Add a crushed or shredded symbol of your craving; if alcohol, add a drop or two to psyllium seeds or dried husks for faster action. Place the mix in a paper bag and dispose of it in the garbage away from your home. • Mix up a liquid using a little husk in water while reciting the name of the person holding you back from happiness. Pour the mix away under a fast flowing tap, washing out the container afterward in hot, soapy water, saying, *It is gone, it is done.*

CAUTION

Psyllium is not for pregnant or breastfeeding women. • It can occasionally cause an allergic reaction. • Psyllium should not be used long term for gut problems.

Pumpkin

(*Cucurbita moschata*) and (*Cucurbita maxima*)

MAGICAL FORMS

large fruit of the gourd, closely related to the marrow, and squash, characterized by hard, grooved orange or yellow rind • a creeping plant producing long vines • cooked as a vegetable or sweetened as dessert • native to Central America but cultivated worldwide, maturing in early fall • magically use the whole pumpkin, flesh, and seeds

PLANETS AND ELEMENTS

Moon/Venus • Water/Earth

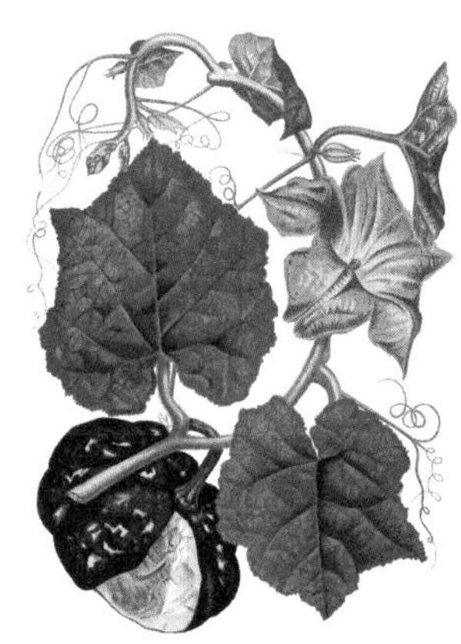

MAGICAL USES

the pumpkin is associated with Halloween and the ancestors, offering protection from all malevolent spirits at this time of the year • Jack o'Lantern was said to have three times refused to cross the river of immortality with the loveliest of the Celtic Morrigan raven sisters and so he was condemned to walk forever through the darkness between worlds carrying his Halloween pumpkin, a warning not to let fear hold back necessary change • magical cookery

HOW TO USE

On Halloween, the old Celtic festival of Samhain, summer's end, marking the beginning of the "darker half" of the year when spirits traditionally roam free, set out carved jack o'lanterns, one on either side of the door, to keep away all malevolent spirits, but light the way home to beloved ancestors. • Make pumpkin pies, often part of a Thanksgiving feast, to welcome all to the table. • Add dried pumpkin seeds (possibly from a pumpkin you have prepared), to prosperity jars with small, gold-colored items and fertility bags filled with dried rose petals.

CAUTION

Pumpkin seed oil has not been fully tested.

Purple Mat

(*Nama demissum* var. *demissum*)

MAGICAL FORMS

a flowering plant, also called desert purple mat • pinkish or purple funnel-shaped flowers, growing in a patch of hairy glandular herbage • found in the southwestern desert of the USA, including the Mojave Desert in Arizona, Nevada, Utah, and southwest California, and Mexico, blooming in desert places from February to May • three inches high • magically use the growing plant for meditation and empowerment and the flower essence

PLANET AND ELEMENT

Sun • Fire

MAGICAL USES

as the flower and flower essence for overcoming fears and phobias • encourages responsible risk-taking emotionally, psychologically, and physically in those who are overcautious • assists in expressing needs, opinions, and feelings rather than hiding them for fear of rejection or ridicule • for being true to the self • developing self-esteem

HOW TO USE

If you cannot work with the flower, which can be very difficult to find, use the image as a screen saver on your computer, smartphone, or tablet. Sip a drop or two of the essence in water while looking at the screen as a reminder that your opinions are valid and you have a right to express and live by them if you know you will be challenged. • Meditate on an enlarged picture of the growing mat of flowers if you need to persuade others to see your point of view. • Use the essence before attempting an activity that scares you, making an empowerment that you have no fear.

Purslane

(*Portulaca oleracea*)

MAGICAL FORMS

Smooth, reddish stems sprawling along the ground • yellow flowers that, depending on rainfall, can appear any time of the year, opening singly in the center of the leaves only for a few hours in the morning if sunny • grows in all continents except Antarctica • golden purslane (*Portulaca oleracea* subsp. *sativa*) with yellow leaves is cultivated mainly as a potted herb but has similar properties • dates back more than two thousand years as a medicinal herb in Europe, Iran, and India, and even earlier as a nutritious vegetable • around 30 CE, the Roman philosopher and naturalist Pliny the Elder recommended purslane as an amulet to keep away sickness and malevolent forces • magically use the whole plant, dried leaves, stems, and seeds

PLANET AND ELEMENT

Moon • Water

MAGICAL USES

for restful sleep • protects against physical, psychological, and psychic attack in potentially dangerous situations • a luck and money charm, especially the yellow leaves (it also brings luck as a potted plant if gold-colored coins are buried in the soil)

HOW TO USE

Add purslane to a sleep pillow to overcome fears of the dark and nightmares, and to drive away malevolent nighttime spirits such as poltergeists and paranormal sexual predators. • Keep a bundle of dried stems with any birth charts to counteract less helpful astrological transitions. • Clear magick mirrors and crystal spheres with a weak infusion and a white cloth to increase clairvoyant sight. • Tie the stems together firmly and hold upright like a wand on full moon night, facing the moon, for past-life visions and messages from the ancestors.

CAUTION

If misused, leaves can be addictive and hallucinogenic. • Not enough is known about the safety of ingesting purslane in pregnancy and breastfeeding, so avoid.

Queen Anne's Lace

(*Daucus carota*)

MAGICAL FORMS

also known as the wild carrot • the ancestor of the orange cultivated carrot (see "Carrot," p. 104), with tiny lacelike blossoms when in full bloom from May to August • beautiful feathery leaves, worn as an adornment in sixteenth-century England • the wild growing carrot is native to temperate parts of Europe and southwestern Asia and believed to have come to the USA with European colonists in the seventeenth century as a medicinal herb • American settlers boiled it in wine • the taproot of the wild carrot, the underground part that is eaten, is generally white, less flavorful, and more spindly than the domestic orange carrot • magically use the seeds as a spice, the essential oil, the taproot, and the growing or cut flower

PLANET AND ELEMENT

Mars • Fire

MAGICAL USES

named after Queen Anne, wife of James I of England and Scotland, born in 1574 or some say the Stuart Queen Anne, born 1665 • it is told the queen, competing with her ladies making lace, pricked her finger and a drop of blood fell in the center of the lace, where there is a red dot in the center of the real lacelike flower • the root cooked and eaten in a flavorful meal increases desire • the seed oil is used to anoint a white candle, diluted in a little olive oil, on full moon night for fertility

HOW TO USE

Place the dried chopped stems and flowers in a sachet in or under your pillow for psychic dreams. • Cut flowers are used in informal weddings or in a bouquet for an anniversary, birthday, or Mother's Day with a gift of lace.

CAUTION

If picking in the wild, beware Queen Anne's lace resembles poison hemlock (*Conium maculatum*). • Do not consume any form of Queen Anne's lace during pregnancy or breastfeeding.

Quince

(*Cydonia oblonga*)

MAGICAL FORMS

also Chinese or Japanese flowering quince (*Chaenomeles speciosa*) • the flowering branches of the shrub in white or pink (*Cydonia oblonga*) • vibrant red and orange colors among the Oriental kind • fruit grows well in California • magically use the dried or fresh blossoms, fruit, and seeds

PLANET AND ELEMENT

Saturn • Earth

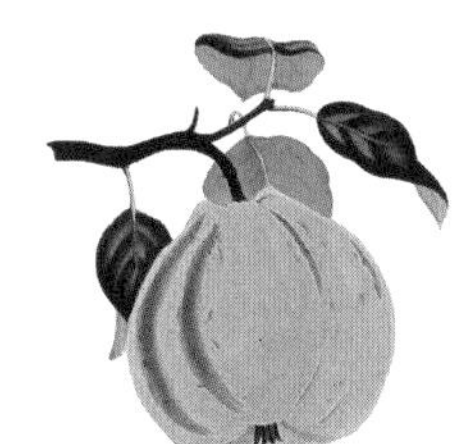

MAGICAL USES

powerful wedding connections dating back centuries as decoration when flowering • the fruit is a token of lasting love, shared by a couple after their wedding, handfasting, or informal garden ceremony or given as a plant to be taken home and set in the garden of the marital home to bring fidelity and happiness • linked with the love goddess Venus, who was given the fruit by her love, Paris; statues often depict her with a quince in her right hand

HOW TO USE

Use the fruit in magical cookery to increase commitment. • Carrying the seeds promises protection from all harm, deliberate or accidental, from ill wishes, and during travel. • Keep dried flowers in a sachet above a pet bed or sleeping area to keep the animal from straying. • Set a quince fruit on a love altar, a rite practiced on the altars of Venus since Roman times, surrounded by a square of four red candles and with a green altar cloth. Burn the candles to call new love or strengthen a love with a present lover, and afterward share the fruit with the lover or eat it alone to absorb the love radiance.

CAUTION

The seeds, particularly in larger quantities, are toxic. • Japanese and Chinese quince fruits are very tart and may cause mouth irritation if ingested raw. • Some species can be eaten raw, however, so check when buying the fruit or the plant.

Radish

(*Raphanus sativus*)

MAGICAL FORMS

also *Raphanus raphanistrum*, the wild radish • root vegetables, usually small, round, peppery, and red, though they can be purple, white, or double colored and oblong • when ready for harvesting they may start to appear above the soil • if radishes flower before they are harvested, they will become progressively bitter • however, they make eye-catching pink, white, and purple cut flowers that magically contain the power of the radish itself • though of Asian or Mediterranean origin, they are now grown worldwide • magically use mainly the root vegetable

PLANET AND ELEMENT

Mars • Fire

MAGICAL USES

in the temple at Delphi, the offering of a solid gold radish was dedicated to Apollo; the beet was silver, and the turnip lead, and so the radish was highly prized • an aphrodisiac • brings prosperity • since it is peppery flavored, adding salt before eating doubles its protective properties

HOW TO USE

To protect against the evil eye, invisibly etch an eye on a radish with the index finger of your writing hand and keep the vegetable with you in a yellow bag or placed facing the direction of the envy if known. • Chop radishes for a meal with a lover, cutting through all that stands in the way of passion, whether lack of libido or a love rival. Stir the chopped radish into salad or cooking, saying, *Think only of me, see only me, be only for me now and till eternity,* to enflame unbridled lovemaking after the meal.

CAUTION

Do not give to potentially volatile people or those quick to take offense. • Avoid eating raw if you have thyroid problems or are taking medication for the thyroid.

Ragweed

(*Ambrosia artemisiifolia*)

MAGICAL FORMS

the scapegoat of the wildflower world, considered an invasive species and major allergen • grows throughout temperate regions of North America and Canada except the far north and increasingly in Europe and the UK because of the warming climate • common ragweed resembles a fern, three to four feet high with rough, hairy stems, leaves, and greenish-yellow flowers • the great or giant ragweed (*Ambrosia trifida*) can grow to seventeen feet • ragweed is a rich source of late pollen for bees, the leaves for caterpillars, and the oil-bearing seeds for birds and other wildlife • ragweed also removes heavy toxic metals like lead from the soil and clears the effects of industrial waste • the pollen season begins between August and September and ends in October or November according to the climate • avoid using the plant magically and drying during this period • at other times, magically use the dried, shredded stems and leaves

PLANET AND ELEMENT

Mars • Fire

MAGICAL USES

drives away fears • use in rituals for environmental survival • for healing the planet and turning loss into gain

HOW TO USE

Burn ragweed (with care) out of pollen season when there has been major pollution, such as an oil spill or a radiation leak, or an area devastated by war or land mines, to send healing energies. • If you are scapegoated by your family or at work, make a tightly sealed amulet bag of ragweed leaves and stems in a biodegradable bag. Bury it deep where nothing grows, saying, *Scapegoat, take my unfair blame, thus I abandon my scapegoat name.*

CAUTION

Do not bring ragweed indoors or handle when it is flowering if you suffer from pollen allergies.

Ragwort

(*Senecio jacobaea*)

MAGICAL FORMS

two to three feet high with multibranched, furrowed stem • short taproot spreading into many roots • glossy green leaves and bright-yellow, flat-topped flowers, many plants growing together • native to Europe, the UK, Ireland, Siberia, northwest India, and parts of western, midwestern, and northwestern USA • magically use the roots, dried flowers, leaves, and stems

PLANETS AND ELEMENTS

Sun/Venus • Water/Earth

MAGICAL USES

protection as an amulet against human and spirit enchantments and binding spells • the root gives the ability to see the fae • faeries were believed to turn ragwort into golden, magical horses to take them to their revels • in medieval times, ragwort was, in myth, adapted into brooms by witches or as part of special flying salves (highly toxic) to fly or astrally project • grows on battlefields, such as the 1746 Scottish uprising at Culloden where many clans died, and wartime bomb sites as symbol of regeneration • associated with both mind travel and increased libido, especially for women

HOW TO USE

Create a circlet of the fresh flowers and leaves from the midsummer, first, and second harvest celebrations, since the plant blooms from June to October. Woven on wire, wear or set as a focus during meditation for visions of other dimensions. Alternatively, hang the circlet on the bedroom wall for passionate sex and sex magick. • Set the dried flowers in a lucky charm bag hung in a stable or trailer for horses in competitions and races, though the plant is poisonous to horses and cattle if overly ingested. • Walk through fields of the golden plant to attract money-making opportunities.

CAUTION

Ragwort is highly toxic to humans if ingested in large quantities.

Rain Tree

(*Samanea saman*)

MAGICAL FORMS

also called the monkeypod tree • different from the flame tree (see p. 229) • originally from Madagascar, now growing in Mexico, tropical and subtropical Australia, and North America, in Florida, Texas, Arizona, and California • flowers in late spring and early summer • the yellow poinciana (*Delonix floribunda*) can be grown potted indoors or trained as a bonsai in most places in the world, though flowering may be more difficult in a pot (worth contacting an exotic flower garden center) • magically use the huge fresh or dried flowers, the growing tree, or your bonsai or potted version

PLANET AND ELEMENT

Venus • Water

MAGICAL USES

because leaves fold up before rain, used for protective rituals • for wise caution and to bring foresight • if you can find the tree, ideal for meditation to see glimpses of the future, especially avoidable hazards

HOW TO USE

Buy the dried leaves online (sometimes called thorn or monkeypod leaves) to add to potpourri for protecting the home against both natural disasters and malevolence. • Buy some small pieces of wood, sometimes called monkey or rain wood, from an exotic wood craft store (it easily splinters) to keep in an amulet bag to hold whenever you have a major decision involving risk but potential advantage so that you will be safe. • Save blossoms or buy from a local store near where the tree grows for using in charm bags to attract abundance and prosperity through viable ventures.

CAUTION

Parts of plant are poisonous if ingested, though not the seedpods, which are sweet and edible inside. • The leaves may cause skin irritation.

Ranunculus

(*Ranunculus asiaticus*)

MAGICAL FORMS

though native to Europe and Asia, it grows through the temperate regions of the USA and Canada • also called the Persian buttercup • some species are wild in the USA, such as the *Ranunculus lyallii*, with big, white flowers • with large round blooms belonging to the buttercup family, ruffled, layered petals in white, pale yellow, pink, orange, or purple • magically use the whole, growing flower, whether in a garden, container, or pot; cut flowers; and fresh and dried petals

PLANET AND ELEMENTS

Sun • Fire/Earth

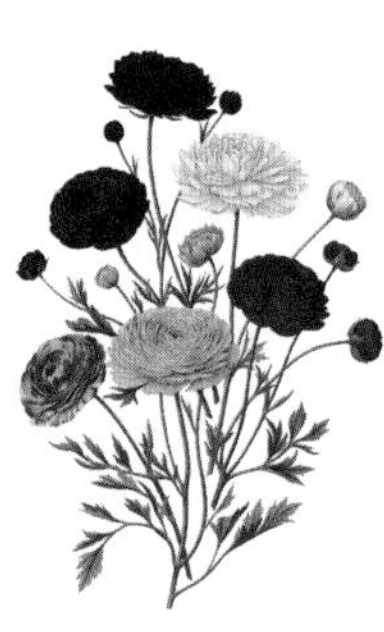

MAGICAL USES

often used in weddings, especially white • as mixed rainbow colors in a more exotic tropical marriage setting • add to garden roses and sweet peas for a country or garden wedding or a handfasting bouquet • each flower contains its own spirit essence and so permission should always be asked before picking them

HOW TO USE

Petals are plucked for love questions, whether *They love me/love me not?* or *Should I speak or remain silent/act or wait?* until the flower is empty of petals and the answer received as the last petal is plucked. • The pink flowers or the ruby-red *Ranunculus tango* are given as a romantic gesture on a special date or for a wedding proposal, accompanied by a ring within the bouquet. • The dried purple flower can be sealed in a purple purse and kept in the glove compartment of a vehicle to shield the occupants from danger, since some flowers may have a protective clawlike form. • *Ranunculus asiatica* is sometimes called Persian crowfoot and for the same reason is planted in or near the home.

CAUTION

Should not be ingested by animals or humans, as all ranunculi are toxic. • Handle with care, and if you have broken or sensitive skin, use tweezers to pluck your petals.

Raspberry

(*Rubus idaeus* var. *strigosus*)

MAGICAL FORMS

also European raspberry (*Rubus idaeus* var. *idaeus*) • originally from Europe and northern Asia • flourishes in any cooler climate • the berries have been eaten since Paleolithic times and were documented by the Romans • the American kind are a separate but very similar plant • magically use the dried leaves in tea, the growing thorny bush in the garden, and the ripe fruit

PLANETS AND ELEMENT

Moon/Venus • Water

MAGICAL USES

Rubus idaeus translates to "the bramble bush of Ida," nursemaid of the infant Greek god Zeus, who pricked her finger on the then-white raspberry, staining it red with her blood • Zeus's mother, Rhea, hid the infant from his father, Cronus, who wanted to swallow him like his brothers to prevent him from taking power, so the raspberry in all its forms has always symbolized protection • a bush in the garden (take care with small children) offers home, home businesses, and family security from all harm • use in love potions

HOW TO USE

Drink the tea or eat the fruit to speed any ventures that are slow-moving or offer to people who are resistant to change and to avoid being ignored or overlooked. • Set the ripe fruit or fresh leaves on an impromptu altar in a forest using a flat rock, then ask the tree mothers for fertility and for the safe delivery of a healthy child and easy childbirth if there have been previous difficulties giving birth.

CAUTION

The leaf tea is traditionally used to shorten labor or for delayed labor but needs expert care and advice in administering.

Rattlesnake Root

(*Polygala senega*)

MAGICAL FORMS

also called Seneca snake root • native from Newfoundland to Alberta in Canada and from New England to Georgia and Arkansas and west to the Dakotas in the USA • named after the Seneca Native North American people who extensively used snake root medicinally and as an antidote to snake bites • magically use the long, slender, narrow roots, whole, dried, chopped, or powdered

PLANET AND ELEMENT

Mars • Fire

MAGICAL USES

in an amulet, protects against false friends, liars, cheats, spite, and malevolent spirits • banishes all harm and guards against accidental pitfalls as well as deliberate malice and financial or romantic scams

HOW TO USE

A decoction (liquid infusion) made with the root or dry powder, when rubbed daily on the bottom of shoes, protects against any who would seek to trip you up mentally, or unscrupulous rivals. • If you rub the decoction on coins and leave them to dry, they will attract more money or opportunities, especially if you are involved in sales or commission work. • Add snakeroot to a jar of olive oil, seal, and steep for six weeks: the protective oil can then be used for anointing door handles and window ledges at home and in workplaces.

CAUTION

Avoid if pregnant, breastfeeding, or if you have gastric problems, and do not take in excess.

Red Horse-Chestnut

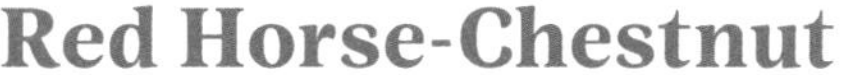

(*Aesculus × carnea*)

MAGICAL FORMS

a hybrid between the common horse chestnut and the American red buckeye • may have occurred naturally in Germany in the 1800s (see "Chestnut Tree," p. 118) • reaching sixty feet high, its erect flowers, from which the flower essence is made, are deep pink to red and appear in late spring • red horse-chestnut grows in temperate USA, the UK, and Europe • the fruit, often called a conker, is brown and shiny and contained in a slightly spiny outer cover • magically use the flowers and the flower essence

PLANET AND ELEMENT

Jupiter • Air

MAGICAL USES

as the growing tree, the flowers, and essence, use for overcoming fears about the well-being and safety of those emotionally close, that may result in parental over-possessiveness of children at any age • for reducing worrying in advance the night before about the problems of the day ahead and conversations that have happened or may happen

HOW TO USE

Sit under the tree in flower and absorb the strength and detachment to deal with your own and others' problems without anticipating disaster or restricting your or their freedom. Take some fallen blossoms home to dry and put them in a green bag with a drop or two of essence to carry to remind you of the peace you felt beneath the tree. • Sip the essence in water throughout the day whenever you feel panic rising. • Add a little essence to almond carrier oil to seal your Third Eye in the center of your brow by massaging it counterclockwise, and to your inner wrist points to calm heart and mind before bed. • Tie conkers to a string and bang them in circles against a wall until they shatter to break circular worries.

CAUTION

As a relative of the horse chestnut, red horse-chestnut should not be ingested. • The nut or conker is poisonous when eaten.

Red Penstemon

(*Penstemon digitalis*)

MAGICAL FORMS

a popular form of the many penstemon cultivars, such as husker red • also known as beardtongue • red penstemon is a bushy, clump-forming plant with erect stems and clusters of bell-shaped flowers in purple, red, pink, or blue, usually with a white throat • purple-red foliage • native to Central America and North America, especially the western USA • *Penstemon rostriflorus*, another popular variety often used to make the essence, originates in southwestern USA with tubular red to orange-red flowers • most penstemon varieties will grow in gardens in temperate zones, including the UK • magically use the whole, growing plant; dried flowers; and flower essence

PLANETS AND ELEMENTS

Mercury/Mars • Air/Fire

MAGICAL USES

for a sense of adventure at any age • increasing stamina and prowess in physical activity regardless of age and ability • for children, brings pleasure in group activities if child is timid and reluctant to join • also for children with disabilities, to help them exceed their predicted potential

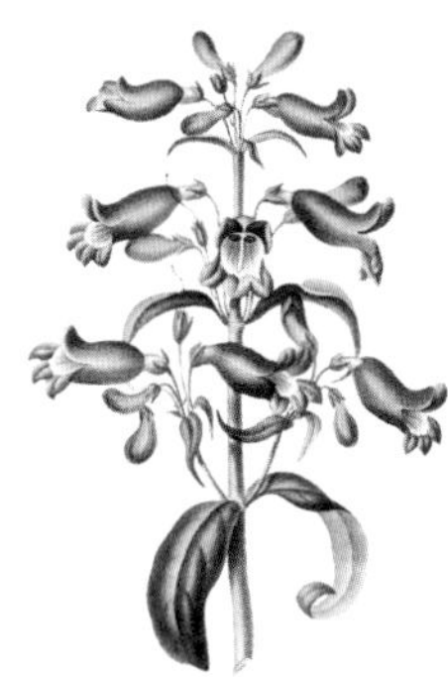

HOW TO USE

For a wedding or commitment ceremony, use penstemon wedding day white flowers with pink buds, blooming summer to fall, to bring happiness and good fortune to the couple. • Use the flower essence daily as you begin or revive any physical training to shed inhibitions and self-imposed limits. • Make a penstemon charm bag of dried flowers, adding a small piece of iron pyrite, hematite, or any iron. • Carry it for courage and perseverance when times get hard.

CAUTION

Some penstemon may resemble foxgloves, which are poisonous. • Do not ingest or apply medicinally without expert advice. • Take care when growing around children and pets.

Red Root

(*Ceanothus americanus*)

MAGICAL FORMS

a white flowering shrub found especially in eastern North America, with long, very deep reddish roots that survive wildfires • popularly called New Jersey tea because the leaves and roots were substituted for tea during the Revolutionary War by the American colonists • the plant grows between twenty and forty inches high • magically use the cut roots, dried leaves, tea (sold as tea bags and loose tea), and flower essence

PLANET AND ELEMENT

Mars • Fire

MAGICAL USES

as a plant and an essence, for avoiding guilt at your good fortune and hiding your abilities so you remain unnoticed • becoming disentangled from feeling responsible for the sorrows of others • removing superstitious fears and being ruled by them or fears of spirits and ghosts • resolves you from feeling at the mercy of fate that all might be taken away because you are undeserving

HOW TO USE

Make the tea from chopped roots, boiled leaves, or tea bags, and add to a floor wash for uncarpeted areas or doorsteps to keep away not only restless spirits but superstition-averting routines that can rule your life. • Use the essence before meeting with people who make you feel responsible for their misfortune. • Use cut and sifted red root, obtainable online and in specialty health stores, with a drop of the essence, for an amulet bag to carry with you as a reminder not to hide your talents or feel guilty about deserved success.

CAUTION

As yet there has not been sufficient mainstream research to pronounce red root safe for ingestion or topical use, so avoid, especially if pregnant or if you have problems related to blood clotting.

Redbud Tree

(*Cercis* spp.)

MAGICAL FORMS

including the eastern redbud (*Cercis canadensis*), California (western) redbud (*Cercus occidentalis*), and the Texas redbud (*Cercis canadensis* var. *texensis*) • the eastern redbud grows in eastern North America from New York to Texas • a small, flowering tree with spring pink or white flowers and heart-shaped leaves • also found in temperate regions of northern Europe including the UK, and in China • western redbud grows wild in south Utah and Nevada and through Arizona and California, and is smaller with rose-colored flowers • the Texan redbud, also more shrublike, is native to Oklahoma and Texas • magically use the growing tree, especially in full flower; dried flowers and leaves; and flower essence

PLANET AND ELEMENT

Venus • Earth

MAGICAL USES

use in rites for blessing land and endangered locations • removes stagnant or overactive earth energies from your home or workplace • for overcoming prejudice • connected with the goddess in all her forms

HOW TO USE

Use the fresh or dried buds on your altar or special place as the central focus for romance and new love rites, afterward carrying with you a few of the flowers in a charm bag. • Scatter dried flowers or leaves over a map of a war-torn zone or area of famine or flood, asking the protection of the Earth Mother. • Use the gold and yellow leaves ritually and as a charm for late-blooming love. • Plant a tree in the yard or visit one on an anniversary with a lover for love that grows and endures through the years.

Relish/Pickle/Chutney

MAGICAL FORMS

relish is composed of various chopped fruits and vegetables • a significant relish magically is sweet relish, that is made from cucumbers (potency), sugar (sweetness), onion (protection), mustard seeds (passion and money), celery seeds (travel), clove (sexuality and learning), and cider vinegar (love and fertility) • a pickle is a relish of fruit or most usually vegetables preserved in vinegar or brine, for example dill pickle or relish (for safe journeys, protection, and prosperity) • the word "relish" comes from the French *reles*, meaning *remainder,* referring to relishes being sometimes made from leftover fruit and vegetables • chutney is usually sweet and spicy, composed of chopped fruits, spices, sugar, and vinegar, cooked in a thick spread (and so with concentrated power) • magically make your favorite relish, pickle, or chutney or read ingredients in your chosen prepared version

PLANETS AND ELEMENTS

Mars/Venus • Fire/Water

MAGICAL USES

when the ingredients are spiced and/or preserved, they represent more lasting strengths and are slower-acting than the fresh vegetables or fruits • they signify modifying views or taking the long-term perspective • in magical plant lore, an alchemical mix in which the whole is greater than the separate parts • for example, sweet relish signifies bringing immense good fortune and happiness to your life

HOW TO USE

If you make your own relishes, pickles, or chutneys, name each ingredient and its magical power as you add it. As you mix them together, name the overall magical purpose. If using a commercial product, put some in a dish, stir well, and name the powers of the separate ingredients and again your overall purpose. • At a celebration or meal with extended family, have a selection of relishes, pickles, and chutneys in a circle on the table. Pass your hands a few inches above the table in spirals, palms horizontal, facing downward, before everyone arrives, asking for the blessings you most desire for those who will be present at the event, not forgetting yourself.

Rhodiola Rosea

(*Rhodiola rosea*)

MAGICAL FORMS

also called roseroot stonecrop, the golden root, or arctic root • a fleshy, flowering plant with thick, oblong leaves, yellow flower clusters, and several erect stems growing from a thick rootstock • the leaves have a waxy coating as insulation against the cold • grows in wild arctic regions of Europe, Asia, North America, Scandinavia, Russia, and Alaska • traditionally used by Russian athletes, astronauts, and the army to increase stamina • Pedanius Dioscorides, the ancient Greek physician and botanist who lived between 40 and 90 CE, first wrote of the plant • magically use the fresh or dried roots, leaves, stems, and fresh or dried flowers

PLANET AND ELEMENT

Jupiter • Air

MAGICAL USES

anti-stress in difficult situations • for self-image problems • those with physically or mentally demanding jobs • fertility • long life

HOW TO USE

Follow the Siberian custom by giving matching roots to a marrying couple so that they will have healthy children. Find twin roots or two large root pieces, plus a smaller one for a baby. Set them in a small basket in your bedroom lined with the dried or fresh rhodiola flowers for three nights before and then on full moon night. On the waning moon, float the basket and its contents along a gently flowing body of water. • Chop roots, mixing with dried leaves, flowers, and stem (if obtainable, or otherwise rosemary) in a charm bag to keep with a photo of a family member. On the morning of a major examination or interview, scatter the contents in an open place to release confidence, memory, and initiative.

CAUTION

Rhodiola can cause irritability and insomnia. • It is not suitable for those with bipolar disorder or other psychological issues, autoimmune disorders, or thyroid problems, or if using anticoagulants.

Rhododendron

(*Rhododendron* spp.)

MAGICAL FORMS

a close relative of the azalea (see p. 43) and also fruiting shrubs such as cranberries (see p. 140) and blueberries (see p. 72) • belongs to the heath family • exotic, bell-shaped flowers in clusters • blooms in spring, with white, yellow, pink, purple, blue, and red flowers, and thick, leathery, glossy leaves • sometimes has twisted, clustered trunks • found in the USA, Europe, the UK, and Ireland as a temperate shrub or tree and a tropical shrub in Asia and Australia • magically use the whole, growing shrub or tree; cut flowers; and fresh or dried flowerheads or petals (handle with care)

PLANETS AND ELEMENTS

Sun/Jupiter • Fire/Air

MAGICAL USES

flower of the fifty-fourth wedding anniversary in accordance with its meaning of supporting one's partner through good times and bad • the pink and white blooms are used in wedding bouquets, sometimes as a single flower, and pink, blue, or purple blooms are sent as congratulations in the flower's Japanese significance as celebrating success and achievement

HOW TO USE

Regarded by the Victorians as a warning flower, rhododendron can be grown in the garden or displayed as cut flowers indoors to guard against those who would deceive, whether unscrupulous relatives, visitors, neighbors, or scams via the phone or computer. • If making a decision where the outcome is uncertain, pluck the petals from a single flower one by one and place them into a bowl (washing hands afterward), asking each petal whether to trust, go ahead, invest, or not.

CAUTION

All parts of rhododendron are poisonous to humans and pets if ingested, though they rarely cause skin irritation.

Rhubarb

(*Rheum rhabarbarum*)

MAGICAL FORMS

thick, reddish, edible stalks of the cultivated plant from the dock family • also can be pink or green • produced in fields, gardens, or in hothouses to force its growth • originally used medicinally, culinary rhubarb is related to Chinese rhubarb (*Rheum officinale* or *Rheum palmatum* are two of the main kinds) whose rhizome has been used in traditional Chinese medicine for more than 2,500 years and in Ayurvedic practices • Chinese rhubarb is not edible except the rhizome but can be grown as an ornamental • both culinary and Chinese grow in the UK and in the USA and cool, temperate zones worldwide • magically use the raw and cooked culinary stalks

PLANET AND ELEMENT

Venus • Earth

MAGICAL USES

the fidelity fruit when baked in pies or stewed to deter a mate from straying and to resolve relationship problems without acrimony • an aphrodisiac if a man has been made to doubt his virility • a happy family fruit, cooked and sweetened particularly to protect children from bullying on- and offline

HOW TO USE

Combine the phallic rhubarb with the female strawberry in a meal before sex magick with partners of either sex or to revive passion in a long-standing relationship (culinary rhubarb is especially good during perimenopause and menopause for rekindling libido). • Grown in gardens, it protects the home against evil spirits and those who would spread dissension, whether disruptive neighbors, ruthless debt collectors, or troublesome ex-partners.

CAUTION

All rhubarb leaves are poisonous, as are the stems of Chinese rhubarb. • Do not use Chinese rhubarb topically or medicinally by ingesting while pregnant or breastfeeding, during menstruation, or if suffering from gout or kidney stones. It should not be used by children. • As a general precaution, use only moderately under expert advice.

Rice

(*Oryza sativa*)

MAGICAL FORMS

a grass seed, rice originated in Myanmar thousands of years ago • over 90 percent of the world's rice is produced in Asia, especially China, India, and Indonesia, with numerous varieties obtainable around the world • magically use the raw and cooked grains of rice and straw

PLANETS AND ELEMENTS

Venus/Moon/Sun • Earth/Water/Fire

MAGICAL USES

it is believed in traditional cultures that rice contains the soul of the nurturing Earth Mother and that benign female Earth spirits dwell within the growing plants • thrown at weddings to attract prosperity, marital happiness, and fertility • a small bag of raw rice grains offers the protection of the earth if you are in an unfamiliar place • if while being cooked a ring of rice forms around the inner rim of the pan, it is an indication that money is coming

HOW TO USE

Keep a rice jar topped up in the kitchen to draw prosperity and happiness to daily life. • Basmati rice—long, slender, and with a floral aroma—is a natural wealth bringer. • Use grains of rice to mark out the initials of you and a love or desired love in the cooling melted wax of a beeswax candle, secured on a flat tray so the wax makes a pool. Cut out a heart around the initials and keep the wax heart in silk until the grains fall out as the wax crumbles. • Buy strong (inedible), dried rice straw online to tie magical knots to bind in prosperity, health, and protection from all harm. Hang the knotted cord near the center of your home. • Cook a meal with jasmine rice (a long-grain rice) while burning or diffusing jasmine flower oil to bring enchantment and romance and encourage commitment in love.

Rice, Sweet or Glutinous

(*Oryza sativa* var. *glutinosa*)

MAGICAL FORMS

also called sticky or waxy rice • from Southeast and eastern Asia and northeastern regions of southern Asia, where it remains very popular for sweet and savory dishes • obtainable worldwide • so named because it sticks together when cooked • short and round grains • sold milled and white, milky and opaque, with the bran removed • if unmilled with only the husk removed, a purple or black color • magically use both the milled and unmilled rice, raw and cooked

PLANETS AND ELEMENTS

Venus • Earth (as white), Mars • Fire (as black)

MAGICAL USES

for romance • domestic happiness • harmonious family gatherings • served at seasonal celebrations with the wish that there will always be enough food, fuel, and clothing for the year ahead

HOW TO USE

Serve white sticky rice for any occasions where you seek loyalty, commitment, or unity with a partner or family. Before serving, empower by stirring invisibly with a spoon on top of the rice, saying the names of those you are uniting. • Use the rice as a dessert, perhaps as the traditional Thai sticky rice with mango (see p. 279), a love fruit for not only kindling romance and passion as part of a love feast, but sweetening the temperaments of difficult, sharp-tongued family members. • Scatter raw black sticky rice on the doorstep and sweep it away to banish a quarrel or ill feeling that has occurred in your home. • Carry a small bag if you have a pressurized or confrontational workplace: each day, dispose of the rice on the way home and leave troubles behind, then replace the following day.

Rice, Wild

(*Zizania* spp.)

MAGICAL FORMS

not rice, but grain from semiaquatic grass producing long, thin husks covered in brown, black, or green that are removed and the grain polished • only the flowering head appears above the surface • traditionally from the wetlands of the Western Great Lakes in North America • found naturally in other parts of the USA, in China, and Hungary • the state grain of Minnesota, where it is still harvested in the Indigenous way in canoes steered with poles • now produced commercially in paddy fields in Minnesota, Wisconsin, Idaho, Oregon, and California • magically use the rice still in its husks and raw or cooked grain

PLANETS AND ELEMENTS

Mercury/Moon • Air/Water

MAGICAL USES

a sacred rice, grown for thousands of years among the Ojibwe people and other Indigenous people of the Western Lakes of Cumbria, called Manoomin or "the good berry" • considered a gift from the Great Spirit and still celebrated at the time of harvesting at late summer and early fall in the Western Lakes • for spontaneous moments • freedom from routine and stagnation • vacations and days away • welcoming unconventional family members

HOW TO USE

Offer raw wild rice in its husks—if possible obtained from the naturally harvested source, in a field or open grassland—to ask for the blessings you need for your personal financial, emotional, or spiritual harvest to occur. • Cook wild rice for special family occasions such as a birth, a commitment ceremony, an anniversary, a graduation, or the homecoming of a traveler to give thanks and to endow future good fortune on the focus of the celebration.

Rock Fringe

(*Epilobium obcordatum*)

MAGICAL FORMS

called the survivor flower, a member of the evening primrose family, blooming in the late summer after other flowers have faded • so called because it clings to rock crevices in high places • its flowers are rose or magenta to purple with four, often perfect, heart-shaped petals and long, thick roots that penetrate rock crevices of the Sierra mountains • native to the western USA from Idaho to California in mountainous areas • rock fringe will grow in gardens and in deep containers to leave room for the roots • magically use the growing and dried flowers and the flower essence

PLANET AND ELEMENT

Saturn • Earth

MAGICAL USES

the plant of clinging on in harsh conditions through inner power and determination • as the flower and flower essence, it helps older people from midlife to regain enthusiasm for new challenges • stimulates a new lifestyle, maybe following one's heart for the first time after redundancy or early retirement to reconstruct life when one path has ended

HOW TO USE

Add a drop of the essence to almond or warmed jojoba carrier oil and massage around the navel area and the solar plexus in the center of the base of the rib cage: this gives the incentive to get up in the morning if you have a midlife energy dip because of being passed over by younger people in your career. • If you can obtain the flowers, dry them and keep them in a purple bag with any new plans or near your computer if you are setting up a self-employment business later in life. When ready to launch your business, or if a new job opportunity appears, take them to the highest place locally, even the top of an apartment block, and let the flowers fly free.

CAUTION

While some Epilobium species are edible and nontoxic, there is not sufficient data about rock fringe to be sure, so avoid ingesting and using it medicinally unless advised by an expert.

Rooibos

(*Aspalathus linearis*)

MAGICAL FORMS

also known as red bush • a broom- or gorse-like bush, with yellow, butterfly-like flowers in spring, grown almost exclusively in the West Coast district of the western cape of South Africa • found mainly in the rest of the world as processed, oxidized leaves used for making a red-colored tea, a caffeine-free alternative to black and green tea with many healing properties • the bush, with its needle-shaped leaves, can be grown, but not easily, in the USA in regions where it is hot in summer and cool in winter, or in containers • the red is similar to honeybush tea • magically use the dried leaves or as tea • occasionally sold as bath products or room sprays (the tea can also be added to the bath)

PLANET AND ELEMENT

Saturn • Earth

MAGICAL USES

long life • determination • courage • seeing and seeking priorities and helping others to cut through irrelevancy and prejudice or narrow-minded thinking • wisdom and acquiring or recalling traditional knowledge, the latter from past worlds • for improving self-image

HOW TO USE

Mix the red and green tea leaves in a charm bag, tied with red and green threads in nine knots, adding three red and three green crystals for attracting good fortune and the impetus and opportunities to seek that luck. • Keep the bag concealed at home or in your business or workspace and hold it before making a courageous move or speculation. • Add different herbs, spices, and flowers that will be increased by the power of your rooibos tea for specific purposes, such as rooibos and vanilla shared with a partner or desired love for commitment and fidelity, mint for money, or eucalyptus and honey for a health boost. • Name your intention and, if for someone else, their name as you stir your brew. • Include milk for abundance and help from others.

CAUTION

Rooibos raises production of estrogen so should not be used if suffering from hormone-related conditions.

Rosalina Tree

(*Melaleuca ericifolia*)

MAGICAL FORMS

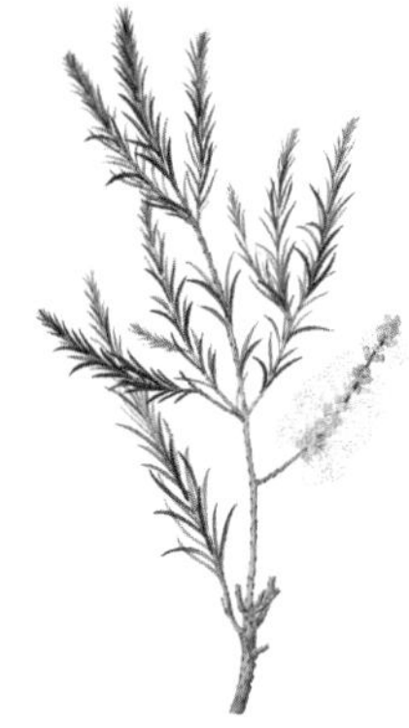

also called the swamp paperbark • tall shrub, which has soft leaves and creamy or yellowish, spiky flowers • found mainly in Australia's northern Tasmania, southern Victoria, and up the coast to northern New South Wales • magically use the oil made from its leaves, which some describe as a cross between lavender and tea tree in fragrance

PLANETS AND ELEMENTS

Moon/Saturn • Water/Earth

MAGICAL USES

as the oil, for calming hyperactivity and workaholic tendencies • since it's very yin, use for counteracting confrontational and constantly irritable people at home or in the workplace • creating sacred, restful space

HOW TO USE

Diffuse oil or use in a water-based room spray if you have hyperactive family members to create quiet times, especially if the family or your partner is sports obsessed, whether watching live in-person or via television. • If your home or workplace is too yang or you have overactive earth energies or constant background noise and artificial lighting, keep dishes of lavender potpourri refreshed with the oil. • Use for personal inhalation with an aroma bracelet, from an infused cotton ball, or an aroma massager ball to stop yourself from being swept along by impulsive financial decisions or unnecessary risk-taking. • Before bed, anoint your Third Eye in the center of your brows, rubbing counterclockwise with the oil diluted in jojoba or coconut oil, or do the same on your inner ankles and wrists to close your activity energy centers before sleep and for gentle lovemaking.

CAUTION

Check with a physician or midwife before using while pregnant or breastfeeding. • Dilute before applying to skin.

Rose

(*Rosa* spp.)

MAGICAL FORMS

genus of beautiful flowering plants, including three hundred species and thousands of cultivars • magically use the whole, growing plant; cut flowers; petals; thorns; oil; and fragrance

PLANET AND ELEMENT

Venus • Water

MAGICAL USES

roses are the most potent love flower • pink rosebud: first innocent attraction and romance • full red rose: passion and fidelity • golden rose: mature love • white rose: love that must not be revealed • in all colors, for increasing psychic powers • money • good fortune • moon spells • magick connected with fertility, motherhood, and children • pets • older people • those who have been abused

HOW TO USE

Cast ten red and white roses, alternating colors, from a bridge into a flowing river or stream to call back lost or absent love. • Burning rose incense or rose-scented candles, or adding rose essential oil and rose petals to bath water will attract love and increase the radiance in your aura before a social event. • Cook for a hesitant lover with rose water, essence of rose hip, or rose hip syrup to arouse desire. • Keep a blood-red rose in a vase in the center of the home and replace it every Friday if a marriage or relationship runs into difficult times. • Yellow roses grown in the garden or kept in the home protect against jealousy from relatives, ex-partners, or love rivals who resent your happiness. • Anointing the Third Eye with a drop of rose oil opens the psychic powers, especially clairvoyance, past-life recall, and the power to see the truth in people's hearts. • Roses in garden attract fey. • Use the thorns to fill protective bottles buried near the doorstep to remove and keep ill intent, earthly and paranormal, from the home. • Anoint candles with rose oil for money, tracing in oil on the side of the candle the amount needed.

Rose, Centifolia

(*Rosa × centifolia*)

MAGICAL FORMS

also called the cabbage rose • see also the rare Grasse rose (p. 385), which is a hybrid centifolia and often called by the same name as the cabbage rose, rose de Provence, and rose de Mai because it blooms in May but only grows in Grasse in France • the classic centifolia rose was brought to Europe by the Crusaders from the Middle East and was developed in its present form as the cabbage rose around the sixteenth century as a cross between the autumn damask and an alba rose • with large, fragrant, globular blooms, cabbage roses resemble, with their many-clustered petals, small cabbages in pink, red, or less commonly white or dark red-purple • cultivated in gardens in the USA, Europe, Morocco, and the UK • considered the best rose for fragrances after its close cousin the Grasse rose, though more widespread • magically use the growing and cut flowers, dried petals, essential oil, and fragrance

PLANET AND ELEMENTS

Venus • Water/Earth

MAGICAL USES

the ultimate gentle healing herb of love and reconciliation, especially good for healing the young, the very old, anyone who has suffered abuse, and the vulnerable

HOW TO USE

Cut centifolia for a spectacular bridal bouquet or venue room decoration with a drop or two of centifolia perfume added to the flowers and the fragrance worn by the bride for a happy day and joyous life ahead. • Meditate on your fragrant cabbage roses while wearing the perfume or a drop of the diluted oil on each of your inner wrist points to open your heart to love, compassion, and forgiveness if you have given up on life and people.

CAUTION

Dilute the oil well before use. • Though the oil is topically considered good for a woman's gynecological problems and skin, it should not be used in pregnancy or when trying for a baby.

Rose, Charlie Brown

(*Rosa rubiginosa* 'Charlie Brown')

MAGICAL FORMS

a miniature rose created from several varieties, with a large number of petals, often more than nine on each flower • blooming naturally in late spring and summer through to winter and so ideal for celebrations of all kinds • grows in the USA as well as the UK and Europe and can be exported from hothouses worldwide • light and pastel brown hues with peach and white undertones • can also be red and gold • each flower is less than two inches wide • magically use the growing rose or cut flowers, empowered and gifted, especially for matters of love

PLANET AND ELEMENT

Venus • Water

MAGICAL USES

Charlie Brown is a flower often given on the nineteenth wedding anniversary • can also be used at weddings later in life to pledge a settled love based around a happy home • for bon voyage when friends or family are moving away or going on a very long vacation or when a colleague or friend is retiring • grow brown roses in your garden or as indoor potted plants and it is popularly said you will never be without a roof over your head

HOW TO USE

The small Charlie Brown roses convey not grandiose gestures but appreciation and loyalty to older relatives, friends, and an established lover. • They are ideal for male couples to exchange or one give the other to convey lasting commitment if words are hard. • Give to someone living alone, whether from choice or because of circumstances, if you know a particular day may be full of sad memories. • If you move, buy a large bouquet of the roses, leave half for the new residents, and take half with you to your new home to transfer your happiness.

CAUTION

Charlie Brown roses have prickles rather than thorns and as such need care around children and pets.

Rose, Cherokee

(*Rosa laevigata*)

MAGICAL FORMS

magically use the growing plant, cut flowers, and fresh and dried petals and stamens

PLANET AND ELEMENT

Venus • Earth

MAGICAL USES

for love after loss • a popular wedding flower where family are on the other side of the world and you or they will be reuniting for the wedding • for following the wedding customs of your Indigenous culture • it is said that the flower grew from the tears shed when the Cherokee Nation was forcibly removed from its homeland more than five thousand miles to a reservation in Oklahoma in 1838 on what was called the Trail of Tears because of the suffering inflicted by this journey when more than seventeen thousand died; the chief prayed for a sign of hope, and it was said that a flower sprang up wherever a woman shed a tear • Cherokee rose became the state flower of Georgia in 1916, naturalized also in Florida, Alabama, and South Carolina • originally planted in northern Georgia around 1780 by Cherokee people • the seven petals coming to represent in later times the seven clans forced to leave their land

HOW TO USE

Use the plant growing up a wall or as cut flowers in a vase in the center of your altar, home, or workspace, as its golden stamens represent a recovery of financial fortunes after a major setback. • Carry the dried petals and stamens as a symbol of hope when you have to unwillingly relocate or lose your home. • Scatter them free on each full moon making a wish for where you most want to be and a safe home, and replace the petals and stamens on the morning after the full moon. • Scatter the petals on a printout of any papers relating to researching your family tree, especially if, through adoption or emigration, you have lost connection with the family.

CAUTION

Beware of the hairs around the seeds just beneath the fruit, which can cause irritation if ingested.

Rose, Cliff

(*Purshia stansburiana*) or (*Purshia mexicana*)

MAGICAL FORMS

cliff rose is a tall, many branched fragrant flowering shrub • *Purshia stansburiana* is a variation of *Purshia mexicana* and is native to southern Idaho, southwest Colorado, Utah, Arizona, New Mexico, South Carolina, and northern Mexico, often on lower elevations • while *Purshia mexicana* is found high in the Rockies, in southwestern USA, the Great Basin, and into Mexico • called cliff rose because many grow on edges of cliffs or perched on rocks • cliff rose flowers are white with many yellow stamens, growing between mid-spring and summer • magically use the wood and the flower essence

PLANET AND ELEMENT

Venus • Earth

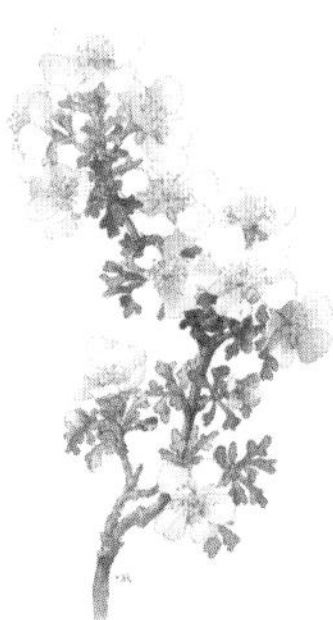

MAGICAL USES

achieving clarity of purpose, especially mental clarity • putting ideas and intentions into action to bring manifestation • for overcoming procrastination and lack of motivation to action or change • to bring spiritual purpose into everyday life

HOW TO USE

Among a number of Native North Americans, prayer sticks, especially for women, were made of cliff rose wood and decorated with feathers to call the spirits, and after use were buried or planted in holes. With respect for rituals dating back thousands of years, we can, in the modern westernized world, make narrow prayer sticks about seven inches long from cliff rose wood, decorate them with feathers, painting symbols of our petitions, or attaching to the feathers biodegradable written prayers, and planting the prayer stick with offerings in a high place. • Use the essence regularly as is or add it to bath and massage oil if you have many good creative ideas consigned to the one-day-maybe space. • Mix the essence with sunflower or almond carrier oil for skin care and massage.

CAUTION

It has not been pronounced safe for ingesting, although the flower essence can be used without worry.

Rose, Crystal Wedding 15th Anniversary

(*Rosa rubiginosa* 'Crystal Wedding 15th Anniversary')

MAGICAL FORMS

a special hybrid species of white floribunda rose created in the UK for the fifteenth wedding anniversary • the crystal wedding rose bush is in the UK an official flower of the fifteenth anniversary (crystal), with cup-shaped white flowers that bloom in clusters by the middle of summer, filling the whole bush with repeat blooming • in the USA, if you cannot obtain a crystal rose, substitute any pure white rose • white floribunda rose, such as 'Iceberg,' is produced by crossing hybrid tea roses with polyantha roses, is similar and has white flowers in small clusters that continue until winter • magically use as a growing plant, in bouquets, and as fresh or dried petals

PLANET AND ELEMENT

Venus • Water

MAGICAL USES

set white roses on your altar or near a photo of a departed loved one and you will hear or see in your mind a message from the other side • burn white rose incense to clear a magical space or if you feel spooked or wished ill

HOW TO USE

A white rose over a door in medieval times indicated whatever was spoken in the room remained secret. • White petals in a charm bag next to your computer or in your workspace will prevent others gaining confidential information about you, replacing the petals every night. • Pluck a bunch of white roses flower by flower, or a single rose petal by petal, if you have a love question, especially if you are worried about betrayal, asking, *Does she or he love me or love me not* for each petal until all are shed. • Keep white roses in your home or workplace if you are unfairly accused so that your innocence will be proven. Pick a petal each day and burn or bury it to lessen the false evidence against you.

CAUTION

The white rose is not considered toxic, but beware of the thorns.

Rose, Damask

(*Rosa damascena*)

MAGICAL FORMS

damask rose is a small, prickly shrub with pink, highly fragrant blossoms with thirty-six petals • native to Asia and mainly grown commercially in Bulgaria, Turkey, and France • can be cultivated in gardens in the USA, the UK, and Europe, especially thriving in a mild, temperate climate • a variety of the oil, rose otto or rose damascene, is produced by steam distillation • rose absolute oil is also produced from the damask rose; it is solvent based and, while beautiful and fragrant, less pure and more economical • contains the same properties as rose otto • magically use the flowers and the essential oil of any kind

PLANET AND ELEMENT

Venus • Water

MAGICAL USES

as the oil, use for romance and fidelity, love, and reconciliation • rose otto or damascena is an expensive but all-purpose oil, and you need to use very little • brings lasting joy and fertility, fidelity, and family joy • burned or used in massage for all forms of love magick and to increase personal desirability • for healing rituals, especially from abuse • also for spells concerning children and babies, the very old and vulnerable, and animals • mixes well with almost every other oil, essential and carrier, and can be substituted for almost any other oil magically

HOW TO USE

Send damask roses in birth bouquets, especially for the birth of girls, weddings, commitment ceremonies, and anniversaries. • Use in flower psychometry for answers to questions of the heart. • Add a few drops of rose oil to your bath before a special date and burn or diffuse it in the background for romance if you have invited a lover to your home. • Diffuse also or add to a humidifier in the home to minimize confrontational attitudes among family members and to reconcile differences with a partner when discussing sensitive, potentially controversial matters.

Rose, Darcey Bussell

(*Rosa* 'Darcey Bussell')

MAGICAL FORMS

cultivar of English shrub rose • a beautiful example of the numerous red roses grown and sold worldwide • special occasion bouquet red roses include the explorer rose and the Rhodos rose • however, all red roses share the same magical powers and symbolism • the English Darcey Bussell rose, named after a ballerina, is considered one of the best crimson roses to grow, with its abundance of flowers blooming in summer and again in fall, also cut and gifted • Rhodos roses, exported from Kenya to the USA and beyond, have bigger leaves than traditional roses, with no thorns • found mainly in bouquets and flower arrangements • magically use the red roses growing on bushes, cut flowers, and fresh and dried petals

PLANET AND ELEMENT

Venus • Water

MAGICAL USES

ancient Greek legend tells that the first red rose grew when Aphrodite's lover, Adonis, was slain by a wild boar • her tears mingled with his fallen blood, a reminder that red roses are a flower of consolation as well as celebration • red roses express love and commitment, formal and informal • a flower for the fifteenth, twentieth, and twenty-sixth wedding anniversaries • for the renewal of vows • scatter dried red petals across a bed to induce passion

HOW TO USE

Buy yourself cut red roses from a florist or garden center and empower them if you are alone on Valentine's Day or a significant love anniversary before using a dating site or attending a social event. • If you have lost your passion for life, give a red rose to everyone you meet, afterward buying new red roses to begin the first steps to manifesting your desires.

Rose, Floribunda

variety of (*Rosa floribunda*)

MAGICAL FORMS

floribunda roses can be found on both sides of the Atlantic or can be shipped worldwide • examples include Rosa Gold Spice, Togmeister, Absolutely Fabulous, and Julia Child • floribunda roses are a modern group of garden roses that are crossed hybrid tea roses with polyantha roses, producing many flowers in large clusters • bloom repeatedly through summer and fall • magically, and for celebrations, use the growing flowers on their upright bushes, as cut flowers, and as petals, both fresh and dried

PLANET AND ELEMENT

Venus • Earth

MAGICAL USES

increasingly one of the most popular golden roses for fiftieth wedding anniversaries • may be named specifically, such as Golden Wedding Rose, Golden Memories, or Precious Gold, whether as a garden gift in the form of a bush or as a bouquet, sometimes with a real rose dipped in liquid gold • used in weddings and love trysts for older couples, especially in retirement • used in protective rituals against spite and jealousy

HOW TO USE

Floribunda roses are natural money magnets, so place them live in a large container, or cut in a vase, to increase prosperity. • To usher in a financial opportunity, add a small magnet and a handful of dried petals to a glass jar, then seal. Each day shake the jar nine times, saying nine times: *Gold and silver I have none, into my life may fortune come.* Each day, add another handful of petals and repeat the same process. When the jar is full, tip the contents into a glass bowl with golden coins and gold jewelry, then leave it where the morning sun shines until the petals fade. • Put the flowers in a vase near the entrance to your home or business or carry the dried petals as a defensive amulet against spite and jealousy.

Rose, Grasse

(*Rosa gallica* var. *centifolia* L. Regel)

MAGICAL FORMS

also known as cabbage rose and the rose of a hundred petals • a complex pink hybrid of *Rosa × centifolia*, also called the Provence Rose or Rose of May • created through plant breeding by the Dutch in the seventeenth century • the true Grasse rose is grown exclusively in the small town of Grasse, north of Cannes in Provence where soil and weather combinations between the mountains and sea make the flower unique • Grasse (the town) is called "the perfume capital of the world" • an annual international rose exhibition is held in Grasse in May • Grasse rose is prized as an ingredient in some perfumes • the extract of Grasse rose is said to be worth more than its weight in gold • magically use the rose water, which you may find online, though rare; otherwise, use a fragrance containing the essence or, alternatively, red or pink rose petals fragranced with a few drops of the chosen perfume

PLANET AND ELEMENT

Venus • Earth

MAGICAL USES

a twin soul symbol for calling in your true mate or strengthening love with them

HOW TO USE

If you can't obtain dried Grasse rose petals, use another fragrant variety of rose and add a few drops of the Grasse perfume, mixing before filling a dream pillow. • At your wedding or commitment ceremony, anoint each other's brow and wrists using a fragrance containing Grasse rose. • If you can obtain the rose water, place it in your bath water to open your heart to love if you have been betrayed or suffered loss. • If the rose water is not available, include a drop or two of a fragrance incorporating Grasse rose into any favorite perfume.

CAUTION

Avoid if pregnant.

Rose, Guelder

(*Viburnum opulus*)

MAGICAL FORMS

also known as cramp bark • guelder rose is not a rose at all but a deciduous shrub either growing wild or as an ornamental garden plant • twenty-five of the 150 species are native to North America, and it also flourishes in Europe • used medicinally to relieve menstrual and other cramps, especially by the Native North American Meskwaki nation, hence also called *cramp bark* • magically use the whole, growing plant; the blossoms, fresh and dried; the leaves, especially in the fall, when a number of species turn red, orange, or yellow; the berries; and the bark

PLANET AND ELEMENT

Mars • Fire

MAGICAL USES

used in magical cookery, especially the berries, for happiness and love in the golden years and for family unity between the generations, especially if sharing a home with older relatives • one of the national symbols of Ukraine, known as *Kalyna* • in Slavic mythology, Kalyna Bridge links the realms of the living and the afterlife • place the plant, especially its white springtime blossoms, fresh or dried, on an altar or séance table • is an enhancer of mediumship and loving connection with the ancestors and guides • beloved by Queen Victoria, it may be speculated that since she reputedly contacted her late husband through mediums, she may have known the plant's s secrets

HOW TO USE

Said to grow wild in ancient woodlands, guelder rose is a marker of the energy tracks on both sides of the Atlantic. • Find a strong twig fallen from a bush and carve into a fork or point. Hold in your writing hand, letting it guide you to indicate the subterranean tracks. • The fall plant provides a magical focus in rituals for men and women entering their wisewomen and wise men stage. • In the same way, guelder rose can help you rejoice in the wisdom of your later years if younger people have made you feel old and useless.

CAUTION

Avoid if pregnant or breastfeeding.

Rose, Nootka

(*Rosa nutkana*)

MAGICAL FORMS

a wild rose on an upright thicket-forming shrub • native to the Pacific Northwest of the USA, from Alaska to northern California and east to the Rockies • also cultivated in gardens in the UK, the USA, Canada, and Australia • often as a hedge • grows three to nine feet tall with fragrant pink flowers in the summer and round, red-orange hips that flourish all winter • rich in vitamins A, C, and E, the nootka rose is a popular folk medicine and most parts are edible (however, check online as, for example, the layer of hairs around the seeds just below the rose hips can cause irritation of the mouth and digestive tract if ingested) • magically use the growing plant, rose hips, cut fresh or dried flowers, and flower essence

PLANET AND ELEMENT

Venus • Earth

MAGICAL USES

helps to experience and express happiness, laughter, and spontaneous fun • especially helpful if the user has experienced abandonment, abuse, or trauma that has closed the heart to life's possibilities, love of life and people, and blessings

HOW TO USE

Make the rose hips into tea or sip the essence in water to become more aware of the positive aspects of daily life and challenges that can become opportunities, seeing the glass as half full rather than half empty. Share with family members or a partner who has retreated into their shell or finds it hard to express joy, trust, and gratitude, maybe because of past or recent events. • Make a hedge of your roses to ensure happiness and positive energies stay in the home and to deter those who come spreading doom and gloom. • Carry the fragrant dried petals with a drop or two of rose absolute essential oil added in a sachet, or float the fragrant petals in a bath in a net to attract optimistic and helpful people and opportunities into your life.

Rose of Sharon

(*Hibiscus syriacus*)

MAGICAL FORMS

see also hibiscus (p. 217), with its own unique properties and significance • a hardy, late-flowering hibiscus with large, trumpet-shaped flowers in blue, red, lavender, pink, violet, or white • flowers from late summer to mid-fall • a member of the mallow family • a shrub without thorns native to Asia that can be trained into a tree up to ten feet • known as the Korean rose, it is the national flower of South Korea • grows worldwide including temperate regions of the USA and Canada and introduced into Syria and the Middle East • named after the fertile plain near the coast of Israel • magically use the bush in situ, cut flowers, and fresh or dried fallen petals

PLANET AND ELEMENT

Venus • Earth

MAGICAL USES

the rose of Sharon is mentioned in the Song of Solomon in the Bible and has gained connection with love and in Judaism and Christianity with divinity, though some argue the biblical Sharon rose is a different plant • use in rituals for love, increasing radiance and healing, twin soul connections, spiritual and religious dedication, and protecting loved ones • an ideal gift for the eighteenth wedding anniversary, the porcelain anniversary, as the growing or cut flowers representing spiritual love

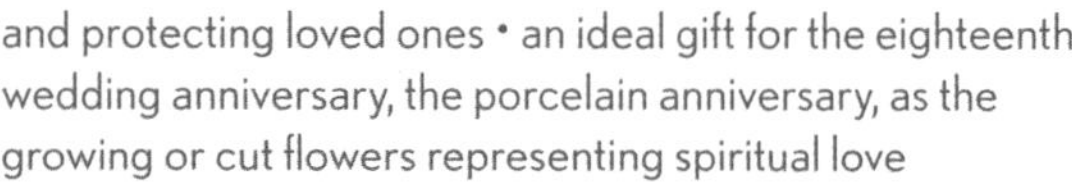

HOW TO USE

In China, the rose of Sharon signifies harmony and unity among families, in India happiness and prosperity, and in biblical times it was planted near homes to keep away evil—growing it in the garden. • Because of its lack of thorns, it is a plant for gentle goodbyes. • Collect fallen petals and set them free from a high, open place or cast them into slow flowing water or a lake where they will sink to let go of a destructive relationship, sorrow, or guilt.

Rose, Pink Pearl Anniversary

(*Rosa* 'Pearl Anniversary')

MAGICAL FORMS

if you cannot obtain this rose variety in the USA or get it shipped, substitute a mother of pearl rose or any soft-pink, shimmering rose • mother of pearl has masses of pearly pink roses with a touch of silver and repeated flowering throughout the summer • more apricot-colored and luminous, with small clusters of roses that bloom profusely from spring to fall • for either, magically use the potted or growing bush and fresh and dried cut flowers and petals

PLANETS AND ELEMENT

Venus/Moon • Water

MAGICAL USES

ideal for the thirtieth wedding anniversary, pearl, perhaps with pearl jewelry slipped into the bouquet • mother of pearl roses are often bought on the anniversary of one's own mother's death or sent to someone still grieving • use either for ocean rituals on full moon • for fertility

HOW TO USE

Collect sea water in a wide glass jar on the incoming tide. Add fresh rose petals from either of the listed varieties or any pink rose, with a single pearl or small piece of mother of pearl as offering to the Sea Mother. On the outgoing tide, tip the contents back into the ocean, saying, *Lady Ocean, Mother Sea, I return what is yours, send what is mine home to me*. Ask for a lost or estranged love to return or a loss of health, happiness, money, or career to be returned on the incoming tide. • Use a pearly or luminous pink rosebud in a vase of water, or growing on a bush or in a pot, to stir an unresponsive love or new romance slow to develop, each day passing your hands above it and calling their name nine times. When the flower unfolds, make a practical move to further the relationship.

Rose, Prickly Wild

(*Rosa acicularis*)

MAGICAL FORMS

encompasses California wild rose (*Rosa californica*); Dog rose (*Rosa canina*), the most common kind of wild roses; and any cultivated rose found growing wild • found in Europe, the UK, the USA (especially in eastern coastal regions), northwest Africa, and western Asia • white or pink wild roses with five petals instead of the multi-petaled rose • with thorny stems, as single early summer flowers, followed by rose hips • magically use the growing bush or shrub, whole flowers, fresh and dried petals, ferocious thorns, and flower essence

PLANET AND ELEMENT

Venus • Water

MAGICAL USES

for unconventional love, breaking barriers of prejudice and overcoming family or community disapproval • use in informal commitment ceremonies and handfasting as part of a wildflower bouquet • for tough love toward a partner or family member behaving destructively or irresponsibly

HOW TO USE

Mix the dried petals or whole flowers and, with care, thorns in a thick cloth bag; keep with a photo of a loved one who is risking danger for altruistic purposes or traveling to distant, wild, or dangerous places. • Cast the contents of a small bag filled with wild rose hips in an open place on a windy day to call a love that seems unattainable because the consequences of being together involve great risk and are causing hesitation on your lover's part. • Add dried wild rose petals to potpourri with eucalyptus and lemon verbena, or make into an infused rose oil, as you would cultivated roses, to add spontaneity to your relationship or family life, as these are the roses of freedom from inhibitions. • Send a bouquet of wild roses with an invitation for a day in the countryside, at the ocean, or at an outdoor sporting activity to someone you secretly admire and would like to know better in an informal setting.

Rose, Tea (Hybrid)

(*Rosa × hybrida*)

MAGICAL FORMS

descended from the original tea rose imported from China • the tea rose hybrid was created in France in the mid-1800s by crossing the traditional delicate tea rose with large, sturdy perpetuals • the Thomas Jefferson Center for Historic Plants in Monticello bears witness to his devotion to the original tea rose • magically use the flower growing on a bush, cut flower, and fresh and dried petals

PLANETS AND ELEMENTS

Venus/Mercury • Water/Earth

MAGICAL USES

carried, especially in white, in a bridal bouquet • the pink is a good anniversary gift, and for an older couple, yellow • the elegant red tea rose, a single, long-stemmed, fragrant rose, is given as a Valentine's Day gift or on any special love occasion to say, *I will love you forever*

HOW TO USE

Out of the huge range of hybrid tea roses, all can be empowered magically for their related purpose, according to the flower's name. • Use in meditation still growing on a bush or by placing cut flowers on the altar, or enchant as a cut flower. • Alternatively, carry the dried petals in a charm bag corresponding to the flower's color. • The Soleil d'Or, created in 1900, is a golden bloom for sun magick and success, as is the yellow Celebrity tea rose, which also increases fame and fortune. • Mix yellow petals from the Midas Touch in a charm bag with gold coins for gambling or speculative money making, or place the bag on top of lotto tickets before lucky numbers are drawn. • The red Veteran Honor tea rose, introduced in 1999 to honor the men and women of the armed forces with a donation to the Veterans Society, can be used for courage or as a gift of respect and appreciation. • Gift any red tea rose for a proposal, engagement, or renewal of vows.

Rose, Tundra

(*Potentilla fruticosa*)

MAGICAL FORMS

also known as the arctic cinquefoil (*Potentilla hyparctica*) • bright-yellow, five-petaled flower with heart-shaped flowers and three-lobed, dark-green leaves covered on the underside in hairs • also flowers in white, orange, and pink, blooming late spring to early summer • range is just below the ice cap, including parts of North America, such as most of Alaska and the northern half of Canada, and the northernmost part of Europe • about three inches tall • often grown as an ornamental because of its hardiness in cooler climes • magically use the whole, growing plant; flowers; and flower essence

PLANET AND ELEMENT

Saturn • Earth

MAGICAL USES

protects against feeling overwhelmed by responsibilities and demands on time and energy • for those who act as mother or father to the world even when not asked or required • restores sense of purpose, energy, and motivation

HOW TO USE

Spritz your aura with a drop or two of the essence in a water spray bottle when you know you will be entering a situation where you will volunteer or accept demands you cannot easily fulfill. • Float small, fresh flowerheads in flat dish of water in your workspace or home office if you lack motivation or energy and have a mountain of tasks or have run out of ideas and have deadlines to meet. • Set them free outdoors when withered and replace.

CAUTION

Beware not to mistake for the poisonous yellow marsh marigold or snow buttercup, whose petals are smooth and leaves hairless.

Roselle

(*Hibiscus sabdariffa*)

MAGICAL FORMS

also called rosella, Jamaican sorrel, or java jute • a close sibling of the delicate hibiscus, but with its own distinctive properties • a flowering plant native to West Africa • grows in the West Indies and Asia, in subtropical and warmer parts of the USA such as Florida, and in other subtropical regions in Australia • woody stems used as a fiber substitute for jute • cranberry-tasting dried calyces • the scarlet cup sepals of the flower • sometimes-white petals are made into a healing and magical brew, bought online or in grocery stores as the loose tea or split tea bags • unlike regular hibiscus, rosella is a form that grows well indoors as well as out • magically use cut in flower arrangements, as tea, and as jute

PLANETS AND ELEMENT

Saturn/Venus • Earth

MAGICAL USES

good luck, prosperity • drink the tea or juice before meditation to connect with higher spiritual energies, especially for blessings • linked to the Virgin Mary and female goddesses, so used in female and mothering rituals and rites of passage or in a bouquet offered as appreciation to mothers

HOW TO USE

Use rosella jute baskets, available online or in specialty stores, for sacred offerings or to strengthen the power of any other herbs or plants placed within them. • Drink rosella tea or juice or use the edible leaves in magical cookery before psychic work to open clairvoyant powers. • Keep the flower (if necessary in loose tea form) in an amulet bag for tough love in times of relationship difficulties or with a photo of an errant family member to restore them to the fold.

Rosemary

(*Rosmarinus officinalis*)

MAGICAL FORMS

also called elf leaf • magically use the dried or fresh herb, leaves, and oil

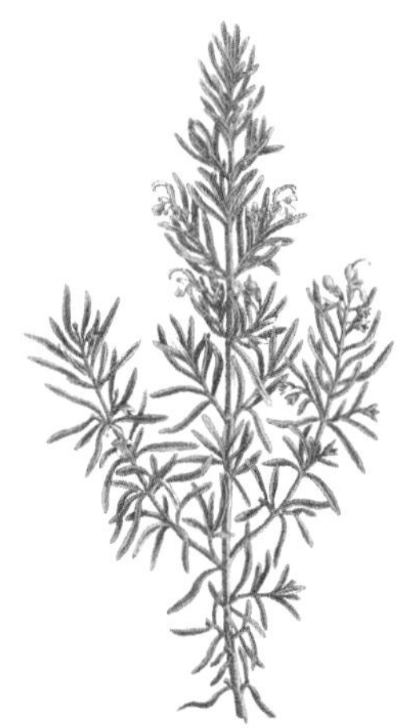

PLANETS AND ELEMENTS

Sun/Mercury • Fire/Air

MAGICAL USES

abundance • anti-theft • attracts nature spirits, especially elves • career • good luck • law • memory and concentration • prosperity • protection against sickness, malice, and nightmares • purification of home and altars • one of the main divinatory herbs, burn to bring answers, love, or absent love • for calling back ex-lovers and keeping absent lovers in mind, when sprinkled secretly around their smartphone • passion • reconciliation with estranged family, friends, and lovers • renewal of vows • study and learning new things • radiance and youthfulness • wishes • herb of Beltane or May Eve and midwinter solstice

HOW TO USE

Add dried herb to charm bags and use to stuff healing poppets or dolls. • The dried or fresh herb can be used to make protective infusions, teas, and beauty-attracting baths. • Burn as incense, especially on charcoal, to remove negativity. • Rosemary can be used in magical powders or as an ingredient in magical cooking and is quite powerful in magical gardening. • It is a perfect ingredient for protective witch bottles. • Burn branches of rosemary for smudging. • Sprinkle the dried or fresh herb on water for scrying. • The branches can be woven into wreaths outside doors for protection of home.

CAUTION

Avoid rosemary if you have asthma, epilepsy, heart disease, or hypertension, or are pregnant or breastfeeding.

Rosewood

(*Dalbergia* spp.)

MAGICAL FORMS

including the endangered tree Brazilian rosewood (*Dalbergia nigra*), Madagascar rosewood (*Dalbergia baronii*), and Amazon rosewood (*Dalbergia spruceana*) • as the pure, rare oil *Aniba rosaeodora*, from the huge *Magnoliid* tree found in South American rainforests • a rose-scented tree, known for its beauteous rings and patterns, prized especially for making guitars • rosewood, especially Brazilian, is almost impossible to be exported because of overuse and many other kinds are also scarce • rosewood trees can be grown in frost-free areas of the USA such as Arizona and southern Florida • magically use Santos or Bolivian rosewood (can be obtained from specialty and exotic wood stores) and the essential oil

PLANET AND ELEMENT

Saturn • Earth

MAGICAL USES

as oil, rosewood counteracts the hyperactivity of modern life • reduces family and workplace histrionics • for reconciliation • strengthens crystal, herb, and flower spells • for quiet sleep • forgiveness of the frailties of self and others • letting the past go • the wood for wands for peace rituals and to further musical talents

HOW TO USE

Deeply relaxing for mind, body, and spirit at the same time, rosewood oil offers a soothing room fragrance, if potential unsettling issues are to be discussed, during or after conflict, to bring compromise. • Rosewood mixes well in a burner or diffuser with jasmine, neroli, and geranium. • Add a drop of rosewood oil before sealing a spell bag or making a wish powder or jar to blend together different needs or wishes. • Anoint your brow or Third Eye before meditation to connect with angels, spirit guides, and beloved ancestors and before a séance, with rosewood diluted in apricot or virgin olive oil.

CAUTION

While it is nontoxic, do not ingest the oil. • Always dilute with a carrier oil before applying to the skin and seek medical advice if pregnant.

Rosewood, Chinese

(*Dalbergia odorifera*)

MAGICAL FORMS

tall tropical tree with small, white flowers that grows in China • classified as a vulnerable species • magically use the essential oil, but because Chinese rosewood is endangered, consider substituting the essential oil with Ho leaf oil, which incorporates oils from the camphor tree and has similar properties

PLANET AND ELEMENTS

Mercury • Air/Earth

MAGICAL USES

increases sexual desire • manifests desires and visions as reality • breaks old emotional patterns, self-destructive habits, and restrictions

HOW TO USE

Diffuse or burn the oil when spiritually or emotionally burned out as well as being physically exhausted or totally dispirited. • Wear infused aroma beads or inhale the oil to keep your enthusiasm and optimism high when people or situations discourage you, and to prevent your being drained by emotional vampires or too many demands on your time and attention. • Add a few drops of the oil plus lavender or chamomile oil to a candlelit evening bath if you are a workaholic or cannot switch off your whirling mind.

CAUTION

Do not use the oil if you are on blood thinners or sedatives.

Rowan Tree

(*Sorbus aucuparia*)

MAGICAL FORMS

known also as mountain ash, quickbeam, or the Tree of Life • grows in eastern North America; Europe; the north and west of England; Wales; Ireland; and Scotland, where, until the twentieth century, it was considered taboo to cut them down • magically use the wood from fallen branches and twigs and the berries

PLANET AND ELEMENTS

Moon • Water/Earth

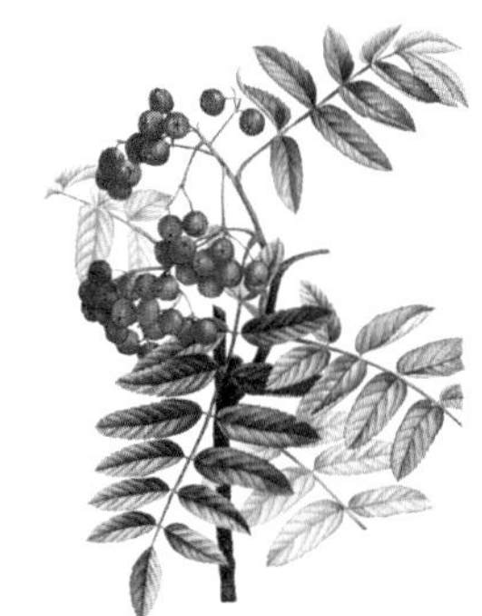

MAGICAL USES

rowan guards households, people, and animals against earthly intruders, psychic and psychological attack, malevolent ghosts, natural disasters, and against self-doubt and bad luck while traveling • in ancient Ireland, Druids of opposing forces would kindle a fire of rowan and recite an incantation over it to summon spirits to take part in the battle and protect their cause

HOW TO USE

Traditionally, matching rowan twigs were fastened in the shape of a cross with red twine. They were then set over the entrances to homes and outbuildings on May 1, to be replaced annually. • Use for extra protection if you fear you have been cursed or wished ill, adding a small wreath of dried berries to the top of the cross, saying, *Mighty tree, protector be, this curse now break, your power shall make, me/us safe. No fear or evil can enter here, begone fear.* • Rowan wands offer safety against malicious elves and are used for marking magical boundaries in ritual circles or around the self, for banishing rituals, and for resisting the manipulation or mind games of others.

CAUTION

Keep unripe rowan berries away from children and pets, though their sour taste tends to be a deterrent.

Royal Poinciana

(*Delonix regia*)

MAGICAL FORMS

associated with the magical phoenix, since the flowers resemble the claw and bright color of the bird that in legend is reborn from the ashes every five hundred years • called phoenix tail in Vietnam • also called flame of the forest or flamboyant tree • national flower of St. Kitts and Nevis and in 2018 adopted as the official tree of Key West, Florida • in Kerala, India, it is called the tree of Calvary because it was believed a small tree stood near the cross and the flowers were stained red with Christ's blood at the crucifixion • magically use the whole, growing tree; fresh or dried flowers; fernlike leaves; and seed pods

PLANETS AND ELEMENT

Sun/Mars • Fire

MAGICAL USES

use flowers and leaves in rituals for regeneration, fame, fortune, increasing radiance, and attracting positive attention

HOW TO USE

Hold your hands against the full-size tree or the potted tree with your hands clasped just above the plant to draw energies to start over and succeed better than before. • Carry the seeds, which are available online from garden centers, in a red bag if you are attending an audition, performing any media work or interviews, making a presentation, or exhibiting your creative products so that your talents will shine through. • To receive answers from the Air, Wind, and Tree spirits, listen to the foot-long or even longer burgundy seed pods that remain on the tree through winter, as they rattle in the wind.

CAUTION

The seeds and seed pods are toxic to dogs, and though the plant has been used medicinally for centuries, there is disagreement whether the seeds, pods, and leaves are toxic for humans to ingest raw, so avoid unless under expert medical advice.

Rubber Plant

(*Ficus elastica*)

MAGICAL FORMS

related to fig and banyan trees • native to southern Asia, where it can reach a hundred feet in its natural habitat • grows outdoors in tropical or subtropical locations including the USA • found worldwide indoors as a houseplant and is mainly used magically in this form • it still can reach six to ten feet • emerald, glossy, oversized, oval, leathery leaves • rarely blooms or has fruit indoors as it needs the fig wasp to pollinate it • magically use the whole, growing plant

PLANET AND ELEMENT

Mercury • Air

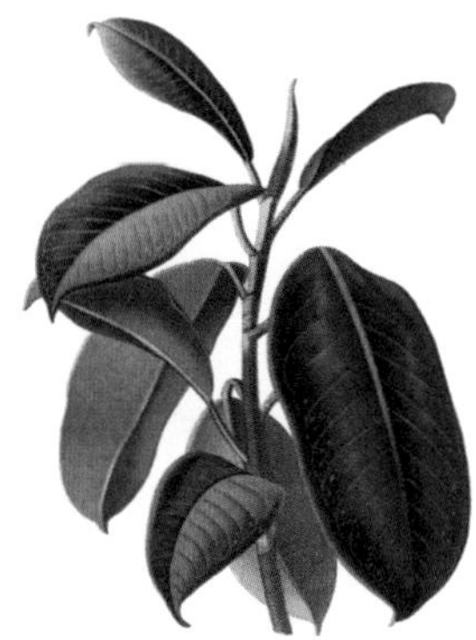

MAGICAL USES

in feng shui, the rubber plant is used to attract prosperity and good fortune • set in corners, the plant removes sharp poison arrows or *sha,* negative energy that can adversely affect harmony and good luck • because the plant cleanses toxins and releases more oxygen than most indoor plants, the rubber plant in the workplace and home eliminates stress, creating fresh energies physically, psychologically, and psychically for focus and increased productivity • ideal for those who suffer from plant allergies

HOW TO USE

Make a mini jungle to create a shield around an open-plan work area to absorb background sounds and to deter gossips or spite. • Buy a ruby rubber plant (*Ficus elastica ruby*) with pink and burgundy colorful leaves, also white and sage green to boost yang energies and bring balance and cheerfulness if you live or work with those who are constantly complaining or playing victim.

CAUTION

Rubber plants are toxic to dogs and cats. • The sap contains latex that can irritate human skin. • If allergic, wear gloves when handling your plant.

Rue

(*Ruta graveolens*)

MAGICAL FORMS

called the "herb of grace" since it was traditionally used in exorcisms from time immemorial • from Roman times considered to keep away the evil eye • Michelangelo and Leonardo da Vinci were reputed to use it • magically use the whole, growing plant; fresh and dried flowers; and oil (with care)

PLANETS AND ELEMENT

Mars/Sun • Fire

MAGICAL USES

healing, protects against illnesses of all kinds and speeds recovery • increases mental powers • love enchantment • banishes regrets, guilt, and anger • improves creativity

HOW TO USE

During a ritual, dip the dried plant in sacred water or spring water and sprinkle areas to be used for rituals and the heads of participants to bring blessings to them. • Set a sprig at the foot or head of stairs leading to dark spooky attics to drive away spirits lurking in the shadows. • Carry an amulet of the dried, chopped herb in a purple bag to overcome unrequited love. • Burn as an incense when action is necessary but fears and inertia dampen initiative; or to resolve issues that are clouded in uncertainty. • Hang dried rue over entrances to drive away earthly malevolence and illness. • Rub olive oil with a drop of rue oil added into a red candle before lighting on full moon, then diffuse the well-diluted oil in water or burn in incense to attract fast, urgent money.

CAUTION

Rue can be toxic in excess quantities. • Contact dermatitis can occur with the plant or oil in some users, especially on hot days, so do a patch test even with well-diluted oil. • Avoid rue totally if you are pregnant or elderly, or if you have liver or kidney problems. • Take care around children and pets, though the bittersweet taste and strong aroma tends to deter them.

Rue, Syrian

(*Peganum harmala*)

MAGICAL FORMS
plant native to the eastern Mediterranean; has spread to western USA and Europe • cultivated because of its beautiful white flowers and fernlike foliage • magically use the growing flowers in a safe place and the flower essence

PLANETS AND ELEMENTS
Jupiter/Mars • Air/Fire

MAGICAL USES
known as the truth serum, use for adults, teens, and children who may find it hard not to embellish, or go into denial to give the answer they think will be acceptable • for knowing who is dishonest and trying to manipulate you or a family member • for overcoming betrayal and learning to trust again

HOW TO USE
Like all defensive herbs, especially those belonging to the rue family, Syrian rue, which has a history in the Zoroastrian fire religion in old Iran, has its perils. • Meditate on the growing flowers in the wild or in a safe place in the garden to clear your mind if you have doubts about people or situations. Guidance will emerge clearly in your mind as images and words. • Use a drop of the flower essence diluted in water to anoint your teenagers' bedroom door knobs, window latches, the handles of any drawers where they keep their smartphones and tablets, and the corners of their computer desk while they are out, if you suspect your teenager is not telling you the truth about their online activities and getting into hot water.

CAUTION
The seeds may cause hallucinations. • Avoid while pregnant or if you have heart or liver conditions. • Only ingest under the strictest medical supervision. • Syrian rue is toxic for livestock when growing wild. • Take care around pets and children if growing near your home, and handle with gloves.

Rush

(*Juncus* spp.)

MAGICAL FORMS
includes soft rush (*Juncus effusus*), hard rush (*Juncus inflexus*), blue rush (*Juncus glaucus*), and the common rush (*Juncus conglomeratus*), as well as rushes outside the genus, including the field wood-rush (*Luzula campestris*), also called sweep's broom • many species of rush are found in North America, including the Baltic rush (*Juncus balticus*), native to lakeside areas; also in western South America, northern England, Scandinavia, and western Europe • soft rush is found in every continent except Antarctica • magically use the whole, growing plants and fresh and dried stems and flowers

PLANET AND ELEMENT
Venus • Earth

MAGICAL USES
for binding knot magick for a limited period • soft rush was originally used for tying hops and when they grew the rush naturally broke • because rushes grow in clumps and there are numerous small flowers on the stem, set a bunch of whole plants in a vase on the altar for a ritual to bring unity to the home, neighborhood, or workplace, drying the plants afterward

HOW TO USE
As described by Shakespeare, rushes were woven into a wedding ring for marriages considered not likely to last. • Make a rush ring for your wedding finger and gently cut it to break the hold of a false or destructive lover. • Scatter chopped green rushes over doorsteps; fresh and green rushes were strewn around wealthy houses after the Easter fires to clear out odors and parasites that accumulated during the winter. • Grow corkscrew rushes (*Juncus spiralis*) in a large pot near the door for ongoing cleansing of the home or home business of stagnant or unhelpful energies.

CAUTION
Rushes are toxic to horses.

Rye

(*Secale cereale*)

MAGICAL FORMS

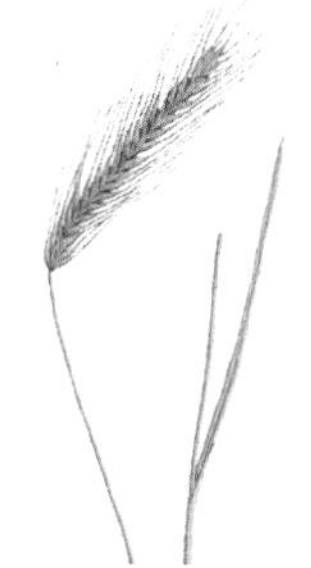

not to be confused with ryegrass (*Lolium perenne*), a different plant • an edible grain used mainly in making bread and whiskey, reaching up to six and a half feet high • the small flowers, borne on spikes, develop into one-seeded fruits or grains with long bristles • its dark color results in a black bread (see "Bread," p. 79) that lasts longer than many other varieties • lighter-colored rye bread is formed by mixing rye with wheat and other cereals • pumpernickel is made from unsifted grains • rye originated in Turkey and was introduced into Europe by the Romans about two thousand years ago • recorded in the USA in the 1600s near Jamestown for distillation purposes and made popular by German settlers for bread and whiskey in the early 1700s, especially in New England as a hardy crop • magically use the dried grain on stalks, the seeds, and as flour or bread

PLANETS AND ELEMENTS

Mercury/Venus • Air/Earth

MAGICAL USES

for love, fidelity, prosperity, and property • soothes quarrelsome folk • for protection, scattered around boundaries and on paths • serve rye bread or cereal to those you love to strengthen the bond

HOW TO USE

Eat rye seeds before meeting someone you want to impress with your wit and speedy responses at work or socially. • Long strands of dried rye can be woven into circlets to bind to protect the home and family from malevolence or can be added to arrangements of dried grasses for the same purpose. • Keep rye flour in the kitchen so that prosperity will enter and remain in the home. • To further a desired office romance, share rye bread with a desirable colleague, adding pastrami for the possibility of raising friendship to more.

Sacred Datura

(*Datura wrightii*)

MAGICAL FORMS

related to jimsonweed (see p. 239) • large, fragrant, white, trumpetlike flowers, growing wild or as an ornamental garden plant • native to southwestern USA and northwestern Mexico, from central California to northern Mexico and east across the southwest to Texas • can be cultivated in the UK and Europe • blooms from April to October • flowers open in the late afternoon until noon the next day, closing in the heat of day • globe-shaped capsules covered with spines, split open to release seeds • magically work with the nontoxic flower essence and, with great care, the poisonous growing flowers in situ (not too near)

PLANETS AND ELEMENT

Mars/Sun • Fire

MAGICAL USES

eases confusion in the midst of changes, especially involving shattered dreams and illusions • called sacred because its hallucinogenic properties are used in Indigenous initiation ceremonies and shamanic rituals • even among traditional practice, it is fraught with danger

HOW TO USE

The flowers will attract sphinx or hawk moths, which are considered messengers from the spirit world and ancestors. If you ask a question, the presence of the moths will result in answers coming into your mind or seen through half-closed eyes. • Alternatively, anoint the Third Eye with a drop of the essence in lavender or almond oil to open a connection with the spirit world. • Wash away a few drops of the essence under a fast-flowing, cold tap to banish hexes, jinxes, and ill wishes. Leave the tap running for five minutes, and afterward clean out the sink after squeezing a final drop of the essence down the drain.

CAUTION

All parts of the plant are poisonous if ingested. • The sap may be an irritant. • The plant is prohibited from being smoked or ingested in some places. • Sacred datura is described as a seventy-two-hour nightmare if used to alter consciousness and has serious and even fatal consequences, especially if tourists experiment with false shamans who employ its use.

Safflower

(*Carthamus tinctorius*)

MAGICAL FORMS

also sometimes called American or Mexican saffron • though grown commercially mainly for its oil and dyes and considered a substitute for the more expensive saffron, safflower has its own unique magical properties in a garden • magically use the whole, growing plant; petals of bright yellowy orange; flowers; seeds; seed oil for enchanted cooking; body oil that can be used on the skin; and essential oil

PLANETS AND ELEMENTS

Saturn/Mars • Earth/Fire

MAGICAL USES

alchemy • attraction and stability in same-sex relationships • protection in love affairs to prevent disillusion • the oil in magical cookery • the body oil, as a carrier oil for essential oils, as a love ingredient

HOW TO USE

Gay men in India traditionally smudge themselves with safflower incense before socializing. If you are an LGBTQ individual or couple, do the same for confidence, and if alone, to find the right love. • Female relatives in India dye the bed sheets of a newly married couple with saffron petals to bring luck and fertility to the couple. • Alternatively, make a sachet of the dried flowers in a dyed yellow bag as a honeymoon gift, especially if the couple want children soon. • To allow passion to grow spontaneously, use safflower body oil mixed with saffron petals or the essential oil diluted in almond carrier oil, and apply sparingly around the base of the spine, outer thighs, and buttocks. • Add petals in a bath sachet or a little essential oil to bath water for the restoration of self-esteem if you have experienced rejection in any area of your life. • Carry nine seeds in a small orange purse if you are seeking a loan or raise.

CAUTION

Do not use flowers, essential oil, or seeds during pregnancy. • Safflower cooking oil is made from pressed seeds and is safe to ingest, but not the pure safflower essential oil, which is made from the petals and should only be used externally when diluted. It can sometimes cause skin irritation.

Sage

(*Salvia officinalis*)

MAGICAL FORMS

see also sagebrush (p. 398) • magically use the whole, growing plant; fresh and dried herb; and well diluted as oil

PLANET AND ELEMENTS

Jupiter • Air/Earth

MAGICAL USES

employment • examinations and tests • fidelity • healing • home renovation • justice, legal and personal • learning over a prolonged period or later in life • long life • luck in games of chance • marriage in the golden years • long-term prosperity through saving • promotions • protection • travel, especially safety at night • Halloween or Samhain • Thanksgiving • New Year's Eve

HOW TO USE

Use sage in anti-evil eye rituals. • To use in candle magick, burn in the flame or roll in beeswax in order to make the candle itself. • Add to charm bags and talismans for specific purposes that must happen in a particular time frame. • Sage can also be used to empower runes. • It is also useful in four elements magick, which can be accomplished by burying some of the leaves and then casting some to the winds. • Burn sage and then cast into the water for success in interviews and major endeavors. • Grow it in healing gardens, or plant to mark protective boundaries of land. • Add the empowered herb to recipes for magical cooking. • Write smoke petitions in the air using an incense stick. • Include sage in wish powders or scratch a wish on a sage leaf.

CAUTION

Sage is not to be taken internally as oil. • Do not use oil when pregnant.

Sage, Clary

(*Salvia sclarea*)

MAGICAL FORMS

magically use all aerial parts, seeds, and oil

PLANETS AND ELEMENTS

Moon/Mercury • Water/Air

MAGICAL USES

encourages optimism and self-belief as well as the strength to go on • restores balance and harmony after stress or a setback • when problems seem insurmountable, brings unconsidered options and assurance all shall be well • repels attacks from ill-wishers • unblocks frozen emotions • for gentle spells of healing and for children and happy family spells • reverses bad luck • increases the effectiveness of clairvoyance, trance work, and mediumship

HOW TO USE

For divination, keep the dried herb in dishes where you read tarot or runes. • For enhanced channeling or meditation, burn or diffuse the oil with lavender. • Use its very protective properties by planting it in the garden or hang the dried herb around the house or placed over door lintels to establish boundaries. • Use in sachets until they lose their fragrance for the workplace and around the home to create a sense of harmony and reduce tendencies toward hyperactivity, replacing tension with gentle energy. • A sachet under the pillow prevents bad dreams and nocturnal paranormal attack.

CAUTION

Not to be taken during pregnancy or if trying to conceive, though the diluted oil is used in massage during labor as pain relief (check with midwife). • Excess inhalation of clary sage can cause tiredness, so driving should be postponed. • The oil should not be taken internally. • Avoid with alcohol.

Sage, Pineapple or Tangerine

varieties of (*Salvia elegans*)

MAGICAL FORMS

a shrub that can grow up to three feet tall, native to the pine oak forests of Mexico and Guatemala • ruby red flowers • cultivated since 1870 in warmer parts of the USA and other lands, though it will grow in cooler climates as an annual plant, being intolerant of frost • also can be grown in pots in a kitchen herb garden • releases a strong pineapple aroma when plant is crushed • related to common sage and mint • magically use the dried and fresh leaves in teas, often sweetened with honey; the cut flowers; and the whole, growing plant in the garden

PLANET AND ELEMENT

Jupiter • Air

MAGICAL USES

new beginnings • transitions • spring cleaning any time of the year in a floor and doorstep wash • blooms in the late summer and early fall and so also part of fall equinox celebrations, reaping the benefits of earlier changes • the red flowering herb can be used fresh or dried as part of a wildflower bouquet or arrangement for enduring love, especially in later years or a later marriage • the leaves are used especially in magical cookery • its energy, which is lighter and brighter than regular sage, brings lasting success through mutual agreement and negotiation

HOW TO USE

Add the chopped, dried leaves to potpourri in the home or workspace to attract abundance and unity and banish inertia, pessimism, and clouded thinking. • Drink the tea to brainstorm ingenious solutions and ways around obstacles, especially caused by the lack of enthusiasm or overanxiety in others.

CAUTION

Though pineapple sage, especially the tea, is used medicinally, avoid in pregnancy, while breastfeeding, and if suffering with diabetes.

Sage, Russian

(*Perovskia atriplicifolia*)

MAGICAL FORMS

tall plant (three to four feet), not scientifically classified as a sage, but rather related to the mint family • silver stems, lavender-blue fragrant flowers on spikes, and gray-green leaves that are aromatic when crushed • native to high parts of central Asia • grows most readily in hot, dry regions, but a tough plant that will also survive colder weather • found in the USA and the UK • magically use the dried or whole, growing plant; flowers; and fresh or dried leaves

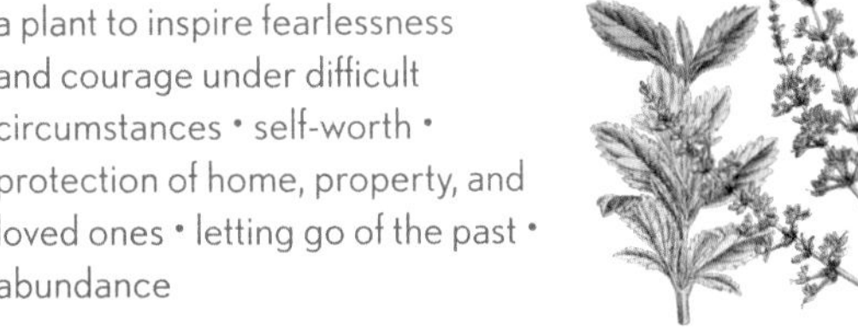

PLANET AND ELEMENT

Jupiter • Air

MAGICAL USES

a plant to inspire fearlessness and courage under difficult circumstances • self-worth • protection of home, property, and loved ones • letting go of the past • abundance

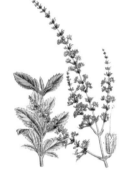

HOW TO USE

Use the leaves and dried flowers that bloom into the fall in potpourri, which will bring family unity and loyalty to stick together through good times and bad. • Adding the dried crushed flowers and leaves to an amulet bag strengthens determination to protect what or who is precious if your home or lifestyle is under threat or if your self-confidence has been shattered. • Add dried Russian sage leaves as smudge in an incense, or as smudge sticks to spiral smoke around doors and window frames to create secure boundaries around your home and to clear away malignant spirits or bad memories lingering from a previous owner. • Grow in the garden to attract prosperity, helpful people, and new sources of income to build or rebuild your finances, overcome debt, and generate a sense of optimism to trigger positive action to find solutions to difficulties.

CAUTION

The leaves and flowers are toxic to some degree and should not be ingested by humans or pets.

Sage, Spanish

(*Salvia lavandulifolia*)

MAGICAL FORMS

herb native to Spain and southern France • a small, intensely aromatic shrub • silvery foliage and above it pale-violet spikes • can be grown in pots indoors or out in many locations • magically use the dried herb as tea, fresh or dried herb in magical cookery, essential oil made from the leaves and flowers or buds, and dried flowerheads

PLANET AND ELEMENT

Jupiter • Earth

MAGICAL USES

for boosting mental and spiritual faculties • focus in examinations • increases memory and mental acuity, especially in older people • cleansing and uplifting home, workplace, and personal energies

HOW TO USE

Diffuse oil with frankincense and peppermint oils or rub on fingers and inhale when it is important to understand as well as recall new facts and methods. • Spanish sage is also helpful if you are getting older and worry about becoming forgetful, and for those studying in later life. • Wear Spanish sage or carry as oil in personal aroma devices to relieve exhaustion. • Dry brush all the nonsensitive parts of your body with a soft bristle brush, followed by a shower, then use Spanish sage oil diluted in a carrier oil like jojoba (see p. 240) for a gentle all-over massage to cleanse yourself emotionally, spiritually, and physically, and to create sacred space around yourself. • Stir the herb into magical cookery if you need to lovingly communicate with a partner or family member without their preconceptions getting in the way.

CAUTION

Do not use Spanish sage if pregnant or breastfeeding, or if taking medication for hormonal conditions. • Use with caution if suffering from diabetes, as Spanish sage may lower blood sugar levels.

Sagebrush

(*Salvia apiana*) and (*Artemisia tridentata*)

MAGICAL FORMS

common name that encompasses both California white or desert sage (*Salvia apiana*) and big sagebrush (*Artemisia tridentata*) • desert sage has the stronger fragrance • a Native North American herb that has entered westernized spirituality • used for smudging using the smoke of an herbal stick with herbs tied in a bundle together or the broad leaves burned loose in a heatproof bowl without charcoal • as well as in Canada and the USA, sagebrush is grown in the desert regions of Australia • sagebrush should be treated with the utmost respect for its sacred tradition and obtained only from reputable sources who do not exploit and over-farm • magically use the dried leaves

PLANET AND ELEMENTS

Jupiter • Air/Earth

MAGICAL USES

for purifying and energizing self, artifacts, or a space for ritual • banishing negativity • for healing to trigger the innate power of the body, mind, and soul for regeneration • for transformation and personal connection with the source of light and goodness • white sagebrush is also good for cleansing and re-energizing the human aura and for cleansing and empowering crystals before and after use

HOW TO USE

To cleanse a room or home after illness or quarrels, or if there are unfriendly spirit energies, carry a dish of burning sagebrush leaves from room to room, wafting the smoke into every corner with your non-writing hand or a fan. • For personal purification before or as part of a ritual, use a lighted smudge stick to honor the four directions, the sky, and the earth with the smoke, then spiral the smudge stick or work with a partner to create spirals around yourself. • To defuse workplace conflicts, smudge around a drawn plan of your workplace remotely from home.

CAUTION

It is best to smudge outdoors if possible; if indoors, make sure the room is very well ventilated.• Do not inhale smoke while pregnant or if suffering from lung or breathing problems.

Salal

(*Gaultheria shallon*)

MAGICAL FORMS

a thicket-forming shrub with deep roots • the shrub may live hundreds of years, the stems and twigs for eighteen years, and the leaves for two to four years, growing at different times • egg-shaped, waxy, glossy, green leaves with a serrated edge • fuzzy, pink or white, bell-shaped flowers drooping from the plant in spring replaced by bluish-black, edible berries • the plant grows up to six feet tall on the West Coast of the USA in Alaska, Washington, and Oregon, and from British Columbia in Canada south to northern California • localized in the UK, where it may be called gaultheria • magically use the flower essence and cut foliage

PLANET AND ELEMENT

Saturn • Earth

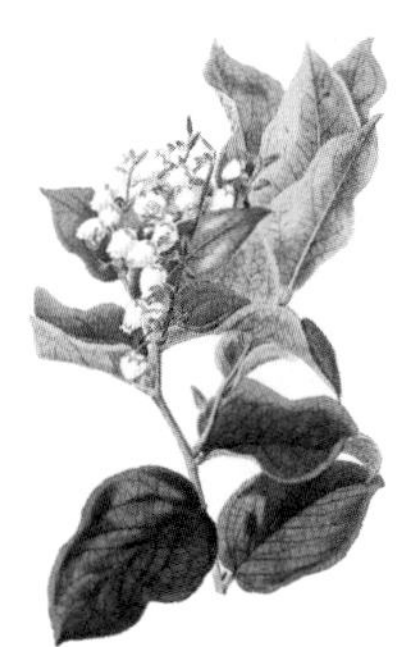

MAGICAL USES

the greenery is a symbol of lasting love and unity through good times and bad • the flower essence reduces unwarranted guilt and aids in letting go of the past, including past lives and forgiving others' mistakes and our own

HOW TO USE

The greenery in flower bouquets and as part of green foliage bouquets carries the message of lasting loyalty and unity. • Add the greenery to a flower arrangement or bouquet to mark starting over, whether as a reconciliation gift or in a wedding or commitment ceremony, formal or informal, when a couple has been together before and parted for a time. • Use salal for second and subsequent marriages and commitments when it has not been easy to come together because of opposition. • Use the essence or greenery when meditating on past lives to discover when you have been with a present partner in earlier times and how you can overcome current problems.

CAUTION

Eat salal in moderation and check with your physician if you are pregnant or taking other medications.

Sandalwood

(*Santalum album*)

MAGICAL FORMS

also called yellow sandalwood • red sandalwood (*Pterocarpus santalinus*), which is not aromatic, is harder to obtain and is no longer legal to sell in some areas because of its scarcity • white sandalwood is a medium-size, partially parasitic tree native to eastern India, cultivated in Southeast Asia and also Australia • has vulnerable status in Asia • magically use the wood chippings, powdered wood, heart wood, wood from the inner tree (especially for love tokens), and essential oil

PLANET AND ELEMENT

Jupiter • Air

MAGICAL USES

associated with ceremonial magick in many cultures from ancient Egyptian times, and in Eastern and Western spirituality, often with frankincense for wealth and connection with higher vibrations • in formal magick, in India, sacred to Lakshmi, whose home was a sandalwood tree • burned as chippings or powdered in healing incense for protection and mixed with lavender incense to call spirits

HOW TO USE

Write or etch a wish on a sandalwood chipping and burn it. • Name individual sandalwood prayer beads on a necklace, not just for the words of sacred chants but dedicating each as a personal blessing or healing needed, and wear for protection. • Burn as incense in mourning rituals to help the soul ascend on the richly scented smoke, ideal if you cannot attend a funeral or acknowledge loss publicly. • Dilute the oil for anointing the Third Eye to prevent malevolence from entering and to open spiritual channels (traditionally red sandalwood paste was painted as a dot on the Third Eye). • Anoint candles and bedposts to enhance sexual magnetism, commitment in love, self-esteem, and a positive body image. • Sandalwood can heighten meditative abilities.

CAUTION

Avoid sandalwood if you suffer from kidney or liver problems. • Dilute the oil well to avoid allergic reactions and choose pure white sandalwood. • Consult your doctor before using if pregnant.

Sandalwood, Australian

(*Santalum spicatum*)

MAGICAL FORMS

a tree endemic to southwestern regions of Australia, whose wood is fine-grained, yellow, heavy, and retains its aroma for many years • Australian sandalwood has a woodier, earthier fragrance than Indian sandalwood • the oil, made from the heartwood, is called liquid gold and is slightly sweet and also woody • magically use incense sticks, essential oil, or perfume containing Australian sandalwood • if you can obtain it, an artifact made from the wood as a protective amulet for the home

PLANET AND ELEMENT

Jupiter • Air

MAGICAL USES

as the oil, Australian sandalwood removes anxiety, clears the mind of fears, and encourages a higher level of consciousness in meditation and yoga • Australian sandalwood has been used by Indigenous people for centuries for healing and adopted into modern herbal medicine against fever, colds, inflammation, anxiety, urinary tract infections, and skin problems

HOW TO USE

The oil blends well with neroli, lavender, rose geranium, or ylang-ylang in an aroma lamp or diffuser for use before bed to have quiet sleep and beautiful dreams. • Burn the incense to connect with angels, guides, and wise ancestors, often producing images in the smoke. • Anoint your bedroom door handles and inner window catches with a drop or two of the oil to keep away fears and specters of the night.

CAUTION

The oil should be well diluted for use on the skin (try a patch test) and should not be ingested. • Check with a physician before using Australian sandalwood medication. • Be extra cautious or avoid it during pregnancy, except in perfumes, soaps, and cosmetics pronounced safe.

Sandarac

(*Tetraclinis articulata*)

MAGICAL FORMS

also known as avar tree • a small cypress-like tree native to northwest Africa and the southern Morocco regions of the Atlas Mountains, the southern Mediterranean, and Malta, as well as drier parts of California • magically use the resin, which appears in translucent, yellowish, hard tears with a balsam-like fragrance, and the essential oil, which is quite rare and made from the resin or, less commonly, the bark and leaves

PLANETS AND ELEMENTS

Moon/Saturn • Water/Earth

MAGICAL USES

burned as resin or oil in home protection, to call benign spirits and make petitions to the deities, angels, and archangels in more formal magick • to give wish powders a spiritual basis • during the days of Jesus, sandarac was called gold and it may have been the gold taken by the wise men to baby Jesus since their other offerings (frankincense and myrrh) were precious resins

HOW TO USE

The Assyrian name sandarac means "as bright as the moon," and so the resin can be cast on full moon fires or burned with moon fragrances such as jasmine and myrrh as incense at celebrations to call the power of the full moon down into the participants. • The oil, when used in a diffuser or burner, will restore harmony after bad news or workplace confrontations that have spilled into the home. • Use sandarac also in the evenings to calm restless children or hyperactive workaholic adults who suffer from insomnia to draw the day peacefully to a close.

Sarsaparilla

(*Smilax ornata*)

MAGICAL FORMS

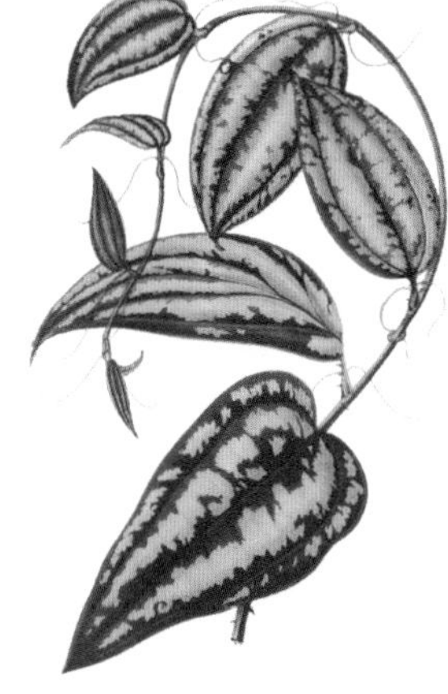

a trailing vine reaching up to sixteen feet, with tendrils, small, greenish flowers, and prickly stems • native to Mexico and the central USA, introduced by the Spanish to North America in 1563 as a suggested cure for syphilis • a major ingredient in a soft drink of the same name in the 1800s made from *Smilax ornata* or *Smilax officinalis*, still available in the Philippines, Singapore, and Australia • originally used in drinks in the UK as a concession to the temperance movement • combined with sassafras in traditional root beer (now made with different ingredients) • magically use the root

PLANET AND ELEMENTS

Jupiter • Air/Fire

MAGICAL USES

for a happy home • brings increased wealth, love, luck, and good health • regarded as an aphrodisiac

HOW TO USE

For acquiring money, powder the root or use it as chips in layers with cinnamon, ginger, and sandalwood, with a layer of coins of five different values, small yellow crystals, or gold glass nuggets at the bottom of a jar. • Carry the root in a charm bag for success in court cases and all legal and official matters. • Burn the chips with frankincense and myrrh resin as a blessing for a new home or one where there has been sickness, a separation, sadness, or money worries.

CAUTION

Sarsaparilla is not regarded as toxic but may unduly increase the strength of conventional medications. • Its effects during pregnancy have not been fully researched, so seek professional medical advice before use.

Sassafras

(*Sassafras albidum*)

MAGICAL FORMS

a tree famed for its aroma and brilliantly colored fall leaves • native to North America • magically use the wood, fallen bark, dried leaves (especially if during fall), and root

PLANET AND ELEMENTS

Jupiter • Air/Fire

MAGICAL USES

prosperity • success through advancement or business • in modern Wiccan and pagan beliefs, triple goddess (maiden, mother, and wisewoman) three-leafed leaf charms and amulets are carried or worn because the tree unusually has three types of leaves growing on the same tree: single, double, and triple lobed, representing the three stages of magical womanhood and phases of the moon

HOW TO USE

Burn dried sassafras root or bark and, if possible, a few dried, shredded fall leaves as part of a recovering-money-after-loss incense mix, including copal, frankincense, and bay leaves. Bury the ashes with a shredded piece of biodegradable paper, naming the amount you owe or need to become solvent again beneath a thriving (if possible) sassafras tree. • Shipped in large quantities back to the Old World as the first export, sassafras became considered a lucky omen on ships. • It is often built into new ships to keep away all harm. • A root in a charm bag is still considered to offer protection during journeys, especially overseas or by sea. • In the Choctaw flood legend, a prophet who tried to warn the people to change their ways was saved from the Great Flood on a raft made of sassafras logs. • Carry the shredded bark in an amulet bag to detect and remove earthly and paranormal malevolence and to ensure that you will be believed when others doubt you.

CAUTION

The use of sassafras, once regarded as a cure-all, was banned in drinks in 1960 as a possible carcinogen and cause of liver damage.

Savory

(*Satureja hortensis*) and (*Satureja montana*)

MAGICAL FORMS

includes summer savory (*Satureja hortensis*) and winter savory (*Satureja montana*) • summer savory is a milder oil and the herb has a more subtle, culinary flavor • plant both for all-around protection • summer savory is an annual plant, flowering in summer then dying in fall, but winter savory is a perennial that can be harvested for much of the year • magically use the whole, growing plant; leaves; flowering tips; and essential oil for both summer and winter savory

PLANET AND ELEMENT

Mercury • Air

MAGICAL USES

both herbs have similar magical properties • summer savory is sometimes associated with St. Julian the Hospitaller in an old tradition and so linked with safe travel and offers a welcome to visitors when planted outside the home • honesty • friendship and playfulness • curiosity to learn new things and to aid memory and fact retention • summer savory rather than winter is an aphrodisiac • magical cookery

HOW TO USE

As a culinary herb, savory, especially summer savory, is an ideal ingredient; you should add wishes and call love as you stir the herb. • Carry the dried leaves of either herb to an examination or test to recall the necessary information and to an interview to persuade the panel or interviewer you are trustworthy and will fit in. • Plant both herbs for happiness in the home, and keep a sachet of dried flowers of summer savory to ensure mutually loving sex and that your partner will create a happy home with you. • Place dried flowers and leaves of both, mixed, over the door to bring absent family safely home.

CAUTION

Dilute well because savory oil or leaves may cause skin irritation. • Do not use if pregnant or if taking blood thinners. • If skin irritation is experienced with summer savory, do not use winter savory.

Saw Palmetto

(*Serenoa repens*)

MAGICAL FORMS

a small palm tree growing to twenty feet, with fans of yellow-green leaves and white flowers • native to North America, growing along the sand dunes of the coasts and from South Carolina to Texas • magically use the dried or fresh berries, which have a nutty vanilla taste, and tea made from the berries

PLANETS AND ELEMENTS

Sun/Moon • Fire/Water

MAGICAL USES

for power and energy and for male potency • empowers anyone, male or female, who is afraid of intimidation, especially sexual predators or bullies

HOW TO USE

Dried berries can be added to a white charm bag for health and vitality, to a red bag for passion, to a pink bag for romance, and to a green bag for money and good luck. • Worn or carried, the berries serve as a male aphrodisiac and fertility charm. • Both sexes should carry a sachet of the dried berries for an increase in confidence and power if facing prejudice of any kind. • Share the tea before lovemaking for increased sexual powers and libido. This is especially helpful in long-lasting male relationships where one partner has lost interest in sex.

CAUTION

Avoid saw palmetto in any form if you have high blood pressure or a heart condition, or are pregnant or trying to become pregnant. • All preadolescent and adolescent males should avoid saw palmetto, as the palm can adversely affect the development of male genitalia.

Saxifrage

(*Saxifraga stolonifera*) and (*Saxifraga oppositifolia*)

MAGICAL FORMS

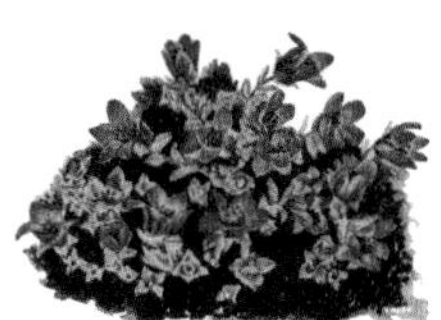

includes both creeping saxifrage (*Saxifraga stolonifera*) and arctic alpine saxifrage (*Saxifraga oppoitifolia*) • the emblem of Nunavut, Canada, and county flower of Londonderry, Ireland • these are two of the eight species of saxifrage in North America and are the most significant magically and medicinally • magically use the whole plant of the alpine variety (which can be grown in a pot; this variety is found in Vermont), the flowering plant, and the leaves of both

PLANET AND ELEMENT

Moon • Water

MAGICAL USES

both varieties link with and assist adapting to the ebbs and flows of life • the alpine variety, whose flowering coincides with the calving of the caribou among the Inuit people, represents fertility and new beginnings, especially when in flower • the *stolonifera*, often called the mother of thousands or creeping saxifrage, signifies not only fertility but spreading influence and ideas to gain authority and recognition

HOW TO USE

Saxifrage translates as "stone break" because the small, kidney-shaped, grain-like bulbils at the base were considered curative for kidney stones. • Dry bulbils on your altar, carving on each a symbol of any impasses you wish to break, and cast them into flowing water. • Since the alpine version endows saxifrage with time-keeping properties, the flowering coinciding with the calving, keep the dried flowers and leaves of any saxifrage under your pillow at times when you are worried about sleeping through an alarm, especially if you have been in a different time zone. • Secure the runners or creepers from between the creeping red and white *stolonifera* for binding magick, especially for fidelity; the purple, starlike alpine form can be used in star magick.

Scabious

(*Knautia macedonica*)

MAGICAL FORMS

also called pincushion flowers • eighty to a hundred varieties, popular ones including Macedonian scabious (*Knautia macedonica*), the long-flowering white scabious (*Scabiosa caucasica* 'Perfecta Alba'), the dwarf or dove scabious, a smaller variation, often a wildflower (*Scabiosa columbaria*), the giant scabious (*Scabiosa cephalaria* 'Gigantea'), and sweet scabious or grandmother's pincushion, another small variety in purple or wine color (*Scabiosa atropurpurea*) • also grows in gardens as a wildflower • small flowers cluster together on a single, often long, wiry stem • prominent stamens emerge from flowers, resembling pins in pincushions • domed flowers bloom from summer to fall in white, blue, red, yellow, and purple • native to Europe, Asia, and Africa and grows well in many parts of the USA • magically use the growing flowers in situ with their stamens; flowerheads; flowers; and seeds

PLANET AND ELEMENTS

Venus • Earth/Water

MAGICAL USES

as cut flowers with the taller stems, for bouquets for weddings and anniversaries • a suggested alternative flower to the dahlia for the fourteenth (opal) wedding anniversary, especially in white • dove or sweet scabious are often called "the devil's bit," as it was told that the devil, jealous of the plant's healing power, bit off half the root • as consolation, all scabiosa have power to ward off evil • carry an amulet bag with dried flowerheads and seeds for protection

HOW TO USE

Tie long stems of cut, fresh flowers together with red thread for binding rituals and mending quarrels or coldness. • Allow seeds to develop in the flowering head pincushion of other still-growing flowers, then dry the flowers with the seeds still inside for a flower arrangement for the home to preserve the unity and harmony restored by the earlier rituals. • Burn dried root chips with agrimony and rue to break any negative magical hold or earthly threats.

Scallion

(*Allium fistulosum*)

MAGICAL FORMS

also known as green or spring onion • originally found in Asia, scallions spread via trade routes to Egypt and from there worldwide as food and medicine • related to leeks, chives, and garlic with onion-like flavor, green leaves smelling like grass, and small, white, onion-fragranced bulbs • the white and green parts are edible • in tea, the chopped white bulb is added to ginger, salt, and sweetener or the chopped leaves and bulbs as a healing broth • scallions form clusters of tiny, fluffy, white flowers in hot climates (may be obtained in farmers' markets or specialty outlets, still attached to the stems) • magically use the cut or whole, growing plant; bulb; leaves; and flowers

PLANET AND ELEMENT

Mars • Fire

MAGICAL USES

clear and honest communication, avoiding misunderstanding and unintentional tactlessness • domestic happiness and nonconfrontational family mealtimes • magical cookery

HOW TO USE

Use in magical cookery or as tea or broth, eating before meeting someone you would like to know better (using breath freshener after, of course) to convey interest without overeagerness. • Use in family cookery with relatives who are quick to take offense. • Grow in a vegetable patch because, like conventional onions, scallions act as protectors against evil, especially paranormal specters of the night. • Scatter the dried, white flowers (which have a fragrance between onions and grass) into flowing water to banish angry words spoken in haste and the effect of those determined to portray you in a negative light.

CAUTION

Avoid scallions if you are taking blood thinners.

Scarlet Pimpernel

(*Anagallis arvensis*)

MAGICAL FORMS

low-growing, small, red, purplish-blue, or dark-blue star-shaped flowers, short stalked with bell-shaped or almost flat flowers • native to Europe and naturalized in North America and many parts of the world • considered invasive in California and the Pacific Northwest • also called the shepherd's weather glass because the flowers open in the morning if sunny and close late afternoon or earlier if they sense rain coming • magically use the growing or dried plant, chopped and hulled dried flowers, and leaves

PLANETS AND ELEMENTS

Venus/Mercury • Earth/Air

MAGICAL USES

drives away deceitful people in matters of love and finance • protects against illness and accidents • the fictitious Sir Percy Blakeney from the 1903 novel *Scarlet Pimpernel* rescues French aristocrats by spiriting them away across the border, revealing the courage and strength of this feisty little plant that is often underrated

HOW TO USE

If grown in the garden, the pimpernel protects against malevolent spells and ill wishes. • Weave the flowers in a circlet with dill and rue, and hang over the door to guard the home against misfortune and unwelcome callers. • Adopt the plant as an amulet when you are taking on corrupt officialdom or workplace bullies. • In an adaptation of an old rite, chopped scarlet pimpernel is used to consecrate the blade of ritual knives, mixed with dragon's blood resin in incense and the knife passed through the smoke. • Carrying blue and red flowers mixed together in a charm bag gives second sight and a telepathic link with birds and animals.

CAUTION

The plant is toxic to humans and pets and should not be ingested, except with expert advice. • The leaves may cause skin irritation.

Schisandra

(*Schisandra chinensis*)

MAGICAL FORMS

an aromatic vine that can extend up to twenty-six feet with cuplike, pale-pink, cream, or white flowers that produce spikes of berries • native to China and cool temperate parts of North America; also found in Russia • its Chinese name, *Wu Wei Zi*, means "five-flavored fruit" or "berry," and was given because it contains all five elemental energies and is an all-healer • used magically and medicinally mainly for its berries, which are made into a decoction tea or, using the seeds, as a stimulating infusion

PLANET AND ELEMENT

Jupiter • Air

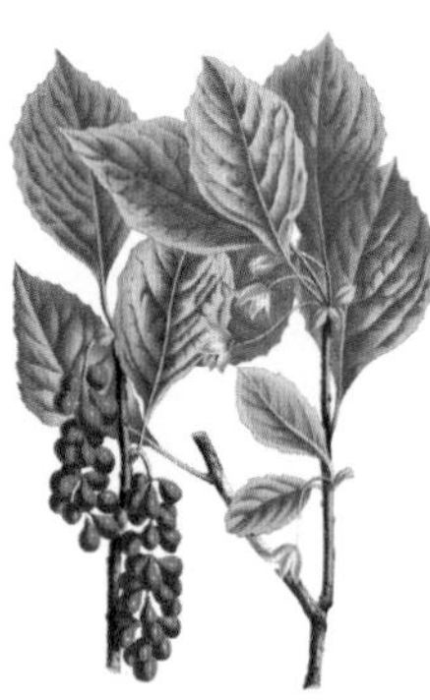

MAGICAL USES

boosts psychic abilities • increases sex drive and fertility in men • for tantric and sex magick • enhances concentration and recall of necessary facts in the present world and memories of past lives • increases mental as well as physical stamina and calms a troubled mind

HOW TO USE

Keep the dried flowers in a small wicker basket with two tiny dolls lying side by side on a love altar until the fragrance fades to call and/or keep your twin soul loving. Then float the basket with the two dolls tied loosely face to face with biodegradable ribbon into a fast-flowing river or the outgoing tide, asking that love between you will always willingly be given and received. • Cut a piece of the fruit-bearing vine and cast it away in a high place to remove the hold of a destructive or unfaithful lover. Eat or make the berries from the piece of vine into tea or juice and drink it to absorb your own power to thrive and find true love.

CAUTION

Plant can cause skin irritation. • Consult a doctor before using if you are taking other medications, and avoid while pregnant, as it can stimulate the uterus.

Scholar Tree

(*Alstonia scholaria*)

MAGICAL FORMS

also called the blackboard tree • an evergreen from the dogbane family • native to the subtropics and tropics of Asia, especially southern India, where it is called pulai wood; Africa; and northern Australia, where it is known as white cheesewood • grown as an ornamental in California and southern Florida • mini traditional blackboards and pencils were once widely made of this wood; you may be able to find some at specialty craft and stationery stores • state tree of West Bengal • magically work with the tree, especially in flower, and the dried and powdered wood or bark (available online)

PLANET AND ELEMENT

Mercury • Air

MAGICAL USES

learning rituals and meditation • in Theravada Buddhism, the first Buddha is said to have used this as a tree for enlightenment • the leaves were once awarded to graduate and postgraduate students at Visva-Bharati University in West Bengal • for environmental reasons, now a single leaf is presented by the chancellor to the vice-chancellor on behalf of the graduating students • the powdered or dried bark or wood can be carried for success in all study, examinations, and writing ventures

HOW TO USE

This tree was given the name of the devil-tree in parts of India and was once linked with the nagas, magical beings with serpent and human features in Hinduism, Buddhism, and Jainism, who can be benign or destructive. • The bark, wood, or leaves of the tree offer protection against all harm, human and spirit, when hung in a bag over the door of the home or workplace. • Sprinkle a little of the powder over a blackboard (you may not be able to obtain the traditional wooden kind) on which you have written what you most want to attain or lose. Leave the board and powder out in a rain shower in a safe place where children or pets will not ingest the powder.

CAUTION

Do not ingest, and wash hands after using the wood, leaves, or bark. • Avoid in pregnancy.

Scleranthus

(*Scleranthus annuus*)

MAGICAL FORMS

called *knawel* in Germany, meaning "tangled mass of knotted stems" • native to Eurasia and Africa • introduced and naturalized in North America and in many temperate parts of the world • two to five inches high • blooms in spring but dies in late spring or early summer, leaving its seeds for the following year • magically use a piece of the dense, fading, tangled mat of plants, which you can grow in the garden or find growing wild on uncultivated land, and the flower essence

PLANET AND ELEMENT

Saturn • Earth

MAGICAL USES

as the plant and flower essence, brings decisiveness, whether choosing between two options or overcoming a general inability to make decisions, that may manifest physically as mood swings, motion sickness, or frequent inner ear and balance disturbances seemingly without physical cause • increases the ability to trust intuition and accept a decision once made rather than agonizing over whether it was the right one

HOW TO USE

Take a piece of the dying plant mat and shred it to remove indecision. If making a choice between two or three options, name each and shred the plant into two or three piles. The last piece determines which option is correct. • Take the essence before and during travel if you suffer from motion sickness or at times when you feel disoriented and dizzy under pressure when events are moving too fast. • Using a drop of the essence mixed with aloe vera, the carrier oil of balance, anoint the middle of your hairline on your crown chakra energy center for clarity of thought, around the solar plexus for determination to decide, and the soles of your feet and behind your knees to steady yourself.

Scorpion Weed

(*Phacelia* spp.)

MAGICAL FORMS

includes *Phacelia arizonica*, *Phacelia distans*, and *Phacelia tanacetifolia* • more than a hundred kinds of scorpion weed grow in Western Australia • may be hard to tell apart • so called because some species of flowers have a curling, scorpion-like tail formation, such as silverleaf phacelia (*Phacelia hastata*) • scorpion weed is found wild in desert, often high places, in the southwestern USA and northwest Mexico • showier kinds such as the purple (*Phacelia tanacetifolia*) are cultivated in gardens in warmer places and used as cut flowers • scorpion weeds bloom pale, bluish pink, purple, bluish white, white, pale and lavender blue, and brighter purple through spring and summer, some until early fall • they can be grown in containers in more temperate climates • magically use the growing flowers, especially the dried scorpion-tailed kind, and the flower essence

PLANET AND ELEMENT

Mars • Fire

MAGICAL USES

the plant and essence for courage, emotional and physical strength, and determination to overcome fears, especially those that are magnified out of all proportion in the long hours of the night • use for speaking and acting in anxiety-provoking situations without worrying about disapproval, loss of love, or condemnation by others

HOW TO USE

Add the dried scorpion tail flowers to an amulet bag to reduce fears of spiteful family members or work colleagues so you can deal decisively. • Sip the essence through the day if you are afraid of making mistakes or being found lacking at work. • If you can obtain the cut flowers, keep them in a vase at celebrations or grow your container plant near the door to prevent jealousy or backstabbing from entering if you must see people who try to make you feel inadequate.

CAUTION

Handle with care, as some phacelia species may cause a skin irritation akin to poison oak (see p. 354).

Sea Buckthorn

(*Hippophae rhamnoides*)

MAGICAL FORMS

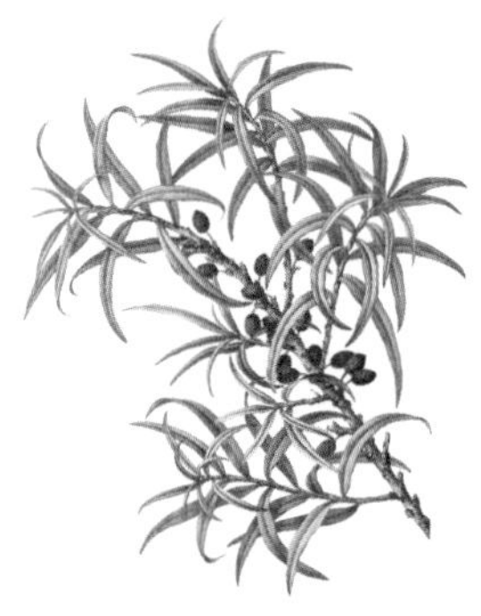

a wild, thorny shrub that can grow up to sixteen feet high • has narrow, silvery leaves and clusters of orange berries, harvested in the fall • indigenous to Europe and Asia, especially Mongolia, where the sour, nutrient-rich berries have been used medicinally and as food for thousands of years • introduced to the Canadian prairies in the early 1930s for sheltering the land and to protect soil erosion • magically use the commercially produced carrier oil made from the berries (in preference to oil from roots and leaves, which has fewer healing properties), the fresh and dried berries, and the growing plant

PLANETS AND ELEMENTS

Moon/Mars • Water/Fire

MAGICAL USES

called "the oil of small miracles," made from the seed oil and also named "the holy fruit of the Himalayas" • empower the oil to enhance radiance and use on skin and hair either alone or with a little almond or jojoba carrier oil • revives optimism and brings solutions for seemingly insoluble situations

HOW TO USE

To make the home safe if there are paranormal disturbances or you have troublesome neighbors, keep a dish of berries or sprigs of the plant with berries attached in a hanging basket where the air circulates and replace when they wither. • The berries, freshly picked or purchased dried, can be kept in an orange charm bag near where you handle home or business finances to attract prosperity and good fortune.

CAUTION

Consult your doctor before using sea buckthorn if you are pregnant or chronically ill. • Take care around the thorns with children and pets.

Sea Lavender

(*Limonium latifolium*)

MAGICAL FORMS

also known as marsh rosemary, statice, and lavender thrift • native to salt marshes and sand dunes in the Mediterranean, where it was once valued for its medicinal and culinary purposes • now grown worldwide ornamentally in gardens as well as wild • prized for their long-lasting color • flowering plants have tall, sturdy stems and a cloud of tiny white flowers with purple, yellow, or pink petals (depending on the variety) that blossom in summer and early fall • magically use the individual flowering plant, a bunch of the flowering plants dried in wreaths or bouquets, and the dried petals

PLANETS AND ELEMENTS

Jupiter/Moon • Air/Water

MAGICAL USES

the flower of memory, a lasting dried or fresh bouquet says, *I am thinking of you*, *Get well soon*, or *Congratulations on your success* • bouquets for remembering departed loved ones, gifted to the bereaved on anniversaries, or placed as a flower arrangement on a grave • sent to an absent or estranged love as a fresh or dried bouquet • dried flowers carried in a sachet can improve memory, whether for examinations or to recall happy memories

HOW TO USE

Cast sea lavender into a river or the ocean with the spoken message, *I miss you* or *Forget me not*, to a lost or past love. • Sea lavender is called "Lethe's bramble" after the ancient Greece underworld river of forgetfulness. • Mix dried sea lavender heads in a sleep pillow with true lavender to recall your dreams and to meet a known or unknown lover on the dream plane (the identity may come as a surprise if it is someone you formerly thought of as just a friend). • Keep the dried flowers, gathered or purchased on vacation, in a vase in your home to recreate or recall a sense of freedom and excitement if you live in the center of a city and feel stifled. • Meditate on a single or group of growing flowers for visions of the ocean and maybe past worlds if you have a seemingly inexplicable longing to live or work on or near the sea.

Sea Lettuce

(*Ulva lactuca*)

MAGICAL FORMS

also referred to as algae and sea essence • attached to rocks or in rock pools if detached • bright green and translucent with ruffled fronds that resemble garden lettuce in shape • found on rocky shores around the world • sometimes a major ingredient in Welsh lava bread and in Japanese and Korean cuisine • magically use the algae on the shore and the essence

PLANET AND ELEMENT

Moon • Water

MAGICAL USES

as a plant and essence, for detoxifying the mind and life as well as physically detoxing the body • acknowledging and healing the shadow side of the self rather than repressing or denying it • leaving behind what cannot be fixed • keep your essence surrounded by shells or water crystals like fluorite or aquamarine to empower it

HOW TO USE

Find sea lettuce that has become detached from the rocks and is in a rock pool below the high tide line. Place on top of it, hidden in its leaves, a pearl or piece of mother of pearl. Name regrets, repressed sorrow, or anger and say, *Lady Ocean Mother sea, take this grievous burden from me.* • Dissolve a few drops of the essence in a glass of water while playing ocean sounds. Tip the essence water gently into another glass of the same size and back again, repeating the action until you feel there is only peace. Afterward, sip the water from the full glass throughout the day. Wash the empty glass under a running tap.

CAUTION

If planning to ingest, use sea lettuce from accredited sources or a cooked product such as laverbread. • Before ingesting, seek medical advice if suffering from thyroid, kidney, or intestinal problems, or if you are pregnant.

Sea Vegetable

MAGICAL FORMS

there are hundreds of sea vegetables, which are edible seaweed that only grow in oceans, not fresh water • includes brown algae (*Phaeophyceae* spp.), green algae (*Chlorophyta* spp.), and red algae (*Rhodophyta* spp.) • especially popular in Chinese, Japanese, and Korean cuisine • wakame (*Undaria pinnatifida*) is one of the most widely adopted sea vegetables worldwide, a variation of kelp found in France, Australia, New Zealand, Japan, and Korea • a major ingredient of miso soup • ogonori (*Gracilaria* spp.) is a red seaweed that grows in Hawaii, the Philippines, China, Japan, and Korea • exported widely for soups, salads, and stews • see also dulse (p. 165), Irish moss (p. 297); kelp (p. 243), and sea lettuce (p. 407) • magically use imported, dried sea vegetables that can be rehydrated in cookery and fresh or dried sea vegetables in rituals and empowerments

PLANETS AND ELEMENT

Moon/Venus • Water

MAGICAL USES

for money magick, preserve in brine or whiskey • gim, or nori (*Porphyra* spp.), a red, dark-purple, or green algae from Korea and Japan, is made into seaweed sheets, eaten split and roasted, for the fair division of assets and for encouraging others to share their resources if they lack generosity

HOW TO USE

Choose a green sea vegetable for the inflow of love, red for a surge of action or energy, and brown or green for all financial gain and to prevent the outflow of money. • Rehydrate your sea vegetables to restore health, optimism, and communication.

CAUTION

Make sure sea grapes, which are widely available, come from a reliable source, as they may, if contaminated, lead to food poisoning. • Check with your doctor before ingesting if pregnant or taking thyroid medication.

Sedge

(*Carex* spp.)

MAGICAL FORMS

genus includes *Carex pendula*, the pendulous sedge, and *Carex hirta*, hairy sedge, which grows wild in the USA, Europe, and Asia • sedges can be bought from garden centers for cultivation in most lands or from craft stores ready-dried for weaving • beautiful and elegant flowering plants, growing along water edges in the wild or planted near garden ponds • typified by triangular solid stems with no nodes or joints • many *Carex* species are evergreen with bronze to gold foliage • magically use the stems and foliage of any sedge and the whole, growing plant in situ

PLANET AND ELEMENT

Venus • Water

MAGICAL USES

for outdoor water magick • for water spirit contact, especially the yellow drooping catkin flowers of the pendulous sedge • also for avoiding illusion in love • since pendulous sedge especially grows in former ancient woodlands and water courses and water is said to hold the human memory, it is an excellent plant for meditation close to the plants • in ancient Egypt, sedge was the symbol of the king of the southern half of Egypt and could form focus for rites for personal or business advancement • in Norse mythology, the nature goddess Freya's chariot, pulled by cats, had hairy sedge wheels

HOW TO USE

Hairy sedge and other well-established sedges aid spontaneous astral travel, especially connected with water and wild places. • Aine, the sun goddess of old Ireland, was offered sedge to bring fertility. • Any strong sedge can be woven into a tiny basket or used to line a ready-made one in which fertility crystals such as carnelian and rose quartz are floated in slow-flowing water to bring a child. • Dry the leaves of any sedge and use them woven together for knot magick to hold the love (willingly) of a desired partner or a partner who has become neglectful. • Tie nine knots in a sedge leaf rope for happiness, money, health, and love, and hang it from a tree near water.

Self-Heal

(*Prunella vulgaris*)

MAGICAL FORMS

also called woundwort • low-growing plant with spikes of violet-blue and reddish to pink flowers blooming from June to September • pointed oval leaves with hairs on the underside • native to Europe, the UK, and Asia, taken to North America by early settlers and now widespread • self-heal now grows in temperate regions worldwide, usually wild, though it can be cultivated • magically use the flowers, stems, and leaves, which can be bought online already shredded for charm bags and spells

PLANET AND ELEMENT

Moon • Water

MAGICAL USES

to heal inner and outer wounds and secret sorrows • traditionally picked for amulets on the dark of the moon, for that which must not be revealed

HOW TO USE

Burn shredded self-heal leaves as part of a healing incense mix with lavender and myrrh resin if there has been lingering sickness in the home that has not responded to conventional treatment. • Make an infusion, strain it, and spray or sprinkle on doorsteps to prevent sickness from entering or lingering if there is an epidemic or winter ills. • Hang a white bag with dried leaves, a few sandalwood chips, and dried sage over the front door to heal sorrows or resentments repressed by a partner, family, or visiting relatives to allow healing words to be spoken. • Bury the dead flowers if you are tempted to share a secret that would cause unhappiness if spoken.

CAUTION

Consult your doctor before using if you are pregnant or nursing. • Self-heal can cause skin irritation.

Senna

(*Cassia* spp.) and (*Senna* spp.)

MAGICAL FORMS

including *Cassia marilandica*, *Cassia senna*, and *Senna acanthoclada* • small, woody shrub with yellow flowers, one of the best-known and used herbal medicines worldwide • native to tropical Africa, there are four hundred varieties growing, including silver cassia (*Senna artemisioides*) in Australia; the American senna (*Senna hebecarpa*), which grows wild through the northeastern USA and southeastern Canada; *Cassia marilandica*, or Maryland senna, in eastern North America; and *Cassia cutifolia*, an ornamental in the far south with bright-yellow flowers • leaves are stronger medicinally and are picked before or while the plant flowers • pods are harvested in the fall • magically use the dried flowers and leaves

PLANET AND ELEMENT

Saturn • Earth

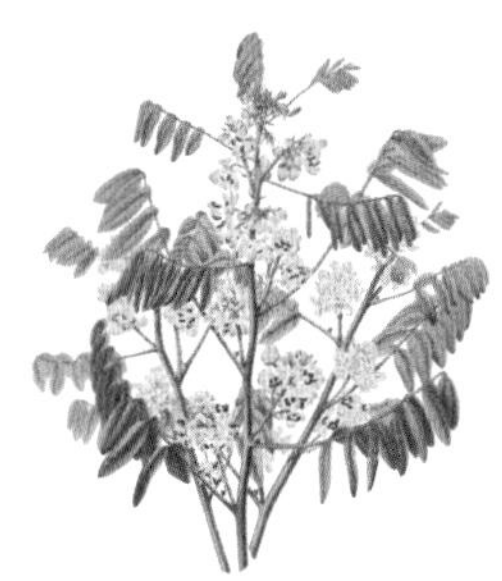

MAGICAL USES

the magical properties of senna are often overlooked • the pods have psychic as well as physical effects in reducing restrictions and obstacles whether to love, success, or happiness

HOW TO USE

For protection, soak senna leaves with cumin and coriander seeds in cold water for nine days, afterward straining the liquid off. Bury the mix in soil near the front door, at the four corners of your home, or in a deep plant pot to banish and keep away malicious energies. • Burn the crushed leaves in incense with a powerful fragrant resin such as frankincense or copal to purify a space or room to clear the air after a major quarrel, refusal, or rejection to revive your power to fight on or accept that you need to find an alternative path if the present one is blocked.

CAUTION

Senna is not recommended for children under twelve. • Do not use if suffering from colitis or without medical advice if pregnant or breastfeeding.

Serviceberry Tree

(*Amelanchier laevis*)

MAGICAL FORMS

also called Juneberry because the fruit first appears in June • small fruit tree or multistemmed shrub with masses of white flowers, one of the first trees to bloom in spring • followed by small, purple, edible fruits and finally red, yellow, and orange leaves in the fall • at least one species exists in every US state except Hawaii, and in every Canadian province • introduced in the seventeenth century as snowy mespilus (*Amelanchier lamarckii* or *Amelanchier canadensis*) from northeast USA to Europe and the UK where it is now naturalized, with white, star-shaped flowers and purple-black, globular, sweet fruit when ripe • magically use the whole, growing tree in situ; berries; flowers; and fresh or dried leaves

PLANET AND ELEMENT

Saturn • Earth

MAGICAL USES

the coming of spring or new beginnings • asking for and receiving the right official or legal help or judgment you need • slows aging

HOW TO USE

The serviceberry tree is known as the time tree because its flowering once coincided (less so now) with the annual returning of the shad fish to spawn up the Hudson River. For this reason, it is also called the shadbush. • Use the blossoms, in bloom if possible or dried if not, to mark a wedding or love-pledging anniversary, a birthday, or a memorial by scattering them with blessings in a place loved by those being celebrated or mourned. • Use the fresh or dried fall leaves on Halloween fires to connect with ancestors. • Invite family, friends, and neighbors for a fall feast where you serve pies, jams, or preserved berries, to plan community events to serve peers who are lonely or disadvantaged. Serviceberry can also be eaten while sharing meals and exchanging practical services such as babysitting.

CAUTION

The leaves and pink or green fruit should not be ingested. • The fruit is toxic to livestock. • Do not eat large quantities of the fruit if you are pregnant nor allow children to do so.

Sesame, Black

(*Sesamum indicum*)

MAGICAL FORMS

sibling of white sesame, which has had the black outer hull removed • from the erect sesame plant that can be over six feet tall with seed pods containing the black seeds that are gathered after the pods have turned brown-black • native to Africa and grown in tropical and subtropical regions throughout the world • can be eaten raw, but more flavorful toasted • magically use the seeds, whole and ground

PLANET AND ELEMENT

Mars • Fire

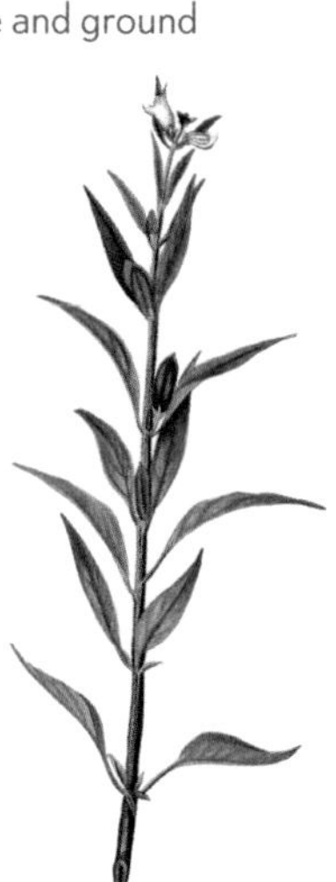

MAGICAL USES

known from the Arabian Nights tales as magical for the words *Open Sesame* revealed the cave with the lamp containing a genie for Aladdin • indicates the power of black and white seeds to unlock previously closed doors of opportunity and find hidden treasure at sales • for overcoming karmic debts • connection with intuition and with the ancestors

HOW TO USE

Burn ground black sesame seeds in incense if you suffer nightmares, especially paranormal ones, or nocturnal attack. • Carry the burning seeds in a pot through the whole home wafting the smoke if there is a hostile or spooky atmosphere in a house or apartment into which you have recently moved. • Eat the black seeds before meditating or carrying out automatic writing to receive messages from the ancestors as they guide your hand to create words in answer to your questions. • Use as an offering to the Earth on anniversaries of the death of family members and on the festivals of the dead in the westernized world from October 31 eve to November 2.

CAUTION

Avoid sesame with nut allergies, diabetes, or low blood pressure and while pregnant or breastfeeding.

Sesame Seed, White

(*Sesamum indicum*)

MAGICAL FORMS

black sesame with the outer hull removed • grows in pods on the sesame plant, which can be over six feet tall, with white to purple flowers • native to Africa and India, and can be grown with care in hot, dry conditions • magically use the white seeds (often in magical cookery) and the cold, pressed, unrefined oil as a carrier oil

PLANET AND ELEMENT

Mars • Fire

MAGICAL USES

open hidden opportunities, especially in career • attracts money when sprinkled on food or baked in bread • eaten for increased libido and fertility • the white cooking oil (also found in black), is made from toasted or roasted seeds to magically bring abundance and energy, and to revive enthusiasm for ventures, especially those involving people sharing the meal

HOW TO USE

Use in a head-to-toe warming massage followed by a bath or shower when you need to be persuasive in money-making ventures or make fast, accurate major decisions regarding speculation. • Mix black and white seeds in a charm bag for the yin and yang connection to find your twin soul or, if you know them already, to awaken soul recognition in the other person. • Also eat the mix before meditating to explore past lives you believe you have shared to understand a connection with someone new with whom you sense immediate recognition.

CAUTION

Blend sesame seed oil with another carrier oil so its distinctive odor does not overwhelm. • If pregnant or breastfeeding, use in moderation after checking for suitability with a physician or midwife.

Shallot

(*Allium ascalonicum*)

MAGICAL FORMS

including the French red shallot (*Allium cepa* var. *aggregatum*) • edible small bulbs from the onion family • the most popular kind in the USA are Jersey shallots, with pale-purple skins with white flesh • red shallots have red skins and purple-tinged flesh • shallots have a taste between onion and garlic • named after the city Ashkelon in Palestine and known historically in ancient Egypt, China, Greece, and Rome • brought to France by the Crusaders • grows worldwide, including Brittany (France), Quebec, Ontario, New Jersey, New Hampshire, and Chile • harvested in the summer • magically use the raw, unskinned bulbs; peeled, raw bulbs; and cooked bulbs

PLANET AND ELEMENT

Mars • Fire

MAGICAL USES

added to slow-cooking dishes to overcome misfortune, self-destructive habits, and phobias, and to avoid repeating mistakes • eaten raw to increase psychic powers and prophetic dreams

HOW TO USE

If you have a small home, hang shallots on a string in your kitchen (those with leaves are especially easy to attach) instead of the larger and more pungent onion. This keeps away all harm, bad luck, illness, and accidents, and preserves a harmonious, welcoming home, whether you live alone or with others. When the shallots start to wither, replace them, but do not use the old ones. • Peel off the golden, red, or brownish-purple skin (you may need several shallots), naming whatever you wish to discard from your life as you peel. Add the peeled shallots to a meal you are cooking, naming each separate clove for what or whom you wish to bring into your life to replace what is being left behind.

CAUTION

Avoid shallots if you have IBS or allergies with symptoms such as asthma, red itchy eyes, or skin rashes.

She-Oak

(*Casuarina* spp.)

MAGICAL FORMS

often called Australian pine, though *Casuarina* is neither a pine nor oak • she-oaks vary in height according to the species of *Casuarina*, from a few feet to more than a hundred feet • *Casuarina* trees have reached Florida and Hawaii and many other frost-free coastal habitats worldwide • flowers and fruit are inedible • *Casuarina glauca* is a prostrate, ground-hugging tree from which the Australian Bush essence is made • endemic in eastern Australia along the coast down to New South Wales, growing in brackish water along banks near estuaries and rivers • magically use any *Casuarina* trees in situ, as bonsai trees, or as flower essence

PLANETS AND ELEMENT

Mercury/Venus • Earth

MAGICAL USES

the trees and the essence remove emotional imbalances in women and overcome fears of infertility that may be blocking natural cycles, especially if conception is slow • for men, to resolve virility issues and soothe relationships with women when there are verbal blockages in expressing love, gentleness, and affection

HOW TO USE

Grow or otherwise obtain a *Casuarina* bonsai (*Casuarina equisetifolia*) in a greenhouse or outside in good weather and then focus on it during meditation, picturing the happy birth of a healthy baby if there are problems conceiving. • Add a drop or two of the essence to a gentle massage oil to ease the body into natural rhythms for healing emotionally related imbalances or for a couple who make love only by ovulation charts.

CAUTION

Do not ingest she-oak remedies; instead, use the essence, which is safe.

Shepherd's Purse

(*Capsella bursa-pastoris*)

MAGICAL FORMS

flowering plant with an erect stem, rosette of basal leaves, four-petaled white flowers, and heart-shaped seed pods that follow the flowers • seed pods look like flat, heart-shaped leather purses • native to Europe and Asia • found through most temperate zones growing profusely in the wild • shepherd's purse accompanied the Pilgrim fathers and other settlers throughout the New World • magically use the aerial parts, seed pods, and shredded leaves, which can be bought online

PLANET AND ELEMENT

Saturn • Earth

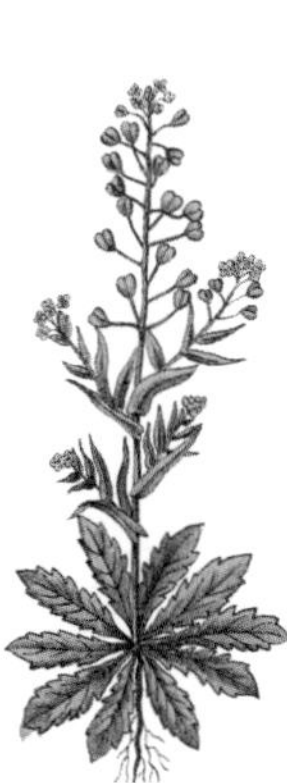

MAGICAL USES

necessary economies, generosity from unexpected sources, mothers or fathers treated badly by their children • use with fragrant herbs or flowers, as some people do not like the scent of shepherd's purse

HOW TO USE

For money and to overcome shopaholic tendencies, burn shepherd's purse with cinnamon, juniper berries, and bay leaves. Carry the cooled ash in a charm bag to ensure money flows in and not out. • Carry an intact, dried seed-pod purse if you are a mother or father who is disrespected by your adult children or ungrateful relatives, especially if you subsidize them. The purse will build up your courage to say no to unreasonable demands. When you feel ready, tip the entire shepherd's purse into the fastest-flowing river you can find or the outgoing tide and speak out to your family members clearly and firmly soon afterward.

CAUTION

Though considered edible and popular in folk medicine, including Chinese medicine, for centuries, use the plant only in moderation. • Before ingesting, check with an expert and be aware that some people are allergic topically. • Do not use if pregnant.

Sicilian Honey Garlic

(*Allium siculum*)

MAGICAL FORMS

so named because of its native origins, the fact that it releases a garlic smell when bruised, and because it has sweet honey nectar for pollinators • clusters of drooping, delicate, bell-like flowers, creamy with stripes of pink and/or green growing on top of a tall, leafless stem with blue-gray, twisted basal leaves • grown as an ornamental as well as for culinary purposes • as a bonus, large, round seed pods, green maturing to brown, stay on the plant into the fall and can be dried for winter decorations • blooms late spring until early summer • native to Turkey, southern France, and Italy, Sicilian honey garlic thrives best in Mediterranean-type climates but can grow in other zones of the USA and in the UK • can be grown potted indoors with care • magically use the whole, growing plant; fresh or dried cut flowers in flower arrangements; and the bulbs for empowering cookery

PLANET AND ELEMENT

Mars • Fire

MAGICAL USES

when grown in the garden or a container, brings protection to the home and premises from accidents, danger, threats, intrusion, and malicious spirits, especially those summoned in a spirit board session or séance • add the fresh or dried cut flowers to a flower arrangement to attract prosperity, health, and above all happiness to the home, neutralizing petty spite and jealousy

HOW TO USE

Make decorations for Thanksgiving and Yule with the dried seed pods by drying the plant with pods attached to attract abundance, named blessings, and fertility in whatever form is needed in the months ahead. • Add the fresh flowers to bouquets for informal marriage ceremonies, woodland weddings, or commitment or renewal-of-vows ceremonies, or if couples are bringing existing children to share in the new relationship, one for each child plus the couple.

CAUTION

Sicilian honey garlic is nontoxic but can be an eye irritant for humans. • It is toxic to dogs and cats in large quantities.

Silk Tassel Bush

(*Garrya elliptica*)

MAGICAL FORMS

rapidly growing bush or small tree with walls of long, silky tassels made of silvery-gray catkins that flower in January and February and remain on the plant into spring after flowering has ceased • the 'James Roof' cultivar has especially long and lasting tassels • long tassels appear only on male plants; the females have shorter catkins but produce purple-brown fruits edible for birds in the summer • dark-green, shiny leaves, grayish silver on the underside, form a backdrop for the tassels • native to Central America and western North America, from southern Oregon to Santa Barbara County in California • grows well in other locations in the USA and in the UK and Europe • the plant can grow up to ten feet tall • magically use the whole, growing plant with catkins; cut flowers in arrangements; and dried catkins

PLANETS AND ELEMENTS

Mercury/Moon • Air/Water

MAGICAL USES

the plant, particularly when containing catkins, flowering or not, acts as protective shield for the home, often grown against a wall • used in wedding bouquets as a token of prosperity and fertility

HOW TO USE

On full moon night, stand in front of a silk tassel bush and turn left and then right, faster and faster until the tassels blur into a silvery screen. Steady yourself and you will receive a message from the Moon Mother and maybe glimpse her face on the silver screen. The next morning, pick a few catkins, dry them, and keep them with tarot cards or other clairvoyant tools for the increase of psychic powers.

CAUTION

Silk tassel bush is nontoxic to humans or pets, but some believe the plant is harmful to horses.

Silver Banksia

(*Banksia marginata*)

MAGICAL FORMS

tree or shrub with yellow, bottlebrush-type flowers that bloom most of the year in subalpine to coastal regions throughout southeastern Australia, with silver underneath the green leaves • grown also in the UK and USA, obtained through specialty exotic flower outlets, flourishing best in a conservatory or a pot • magically use the living tree, dried flowers on stems (available online), and tree essence

PLANETS AND ELEMENTS

Moon/Sun • Water/Fire

MAGICAL USES

for protection of all kinds • to let go of sorrow, anger, grief, fear, destructive habits, or relationships, as well as the tendency to blame others for personal setbacks • for rituals of personal power

HOW TO USE

Carry the bottlebrush-type flower held diagonally upward, shoulder height, as you walk around a room or your whole home, the back of the building to front. First, pass the flower through your own aura space around and above an extended arm's length in the area of your head and shoulders. When you have finished moving the flower in a spiral around the whole house or room, leave it outside the front door. Do the same to cleanse a ritual circle or sacred space of all stagnant or unhelpful energies. • Meditate on the flowering tree or potted plant or a dried flower arrangement, drawing in the yellow light toward your solar plexus, your inner energy center of personal power at the bottom center of your rib cage. Exhale outward all doubts, cravings, and fears until you feel full of golden light and confidence. • Add a few drops of the tree essence to pure water and spray around your workspace before colleagues arrive to remove competitive or confrontational energies.

Silver Bell Tree

(*Halesia diptera*)

MAGICAL FORMS

also called the snowdrop tree • with two-winged fruits, although some species have four-winged fruits • not to be confused with snowbell, which belongs to the styrax family • small tree or shrub native to the southeastern USA; flourishes from Virginia to Florida, west to Illinois, and is cultivated in other locations • clusters of bell-shaped, white flowers followed by distinctive winged fruits and leaves that turn yellow in the fall • cultivated also in Europe and Great Britain • magically use the whole, growing plant; flowers; and fruit

PLANET AND ELEMENT

Moon • Water

MAGICAL USES

mainly used as a source of spiritual joy and release of the inner child • the flowers are said to be the home of the fey and the winged fruit is said to be the way nature spirits travel to their winter homes in the fall

HOW TO USE

Create a nature garden or altar around your silver bell tree and leave offerings of fey crystals to the nature spirits, such as chiastolite, staurolite, lodolite, rutilated quartz, or small fruits. • Meditate on the growing tree for visions of the fey folk, especially around fey activity times such as Walpurgisnacht (April 30), also called Beltane or May Eve, the beginning of the old Celtic summer. • It is also possible to see the fey folk on Midsummer Eve and Halloween after meditating on the growing tree. • It is said that the settlers brought fey folk with them from the Old World and these incomers still jostle for place with the indigenous fey.

CAUTION

Most sources do not mention toxicity for humans, cats, dogs, or horses; however, the Royal Horticultural Society of Great Britain suggests silver bell tree may potentially be harmful. • Due to lack of evidence to the contrary, do not ingest. • Take care with children if you have it in a fairy garden. • Wear gloves if you experience any skin irritation.

Silver Leaf Tree

(*Acer saccharinum*)

MAGICAL FORMS

also called the silver maple or silverleaf maple • the growing leaves have a silvery underside • the sap is refined into maple syrup that tastes like butterscotch • the silver leaf tree is found throughout the northeastern and midwestern USA and in southern Canada, the UK, and parts of Europe • magically use the whole, growing tree; fresh leaves; and syrup

PLANETS AND ELEMENT

Moon/Venus • Water

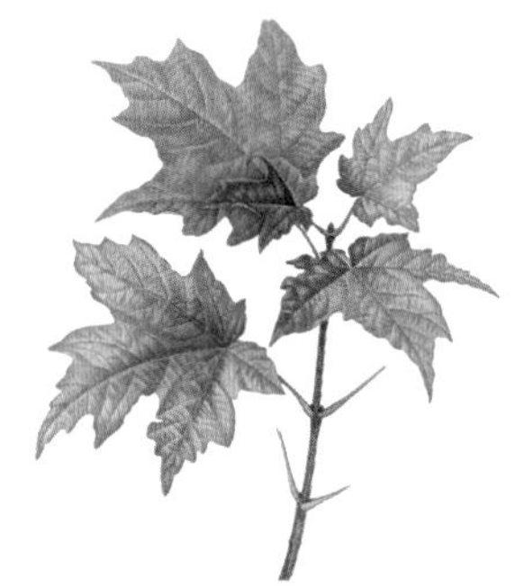

MAGICAL USES

reduces air pollution • fresh leaves are used magically in ritual and divination • use in moon magick, working with the three main phases of the moon and in maiden, mother, and crone ceremonies

HOW TO USE

Meditate directly beneath this tree, reaching your arms up to fill your aura with silver on a full moon. It is especially lucky if you can see the moon through the branches. Afterward, ask the Moon Mother for what or whom you most need and bury three small pieces of silver beneath the tree. • Sit under a silver maple and ask a question, listening to the rustle of the silver-tinged leaves to give your answer, through awakening your psychic, clairaudient, or hearing ability. Afterward, focus on one area of leaves, looking directly upward where you can see nothing but silver. Close your eyes, open them, blink, and allow your clairvoyant senses to create an image in the leaves or your mind to further explain what you heard.

CAUTION

Leaves and twigs that have fallen off the tree and decayed or dried become toxic if ingested by pets or livestock. • Do not work with the tree if you have a pollen allergy to any species of maple tree, sycamores, chestnuts, or lychees. • Silver leaf tree can occasionally cause skin irritation.

Silver Mound

(*Artemisia schmidtiana*)

MAGICAL FORMS

also called angel's hair • named after Artemis, the ancient Greek moon and huntress goddess, as are all the Artemisia plants • a cultivar of Artemisia, of which there are two hundred kinds, including wormwood, sagebrush, and mugwort • native to Japan and growing in temperate regions of the USA and Europe • forms a soft, silky, feather-like cushioned mound or dome, about a foot tall, with glistening, white, silver-green foliage, and finely divided individual leaves that give the plant a starry appearance • magically use the whole, growing plant in situ (in the garden or outdoor containers); the cut foliage as part of dried or fresh flower arrangements; and the leaves shredded and mixed with the dried, yellow, often disregarded summer flowers

PLANETS AND ELEMENTS

Venus/Moon • Earth/Water

MAGICAL USES

a plant for the sixteenth (wax) wedding anniversary • a gift for keen gardeners or as part of a bouquet of creamy or silver flowers • as the plant, used for meditation to connect with angels, especially moon angels, and on starry nights with other dimensions, particularly if you are a Star Soul • the cut dried leaves, plus dried yellow flowers (optional) can be made into a money-bringing sachet, even more powerful combined with 'Ever Goldy', a cultivar with golden leaves

HOW TO USE

Carry out full moon rituals close to growing silver mound or by circling around a container of the plant in moonlight. • Bury silver-colored coins (the color and metal of the moon) in the dirt of the plant as an offering. For each offering, ask Mother Moon for what you most desire by the next full moon. • Light twin beeswax candles and scatter the shredded leaves in circles around the lit candles to call romance or strengthen existing love, asking that the love known or unknown will be lasting.

CAUTION

Silver mound is toxic to people and pets if consumed.

Skullcap

(*Scutellaria* spp.)

MAGICAL FORMS

genus of plants commonly known as skullcap, including *Scutellaria lateriflora*, American skullcap • a native North American herb adopted by the early colonists who called it Quaker bonnets • the name *skullcap* refers to the military helmets worn in medieval times because the flowers have distinctive upper and lower lips that resemble miniature medieval helmets • this recognizes skullcap as an herb of honor • magically use dried and fresh aerial parts • often used powdered in magick

PLANET AND ELEMENT

Mercury • Air

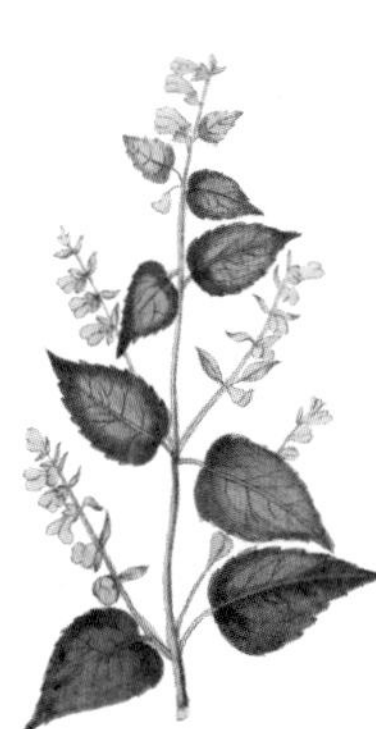

MAGICAL USES

fidelity • prosperity • restores balance after psychic or psychological attacks • acts as a shield against further threats • increases the power of other herbs, crystals, and spells in ritual for women's mysteries, especially connected with the menstrual cycle

HOW TO USE

The blue, pink, or purple flowers are exchanged in handfasting rituals or commitment ceremonies. • Skullcap is often called the workaholic herb because it is burned in incense to encourage meditation and states of mindfulness. • Sprinkle the powdered herb in a circle around a partner's shoes to keep them faithful when traveling away from home. Sweep up the herb circle and set it free outdoors to blow away desire while your partner is absent. Alternatively, add just a pinch to each shoe.

CAUTION

Though used medicinally in the Western world and still part of traditional Chinese and Ayurvedic medicine, Chinese skullcap can cause a drop in blood sugar so should be taken with care. • Any skullcap should not be ingested or inhaled during pregnancy, if attempting to become pregnant, or while breastfeeding.

Snapdragon

(*Antirrhinum majus*)

MAGICAL FORMS

flowering plant • reputed to have been planted on the graves of dragon slayers • magically use the cut or whole, growing plant; flowers; and seeds

PLANET AND ELEMENT

Mars • Fire

MAGICAL USES

use for overcoming intimidation • returns hostile energies to sender • reduces anger, especially directed inward toward the self • used in dragon rituals, especially concerning the acquisition of wealth and working with elemental spirits in magick

HOW TO USE

Wearing or carrying the flowers in a sachet gives the ability to know if people are speaking the truth, while seeds threaded on a necklace keep enchantment away. • For formal rituals to remove a hex or curse, set snapdragons in a vase in the center of an altar with pure-white candles and a white cloth and a mirror facing outward to reflect back all harm. • Keep snapdragons on a table reflected in a mirror that faces the front door to send back out any malevolence or negativity that enters. • This also helps at the end of the day if family returns home stressed. • Burn the flowers in an incense mix in the room where you will be reading tarot cards or performing other forms of divination to open the psychic channels. • Keep a sachet of snapdragon with you if you are cursed or feel malice toward you. As the person who is directing ill will at you walks away, scatter the snapdragon on the ground where they were standing.

CAUTION

Snapdragon is not for internal use. • Do not use black snapdragon (*Digitalis obscura*), as this is very toxic.

Snowdrop

(*Galanthus nivalis*)

MAGICAL FORMS

the wild or cultivated variety is known as *Galanthus elwesii*, the giant or greater snowdrop • related to amaryllis and daffodils, the common variety is a tiny plant with one small, bell-like, white flower on a leafless stalk that opens into six petals, three outer and three inner • native to southwestern Asia and eastern Europe and naturalized in the UK and eastern North America • among the first flowers to bloom in spring, snowdrops are also called the Bells of Candlemas or the fair maids of February • the flower of the pagan Imbolc or Christian Candlemas festival • though the snowdrop was not recorded in the UK until the eighteenth century, it has become grafted onto the Candlemas or pagan festival • magically use the whole, growing flower and fresh and dried closed and open petals

PLANETS AND ELEMENT

Moon/Venus • Water

MAGICAL USES

new beginnings, especially in relationships • in meditation or as a dried flower charm from ancient Greek times, clears the mind of troublesome thoughts, manipulation, and power games • also use to overcome fears of spirit possession • gifted with other early flowers for sympathy after any loss or bereavement and to offer hope for the future • it is said as Eve wept after being banished from the Garden of Eden, an angel transformed the snow into snowdrops

HOW TO USE

Bring the first snowdrops into the home—the old superstition that it was unlucky to bring snowdrops into the house has long been abandoned. • Light a circle of white candles around the vase of snowdrops on February 1 and 2, or as soon as the first snowdrops appear, asking for the blessings of new beginnings in the ways most needed for yourself, loved ones, the community, and globally. Leave the candles to burn through, with the flowers in position until they fade.

CAUTION

Snowdrop is toxic to pets and to humans if ingested in large quantities. • It can cause skin irritation.

Snowdrop, Three Ships

(*Galanthus plicatus* 'Three Ships')

MAGICAL FORMS

a variety of Christmas or pleated snowdrop • originated in eastern Europe, seen growing in the fields in the aftermath of the Crimean War • first discovered in the UK in 1984 growing under a cork oak tree in Suffolk in the east of England • noted for their unusually early flowering, typically by Christmas day instead of the usual February blooming of the other snowdrop, *Galanthus nivalis* • the name reflects the old carol from the seventeenth century, "I Saw Three Ships" • a clump-forming, bulbous plant with white, rounded, pleated flowers and a honey fragrance • can be cultivated in North American gardens in cooler regions • some snowdrops bloom as early as Veterans Day in the USA on November 11 as a sign of peace • magically work with the growing Christmas snowdrop in the garden or in pots, and the cut flowers, though they will not last long unless dried

PLANET AND ELEMENT

Venus • Earth

MAGICAL USES

the Three Ships snowdrop blooms close to the midwinter solstice as well as Christmas, so is the herald of lighter days slowly returning and therefore has become a symbol of hope, survival through hard times, reconciliation for all estranged, and light in emotional darkness

HOW TO USE

Walk among the Christmas snowdrops or use your potted plants if in bloom and ask for the new beginnings you need in your life, burying two or three snow or milky quartz crystals, white howlite, or snowflake obsidian beneath their roots as an offering to the approaching new year, one for each new beginning you seek. You can do this on New Year's Day morning if they are blooming. • Dry or press the flowers and carry them in a charm bag until you see the first snowdrops of spring to keep faith with your springtime plans.

CAUTION

Three Ships snowdrop is harmful if eaten. • Wear gloves when handling it. • Take care around children and pets.

Soapberry

(*Shepherdia canadensis*)

MAGICAL FORMS

also called buffaloberry • not to be confused with the soapberry tree (*Sapindus* species) • a hardy adaptable plant or shrub found in North America, from Newfoundland to Alaska, south to British Columbia, New York, and New Mexico, and in the UK and parts of Europe • grows to eight feet • blooms yellow from late- to mid-spring • produces bright-red, fleshy berries • magically work with the tree in situ, berries, and flower essence

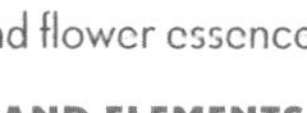

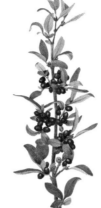

PLANETS AND ELEMENTS

Venus/Mercury • Water/Air

MAGICAL USES

to banish fear of using your own power • for avoiding using power inappropriately or inconsistently • releases fears of the untamed forces of nature and encourages spontaneous expression and actions

HOW TO USE

Mix the berries (not too many) with an equal amount of water and whip the mix until you have a soapy foam, hence its name. Rub a little foam on your hands and wash away the soap foam under a warm running tap, naming what you wish to cleanse from your life, particularly suppressed negative feelings, until all have gone. • Use the essence for at least a week before going on a wilderness trek or work team-bonding survival exercise if you prefer city life or if you find it hard to be spontaneous and ignore consequences of a desired but risky action. Sip the essence throughout the experience to feel the power of nature and your own wild self surging through you if you are naturally overcautious.

CAUTION

The fruit is bitter and contains toxins that are broken down by the body, especially in cooking, but should only be consumed cooked in moderation with sweeteners. • Avoid the berries if you are pregnant or suffering from chronic conditions.

Solomon's Seal

(*Polygonatum biflorum*) or (*Polygonatum odoratum*)

MAGICAL FORMS

also called King Solomon's Seal • native to North America • associated with King Solomon, a powerful magician, who, it is said, possessed a ring that enabled him to summon and control every spirit in the cosmos • Solomon's Seal was so named by ritual magicians because when the plant dies in the fall and the stalk falls from the root, the remaining scar is shaped like a Star of David, also known as the Seal of Solomon • in addition, it was known as a plant that enhanced magical powers • magically use the whole, growing plant and roots

PLANET AND ELEMENTS

Saturn • Earth/Water

MAGICAL USES

protection • exorcism • banishes all negativity and hostility • guards the home • use as sacred offerings • for wisdom • leadership • success • power • authority • making the right difficult decisions and embracing necessary change • use the wise plant at the fall equinox to accept what did not work

HOW TO USE

Burn an incense made of the powdered roots to drive away malicious spirits. • Among Native North American people such as the Cherokee, the smoke cleansed their dwellings. • Solomon's Seal attracts powerful but benign elementals to aid spells, especially to break bad habits and influences and to ritually exorcise evil. • The smoke or a root infusion consecrates the athame (ritual knife). • Hang a fifth of a root high in a brown bag in each of the four corners of the home to act as a guardian. Dry and powder the final fifth of the root, then scatter it to the four winds to ask for the help and support you need to minimize unwelcome change and call new opportunities.

CAUTION

All parts of the adult plant except for the roots are usually regarded as toxic, especially the berries. • Avoid Solomon's Seal if you have low blood sugar or diabetes and while pregnant.

Sorrel

(*Rumex* spp.)

MAGICAL FORMS

herbaceous plant • you can use any kind of sorrel, as the properties are very similar, but wood sorrel (*Oxalis acetosella*) is the most commonly noted in occult books • good in a wildlife rather than formal garden, as it can spread • magically use the whole, growing plant; flowers; and dried and fresh leaves

PLANET AND ELEMENT

Venus • Water

MAGICAL USES

heals sorrow and heartbreak • for gentleness and kindness • affection • rebuilding after loss • regeneration

HOW TO USE

Sorrel is also sometimes called fairy bells and so brings good fortune if planted in the garden, where it is said to give sight of nature essences. • It is believed to assist the sick to regenerate their self-healing powers if placed in their bedroom. • Stuff the dried leaves and flowers in poppets to absorb negativity when hidden as a household guardian near an entrance. Replace when the tangy, sharp fragrance fades, throwing the herbs into running water. • Because of its strong earth energies, sorrel is often used in Mother Earth rituals for healing despoiled places and the planet.

CAUTION

Though sorrel has been used in cooking and medicine by some practitioners for centuries, it is considered toxic if consumed in large quantities. • Avoid all sorrel if pregnant or suffering from gout or kidney stones and be extra careful around pets, particularly cats, if growing it.

Sourwood Tree

(*Oxydendrum arboreum*)

MAGICAL FORMS

ornamental tree often growing in the shade of other trees, with flowers that resemble lily of the valley, but are not poisonous • bright-red leaves in the fall • famed for its honey • native to the Appalachian Mountains, growing on the eastern seaboard of North America and as far south as Louisiana • does not grow wild outside North America, but can be cultivated in sheltered places in Europe, especially France, as well as the UK • initially best in a pot if not in the USA • state emblem of Tennessee • magically use the leaves as healing tea to encourage kindness in others; living tree, especially when flowering or in the fall; and fresh and dried flowers and bark

PLANET AND ELEMENT

Moon • Water

MAGICAL USES

use the honey and flowers ritually for sweetening bad-tempered people and for overcoming discouragement • for rites of passage, especially into the wisewoman phase, to embrace wisdom and not mourn the loss of youth

HOW TO USE

Sourwood tree is said to be the honey of angels; eat the honey before meditation to make connection with your guardian angels and receive messages. • Stand beneath the tree during fall in the wind and catch the leaves until your hands are full (or pick from the ground). Take the leaves to an open place and release them with wishes for the months ahead for health, prosperity, and abundance. • Set the fresh flowers on your altar until they fade, casting them into running water to let go of regrets.

CAUTION

Consult your doctor before ingesting any part of the tree if pregnant.

Soybean

(*Glycine max*)

MAGICAL FORMS

see also edamame (p. 167) and beansprouts (p. 57) • an erect, branching legume often more than six and a half feet tall • produces edible beans within pods, in yellow, green, black, bicolored, or, if commercially cultivated, mainly brown or tan • one of the cheapest, most readily available, and healthiest sources of protein, with no starch • sacred to ancient Chinese and Japanese agricultural deities, the Chinese emperor Yan declared it one of the five sacred plants in 2583 BCE • first cultivated in China seven thousand years ago • introduced into the USA in 1804 and now popular worldwide • magically use the raw or cooked beans

PLANETS AND ELEMENTS

Sun/Venus/Moon • Fire/Earth/Water

MAGICAL USES

magical cookery • add soy sauce (fermented beans in salt water) to dark-green foodstuffs to protect your finances, or add to tomatoes for kick-starting, improving, or maintaining a good love life

HOW TO USE

Eat a soy or tofu meal on full moon night to heighten your psychic awareness. Then scatter raw beans along a path facing the moon or toward a pathway of light on the sea to feel your ancestors walking beside you. If you need answers, count each bean as you drop it for yes/no/act/wait/speak/be silent/go/stay questions. When you have your answer, you may hear and see images in your mind from a beloved ancestor, explaining and expanding the answer, and may feel their reassuring touch.

Spearmint

(*Mentha spicata*)

MAGICAL FORMS

sweeter and less strong than peppermint and a different plant from peppermint with much less menthol, elongated leaves like spears, and, like peppermint, purple-pink flowers • magically use the herb, leaves, and growing, fresh, and dried flowers

PLANET AND ELEMENT

Venus • Water

MAGICAL USES

attracts money • healing • for a happy home • much gentler than peppermint in reconciling rather than escalating conflict • protection and peaceful sleep • for abundance entering and remaining within the home • concentration and memorizing new information, especially if nervous • magical cookery

HOW TO USE

Use in or as part of a sleep pillow to protect against nightmares and paranormal attacks through the night. • Roll a beeswax candle in dried spearmint until some sticks; name what it is you need as accurately as possible (including time frame), then light the candle. • Plant outside the home and keep in pots in the kitchen to encourage savings. • Use in a floor wash after a family quarrel or misfortune to bring reconciliation. • Chew as empowered gum and give to teens to deflect bullies rather than provoking confrontation.

CAUTION

Avoid taking mint internally if using immunosuppressant medicines or medication for high blood pressure, or if treating heart problems.

Spelt

(*Triticum spelta*)

MAGICAL FORMS

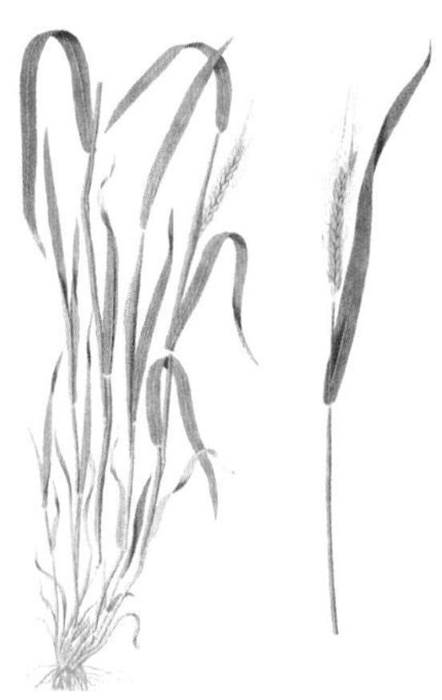

an ancient whole grain related to wheat, barley, and rye that has been cultivated as a food staple from Neolithic times to the Middle Ages in Europe, still popular in Spain and Central Europe and increasingly elsewhere as a health and organic food • introduced into the USA in 1890, primarily cultivated in Ohio, and regaining its place in the UK • may have been a natural hybrid form of wheat and goat grass • magically use the grain on its stem, ground spelt as flour, and in magical cookery

PLANET AND ELEMENT

Saturn • Earth

MAGICAL USES

in flour, as a rice substitute, as whole wheat bread, or as fermented sourdough bread, add to meals for wise budgeting and to slow the outflow of money • shaped as pasta for a stable, uneventful period after chaos or unwilling change • in a vase arrangement with other grains placed on steps to welcome health and security of property and assets into the home or business

HOW TO USE

To encourage economy and savings if money seems to flow out too fast, add nine gold-colored coins to a small bowl of spelt flour so they are buried. Leave them for a week and then shake off all the spelt and wash and dry the coins. Make these the start of a savings plan or keep in a yellow pouch not to be spent. • If a sudden economic crisis looms, make spelt bread and share it to encourage the return of the flow of abundance.

Spikenard

(*Nardostachys jatamansi*)

MAGICAL FORMS

also includes ploughman's spikenard (*Inula conya*) • American spikenard (*Aralia racemosa*), mainly in northeastern USA and eastern Canada • Californian spikenard (*Aralia californica*) • Japanese spikenard (*Aralia cordata*) • a flowering plant from the honeysuckle family • used to create a ceremonial perfume • magically use the perfume, especially in formal rituals as from biblical times (mentioned as a precious fragrance in the Song of Solomon and the Gospel of Mark); in incense; as essential oil; and, more informally, as the shredded leaves and plant

PLANET AND ELEMENT

Mars • Fire

MAGICAL USES

roots of ploughman's spikenard (which is native to Europe, Caucasia, Iran, and Algeria) were hung in ploughmen's and other agricultural workers' huts to sweeten the air and deter fleas • use any spikenard for good luck and protection against contagious diseases and noxious human influences • for fidelity • spiritual enlightenment • called the herb of the student for conventional and spiritual study

HOW TO USE

For love, mix with sweet woodruff (Master of the Woods) and scatter subtly as a finely ground wish powder (made by adding arrowroot or cornstarch) on a path where you know your prospective lover will pass. • Anoint an unlit white candle with the essential oil, diluted in pure olive oil, before meditation, divination, or mediumship. • Place a drop on your Third Eye or brow energy center to open your clairvoyant powers to see other dimensions, as well as the future, and to receive messages from guides and beloved ancestors through allowing your hand to write automatically in green pen on white paper.

CAUTION

Dilute the oil before applying to skin; do not ingest the oil.

Spilanthes

(*Spilanthes oleracea*)

MAGICAL FORMS

also known as *Spilanthes acmella* • a bushy herb with dark, bronze leaves, petalless pompom flowers blooming from midsummer to early fall • usually yellowy gold with red centers resembling an eyeball, "eyeball plant" being one of its names • also called the toothache plant because when the flower is chewed, it dulls tooth pain and relieves infection • native to the Americas, originally Brazil, grows in Florida and sunny, warm spots in less tropical environments, and also in containers • magically use the growing or picked fresh flowers, dried flowerheads, and chopped leaves (available online or in health stores)

PLANETS AND ELEMENTS

Mars/Moon • Fire/Water

MAGICAL USES

the resemblance of the flower to the eyeball stimulates clairvoyant sight • the flowerheads dried in amulet bags give vision into others' motives • the growing plant, especially in flower or, though not fragrant, the crushed leaves or flowerheads added to potpourri in the center of the home, protects against burglars, unwelcome visitors, and intrusive neighbors

HOW TO USE

Because it is recognized as a physical aphrodisiac, make tea from the fresh or dried flowers, adding honey, to share before lovemaking. • Garnish a love meal with the flowers that cause a frisson when chewed to persuade a reticent lover to speak romantic words. • When an intimidating, overbearing person is coming to your home or business, scatter the chopped leaves across the doorway and sweep outward to create a barrier of protection around you. If you suspect the person is untrustworthy, hide eye flowers around the premises to alert you to double-dealing.

CAUTION

Avoid spilanthes if you have an autoimmune problem or are allergic to daisies, and do not use for prolonged periods. • Consult a doctor before using if you are pregnant or breastfeeding.

Spinach

(*Spinacia oleracea*)

MAGICAL FORMS

Leafy, dark-green plant cultivated as a vegetable • originally from west and central Asia but extensively produced and eaten in northern Europe and the USA and where there is cool weather • a fast-growing plant that transitions from seed to maturity in six weeks • will regrow after harvesting if inner young leaves are left alone • six to twelve inches tall and wide • eaten raw and cooked • will grow in containers • magically use the plant in situ and the harvested vegetable, raw or cooked

PLANETS AND ELEMENTS

Jupiter/Moon • Air/Water

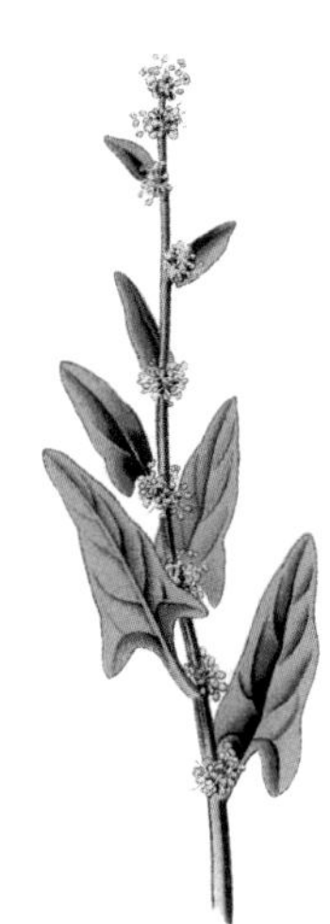

MAGICAL USES

for stamina and perseverance to push through unwelcome but necessary situations • for the swift and satisfactory resolution of challenges and opportunities • considered lucky if grown in gardens or containers

HOW TO USE

Eat empowered spinach on the full moon for improvements in finances by the following full moon. • It is essential with spinach magick that practical action is taken immediately after a spell or empowerment. • Color pasta and bread with spinach juice when there is a lack of enthusiasm or people are stuck in their ways. • Empower small magical tools, special crystals, oils, and sealed sachets of herbs in a bundle of tied spinach leaves on the crescent moon to increase their power. • Generally, spinach magick involves eating the spinach to absorb its energizing powers rather than ritually.

CAUTION

If eaten in excess, spinach can lead to kidney stones from iron and fiber overload. • Care should be taken if using blood thinners because of spinach's high vitamin K content.

Spirulina

(Arthrospira platensis)

MAGICAL FORMS

blue-green algae that grows in fresh and salt water • traditionally used by the Aztecs in Mexico and Indigenous people of Lake Chad in Africa • cultivated in the USA, Malaysia, India, and China • NASA discovered spirulina could be cultivated for astronauts in space as a super nutrient • the blue-green powder is pure algae strained, washed, and dried, without any additions or anything taken out • magically work with the organic powder, which lasts up to two to three years if unopened, and three months once unsealed • alternatively, obtain live culture from a recognized spirulina grower and cultivate your own, which can be consumed magically, raw or cooked

PLANET AND ELEMENT

Moon • Water

MAGICAL USES

absorb health, energy, and good fortune, or whatever is most needed when luck has been bad or there has been lingering illness or sorrow, by empowering spirulina powder as you add and mix it in water, food, or smoothies, and drink or eat it

HOW TO USE

Spirulina powder is a useful magical ingredient for purification work and for calling health and healing on an astral or spiritual level for those who do not wish to physically ingest the algae powder. • For purification rituals, add a small amount of the powder to water, well stirred by all present and accompanied by blessings, then sprinkle to create a protected ritual circle area (outdoors or not on carpets or near furnishings). • The powder (not the live culture, which could interfere with ecosystems) or mixed-in water can be cast on the outgoing tide or fast-flowing river as offerings to take away what is causing harm or self-destructive habits.

CAUTION

Occasionally ingesting spirulina can cause allergic reactions, so take cautiously. • Avoid while pregnant or breastfeeding, or for children, until more verifiable research has been carried out.

Spruce Tree

(*Picea* spp.)

MAGICAL FORMS

coniferous trees, all of which are evergreen • the tallest spruce (*Picea sitchensis*) grows along the Pacific coast from Alaska to North California, and in the UK and Europe • Colorado blue spruce (*Picea pungens*) is found in the western USA, its waxy coating on needles creating blue-gray foliage, and sometimes bright-blue needles • Norway spruce (*Picea abes*), which can live for a thousand years, is widespread in the UK and Scandinavia and native to mountain areas in Europe • magically use the bark, as well as the growing tree and branches, most with the needlelike leaves and cones still attached

PLANET AND ELEMENT

Saturn • Earth

MAGICAL USES

the Norway spruce became popular in the UK when Prince Albert, Queen Victoria's husband, decorated it for Christmas in the German fashion with candles, candies, and ribbons • at any time of the year a spruce tree outdoors decorated with solar lights, or indoor with battery lights on a green branch, is a reminder that emotional light, both psychic and psychological, will return and better times will come • in parts of Germany on New Year's Eve, fresh spruce branches were cut and nailed to the door to symbolize the renewal of life, brought by the New Year

HOW TO USE

According to Hopi wisdom, a medicine man, Salavi, transformed himself into a spruce tree so that he might continue to serve and guard over his people beyond his lifetime. • On the other side of the world as the mother tree, associated with Druantia, the Gallic fir or spruce Mother Goddess, Mother Spruce sheltered wildlife and her new-growing saplings. Sick children were set beneath the tree to be relieved of their illness as the Mother tree absorbed and transformed it. • Spruce wood will, over the years, build up its power, even after it has physically crumbled.

CAUTION

As a precaution, avoid ingesting during pregnancy.

Spruce Tree, Black

(*Picea mariana*)

MAGICAL FORMS

hardy, native from Pennsylvania, north to Newfoundland, and across Canada to Alaska • narrow and conical, sweeping to the ground • grows also in northern parts of the UK and northern Europe • magically use the growing tree, also found as a bonsai; the cones; and the oil, which is extracted from the dark green needles

PLANET AND ELEMENT

Jupiter • Air

MAGICAL USES

bringing balance to everyday life • beginning the day, focused and calm • maintaining balance during the day, ending it quietly • transforms negativity to positive thoughts • fertility

HOW TO USE

Sit close to the tree at dawn and sunset, looking upward and traveling astrally to the stars and what were believed in some northern cultures to be the light and fire of the ancestors. • Burn or diffuse the oil on cold, gloomy days and evenings to be filled with the vibrant life force of the forest, even in a city. • Keep a dish of cones in the center of the home, and every morning hold the dish, making a wish or expressing a need or blessing for the day ahead. Carry a cone with you, chosen with closed eyes, as a reminder, and then hold the dish again, adding back your day cone after the working day has ended to bring resolution. • For fertility and conception, on full moon night, choose another seemingly random cone from your dish. Insert a long ornamental pin to represent conception into the cone. Set them, joined, on the bedroom window ledge in the moonlight. The next morning, keep the cone with the pin inserted safely wrapped in silk in a drawer until the next full moon. Repeat if necessary with the same cone and pin as anxiety can block conception until you relax into the monthly cycle.

CAUTION

While regarded as nontoxic, consult your physician or midwife before using black spruce in later pregnancy and while breastfeeding and if you have a chronic medical condition.

Spruce Tree, Siberian/ Serbian

(*Picea obovate*) and (*Picea omorika*)

MAGICAL FORMS

Siberian spruce (*Picea obovata*), a subarctic, pyramid-shaped, coniferous tree native to Siberia, grows from northern Scandinavia and Russia to East Asia • grown as an ornamental, reaching the UK in 1908 • found in snow forests in the USA and in inland Canada • can be cultivated in cooler regions in the USA, especially in gardens in its dwarf variety, and is found in arboretums • the Serbian spruce (*Picea omorika*) is a slender, spire-like tree native to southwest Serbia and Bosnia but is endangered there • it is theorized that the Serbian spruce may have reached the USA via the Bering land bridge millions of years ago • cultivated, though not extensively, in the USA, where there are cool summers • magically use the trees in situ, the cones of either, and flower essences made from *Picea omorika*

PLANET AND ELEMENT

Jupiter • Air

MAGICAL USES

for strengthening yang energies if they are low, sit close to or against the trunk of either tree • replaces lack of assertiveness with developing a proactive approach to people and life

HOW TO USE

Add the needles of either tree or the fallen, crumbled bark to incense mixes for raising psychic energies. • Sitting with the trees in situ, or taking the essence before meditation, can connect you with fiercer forest spirits for seeking courage in difficult situations. • Sip the essence in water daily to build up your proactive energies to express yourself calmly and with authority if you feel intimidated at work or by family members who override your opinions and wishes. • Also use to raise your profile if you are unofficially restricted by ageism, sexism, or your ethnic background.

CAUTION

Since modern research does not yet confirm safety, avoid ingesting during pregnancy, while breastfeeding, and if taking regular medication. • If in doubt, check with an expert, as some people are allergic to the needles when ingested.

Spruce Tree, Sitka

(*Picea sitchensis*)

MAGICAL FORMS

largest and tallest of the American spruces • a narrow, conical, coniferous tree (see "Spruce Tree," p. 423) • grown extensively in temperate regions across northwestern American forests and the northern hemisphere, including Europe • can reach 165 feet • magically work with the whole, growing tree; needles; and flower essence

PLANETS AND ELEMENTS

Jupiter/Mars • Air/Fire

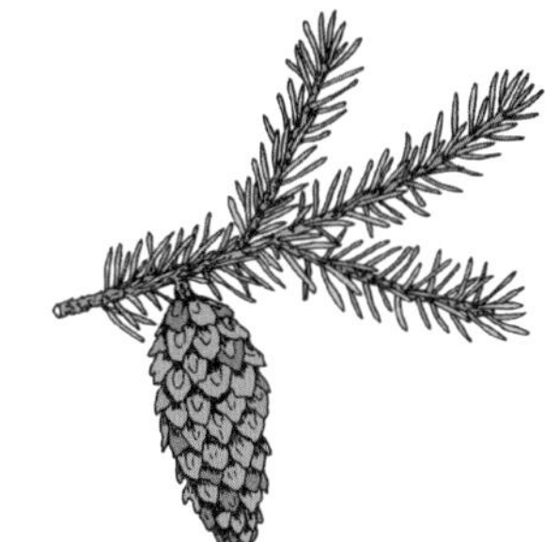

MAGICAL USES

strengthens and balances the animus in anyone where there is reluctance or fear of expressing personal power, needs, and opinions

HOW TO USE

Create a protective dark glass jar for the home by mixing salt with the needles (pack layers of salt alternating with needles, optionally adding a drop or two of the essence. Seal the jar, shake it nine times, and thereafter nine times weekly on Thursday, the day of Jupiter, for increased authority, or Tuesday, the day of Mars, for extra power. Keep the jar on a high shelf or out-facing window ledge for a year and a day and then replace. • Use the plant to make a small smudge or smoke stick. Smudge yourself, wafting the smoke with a feather or fan to fill yourself with confidence when you need to take center stage in any venture or speak out for a principle. • Since guitars and pianos are crafted from Sitka spruce wood, a small piece of the bark of the tree is sometimes carried in a yellow bag to auditions, competitions, and performances by musicians, composers, and singers.

CAUTION

As a precaution, avoid the smoke from smudging, and do not ingest any part of the tree if you are pregnant.

Squash Blossom

flower of (*Cucurbita pepo*)

MAGICAL FORMS

edible flower of the zucchini, pumpkin, and winter and summer squashes of all kinds • blossoms male and female on the same plant (when picked they will last two to three days in the refrigerator) • squash blossom imagery dates back to cave art and the plant, actually a fruit, has traditionally been eaten or made into bread for centuries by the Indigenous people of southeastern America • magically use the fresh cut blossom and flower essence

PLANET AND ELEMENT

Moon • Water

MAGICAL USES

squash blossom necklaces containing silver, turquoise, and wooden beads called "the beads that spread out" because they are shaped to resemble squash blossoms were first created in the late 1870s or early 1880s by the Navajo • by the early 1900s, the Zuni, Hopi, and Pueblo people were also crafting the necklaces, recalling the importance of squash as a means of sustenance • the ultimate flower for magical cookery and as a decoration on food for abundance and to increase intuitive awareness • use the male and female blossoms for sex magick and commitment rituals (female squash blossoms have a stigma-like star or pincushion inside like a small embryonic fruit; the male ones have long, thin stems and a stamen, coated with pollen)

HOW TO USE

The squash blossom necklace features a single turquoise nugget suspended from the bottom, called the *Naja*, which represents an unborn child in the womb. • Encircle a male and female squash blossom tied together within a squash blossom necklace on full moon night to conceive a child. • Spray squash blossom flower essence in water around your aura energy field before going out socially or to work if you are worried about your body image or feel stuck in the same routine. • At Halloween or Samhain, carve a squash instead of a pumpkin, so that there will be sufficient resources in the winter ahead and to protect against the restless spirits who roam that night and the two days after (the Days of the Dead).

Squash, Winter

(*Cucurbita moschata*)

MAGICAL FORMS

flowering plants, indigenous to the New World pre-settlers, winter squash has been grown for five thousand years • marrows and pumpkins share a common botanical heritage belonging to the *Cucurbita* family • each kind of squash, however, has its own unique qualities, defined partly according to whether it is a winter or summer squash • winter squashes grow on vines and include acorn, delicata, Hubbard, and buttercup squashes • though harvested in early to late winter, winter squashes have a much longer postharvesting life than summer squashes, have a far harder skin for storing through the long winter months, and grow on vines rather than bushes like summer squash • see marrow (p. 284) for an example of summer squashes; also see squash blossoms (p. 426) • magically use the whole, raw winter squash and the cooked squash once the rind is cut away

PLANETS AND ELEMENTS

Moon/Venus • Water/Earth

MAGICAL USES

use winter squashes, with their tough rinds and long-lasting qualities, for longer-term magical ventures • the hard rind of the winter squash offers protection against restless spirits and hyperactive people who stir up chaos • for the acquisition of solid resources rather than immense wealth

HOW TO USE

Set a winter squash on your harvest equinox altar as the central focus to represent the slow growth of what has been worked toward in the earlier months, especially if slow to materialize. Preserve it until Thanksgiving or Yule to give thanks for what has been achieved. • Alternatively, at Halloween, remove and shred the rind of a winter squash, mixing it with money herbs such as dried basil, parsley, patchouli, and rosemary, and ancestral herbs like sage and thyme, then burn the mix on the Samhain fires to honor the ancestors and ask that they will ensure sufficient resources through the winter. Eat your winter squash as part of the feast.

CAUTION

Avoid eating butternut squash if on beta blockers.

St. John's Wort

(*Hypericum perforatum*)

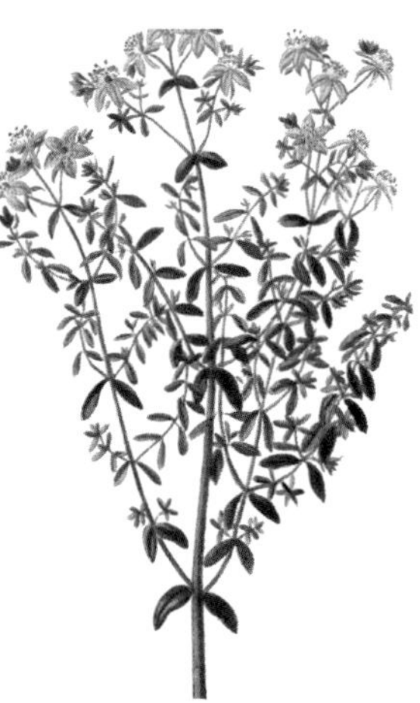

MAGICAL FORMS

flowering plant • magically use the whole plant and all the parts aboveground, especially the fresh and dried tops and flowers

PLANET AND ELEMENT

Sun • Fire

MAGICAL USES

used mainly for courage • invincibility • power • prosperity • authority • one of the four protective herbs, the others being clover or trefoil, vervain, and dill

HOW TO USE

St. John's wort is the ultimate druidic herb of the summer solstice, and so merits a place in a sun garden. • St. John's wort did not acquire its present name until Christian times, when its magic was transferred to Midsummer Day, the feast of St. John on June 24. • Ironically, though it should not be taken internally if trying to get pregnant, the plant has been used by women for centuries as a charm in fertility rituals when picked at midnight on Midsummer. • Keep the flowers and leaves in a sealed jar near a window to banish malevolence, earthly and otherwise, from the home, having passed the jar through a sun incense such as frankincense (keep the jar where children and pets cannot touch or ingest the contents).

CAUTION

Since the berries and flowers are toxic, grow out of the reach of small children and pets and do not ingest the raw plant. • Do not use in pregnancy, while breastfeeding, or when taking antidepressants or medication for a chronic condition.

Star Anise

(Illicium verum)

MAGICAL FORMS
an ancient herb and spice regarded as magical and sacred, especially in the star pod form • though naturally a large tree, star anise can be grown in pots and containers or cut back regularly as a hedging plant in a moderate-size garden • magically use the whole, growing plant; star-shaped seed pods, from the fruit of the tree before it ripens; and egg-shaped seeds within the pods that are dried in the sun and have turned brown

PLANET AND ELEMENT
Jupiter • Air

MAGICAL USES
a luck bringer • increases psychic awareness, especially telepathic abilities • enables truth to be discovered • empowers altar and formal ritual work (place a star pod in the corners of the altar to attract higher spirits) • star magick • magical cookery, especially using enchanted, powdered, licorice-flavored seeds

HOW TO USE
Burn seeds in an incense mix to increase clairvoyance before divination or inhale the fragrance for visions. • Keep a seed in every corner of each room or your workspace for good fortune and protection from all malice. • Star anise is associated with wishes on the crescent moon; when the full moon enters your zodiac sign each month, cast the seeds into flowing waters or from a high place as you make your wish. • Thread the seeds, along with nutmegs, onto a necklace for astral projection and connection with star beings. • Attach a seed to a pendulum for accurate dowsing, or make yourself a pendulum using a large seed—this is especially good for finding lost objects or buried treasure.

CAUTION
Do not use Japanese star anise, *Illicium anisatum*, which is highly toxic.

Star of Bethlehem

(Ornithogalum umbellatum)

MAGICAL FORMS
blooms white with a green stripe and petals in a star formation for several weeks in May or June • especially lucky if you see one blooming at Christmas or Easter • with ten to twenty starlike flowers per stem less than an inch across, opening late morning and closing at sunset or if it is cloudy • native to the Mediterranean • naturalized in North America, where it has escaped from gardens and become invasive in some states • magically use the growing and cut flowers, dried flowerheads, and flower essence

PLANET AND ELEMENT
Venus • Water

MAGICAL USES
so named because it resembles the original star of Bethlehem that guided the Magi • in some legends the star scattered across the earth in millions of pieces to grow as the flower • part of the Five-Flower Rescue Remedy and also as an individual essence to counteract bad news, shock, loss, dismissal, rejection, or physical trauma such as a fall or accident, whether present or past • to overcome fear of speaking in meetings or seminars • for pets who have been attacked or are naturally anxious because they left the litter too soon or have experienced rough handling

HOW TO USE
Use in wedding bouquets and as table decorations for lasting happiness. • Display cut flowers for celebrations for milestone events for those who are achieving their destiny. • Make a sun, moon, and star garden with the Star of Bethlehem representing the stars to keep health, wealth, good luck, and happiness flowing through your home. • Take the essence in water or under your tongue daily after a traumatic experience until you feel your equilibrium returning.

CAUTION
The plant is toxic if ingested by humans or pets, so only use with expert advice. • Do not use if pregnant.

Starfruit

(*Averrhoa carambola*)

MAGICAL FORMS

trees with curving branches and lilac-purple blossoms, up to thirty feet tall, growing ornamentally as well as for fruit • tropical fruit, sweet (the small, pale-green variety) and sour (the larger, yellow form), both with edible skin • when cut in cross-section, both kinds are shaped like five-pointed stars • native to Southeast Asia and India, but cultivated in many tropical lands • eaten raw or cooked • dwarf varieties can be grown in containers and brought indoors in winter • harvestable fruit from June through February • magically use the fruit, especially cut to reveal its star shape and its seeds

PLANET AND ELEMENT

Mercury • Air

MAGICAL USES

the fruit is served at seasonal magical celebrations and at the time of major planetary, meteor, comet, and stellar phenomena • symbol of good fortune and prosperity, absorbed when eaten • in Malaysian custom, place a bowl of the uncut fruit in the center of the home for the same purpose

HOW TO USE

As the stars come out, make the washed, dried seeds (edible but bitter) into a star shape on the ground and step across it nine times without touching the seeds to bring yourself immense good luck at an interview, audition, performance, or whenever you need to shine. Say nine times as you step, *Star shine, be mine, that I may brilliant be, for all to see.* Collect the seeds and carry them in a gold bag when you get your big chance.

CAUTION

Starfruit is toxic to dogs and cats. • Avoid if you have kidney disease, are pregnant, or take regular conventional prescription medicine.

Stephanotis

(*Stephanotis floribunda*)

MAGICAL FORMS

also known as Madagascar jasmine • grows in gardens in warm parts of the world such as Florida, otherwise as a houseplant or in a container to be brought indoors or to the conservatory in colder days • native to Southeast Asia and Madagascar • not jasmine but has a similar scent and color • can grow very tall with green, glossy leaves and clusters of star flowers on a vinelike shrub • magically use the cut flowers or dried and fresh blossoms

PLANET AND ELEMENT

Venus • Earth

MAGICAL USES

often called the wedding flower or bridal veil flower, it is scented, waxy, and white: a symbol of wedded bliss • used for decoration as well as in a bouquet in formal or exotic weddings • the flower brings good luck, especially to a bride • gifted for engagements, Valentine's Day, or Mother's Day • a funeral flower for a beloved relative, friend, or partner on the anniversary of their death • attracts lovers by increasing radiance

HOW TO USE

Stephanos means "crown" or "wreath" in ancient Greek. String together flowers to make a crown and set in the middle of an altar in rituals for success, leadership, authority, or promotion. Afterward, hang the wreath outdoors on a blossoming tree or shrub or the tallest branch you can reach on a tall tree. • Inhale the fragrance to open your psychic senses, especially clairsentience, before divination or magical rituals and to travel while meditating on the plant to distant and past lands, especially the old lost world of Lemuria, linked with Madagascar, source of ancient Indigenous wisdom in many lands. • Scatter the petals on a map or brochure of where you want to travel, whether by yourself or with a lover or friend. When they fade, tip the flowers in the direction you wish to travel.

Stevia

(*Stevia rebaudiana*)

MAGICAL FORMS

also called sweet herb • small herb from the chrysanthemum family, native to Brazil and Paraguay • popularly grown in Japan, the USA, Kenya, Europe, China, and other places where it is warm with minimal frost • magically use in cooking and tea made from fresh or dried green leaves • far sweeter than sugar, the processed white powder can also be empowered magically

PLANET AND ELEMENT

Venus • Water

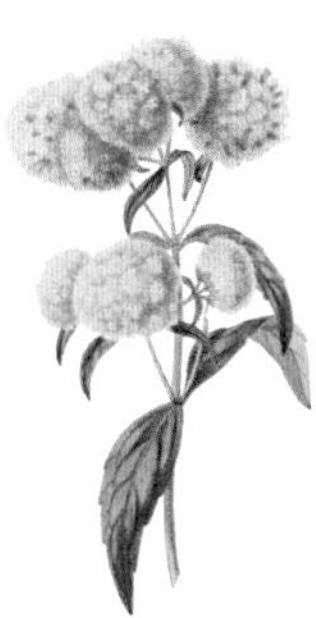

MAGICAL USES

grow stevia in gardens or in pots to deter negative or hostile visitors • served as herb tea, good with bitter herbs or substituted as the processed white form for sugar in drinks to sweeten critical relatives or complaining neighbors

HOW TO USE

Use in enchantment rituals, drink as tea, stir into a drink with a wish, or carry the dried leaves in charm bags (you can use the loose tea if necessary) to increase radiance and charisma and attract the positive attention of a desired person. • Set a potted stevia plant in your workspace or workplace if colleagues or a manager are abrasive or sarcastic. • Stir stevia nine times clockwise when sweetening drinks for sour workmates (with their permission), repeating nine times as you stir it, *May you sweeter be, that we may work in harmony.*

CAUTION

Stevia is considered safe in moderate quantities, even in pregnancy, but be cautious about ingesting homegrown stevia or leaves.

Sticky Monkey

(*Diplacus aurantiacus*)

MAGICAL FORMS

a shrub two to three feet tall, its sticky leaves containing resin • trumpet-shaped flowers, resembling a grinning monkey, flowering late summer in salmon orange, yellow, or orange-red • grows naturally in the southwestern USA, and especially in the Pacific Northwest • cultivated in gardens and national parks • can grow indoors in cooler regions • becomes dormant in the hottest weather or in drought but revives again • magically use the whole, growing plant; dried flowers; sticky leaves; and flower essence • see also its close cousin, the scarlet monkey flower (p. 289)

PLANET AND ELEMENT

Sun • Fire

MAGICAL USES

as the plant and the flower essence, for making sexual pleasure part of a deep, caring relationship • overcoming repressed sexual feelings and intimacy • deterring predators who use sexuality as a form of control • for relationships that survive difficult times

HOW TO USE

The flower closes when touched by an insect. • Spritz your workspace with a few drops of the essence in a bottle of water to create an exclusion zone around your aura energy field to deter inappropriate remarks or touching. • Grow the sticky plants indoors or out at home for encouraging loving intimacy or attracting a partner who will be both caring and passionate.

CAUTION

Consult your doctor before using while pregnant.

Stonebreaker

(*Phyllanthus niruri*)

MAGICAL FORMS

also called chanca piedra • a low-growing herb • native to tropical rainforests in South America, also to India and in tropical regions elsewhere including the USA and Australia • thin, leaf-covered branches with seed pods that grow under the leaves as small, green flowers • magically use the dried, chopped herb, sold also as tea

PLANET AND ELEMENT

Moon • Water

MAGICAL USES

use at work and in the community to break through opposition due to ageism, sexism, and ethnic prejudice • for achieving a major ambition when you have to take a test or examination, be interviewed, or perform a practical demonstration of your skills • for a fast promotion

HOW TO USE

Use the dried tea or chopped herb in charm bags when you know you will face hidden or open bias. Afterward, make it into an infusion by straining and pouring the liquid under a fast-running tap and then replacing the mix. • Use before a special opportunity to display your talents or go for a promotion, when you will need luck as well as skill: add favorite lucky charms, lucky heather, and/or a four-leaf clover to the chopped herb mix (to keep in a small, sealed, clear glass container on top of sample test papers, printouts of invitations to attend, copies of applications, or a picture of someone who has succeeded spectacularly in your chosen field). Set in a sunny spot until you have the results.

CAUTION

Seek advice before ingesting if you are taking medication to lower blood sugar or pressure, are undergoing lithium treatment, or are taking blood thinners. • Do not use while pregnant or breastfeeding, and do not use on children.

Stonecrop

(*Sedum* spp.)

MAGICAL FORMS

sedum or stonecrops in their many varieties are found on almost every continent, characterized by small, star-shaped flowers • English stonecrop (*Sedum anglicum*) is native to the UK and Europe but grows in North America • grows wild (though it is endangered) and is cultivated in gardens • *Sedum anglicum* is low growing and mat-like, only a few inches tall, clinging to rocky terrains in the wild, and surviving in inhospitable landscapes • white flowers, tinged with pink, blooming in later summer • may also be yellow • magically use the whole, growing plant; dried, chopped flowers and leaves; and flower essence

PLANET AND ELEMENT

Moon • Water

MAGICAL USES

as the plant and flower essence, for times of transition to release blockages rooted in fears of change and leaving the comfort zone • for flowing with inevitable changes • the plant is used in love spells and carried in a charm bag to call new love and friendship after a period of loneliness

HOW TO USE

A protective plant, stonecrop can be kept in hanging baskets outside the front door where the air circulates to keep away all harm and danger. • In medieval times, it was believed if stonecrop grew naturally on a low roof, the home would be protected from storms, lightning strike, and fires. • When you move homes, take your hanging baskets with you and attach them to the front of the new house to transfer the best of the old life if you were reluctant to move. • Put a few drops of the essence in a humidifier or spray the rooms of a new dwelling, your present one, or workplace if you are experiencing life changes you did not seek.

Storax Resin

MAGICAL FORMS

resin made from the sap of the Levant storax, *Liquidambar orientalis*, and the American storax, *Liquidambar styraciflua* • the *orientalis* is from southwest Asia Minor, especially Turkey, and the *styraciflua* has grown in Honduras and farther north since Mayan times; it also grows in North America and Europe • storax, a viscous, gray-brown liquid, is extracted from the bark that is removed from the tree and hardens • an offering to the Greek gods, used for many centuries in incense and perfumes • related to benzoin, which is also a styrax derivative; the two are different though often confused • also sometimes called styrax resin • magically use as a resin, in powder form to burn on charcoal, and as styrax or liquidambar essential oil

PLANETS AND ELEMENTS

Mercury/Sun • Air/Fire

MAGICAL USES

to overcome grief, anger, guilt, and resentment • for finding a new path • removing obstacles • discovering the truth • in ceremonial magick, especially related to the ancient deities

HOW TO USE

Use as an offering to the wise ancient Egyptian god Thoth, forerunner of the ancient Greek healer Hermes and messenger god or their successor the Roman Mercury. • Burn as incense or light a yellow candle anointed with the diluted oil to petition Mercury for help with business, communication, all swift-moving matters, learning, travel, healing, and protection against trickery, as well as uncovering lies. • Light the incense to empower opals and turquoise gems.

CAUTION

Styrax or liquidambar has been banned by the IFRA (International Fragrance Association) due, it is said by some, to faulty data. • Dilute any styrax-related oil well, and make sure it is from a reliable source; do a patch test before using topically. • Avoid if pregnant.

Strawberry

(*Fragaria* spp.)

MAGICAL FORMS

including *Fragaria ananassa*, perhaps the most popular kind, and wild strawberry (*Fragaria vesca*) • wild strawberries were harvested as long ago as 3000 BCE and were often transplanted into gardens in Shakespearean times • magically use the whole, growing plant; fruit; flowers; and seeds

PLANET AND ELEMENT

Venus • Water

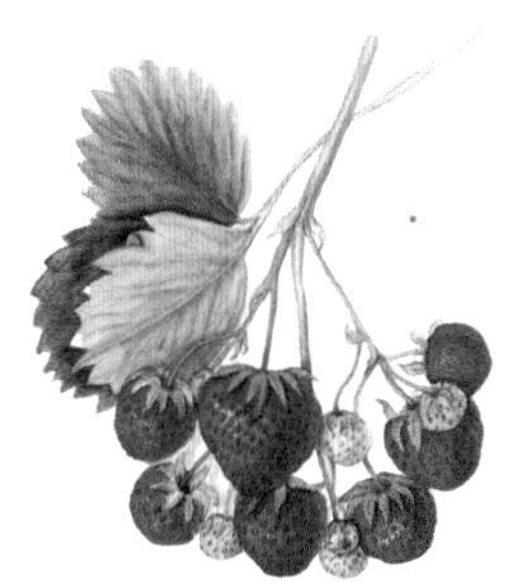

MAGICAL USES

romance • persuasion in love • good fortune • forbidden love • passion • calling new or first love into your life • magical cookery to enchant a lover • festival food of Lughnasadh or Lammas, the first harvest

HOW TO USE

Leaves and seeds were traditionally carried in a sachet for good fortune and by women going into labor so that the experience would be peaceful and their child good-natured and loving. • However, strawberry leaves left on strawberries as a gift could indicate the desire for an extramarital affair with the recipient. • Strawberries, especially those with two fruits attached to a single stem, were exchanged between lovers and eaten as both an aphrodisiac and a fertility symbol before lovemaking. • Crushed fresh strawberries or strawberry leaf tea is a love potion in a bath, sprinkled around the home, or shared with a lover. • Around 2600 BCE, the Chinese Yellow Emperor used weak strawberry tea to counter effects of aging. Strawberry-infused products are still considered beautifiers.

Strawberry Tree

(Arbutus unedo)

MAGICAL FORMS

not related to actual strawberries • large bushy evergreen, native to southwestern Ireland, southern Europe, and Asia • grows in the UK, parts of northern Europe, and on the West Coast of the USA • pink or white bell-shaped flowers • flowers and fruits that resemble strawberries (some consider not as tasty) appear on the tree at the same time, between September and November • with its associations with Old Ireland, this arbutus is especially lucky for those of Celtic origin living in the New World • magically use the whole, growing plant; leaves; branches; flowers, fresh or dried; and fruit, fresh or dried (often in magical cookery)

PLANET AND ELEMENT

Mars • Fire

MAGICAL USES

from ancient Greek and Roman times, recognized for its powerful defense of the young and vulnerable, with a mix of leaves, fresh flowers, and fruit in a short-term amulet bag (make sure they are dry) or the dried flowers and leaves for a longer-term protective bag

HOW TO USE

Find or create a branch with three berries (some say three flowers as well) to bring good luck to the home. • Fresh or dried cut flowers with leaves are traditionally set on a grave to guide the deceased to the afterlife and thereafter on anniversaries. • Plant the bush in the garden for banishing and keeping malevolent spirits from the home. • A cut display of flowering fruiting branches in the center of the home will clear a hostile atmosphere or if there has been sickness. • Share the cooked fruit in a jelly or jam preserve with a lover so that love will be true.

CAUTION

The overripe berries can cause drowsiness.

Sugar Cane

(Saccharum officinarum)

MAGICAL FORMS

grass plant growing between ten and twenty feet high • sugar cane was first brought to the Americas via Brazil in the fifteenth century by Portuguese traders • you can purchase fresh, thick-jointed, stalk sugar cane, akin to bamboo • unrefined sugar • magically use the green, grass-like form that can be planted in gardens

PLANET AND ELEMENT

Venus • Water

MAGICAL USES

for love and sex magick spells • protective when, as unrefined sugar, it is scattered around boundaries (not indoors or it will attract ants) to drive away evil and remove evil intentions or entities • used in magical cookery or to sweeten bitter herbs in teas if critical relatives or complaining neighbors are coming

HOW TO USE

When you need money, take a jar with a lid and add three gold-colored coins or three tiger eye crystals, three cinnamon sticks, and (if you can get them) nine pieces of green sugar cane—if not, use nine sugar sticks. Almost fill the jar with dissolved, unrefined sugar water (boil and allow to cool) and a little sweet or spiced wine, then seal. Shake the jar nine times every day for nine days and then bury the contents in a hole. • Surround the written name of someone you wish or need to impress, making a circle of green foliage around the paper or placing a dish of chopped sugar stalks in the center on top of the paper. At each corner, light a green candle. When the candles are burned through, ignite the paper safely and cast the greenery or sugar stalks into running water, repeating the words.

CAUTION

Green sugar cane should not be eaten while pregnant.

Sumbul

(Ferula sumbul)

MAGICAL FORMS

large, taprooted herbs of the giant fennel family with small white, yellow, and purple flowers • found primarily around the eastern Mediterranean, in Uzbekistan, Russia, India, and southeastern Siberia • may grow up to eight feet high • the root has a musk-like smell • a good substitute for the love properties of conventional musk that comes from the scent glands of an animal and is no longer considered ethical • magically use the cut or powdered root, occasionally found as an extracted resin

PLANET AND ELEMENT

Venus • Earth

MAGICAL USES

for good luck, keep the shredded or powdered root with lottery tickets • use in a charm bag carried during gambling or speculation and for auditions for talent and reality shows • for attracting love and increasing sexual magnetism • quite hard to obtain, but the cut root is available online in the USA and for shipping elsewhere

HOW TO USE

When love seems elusive or a lover neglectful, burn the powdered or ground root that contains resin in a love incense mix with frankincense, lavender, and rosemary. • Also carry the shredded or powdered root in a charm bag when you go out socially or next meet your lover to arouse their interest. • The chopped root, generally sold in pieces two to three inches long, can be kept in a bag with tarot cards, runes, or a crystal ball to enhance the psychic powers of the user. • Sumbul also acts as a gatekeeper if placed loose on the divination or séance table so only good spirits can enter during mediumship, magick, or divination.

CAUTION

The leaves and root should not be used while breastfeeding and there is not enough evidence to guarantee safety while pregnant, so consult with your doctor before using.

Sundew

(Drosera rotundifolia)

MAGICAL FORMS

also called round-leafed sundew • insectivorous plant • spoon-shaped leaves that exude sticky fluid through long, purple or red hairs • sundew traps insects; when an insect lands on the leaf, it becomes caught in the sticky sap and the leaf closes • named from *Ros solis*, Latin for "dew of the sun," because the plant was from early times believed to retain dew even in full sunlight, which was in fact the sticky sap glistening • considered in the sixteenth and seventeenth centuries to dispel melancholy • like sunflowers, sundew turns in the direction of the sun • Charles Darwin was so fascinated that he devoted 284 pages of his book on carnivorous plants to experiments with sundew • magically use the whole, growing plant; leaves; and stamens

PLANET AND ELEMENT

Venus/Sun • Earth/Fire

MAGICAL USES

anti-debt rituals • to silence or disarm criticism and intimidation • for safe travel • keeps predators and malevolent spirits from your home and you from psychic attack

HOW TO USE

Transfer fresh leaves with sticky stamens to a red bag. Carry when you meet those who will take advantage of your good nature, for a relationship where you fear dishonesty or betrayal, for untrustworthy people, or if you are going to an unsafe place. Replace when the leaves dry or crumble. • If you are planning on taking a risk and there are a number of insects flying close to the plants, observe if they fly away or how many, if any, are caught, which would suggest the likelihood of success in getting away with a gamble. • Bury where nothing grows the number of dried red, pink, or white flowers as you have hundreds or thousands of dollars of debt, for example five flowers for $500, $5,000, or $50,000 owed. Place a heavy stone on top, saying, *Rise no more to haunt me.*

CAUTION

Sundew is nontoxic, except in large quantities. • Do not use if pregnant.

Sunflower

(*Helianthus annuus*)

MAGICAL FORMS

flowering plant known for growing to face the sun • magically use the petals, dried and growing flower, seeds, as a carrier and cooking oil, and as incense

PLANET AND ELEMENT

Sun • Fire

MAGICAL USES

happiness • success • self-confidence • granting wishes • fertility • anti-scam • long life • health • prosperity • good fortune • a fae and midsummer oil and incense

HOW TO USE

If you are a woman who wishes to conceive, eat the seeds during the waxing moon. • Alternatively, add a handful of seeds to a jar by the bedside each day from crescent to full moon. On the full moon, scatter a quarter of the contents of the jar to the winds, then eat a quarter in the days ahead, float a quarter on running water, and bury a quarter beneath a thriving plant. • A circlet of sunflowers worn at a handfasting or a necklace of dried heads on Midsummer Eve brings fertility because each flower contains numerous seeds. The next day, give to your partner as a sign of transferring potency. • Use the oil to anoint candles and sacred objects. • Cleanse the ritual area or the self with seed tea. • Use in oil scrying on water. • Plant around the garden to bring good luck and prosperity. • Use the empowered cooking oil in magical cookery for ongoing health and vitality and family celebrations.

Sunflower, Mexican

(*Tithonia rotundifolia*)

MAGICAL FORMS

unlike the common sunflower, a distant relative, the Mexican sunflower, is a flowering shrub with numerous large daisy- or marigold-like blooms with fiery colors—red-orange (*Tithonia rotundifolia*) and yellow or yellowy orange (*Tithonia diversifolia*) • bloom from midsummer through fall • can grow up to eight feet high • naturalized in North and South America and Mediterranean Europe, though it will grow in cooler climes, just not as tall or lasting longer than the season • magically use the growing and cut flowers; flower petals; flowerheads, fresh or dried with the yellow inner disk and golden, orange, or red rays; and dried seeds

PLANETS AND ELEMENT

Sun/Mars • Fire

MAGICAL USES

early Spanish explorers discovered the Mexican sunflower and brought it back to Europe in the 1500s • by 1700 it had reached the USA, and Thomas Jefferson later planted it in his Monticello garden • a suggested twenty-third anniversary bouquet, especially in its dwarf varieties, such as Fiesta del Sol, because of its meanings of loyalty and deep love • for exotic weddings

HOW TO USE

Keep the cut flowers in the bedroom during sex magick rites. • Meditate on the cut or growing flowers for visions of past worlds, especially if you feel connection with Central American ancient cultures. • Carry a small bag of the seeds from the crescent moon for the lunar month to boost your personal power and charisma if you are naturally reticent or others overlook you. On the following crescent moon, replace the seeds.

CAUTION

Generally Mexican sunflowers are regarded as nontoxic to humans or cats, though dogs may have problems, and there are questions about the safety of the seeds. • Until more research is carried out, check with your own physician or herbalist. • As a precaution, avoid in pregnancy.

Survivor Tree

MAGICAL FORMS

the Callery pear (*Pyrus calleryana*) that survived the 9/11 Twin Towers attack is known as the Survivor Tree • in October 2001, the burned and badly damaged tree was discovered in the destruction at Ground Zero and taken by the New York City Department of Parks and Recreation, returning healed to the 9/11 memorial plaza in 2010 • new, smooth limbs were growing from the gnarled stumps • each year, seeds are given to three communities who have suffered and overcome a tragedy, for example to Little Rock, Arkansas, in 2023 after the community was hit by tornadoes • magically, visit the 9/11 memorial tree or one of the sites where the seeds have been planted • alternatively, plant a tree in your area or in your garden, and as you plant it, name those who have survived or had to rebuild their lives after a personal, family, community, national, or international tragedy

PLANET AND ELEMENT

Venus • Water

MAGICAL USES

any tree can become a survivor tree to commemorate a lost loved one or major sorrow; if possible, plant near a grave instead of wreaths of cut flowers that will decay, to visit on anniversaries • gain strength from having survived and brought good out of bad

HOW TO USE

Bury a stone beneath the roots of a tree outdoors or a potted palm or bonsai indoors on which you have invisibly etched requests for relief or thankfulness that you or the family have survived a tragedy. • Add special thankfulness symbols to your thanksgiving tree for the resolution of a family problem. • Scatter the fallen blossoms of your survivor tree or the fall leaves to the winds, whether one you have planted or found growing wild, giving thanks for the strength to go on. • If your survivor tree has edible fruit, eat it to absorb the healing of the tree to endure.

Sweet Cicely

(*Myrrhis odorata*)

MAGICAL FORMS

tall herb • flowers May through June, giving way to dark-brown fruit • magically use the leaves, flowers, and oil

PLANET AND ELEMENT

Jupiter • Air

MAGICAL USES

encourages mediumship, contacting deceased and restless spirits and beloved ancestors • plant of elves; combined with fennel (see p. 176), protects against malicious elves and their arrows • improves clairvoyance and seeing nature beings • named after St. Cecilia, the third-century Roman martyr, and so associated with altruism, developing musical gifts, and musicians • magical cookery

HOW TO USE

Sweet Cicely is believed to predate Christianity as the herb of the goddess of summer. • The dried flowers and leaves are burned as an incense to bring happiness to the home and all therein. • Burn or diffuse the oil indoors on cold, wet days to lift the energies and bring a touch of summer all year round. • Dry and tie strong whole plants to make an asperging rod to regularly sweep from the doorstep to the edge of your boundaries to remove any accumulated negativity, sickness, or sorrow. • The pollen-rich flowers attract bees and butterflies, naturally call abundance and wealth, and grant wishes once they bloom. • The flowers are used to decorate the midsummer altar and as midsummer offerings to the goddesses of flowers and of plenty.

CAUTION

Sweet Cicely can be mistaken for the larger poisonous giant hogweed or even hemlock if taken from the wild. • Do not use the oil while pregnant or ingest it at any time.

Sweet Everlasting

(*Pseudognaphalium obtusifolium*)

MAGICAL FORMS

also known as rabbit tobacco • used magically like other flowers with similar names as dried bouquets or arrangements • called everlasting because they retain color and form when dried • magically use the small, clustered, white and yellow flowers, usually with fuzzy silvery foliage, in rituals and amulets

PLANET AND ELEMENT

Saturn • Earth

MAGICAL USES

growing around the home or more usually as dried arrangements in homes and businesses for long life, survival of a business, long-term health, healing, and to preserve youthfulness of all living or working there • treasured by the Cherokees and people of the southeastern nations, ritually, in sweat lodges and medicinally • the smoke drives away evil spirits • once substituted for tobacco by the Native Americans and Europeans

HOW TO USE

Cast the blossom on incense, a hearth, or an outdoor bonfire to bring blessings and to communicate with the spirits of the earth and water. • Dried leaves and flowers can be chopped and burned in a bowl. Waft the smoke with your hand, a fan, or a feather to cleanse a space, ritual tools, oneself, or another person or group. • Alternatively, make into an infusion and inhale the steam to connect with the ancestors and find messages from wise guides and the otherworlds in images rising from the steam. • Place in a pillow or hang dried over the bed for calm, peaceful, and rejuvenating sleep.

Sweet Flag

(*Acorus calamus*)

MAGICAL FORMS

also known as calamus • includes American sweet flag (*Acorus calamus* var. *americanus*) • an aquatic plant with yellow flowers, resembling the flag iris in appearance • native to India • magically use the whole plant in situ for meditation; the rhizome, whole or powdered (available online from botanical stores, even within the USA); and the seeds

PLANET AND ELEMENT

Mars • Fire

MAGICAL USES

historically the rhizome was considered an aphrodisiac and to increase potency in ancient Egypt and India • for use against bullying, intimidation, domestic violence, and psychic/psychological manipulation

HOW TO USE

Hide the seeds or rhizome in an amulet bag in a drawer if you face intimidation in the workplace or from an angry partner or adult children still at home while seeking help. • Carry it in your pocket in a thick fabric bag if you travel alone late at night. • Keep a rhizome and dried lavender in a sealed healing amulet bag with a picture of someone who is sick or suffering. • Hang a rhizome over the kitchen door so that there will always be sufficient material resources within the home. • Keep a rhizome in a red bag beneath the mattress to increase libido and sexual prowess.

CAUTION

Though a feature of Ayurvedic and Chinese medicine and previously used medicinally in the USA, Europe, and the UK, the sale of calamus in food and medicine is restricted in some countries, including the USA, as some calamus is highly toxic if ingested. • Use magically with care. • Keep your calamus amulet in a sealed bag, wearing gloves or washing your hands after handling.

Sweet Gale

(*Myrica gale*)

MAGICAL FORMS

also called bog myrtle • low-growing, bushy shrub two to four feet tall • native to northern and western Europe, especially Scotland, in wetland habitats • indigenous to the Adirondack Mountains and throughout Canada and northeastern USA, also in Washington, Oregon, and New York • clusters of small yellow and brown catkins appear before the leaves from spring to early summer, followed by berries, eaten by birds • magically use the dried, aromatic leaves that can be purchased online; the essential oil; and the flower essence

PLANET AND ELEMENT

Mercury • Air

MAGICAL USES

for releasing and healing emotional blockages and pain leading to defensiveness in communication and offloading blame or guilt • creating positive meaningful interactions and relationships, especially within love partnerships • reputedly used by Viking berserkers, fierce warriors who knew no limits, to give them total fearlessness

HOW TO USE

Tea made from the leaves aids dream recall and prophetic dreaming. • Use essential oil from the aromatic leaves and branches, diluted in jojoba or grape-seed carrier oil or bought already diluted in the carrier oils, for massage to increase natural radiance and youthfulness and enhance emotional openness in love. • Sip the essence in water if you need to clearly express your feelings without fears of vulnerability and to protect yourself against accusations so that you are neither villain nor victim.

CAUTION

The oil is highly toxic if ingested, as is the plant in large doses. • The plant and its products are unsafe to ingest during pregnancy or while breastfeeding.

Sweet Joe Pye Weed

(*Eupatorium purpureum*)

MAGICAL FORMS

also known as gravel root • can grow up to seven feet • whorls of pointed oblong leaves and clusters of purple-pink vanilla-scented florets, in a soft cloud towering above other plants • blooms in late summer, early fall, and through the winter • has seed-tops • native to eastern and central North America • grows through most of the USA and also in Europe and the UK • named after the Native American who used the root to cure New Englanders of typhus • considered among Native North Americans to have at least fifty curative uses • magically use the growing plant; the cut flowers, fresh or dried; and, most commonly, the root

PLANET AND ELEMENT

Jupiter • Air

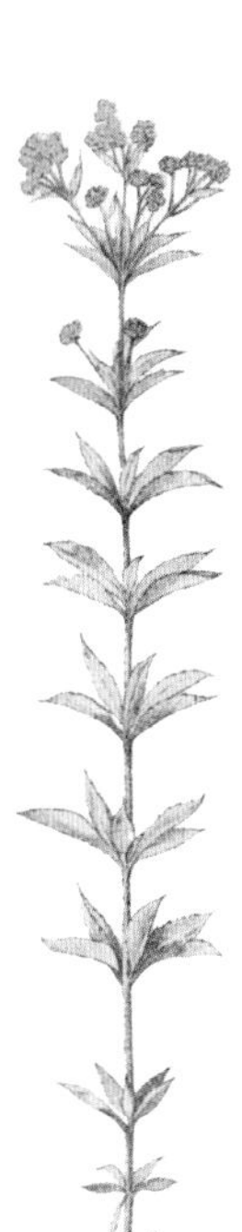

MAGICAL USES

for all employment matters, such as asking for a salary increase or promotion, or for applying to new jobs

HOW TO USE

Carry the root or the seed-tops in a charm bag for luck in gambling and speculation, and keep with lottery tickets. • Keep the root in a charm bag in the workplace to foster coworkers' respect for you and your professional achievements. • Have a cut fresh or dried flower arrangement in your home for entertaining those you need to impress socially, whether of high status connected with your work or a partner's, future relatives, acquaintances, or new neighbors.

CAUTION

Avoid if pregnant or breastfeeding.

Sweet Tea Vine

(*Gynostemma pentaphyllum*)

MAGICAL FORMS
also called jiaogulan, as well as the immortality herb • male and female pale-yellow flowers that appear on separate plants invariably growing close together • green, serrated leaves • a climbing vine with curling tendrils, native to the mountains of Asia and thickets in Japanese forests • grows well in warmer parts of the USA and other regions or cooler areas as an annual plant • used in making healing teas that purport to restore energy and bust stress • grown indoors as a trailing pot plant • magically use the whole, growing plant; tea; stems; leaves; and flowers

PLANET AND ELEMENT
Saturn • Earth

MAGICAL USES
anti-aging • the tea is consumed before rituals and empowerments seeking slow growing, long-lasting manifestations • in magical cooking with the sweet, young stems and leaves, for reassuring insecure people, lasting love, friendship, and financial and property security

HOW TO USE
Grow your immortality herb up a trellis in the garden or in a pot if you have found your ideal home or job and want stability or if you share the home with different generations, to promote mutual benefits. • Create a leaf amulet to carry, hang over the front door, or hide in your workspace (using loose tea if necessary) if you are threatened with eviction or redundancy or you have been asked to relocate and are unwilling. • Use the trailing vine stripped of leaves or flowers for knot magick, tying knots for what or whom you wish to lose from your life and hanging it in a high branch of a dead tree until it withers.

CAUTION
Sweet tea vine should not be taken with immune-suppressing medication. • Use in moderation. • Seek expert advice before using if pregnant.

Sweet Woodruff

(*Galium odoratum*)

MAGICAL FORMS
square stem, whorls of narrow leaves, and fragrant, small, white flowers that appear in spring and early summer • native to Europe and the UK and also found in Asia and Africa, in most Canadian provinces, and every state in the USA except Hawaii • magically use the aerial parts, often dried and shredded, and flowers, especially when blooming

PLANET AND ELEMENT
Venus • Earth

MAGICAL USES
the leaves when dried have the fragrance of newly mowed grass • traditionally set between clothes to sweeten them or scattered among rushes on floors after winter • in legend the herb lined the manger of baby Jesus • in parts of Europe and the UK, Maiwen, made of sweet woodruff steeped in wine, was drunk during Mayday celebrations (still obtainable), a herald of the coming summer and better times • in medieval times, sweet woodruff was brought into churches on Whitsunday and St. Barnabas Day on June 11 to bar evil from entering • brings victory in sports, career, and challenges when carried in fragrant sachets • visions of the fey while walking among the plants • for happiness, especially in LGBTQ relationships • a lucky charm for those who work on the land or spend time in nature

HOW TO USE
Carry the shredded, dried plant in a leather amulet bag for personal protection. • Add the dried, vanilla-scented, star-shaped flowers to potpourri to keep away danger and malevolence from the home or workplace. • Cast the shredded aerial parts over open land or burn as incense to bring justice in family, social, or community matters when you are unfairly blamed.

CAUTION
Do not ingest if taking conventional medication for circulation or during pregnancy.

Sweetgrass

(*Hierochloe odorata*)

MAGICAL FORMS

sometimes called holy grass, Seneca grass, or vanilla grass because of its sweet, vanilla-like fragrance when burned • known as the hair of the Earth Mother • made into a coil, often braided, in the fields as it is picked and then dried • usually braided in three strands for mind, body, and spirit, united in the coil in a knot • also found in loose strands, dried for an incense dish • native to much of northern Eurasia and North America as far north as the Arctic Circle • magically use the fresh or dried grass and braided or growing free

PLANETS AND ELEMENT

Moon/Saturn • Earth

MAGICAL USES

contains very powerful Earth energies • sweetgrass is burned as an incense offering for personal and home blessings • the coil in a dish is employed as a smudge, using your hand or a fan to waft the smoke or swirled with care; purifies the aura and cleanses ritual objects, ceremonial areas, and sacred spaces • burned as incense for past-life recall through inducing a state of meditation • worn as protective amulet or placed in a dream catcher for women's spirituality and magical work • a gentle purifier of grief, sorrow, and abuse • sweetgrass coils can also be wrapped around special artifacts when they are not in use

HOW TO USE

Sweetgrass braids are hung in doorways or on altars to attract good spirits to ceremonies and into the home. • Before rituals, cedar and sagebrush may be burned first to remove malicious entities or energies. • If smudging, ask the Great Spirit or your own source of goodness and light for whatever it is you need, afterward leaving an offering. • Ask also for beauty and blessings to enter your life as you sit with your dish of smoking sweetgrass by candle or moonlight, visualizing the smoke being transformed into silver light and connecting with the flow of the earth and moon.

CAUTION

As an Indigenous sacred substance, sweetgrass should be used sparingly and with respect and purchased from an ethical source, not taken from the wild.

Sweetgum Tree

(*Liquidambar styraciflua*)

MAGICAL FORMS

grows in southeastern North America as far north as New Jersey, also in Mexico and Guatemala • between sixty and a hundred feet tall with fragrant resin from the bark (see "Storax Resin," p. 431) • star-shaped leaves that turn bright red, orange, yellow, and purple in the fall and smell of storax when crushed • large, hard, spiky balls that develop from the globular, yellowish-green flowers in April to May and release winged seeds • magically use the dried leaves; the growing, full-size tree in situ; as a bonsai with its beautiful, textured, gray bark as it matures; and the brilliant fall leaves

PLANET AND ELEMENT

Jupiter • Air

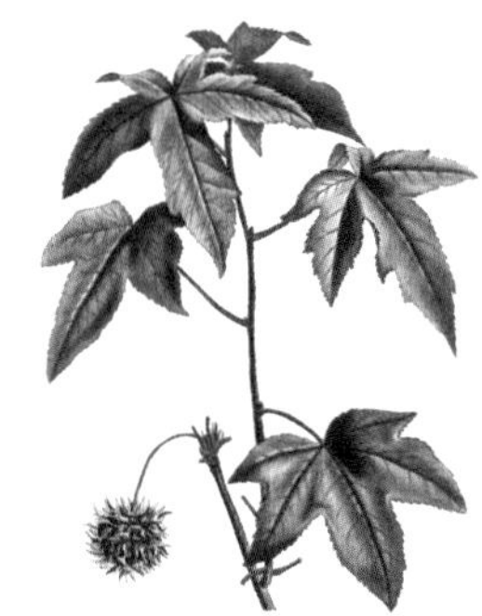

MAGICAL USES

the dried leaves of the full-size tree in potpourri or incense • the bonsai tree as a centerpiece in an indoor garden or outside in warm weather for celebrating and easing the smooth passing of the seasons • adorn the bonsai encircled with flowers at keynote birthdays and anniversaries, especially in the middle and golden years, to bring good fortune and focus on opportunities still available given the wisdom of experience

HOW TO USE

Find a large tree with a hole in the trunk, press inside a written petition to the Tree spirits, and seal the hole, using the leaked resin and/or a small piece of fallen bark. • Meditate on the bonsai, especially with its fall leaves, for ways of moving on if a relationship has ended or is ending or there has been redundancy or unwilling early retirement and you wish to leave without regrets. Cast a single fall leaf into the wind and preserve another until it fades.

Sycamore Tree

(*Planatus occidentalis*)

MAGICAL FORMS

including the American sycamore • long-living, massive tree with a divided trunk • brown seed balls releasing tiny, winged, fluffy seeds in spring • magically use the whole, growing tree; wood; bark; seeds; and seed balls

PLANET AND ELEMENTS

Mercury • Air/Earth

MAGICAL USES

the deep extending roots, huge trunk, and spreading branches of the sycamore have linked it with the underworld, earth, and heavens in ritual and meditation for shamanic journeying • in ancient Egypt, the sycamore was the manifestation of the sky goddess Nut, mother of the deities, and the mother goddesses Isis and Hathor • Isis was frequently depicted standing beneath a sycamore tree • Hathor was called the Lady of the Sycamore, the ancient maternal links strengthening the connection of the tree with fertility

HOW TO USE

Make a wand for rituals involving action, change, insight, and movement. • The balls filled with the seeds can be released outdoors to spread fertility: tap a seed ball with the wand before splitting it, especially if a lack of love or low sperm count is an obstacle to conception. Be careful to not ingest any seeds as they fly. • The flaking bark that earned the sycamore the name "ghost tree" among Native Americans because of the white and gray patches on the trunk gave it the significance of transformation and shedding the redundant and destructive. • Write or etch on the back of a large piece of bark that has fallen from the trunk a wish to be fulfilled that may take time. Attach it with red string or wedge it into the cleft in the trunk, where it will be sheltered to prevent obstacles or unhelpful people standing in your way. • A sycamore is a tree that stands firm in rain or storm; sit beneath the cleft in a rainstorm to absorb the strength and endurance of the tree if you are wavering in your life purpose.

CAUTION

Seeds and seedlings are toxic to humans and animals, especially horses, if consumed.

Tamarind Tree

(*Tamarindus indica*)

MAGICAL FORMS

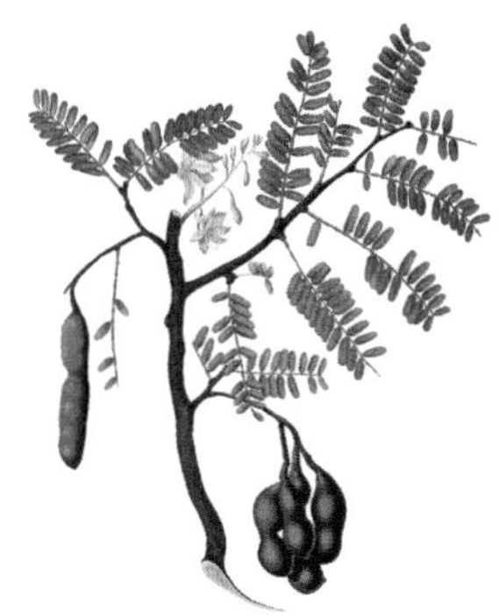

evergreen tree growing up to eighty feet high • orange-yellow flowers and brittle, gray-brown seed pods (the fruit contains up to twelve round seeds embedded in edible pulp) • originally from Africa and naturalized throughout Southeast Asia, including Thailand, India, and China; also in Mexico and the Caribbean • magically use the whole, growing tree; pods; fresh and dried leaves; fruit; and seeds

PLANET AND ELEMENT

Sun • Fire

MAGICAL USES

for love, especially new love and the rebuilding of trust • balancing yin and yang energies within the self • harmony • welcoming benign spirits • fitness regimes • restoring a positive body image

HOW TO USE

Carry the seed pods, available from specialty grocery stores or online, in a white charm bag while on a date or at a social event to make yourself irresistible in love, if you have lost your confidence. • Feed a lover a dish containing cooked tamarind (empower a commercial product with your intention if you wish) as an aphrodisiac and to relax your own inhibitions. • In Indian mythology, the tamarind tree is the tree of knowledge, sacred to Lord Ganesh. • The seven sages, the Saptarshi, learned their knowledges of the Hindu scriptures, the Vedas, while sitting under a tamarind tree, and in hot countries its shade often proves a gathering place for teaching.

CAUTION

Eat pulp and seeds in moderation, and avoid if taking ibuprofen regularly or if you are allergic to legumes.

Tamarisk Tree

(*Tamarix ramosissima*)

MAGICAL FORMS

also called salt cedar • a small, hardy tree with slender branches, plumelike foliage, and numerous pink to white flowers on long spikes, blooming from March to September and sometimes into the fall • relatedly, the French tamarisk (*Tamarix ramosissima*) grows from southern Russia right through most of temperate Asia • both trees have similar magical properties • cultivated in Europe since 1885 and popular in gardens • grows across the western USA, along with other species of tamarisk, where it became naturalized by the 1800s and is often considered invasive • magically use the fresh and dried leaves, dried flowers, and branches or twigs (found fallen unless you have permission to cut the tree)

PLANET AND ELEMENT

Saturn • Earth

MAGICAL USES

rebirth, protection, purification of toxic influences and situations and of malicious spirits • in the Bible regarded as the covenant between God and humans • the body of the slain Egyptian god Osiris was kept safe in a chest inside a tamarisk tree

HOW TO USE

The tamarisk tree has been used for thousands of years to remove malevolent or restless ghosts. Leaves from a branch are scattered in all directions in the place where the presence(s) are most strongly experienced. • Hang a branch woven with silver and gold ornaments (or ornaments painted silver and gold), as well as fresh leaves and flowers, over the entrance to guard against physical storms and emotional disruption within the home. Replace the flowers or leaves when faded. • The Israelites believed the smoke kept away snakes. • Burn the wood chips or dried leaves as part of an incense mix to create a protective barrier around you against human snakes in your life.

CAUTION

Consult your doctor before ingesting if pregnant.

Tangerine Tree

(*Citrus reticulata*)

MAGICAL FORMS

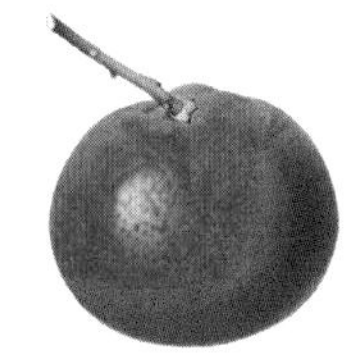

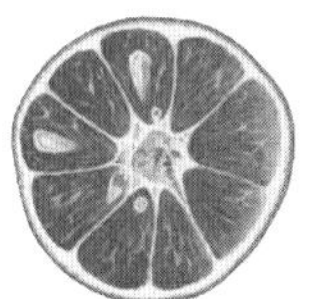

a cultivar of mandarin; the botanical names and magical properties are often interchangeable • a small evergreen tree with thorns • small, easily peeled fruit • fragrant blossoms • the mandarin tree was brought to Europe from its native south China and Asia in 1805 and to the USA in 1845, where it was renamed *tangerine* • tangerines grow in Texas, Florida, California, and Guinea • magically use the blossom, thorns, and essential oil • both tangerine and mandarin essential oil are extracted from the peel of the ripe fruit, though tangerine is used less in perfumes

PLANET AND ELEMENT

Sun • Fire

MAGICAL USES

well-being • makes anything seem possible • creative ventures • breaking safely through spiritual barriers in meditation • balances the body, mind, and spirit's psychic energy centers and aura field • the thorns, when included in protective bottles, will defend against spite from those who are physically vulnerable or very old

HOW TO USE

Use the flowers at the wedding of someone getting married young or the birth of a baby earlier in life. • Diffuse the oil with other citrus oils in the home or workplace to maintain optimism and protect against psychic and emotional vampires.

CAUTION

Tangerine is generally considered safe in pregnancy in later trimesters, but check with an expert, as it is possibly phototoxic. • Dilute oil well if you have sensitive skin. • Tangerine is often given in a very diluted massage mix for older children if they are anxious.

Tansy

(*Tanacetum vulgare*)

MAGICAL FORMS

also called bitter buttons or cow bitter • a tall, stemmed herb, topped with green leaves and yellow, button-like flowers blooming from July to September and a camphor-like scent • native to Europe, the UK, Asia, and mountainous regions of Australia and Japan • naturalized in the northern USA and Canada, grows wild in many parts • magically use the whole, growing plant; the cut plant, fresh or dried; and the aerial parts, dried and shredded

PLANET AND ELEMENT

Venus • Water/Earth

MAGICAL USES

health, long life • associated with Hebe, Greek goddess of eternal youth • conception and pregnancy • invisibility against potential danger when carried in an amulet bag • new beginnings

HOW TO USE

Add the chopped, fresh tansy herb to a protective bottle with powdered ginger and cinnamon, iron nails, and sour red wine as protection against unfair treatment by courts, the IRS, or security services. • Hang a fresh plant over the door if there is sickness or misfortune in the home. After a week or if it fades sooner, burn it outdoors to remove all ill health and bad luck. • Set shredded or powdered tansy, including the flowers if possible, inside an empty eggshell, carefully cut in half. Tie the two halves together with red twine and bury it beneath growing tansy or another thriving herb on full moon night if you want to conceive a baby (handle the herb with care if there is a chance you may be pregnant already).

CAUTION

Leaves and flowers are considered poisonous, especially in larger quantities. • Avoid during pregnancy. • The plant and essential oil are subject to restrictions medicinally in several countries and should be ingested or used on the skin only under professional supervision.

Tansy, Blue

(*Tanacetum annuum*)

MAGICAL FORMS

often called blue chamomile • the now-rare flowering plant is known for its essential oil • yellow flowers produce bright-blue oil due to a chemical reaction, giving it the name blue tansy • blooms from August to October • native to Morocco and the Mediterranean and, though not native, can be cultivated in the UK, Ireland, and other parts of Europe • now found along the northwestern coast of North America, from northern Oregon to southern British Columbia, northern parts of Nevada, and New Mexico • fernlike leaves with white hairs covering them • magically use the essential oil or the growing plant, if you can obtain it for your garden

PLANET AND ELEMENTS

Venus • Water/Earth

MAGICAL USES

opens the psychic Third Eye for clairvoyance, prophetic dreams, and divination • soothes an anxious mind and spirit as well as quieting restless but harmless spirits lingering in the home or workplace

HOW TO USE

Burn or diffuse the oil in your home or workplace or grow the plant in the garden to protect against psychic attacks, mind control, and negative entities and to prevent hostile people from entering. • The smoke of the diffused oil, if wafted (carefully) with a feather, purifies artifacts, spaces, and the aura.

CAUTION

Unlike tansy (*Tanacetum vulgare*), whose flower is similarly yellow (though some have blue in the flower), blue tansy is nontoxic. • Dilute blue tansy oil well. • Do not take before the second trimester of pregnancy, and then only with medical advice thereafter. • Blue tansy stains clothes and the skin blue. • Do not ingest the oil or use if taking medication.

Tarragon

(*Artemisia dracunculus*)

MAGICAL FORMS

common name for herb that also encompasses French tarragon (*Tagetes lucida*) and Mexican or Spanish tarragon (*Taetes lucida*) • magically use the dried or fresh herb, leaves, well-diluted oil, and fresh or dried bright-orange or yellow flowers

PLANETS AND ELEMENTS

Mars/Mercury • Fire/Air

MAGICAL USES

dragon herb associated with courage and protecting what is precious • anti-spite and -abuse • banishes evil spirits • for career success, especially against unfair competition • confidence • focusing on new targets • increasing libido • linked also with serpents, shedding the redundant for new life • prosperity through seizing opportunity • regeneration in any and every aspect of living

HOW TO USE

Use in all dragon rituals, incorporating gold to draw unexpected money. • Use flowers to create an infusion or add drops of the oil in water for floor wash, applying to the doorstep to deter unwanted visitors and cleanse bad atmospheres after external threats such as debt collectors. • Add to magical cooking to stimulate libido and passion in your lover. • Tarragon salt twists or sachets in your office desk or briefcase will help with your career if you are undervalued or job hunting. • Use as part of a defensive incense mix to strengthen determination to not be defeated. • Plant in defensive and/or prosperity gardens. • Use in water scrying (for this purpose, best as dried herb or dried and chopped flowers).

CAUTION

Do not ingest significant quantities of tarragon, and avoid the aroma, if pregnant, as well as when menstruation is heavy.

Tea Plant

(*Camellia sinensis*)

MAGICAL FORMS

the dried leaves or leaf buds are used in what are called the five true teas: black, green, white, oolong, and pu'er • their flavors and qualities vary according to their processing method • magically use the whole, growing plant; fresh or dried leaves; and brewed as tea

PLANET AND ELEMENT

Moon/Mars • Water/Fire

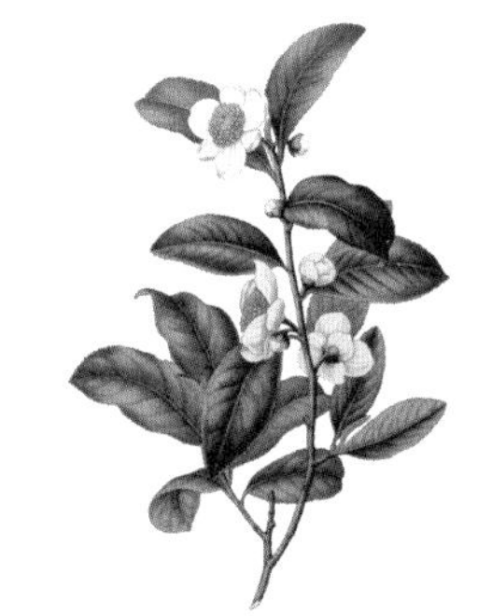

MAGICAL USES

for tea leaf divination, notably in the form of Earl Grey, black tea with added bergamot • the true teas are also used as a base for herbal and floral infusions and decoctions • however, each true tea has its own unique magical and health-giving properties as a drink to absorb, share, or offer to others • can also be added to protective floor washes or sprinkled to create magical boundaries

HOW TO USE

Drink black tea to attract and share good fortune. • If brainstorming new business ideas, draw money by surrounding your pot or cup of tea with Chinese divinatory lucky coins before drinking (also works with green tea). • To introduce stability to a volatile situation, empower or bless the tea. • Drink green tea during tea ceremonies as part of a spiritual group activity or meditative experience. • White tea that brews golden can be shared before lovemaking for increasing fertility by the light of the full moon if anxiety seems to be blocking conception. • Drink oolong tea to restore self-esteem and to awaken psychic powers before tarot reading or mediumship. • Pu'er tea should be offered in the workplace if ageism is an issue.

Tea Tree

(*Melaleuca alternifolia*)

MAGICAL FORMS

tree or tall shrub from the myrtle family, native to Australia, especially northern New South Wales and Queensland • its essential oil, made from leaves and twigs, is traditional to the Australian Aboriginal people as an all-healer • used widely in Europe, Britain, and the USA as a healing and cleansing essential oil, especially for skin problems • will grow in swampy tropical and subtropical areas of North America and indoors worldwide in a pot with care and enough moisture and sunlight • magically use the essential oil; the dried leaves; and the whole, growing, potted plant or tree outdoors if in the right climate

PLANET AND ELEMENT

Mercury • Air

MAGICAL USES

protection against psychic attack and emotional vampires • removes threats from entities and curses • relieves spiritually based ailments and hostile atmospheres

HOW TO USE

Use tea tree oil in a diffuser or burner to clear away sickness, misfortune, quarrels, and confrontational visitors from the home or home business. • Creates a psychic barrier against spite, gossip, or unfair criticism if you are expecting a confrontational or emotionally needy relative or neighbor to call. • Grow the tree in a garden or set a dried flower or leaf arrangement or the potted plant in the center of the home to repel and remove any malevolent or restless spirits, or if your home is built on negative overactive or overly sluggish earth energies.

CAUTION

Dilute the oil well if using on the skin, and do not ingest the oil or any parts of the raw tree. • If you have a potted plant, take care that it is safely away from small children or pets.

Teak Tree

(*Tectona grandis*)

MAGICAL FORMS

native to Asia, from tropical India to Vietnam, into Central and South America and to a lesser extent tropical North America • the wood was first imported to Europe in the early 1800s • magically use the old, pale-gray bark after it has peeled off on the ground, if you can find a teak tree growing wild on vacation or a cultivated one with permission (there are often restrictions due to over-exploitation) • if you have no access to a tree, use teak wood from craft stores and specialty wood suppliers in the USA, England, Europe, or Asia • purchase pre-loved teak furniture

PLANET AND ELEMENT

Jupiter • Air

MAGICAL USES

used in boat building two thousand years ago in Old Egypt on the trade routes between India and the Roman Empire, teak wood, shredded bark, or a small wooden item is an ideal travel amulet or charm for trading overseas (a teak ball can represent the world) • a small statue as a gift at wise man or wisewoman rituals • protection against emotional and financial parasites

HOW TO USE

Seek an antique or yard sale teak table as your altar or special place to add stability and protection to rituals. • Choose a new or pre-loved teak statue that symbolizes your needs or strengths: a dragon, matching hearts, or a bird for the center of your altar as a focus for ritual. • Make or buy a teak wand for healing and to resist emotional or financial pressures by surrounding yourself with a circle of strength and resistance to manipulation. • Write invisibly on bark what you wish to shed, and then bury it.

CAUTION

Teak is nontoxic, but untreated wood may irritate sensitive skin. • Always seek a reputable source for this over-logged wood.

Thistle

(*Cirsium* spp.)

MAGICAL FORMS
numerous thistle varieties, for example the bull thistle, *Cirsium vulgare*, originally an import from Eurasia, now naturalized through much of the USA and Canada • magically use the whole, growing plant; dried flowerheads; leaves; and stems with prickles attached

PLANET AND ELEMENT
Mars • Fire

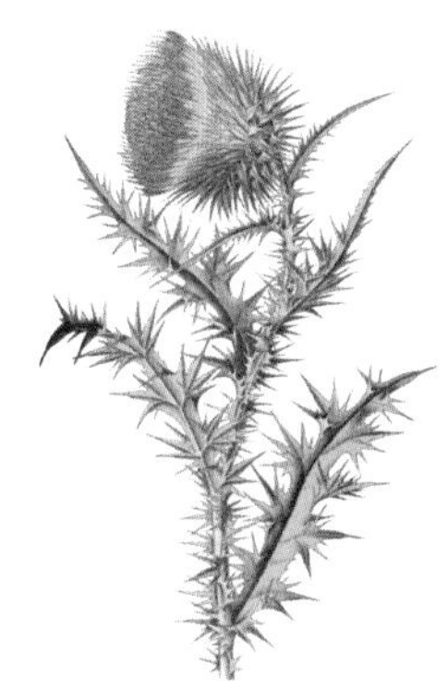

MAGICAL USES
grown in a pot on the doorstep, thistles keep away malicious spirits and divert negative earth energies • most famous is the tall Scottish thistle, *Onopordum acanthium*, also now found in the USA and Australia, traveling with colonists from the UK to the New World • this became the emblem of Scotland from the 1200s, often topped with a crown, because it is told Norse invaders raided a Scottish encampment stealthily by night • one stepped on a thistle and his cries woke the encampment who were able to defeat the Norsemen • the Scottish thistle is used in rituals for defeating seemingly impossible odds

HOW TO USE
Carry a dark-purple amulet bag containing dried flowerheads to prevent ill wishes, curses, and jinxes from taking hold. • For healing animals, whether pets or wild, surround a photo of the creature with a red thistle in all four directions with four white candles. Carefully move the thistles with a wand tip until they are in the center of the photo. Extinguish the candles and discard the thistles from the photo outdoors to remove the sickness or pain.

CAUTION
Handle thistles with care. • Eating the green coating on the plant may cause digestive problems in pets and some livestock.

Thistle, Blessed

(*Cnicus benedictus*)

MAGICAL FORMS
also known as holy thistle, or St. Benedict's thistle because it was grown in monastery gardens and the Benedictine Order was said to build their monasteries on ley lines • found also as star thistle in the USA • best in wildlife gardens • believed to indicate fertile soil • magically use the cut or whole, growing plant; leaves; flowering heads; and spikes

PLANET AND ELEMENTS
Mars • Fire/Earth

MAGICAL USES
purification of ritual areas • breaking hexes and curses • like all thistles, fiercely deters thieves, intruders, and harm to the home and family • an ideal companion magically with barberry, Glastonbury thorn (see p. 199), or indeed any herb names containing the words *holy* or *blessed* or with religious associations such as our lady's milkwort (see "Lungwort," p. 273)

HOW TO USE
Carry the chopped plant, including spikes, in a small thick cloth bag if you are going into a hostile environment or if ghost hunting in a place where there has been a tragedy or evil deeds. • Mix the leaf and flowering head tea with sacred salt and holy water and sprinkle to send an unfriendly spirit to the light in the room(s) where you most feel its presence. • Before meeting your coven, if you sense that one of its members is secretly behaving destructively, make sure to bring the plant in any form. • If planted near the entrance (in a place where children cannot get to it and hurt themselves), it brings vitality and strength and keeps away debt, poverty, and those who would cheat or sell you short.

CAUTION
Avoid medicinally while pregnant or lactating and with very small children.

Thistle, Milk

(*Silybum marianum*)

MAGICAL FORMS

distinguishable from other thistles by its white veins on the purple flowers • used medicinally as milky sap from stems and seeds • magically use the seeds and dried flowers

PLANET AND ELEMENT

Mars • Fire

MAGICAL USES

defensive of animals or pets, pregnant women, mothers, babies, and children because of its link with the Virgin Mary • it is told that Mary was feeding baby Jesus in the shelter of thistles when her milk fell on the plants, spotting them forever white • increases maternal love and nurturing • can be grown as part of a protective garden and to heal polluted land

HOW TO USE

Carry the empowered dried flowerheads or seeds in a charm bag as a curse- and hex-breaker and to induce fertility. • To banish addictions and bad habits, burn as incense with any or all of mullein, frankincense, hyssop, sandalwood, and chicory, or carry as a protective sachet. • The dried flowers can also be carried to reduce sadness or hung high in the nursery in a safe place to keep a new parent devoted to the family and to prevent straying.

CAUTION

Avoid ingesting in pregnancy and if breastfeeding, though some sources say it increases breast milk (consult your physician).

Thistle, Star

(*Centaurea solstitialis*)

MAGICAL FORMS

also called St. Barnabus's thistle • bushy wildflower with beautiful yellow flowers • growing two to three feet tall with sharp bracts protecting the flowers and spiny stems • native to Europe, especially the Mediterranean, and also Asia • introduced into Australia, Argentina, Chile, and western North America, where it has become invasive, though a valuable pollinator and restorative for the soil • rare in the UK except in Kent • magically use the whole plant, chopped and dried, including the spines, and flower essence

PLANET AND ELEMENT

Sun • Fire

MAGICAL USES

St. Barnabas, the first-century saint who founded the Cypriot Orthodox Church, sold all his worldly goods and is known as an icon of generosity • the plant flowers around his saint's day, June 11 • the plant and flower essence overcome fears of not having sufficient resources, causing the withholding of money, praise, and affection • encourages generosity and the ability to receive from others, which many givers find difficult

HOW TO USE

Use the essence in water or under your tongue if you are raising money for charity, if you are trying to persuade a partner to be more open with their resources and affection, or if you find it hard to accept gifts and praise from others. • Star thistle is a fiercely defensive plant, especially protective against storms, fire, and danger. • Burn whole plants or the chopped, dried leaves with thorns in an outside fire, especially on any sun festival or seasonal change point.

CAUTION

The plant is toxic to humans, pets, horses, and livestock.

Thunder God Vine

(*Tripterygium wilfordii*)

MAGICAL FORMS

also called Lei Gong Teng • a climbing vine growing in the Chinese mountains and in Myanmar • white flowers and red, three-winged fruit • magically substitute a less toxic white flower in a dedicated space in the home or use a printout of the plant's image—thunder god vine is not safe to handle and should not be used physically

PLANETS AND ELEMENTS

Jupiter/Mars • Air/Fire

MAGICAL USES

dedicated to thunder and storm deities found in different cultures, including the Chinese Lei Gong, who carried a drum and mallet to produce thunder and hurled thunderbolts at those who wasted food • depicted with a blue body, bat wings, and claws • can be honored more benignly from his original avenging role to protect the innocent and vulnerable

HOW TO USE

Thunder god vine is not a safe plant to have around, but a statue and/or printout of the Chinese deity and the plant can be substituted to keep vulnerable family members safe on journeys and to protect the home against lightning strikes, floods, and thunderbolts. • Create a special space for the statue and/or deity or plant image printout with offerings of nontoxic white flowers, lighted white candles, and dragon's blood or any spice incense, especially on Thursday, which is the day of thunder gods, or before a hazardous journey, in the Chinese thunder god's special indoor space.

CAUTION

The leaves, flowers, outer skin of the root, and the honey are poisonous. • The Chinese folk name for the vine is "walk seven steps and die."

Thyme

(*Thymus vulgaris*)

MAGICAL FORMS

herbaceous plant often grown for culinary use • magically use the dried and fresh herb and flowers

PLANET AND ELEMENT

Venus • Water

MAGICAL USES

ability to see nature spirits • anti-curse • clairvoyance • clairsentience • courage • good health, especially in older people • healing • increasing charisma and attracting love • peaceful sleep • lasting prosperity • renewed energy • to counteract IRS or taxation problems • for success on tests and examinations, especially driving tests • smudging • water scrying

HOW TO USE

Add thyme to charm bags. • Grow empowered protective pots of thyme in hostile workplaces. • Grow outside as part of a prosperity garden. • Use in Mother Earth rituals for restoring despoiled and threatened land. • Use in purifying baths (especially with marjoram, see p. 283). • Put thyme in a sleep pillow to prevent nightmares or for prophetic dreams. • Use infusions or teas to cleanse a ritual area or home with bad atmosphere, purifying artifacts containing bad or sad energies and removing paranormal energies.

CAUTION

Thyme is generally considered safe; in excess it can cause skin allergies.

Thyme, Lemon

(*Thymus × citriodorus*)

MAGICAL FORMS

culinary herb, native to the Mediterranean basin • grows well in many states of the USA, Europe, the UK, and Asia • small and woody with clusters of tiny, pale-pink flowers • intense lemon fragrance • used medicinally, cosmetically, and in essential oil • magically use the growing yellowy-green plant in situ or in magical cookery, the fresh and dried leaves, and the oil

PLANETS AND ELEMENTS

Saturn/Mercury • Earth/Air

MAGICAL USES

prevents nightmares • gives awareness or visions of house guardians and protective house spirits • for success on tests or examinations, if you have previously failed or are studying later in life

HOW TO USE

Use the oil (gentler than conventional thyme oil) in a diffuser in your workspace or home if you are finding it hard to keep up with younger people. • Grow the plant in a pot and endow it with the confidence and energy you need for a new business after redundancy or early retirement by surrounding it with a square of burning tea lights. • Bury a picture of your front door in the pot if you want to attract customers to a home-based business and welcome prosperity to your home. • Inhale as you drink lemon thyme tea (mixed, if you wish, with green tea) to increase your psychic awareness before divination, especially if using psychometry (psychic touch).

CAUTION

Dilute the oil well if applying to the skin, and be cautious if you have a hormone-related condition. • Avoid the oil in pregnancy.

Thyme, Orange Balsam

a variety of (*Thymus vulgaris*)

MAGICAL FORMS

gray-green leaves with scent of oranges and balsam • most fragrant just before flowering (though smells more of orange than of balsam) • fresh or dried pink or white flowers • orangelo thyme is another newer variety of thyme that has a similar scent and benefits • magically use the whole, growing plant; cut or dried herb; and as tea using the dried leaves

PLANET AND ELEMENT

Sun • Fire

MAGICAL USES

increases self-esteem • sense of well-being • for rituals, especially for fertility when anxiety blocks manifestation • a combination of the confidence and joy of orange, the healing and invigorating energies of balsam, and the prosperity and focus of thyme

HOW TO USE

Grow orange balsam thyme or orangelo thyme in your garden or kitchen pot garden or add the dried herb to potpourri to remove lethargy and inability to act on plans and to counteract negative, sluggish Earth energies beneath the home or workplace. • Drink the tea for the incentive and drive to put plans into motion, especially for business, or to embark on a long training leading to eventual rewards and status. • Carry the dried leaves in a charm bag for the motivation to complete tedious but necessary tasks and inspire others. • Use as a charm for late blooming love when relatives cast doubts on motives and advisability, especially where money is concerned.

CAUTION

Thyme is regarded generally as safe in amounts used to flavor food, but avoid if you are suffering from hormone-related conditions.

Ti Plant

(*Cordyline terminalis*)

MAGICAL FORMS

also called the good luck plant, or Ki in Hawaii • tropical plant with colorful, palmlike leaves, growing outdoors up to ten feet in the Hawaiian Islands and tropical zones of the USA and the world, including Asia, Australia, and the Pacific Islands • popular as a houseplant in more temperate areas • magically use the whole, growing plant; smooth, swordlike leaves; and, in spring, the small, star-shaped, fragrant flowers, fresh or dried, though the plant rarely blooms indoors

PLANET AND ELEMENT

Jupiter • Fire

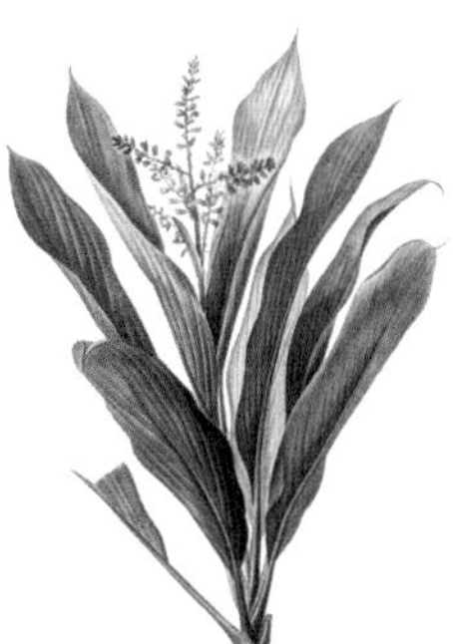

MAGICAL USES

for all sea journeys, hazards, and fears on, in, or over water, as well as for vacations overseas • for good fortune, placed on altars • leaves can be used to wrap sacred offerings (traditionally left at Hawaiian *heiau* temples)

HOW TO USE

Green-leafed ti plants, outdoors or as houseplants, form a protective barrier against human malice and mind control, paranormal entities, psychic attack, and intrusion. • Many practitioners consider the red-leafed variety to be unlucky. These can be shredded and buried or cast in the ocean to break curses or when fierce defense is needed. • Dried green leaves or blossoms, sealed in a purple bag, are hung inside the bedroom door or over the bed to drive away nightmares. • Place five coins beneath an indoor ti plant pot to grow wealth, where there is bright but indirect sunlight. • Ti plants are considered to contain guardian spirits and so are used shamanically to heal and retrieve soul loss when part of the self needs to be restored to bring back health.

CAUTION

Ti is moderately toxic to pets. • Do not ingest the raw plant. • The growing plant should be kept away from small children. • Use caution if pregnant.

Tienchi

(*Panax notoginseng*)

MAGICAL FORMS

also called Chinese ginseng or sanchi • flower grows wild only in the Yunnan and Guang Xi Provinces of China, with tiny green buds that are harvested every three years • very rare and expensive • found in specialty tea stores, Asian culinary stores, and online • the dried flowers, resembling small broccoli heads, are sold as loose tea • the roots are used in Chinese medicine • magically use the buds, dried flowers as tea, and roots

PLANET AND ELEMENT

Venus • Water

MAGICAL USES

as tea before meditation, spiritually uplifting • as an antidote to a 24/7 frantic lifestyle • for triggering self-healing processes and reducing stress

HOW TO USE

Drink the tea, empowering it as you stir it, with the power to calm yourself or share with others who are confrontational, hyperactive, or workaholics. • Carry the root in a charm bag to give you the strength and focus to deal with chaotic situations or to make snap decisions when the outcome is crucial. • The dried tea (must be kept dry) can be added to a small, sealed jar in the kitchen to prevent accidents caused by being hasty and careless.

CAUTION

Avoid if pregnant or suffering from diabetes or heavy menstruation.

Tobacco

(*Nicotiana tabacum*)

MAGICAL FORMS

also flowering or white tobacco (*Nicotiana sylvestris*) • shrubs with long, tubular flowers in white, pink, purple, yellow, and green, blooming from summer to the fall, opening in the evening and at night, releasing an incense-like fragrance • *Nicotiana sylvestris* has flowers like shooting stars • for this reason, tobacco flowers are grown in gardens in warm places ornamentally, as well as cultivated for the leaves commercially as *Nicotiana tabacum* for cigarettes • indigenous to the Americas and the tropics, but now grown worldwide • for safety, magically use tobacco-based fragrances; they are remarkably fragrance- and incense-like and do not smell of cigarettes

PLANET AND ELEMENT

Mars • Fire

MAGICAL USES

used shamanically, especially in South America and by some North American nations to bring visions of spirits • for astral travel and ceremonially in peace ceremonies • however, in the modern world the toxic and addictive effects of tobacco used socially, such as *Nicotiana tabacum*, have deterred many magical practitioners from inhaling tobacco or using it in incense

HOW TO USE

The crushed flowers, leaves, or blossoms can be scattered in flowing water before a hazardous journey and to prevent nightmares, especially paranormal ones. • Anoint your Third Eye in the center of your brow with any tobacco-based fragrance before meditation to connect with the spirit world or before automatic writing if you seek to receive written messages through your hand being allowed to write freely, guided by a beloved ancestor.

Tomato

(*Solanum lycopersicum*)

MAGICAL FORMS

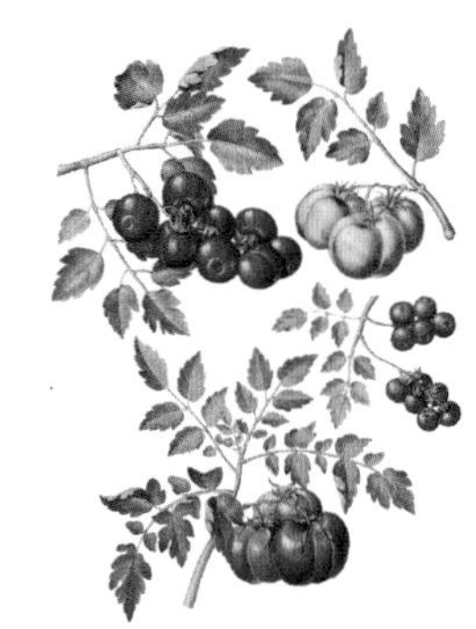

a branching vine with small, five-petaled, yellow flowers becoming green berries that ripen into red, yellow, purple, and orange fruits • the world's most popular fruit • native to Peru, and introduced to Europe in the sixteenth century by Spanish colonists where tomatoes were first grown as ornamentals and the eighteenth century by Italian settlers to the USA • especially adopted into Italian and Spanish cuisine and cultivated worldwide • harvested July through the fall • magically use the fruit raw and cooked, as well as on the vine

PLANETS AND ELEMENTS

Venus/Sun • Water/Fire

MAGICAL USES

tomatoes were once called *pommes d'amour*, love apples • the love connection remained in Europe until the beginning of the twentieth century, to be replaced by a more general meaning of health and money and for wise investments • an aphrodisiac when combined with arugula (see p. 35)

HOW TO USE

Place a ripening tomato on the window ledge to keep sickness from the home, and add one to a shelf near a heat source or a fireplace for ongoing prosperity. • Eat raw tomatoes for fertility and abundance. • A dish of tomatoes at different stages of ripeness on the kitchen table, replaced regularly, brings good fortune and calls family members home in harmony. • Tomatoes are twice as lucky if grown in the garden or as indoor tomato plants and used when ripe in family meals.

Tomato Sauce and Ketchup

MAGICAL FORMS

made from the tomato • the sauce, even if pure tomato, takes on a meaning different from the pure, whole tomato, through its creation • you can, if making a sauce at home, add ingredients to endow the tomatoes with the extra qualities you need; for example garlic for protection or the grounding and calming effects of pasta • tomato sauces are eaten extensively throughout Europe, especially Italy, France, and Spain, and in North America and Mexico • worldwide, tomatoes are made into ketchup as a condiment • ketchup is made from tomatoes, sugar, vinegar, salt, and spices, including allspice, onions, garlic, and mustard, and so offers enthusiasm, energy, and goodwill to the eater • magically empower your ketchup for bringing laughter and happiness and tomato sauces for unity and blending people and situations

PLANET AND ELEMENT

Venus • Water

MAGICAL USES

especially if homemade, both tomato sauce and ketchup can be used for making positive changes in life • for fun, leisure, and spontaneous events, and spur-of-the-moment decisions, especially in love, family matters, or finances • in a fast-food outlet, the tomato ketchup sachets can be empowered by holding them and speaking wishes in your mind

HOW TO USE

When you obtain a new bottle of ketchup, hold the bottle between your hands and fill it with images of previous and anticipated good times and experiences, goodwill, and optimism. • If there has been a family quarrel or whenever you feel those using it are downbeat or irritable, empower the bottle by lighting a red candle next to it for a few minutes so the light reflects into the contents. • With a sauce, whether homemade or commercially produced, stir it clockwise before serving, saying, *Mix and blend, bring loyalty and unity and a harmonious mealtime send.*

Tormentil

(*Potentilla erecta*)

MAGICAL FORMS

creeping, usually wild plant, covered with down and many four-petaled, yellow flowers • grows May to September • native to temperate regions of Asia, the UK, and Europe and introduced to eastern parts of North America • magically use the aerial parts, especially the dried leaves; fresh and dried flowers; and dried root

PLANETS AND ELEMENTS

Mercury/Sun • Air/Fire

MAGICAL USES

the dried, trimmed root as a wand offers protection when practicing mediumship • keeps evil entities from the home when the dried aerial plant is hung over the doorway woven on a circlet of wire, tied with white twine, and replaced when it fades or becomes ragged • the fresh flowers in the garden or cut in the home (dried to last, if desired, when out of season) encourage enduring faithful love

HOW TO USE

Make an infusion and sprinkle around tarot cards, runes, or any other divinatory tools before and after use. • Keep a dried sprig wrapped in white silk with your crystal ball so that it will allow its inner spirit to speak. • Use the root, which usually has one to three branches at the larger end and is the width of a person's finger, as a dowsing rod. • Hold the root by the opposite end to the branches, horizontally, to detect subterranean energy lines in the home and on land and to find lost items or buried minerals when the root dips down and vibrates.

Trailing Arbutus

(*Epigaea repens*)

MAGICAL FORMS

also called Mayflower • trailing ground plant, with small white early spring flowers • native to woodlands in the eastern half of North America and west up to northwestern Canada • introduced to Europe and the UK sometime before the Victorian era, where it was originally given religious significance • magically use the dried flowers, a fragrant item for spell bags, or the chopped and dried flowers and leaves

PLANET AND ELEMENT

Saturn • Earth

MAGICAL USES

of significance to the Ottawa Indigenous people who tell in a version of an old legend: the spring maiden, when winter would not give way to spring, transformed Manito, god of winter, into the white spring flower, a sign for the Pilgrim Fathers that the better weather was coming • official flower of Massachusetts and the province of Nova Scotia • flower of loving devotion to one person • for weddings and births, adult baptisms, religious initiation rites

HOW TO USE

Mix the cut fresh flowers with larger white flowers in a bouquet for someone dedicating themselves in a religious or spiritual ceremony, such as an adult baptism, confirmation, or bar mitzvah/bat mitzvah. • Keep the dried flowers as part of a charm bag with other dried spring flowers for new beginnings after a loss or setback or a long illness, until the fragrance fades.

CAUTION

the plant is nontoxic but not to be ingested, including the white berries. It is not commonly used medicinally.

Treasure Flower

(*Gazania rigens*)

MAGICAL FORMS

also called the gazania • cousin to the Gerbera daisy and the African daisy • called "the treasure flower of South Africa" because of its rich, glowing colors including gleaming gold, orange, and white, and in other forms red or with mixed or striped colors • native to South Africa and the southwestern tip of Africa • an ornamental plant that thrives in warm places, in a pot indoors, or brought indoors during the winter in cooler areas • naturalized in the Mediterranean regions of Europe, the UK, parts of the USA, and Australia • magically use the whole plant growing in gardens, pots, containers, or hanging baskets; cut flowers; and fresh and dried flowerheads (with intact disk florets at the center)

PLANET AND ELEMENT

Sun • Fire

MAGICAL USES

for exotic beachside weddings, congratulatory bouquets, and a way of saying *I treasure you/your company* • for the twenty-third (silver plate or imperial topaz) wedding anniversary, particularly appropriate with its silvery-green foliage, often tinged with blue • a symbol of and focus for rituals for prosperity and good fortune

HOW TO USE

Grow the plant in a garden or in a pot at home or at work to attract wealth, recognition, and good fortune. • Tape a sachet of dried petals to the back of any precious artifacts or a jewelry box to keep them safe. • Since the flowers close at night or if overcast, carry out a two-part evening and morning ritual near the flowers for a return to health or of lost fortunes. • Bury a golden crystal in a waterproof bag in the soil beneath the closing flower (ideally a small golden topaz or golden citrine) to be dug up and carried in the morning through the day, repeating the ritual for a week.

CAUTION

Ingesting these flowers may trigger gastrointestinal problems, so seek medical advice before doing so.

Trillium

(*Trillium* spp.)

MAGICAL FORMS

a member of the lily family • grown over much of the USA and temperate parts of Asia, with more than forty species, thirty native to the USA and ten in Asia • magically use the cut or whole, growing plant, with three wavy leaves backing three petals; root or rhizome, usually unearthed after the leaves fall; and petals and leaves, not usually used separately because splitting them might damage the plant

PLANET AND ELEMENTS

Saturn • Earth/Air

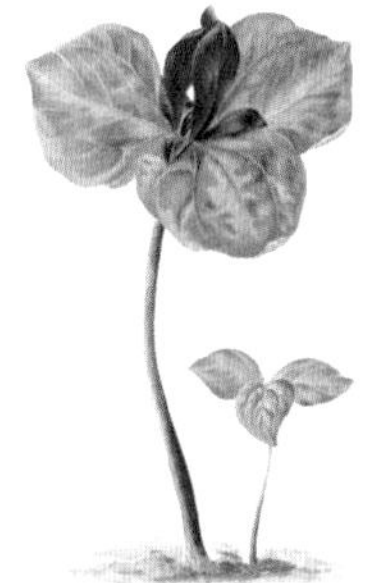

MAGICAL USES

for working magically and spiritually with threes for rites of passage: the Christian Trinity, the three phases of the moon, and the Maiden, Mother, and Wisewoman stages • the root or three dried flowers still on leaves, used as a charm to attract money, luck, and love • for formal magick where precision is needed • in spells to improve accuracy for detailed complex tasks • the first sightings of the growing plant wild or increasingly in gardens is regarded as a sign of spring and a time for new beginnings and wishes • to some Native Americans and western practitioners, the first sighting is an occasion for offerings to the Earth Mother, who gives her lifeblood to protect her people

HOW TO USE

Use empowerments, holding your hands around but not touching trillium, to absorb its unique spiritual powers. • The growing cut or dried plant or root brings courage and the power to thrive in difficult situations. • The large, white, flowered trillium, state emblem of Ontario and Ohio, with its yellow center representing the sun, overcomes fears and panic. • Trillium brings balance and strengthens the awareness of being a spiritual being in a physical body.

CAUTION

Roots and berries may be toxic if ingested. • Do not take while pregnant without consulting with a medical expert.

Trillium, Red

(*Trillium erectum*)

MAGICAL FORMS

the source of a powerful ingredient in spellwork called Dixie John, Southern John, or beth root • used for hundreds of years by Indigenous people and called the birth (beth) root because it was used to assist labor • red trillium is a flowering wildflower plant, with a single, maroon-white or yellow-white flower blooming April to May and upright stem • an earthy, slightly acrid smell • foliage dies back in late spring • native to eastern North America, especially Kentucky, Indiana, Tennessee, and Ohio, but can grow in the UK and Europe • magically use the rhizome and root, harvested in the fall • the root can be bought commercially whole, shredded, or chopped from magick and specialty herbal stores and online

PLANET AND ELEMENT

Mars • Fire

MAGICAL USES

marriage proposals • passion • making you irresistible to a lover • good fortune

HOW TO USE

Carry a whole root in a green charm bag to bring you luck, especially in love. • Knot nine long root hairs and add dried violet leaves, dried rose petals, and dried yarrow leaves in a charm bag hung over your bed to keep a love faithful. • Add Southern or Dixie John root to High and Little or Low John the Conqueror (galangal) roots in less positive magick to control another person against their will by using emotional manipulation. • If you suspect you are being psychologically or psychically compelled, break a root into pieces with a knife or another implement with an iron blade, then bury the pieces at the end of a dead-end road.

CAUTION

Red trillium is not recommended to be ingested during pregnancy without strict supervision and for others only to be ingested with caution, though the leaves are considered edible. • The root may cause skin irritation.

Tuberose

(*Polianthes tuberosa*)

MAGICAL FORMS

flowering perennial plant • magically use the whole, growing plant; white, waxy flowers that bloom at night, fresh and dried; flower essence; and oil, which is very expensive and sometimes blended with jasmine, frankincense, or sandalwood

PLANET AND ELEMENT

Moon • Water

MAGICAL USES

night and moon magick (called the Night Queen for this reason) • reconciliation • messages from ancestors • as an aphrodisiac • for receiving news and reconnection, especially from overseas • sexual ecstasy • as the creamy double-flowered variety called the Pearl, twin soul connections • flower psychometry

HOW TO USE

Anoint red candles with the oil (diluted in almond oil) before lighting the candles for increased passion, to call a twin soul, and for sex magick. • Burn the oil in the bedroom before a lover arrives. • Anoint pink candles for romance. • In a diffuser, the oil (or, alternatively, a vase of the flowers) will open the barriers between dimensions for meditation, divination, and contact with the ancestors. • Send a beautiful, single- or double-flowering tuberose to rekindle a love affair with a simple message of devotion. • Use an international delivery service and order a bouquet containing tuberose if your love is far away. • Anoint your brow with a fragrance containing tuberose or, alternatively, inhale the flower to draw the opportunities for bringing wealth into your life through your own talents.

CAUTION

Tuberose is mildly toxic if ingested. • Take expert advice before using if you are pregnant or have a chronic condition.

Tulip

(*Tulipa* spp.)

MAGICAL FORMS

of Byzantine and Turkish origin (tulip means *turban*, and they were traditionally worn on turbans for power and protection) • the design appeared on Byzantine pottery as far back as 2000 BCE and spread across Europe, especially to Holland, in the medieval period when tulip bulbs were at one time valued more highly than gems, eventually becoming the national flower • tulips are the flower most sold in the USA (175 million tulip stems were sold in 2022) • tulips arrived in the USA with traders from Turkey in the sixteenth century and were fully established by the first Dutch settlers • magically use the growing plant, indoors and out; cut flowers, fresh and dried; petals; and flower essence

PLANET AND ELEMENT

Venus • Earth

MAGICAL USES

pink or white tulips for finding the perfect lover • red for acknowledging commitment • yellow for unrequited love • also a powerful fertility symbol • white to conceive a child • red for a safe pregnancy and healthy infant • yellow for blessings on parents and child after the birth

HOW TO USE

Give or send pink tulips as a flirtation when you want the other person to make the first move. • Grow tulips in a garden to attract peace, abundance, and prosperity. • Hold a white or purple tulip at a 45-degree angle an inch or so from your body, then pass it a few centimeters around your head and the front of your body to cleanse your aura energy field of the doubts, criticisms, and inadequacies others have loaded upon you. • Whenever you are exhausted or dispirited, breathe more slowly and deeply than usual while placing your hands, palms flat and fingers pointing downward, above cut or growing tulips. Continue to slow your normal breathing rhythm and inhale the life force of the tulip, using a soft color for calm and a vibrant one for vitality. • Visualize yourself exhaling misty, gray light to be absorbed by Mother Earth. Afterward, thank your tulip(s) with extra care.

CAUTION

Tulip bulbs are toxic to humans and pets if ingested.

Tulip Tree

(*Liodendron* spp.)

MAGICAL FORMS

includes the American tulip tree (*Liriodendron tulipifera*) and Chinese tulip tree (*Liriodendron chinensis*) • the American tulip tree has flowers with yellow-orange stamens that are upright and tulip-shaped all over the tree, fading on the tree as the leaves turn butter yellow (the Chinese variety are a paler yellow) before falling • among the oldest flowering trees on earth, the tulip tree lived in Europe before dying out in the last ice age • fossils from the tree were first discovered seventy to a hundred million years ago • it now flourishes in eastern North America from Ontario to Florida • introduced into Britain in 1688 • in London's Kew Gardens, a tree planted in 1770 is still thriving • the Chinese tree, native to China and Vietnam, where it grows on mountain slopes, was introduced into Europe in 1901 • magically use the whole, growing tree, especially in flower; dried tulip-like flowers; and leaves

PLANET AND ELEMENT

Venus • Earth

MAGICAL USES

connection with the ancestors and past lives, transition into the unknown • accessing psychically the wisdom of the past

HOW TO USE

Gently shake the seed pods containing the seeds or the loose seeds in a gourd or rattle to induce a light trance to link with your own past lives, the world of your ancestors, and ancient times, with a message for you or images in your mind, relevant to your present life. • Because they contain the energies of the ancient trees, cast the dried, fallen flowers and/or the leaves as they change color and start to fall onto a bonfire to welcome the darker days and to release what did not work out or projects and situations that must lie fallow for a few months until spring returns.

CAUTION

All parts of the tulip tree are poisonous to ingest.

Turmeric

(*Curcuma longa*)

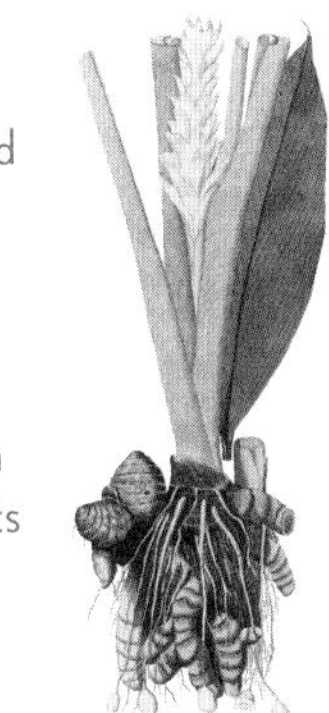

MAGICAL FORMS

an all-healer herb belonging to the ginger family • native to the Indian subcontinent and Southeast Asia • grows in warmer climates in the USA such as Hawaii and California • used in Ayurvedic medicine and cookery for thousands of years • magically use the rhizome or roots, which can be bought from specialty grocery stores and in supermarkets as the yellow culinary spice

PLANET AND ELEMENT

Mars • Fire

MAGICAL USES

detoxing • energizing • enhanced memory • for acquiring wealth and recognition • connection with Mother Earth • for rituals easing transitions of womanhood • the spice is popular in Hawaiian magick for purification • make restorative tea using the powder or chopped roots, often with a cinnamon stick, lemon, and milk • for flavoring food in magical cookery

HOW TO USE

Stir into food or drink the tea, again stirring it while stating its specific purpose related to drawing health and prosperity into your life. • Sprinkle the liquid tea or the powder mixed with salt and pepper in a circle outdoors to create protection around you when carrying out banishing rituals to break curses and ill wishes. • Cut the rhizome into small pieces in a dish during the ritual and cast as far as possible outside the circle at the four directions, while standing within, saying, *Banished be, your power destroyed* [name if you know the perpetrator], *henceforth your malice I do avoid.* Beware sprinkling the powder on indoor surfaces, as it stains. • Hang an individual root in a bright-yellow charm bag on the outside of a drain pipe so every time water passes down inside the pipe, your turmeric amulet clears your home of all malevolent influences, sickness, and misfortune.

CAUTION

Check with a physician before ingesting if you are taking regular medication for chronic conditions.

Turnip

(*Brassica rapa* var. *rapa*)

MAGICAL FORMS

an edible root vegetable, the swollen base of the stem • generally white on bottom and purple on top • originally wild in northern Europe spreading to Asia, though spindly there instead of round • mentioned by Pliny, the first-century BCE philosopher, as one of the most important cultivated vegetables • earlier than the potato, turnips were the staple diet of the poor • planted by colonists in Virginia around 1609 and in Massachusetts in the 1620s • adopted by the Native Americans • now used mainly in regional cooking in the south of the USA as turnip greens, though increasingly popular again organically produced in cool temperate regions • magically use the whole, uncooked turnip or peeled and cooked turnip

PLANET AND ELEMENT

Saturn • Earth

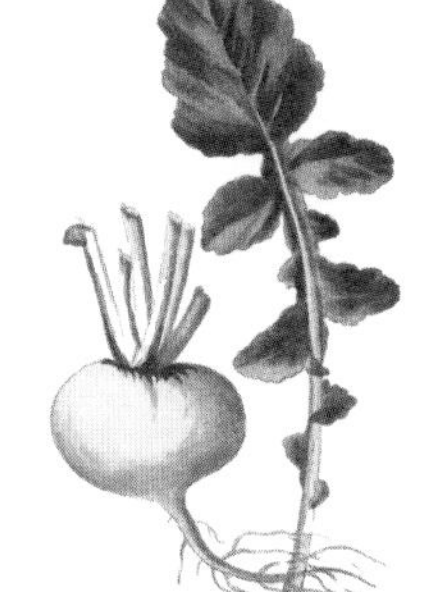

MAGICAL USES

primarily a symbol of protection and removing what is not productive from our lives to make room for what is • forerunner to the Halloween pumpkin, hollowed out and candles lit inside, placed in windows and on either side of the door to scare away the restless spirits believed to walk on this night and welcome the ancestors • Irish immigrants in the USA replaced them with the more readily available Halloween pumpkin • in folklore, seventh-century saint, St. Botolph is called "the old turnip man" and is patron saint of farmers • he drove evil spirits from the marshlands of Suffolk (East Anglia) and drained the swamps so they could be cultivated, presumably with crops including turnips

HOW TO USE

Add to cooked dishes to prepare for a gentle ending whether involving a relationship or any natural transition such as retirement or adult children leaving home. • Keep a whole turnip in a vegetable rack in the kitchen to absorb danger or malice, prevent accidents, and protect the home. When it goes soft, bury it away from the home or add to compost.

Tweedia

(*Oxypetalum coeruleum*) or (*Tweedia coeruleum*)

MAGICAL FORMS

known as blue tweedia or blue milkweed • blue or white, star-shaped flowers that scramble and weakly twine • native to Brazil and Uruguay but grown increasingly in North America • magically use the cut or whole, growing plant with its heart-shaped leaves and fresh and dried blossoms

PLANET AND ELEMENT

Jupiter • Air

MAGICAL USES

a candidate for the bridal superstition to carry *something blue* as a promise that love will be true • also used for wedding venue decorations and boutonnieres • small, so not overpowering, but signifies unfolding step by step lasting happiness and harmony • very popular for DIY wedding bouquets and weddings or handfastings • for butterfly (though not the monarch butterfly like other North American milkweeds) and bee magick • for Star Souls and connection with Light Beings from other dimensions and angelic powers

HOW TO USE

If you have access to a wall-climbing tweedia plant, meditate on it as an upward path to astrally project yourself to other dimensions. • Also work with the cut flowers, their five petals forming a star, moving in your mind along a fragrant blue pathway to connect with your guardian angel. • Dry five flowers and carry them in a blue bag to interviews, auditions, performances, and any attempts to attain fame and fortune, using the petals for one occasion only, saying in your mind five times, *Five times five, my power is alive*. Afterward, replace them, returning the spent ones to the earth.

CAUTION

Tweedia produces mildly toxic sap that should not be ingested. • Some people cauterize the stems before use for this reason, but others believe this hurts the flower magically.

Ugli Fruit

(*Citrus × tangelo*)

MAGICAL FORMS

also known as the Jamaican tangelo • fruit grown on a unique form of the evergreen tangelo tree, growing fifteen to twenty feet tall • originally found in Jamaica • white, fragrant flowers, producing fruit that is a cross between a Seville orange, grapefruit, and tangerine • sweet, tangy, and aromatic • teardrop shaped, with a wrinkled, pitted, yellow-greenish skin and juicy flesh • cultivated in the USA in Arizona and southern Florida, but will grow in climates similar to southern California and indoors or under glass in cooler climates • seasonal from December to April, ugli fruit is sold in the USA, Europe, and the UK between November and April and sometimes from July to September • magically use the whole, growing tree and the fruit

PLANETS AND ELEMENT

Saturn/Venus • Earth

MAGICAL USES

eating the fruit brings to the fore hidden talents and success that puts any detractor in their place • for confidence in situations where glamor and appearance are valued over character and expertise • for protection if social media trolls victimize anyone visually, emotionally, or physically different

HOW TO USE

Eat ugli fruit before going into an environment to defy any who try to make you feel inferior or unattractive. • Because ugli fruit is unique, from a tree created by accident from two different species, add the fruit to desserts when you are introducing new stepfamilies to each other or when people from different religious, ethnic, or cultural backgrounds need to understand the others' points of view and live or work together.

CAUTION

If you are on medication, check with your physician before ingesting.

Unicorn Root, False

(*Chamaelirium luteum*)

MAGICAL FORMS

also called the helonias root • flowering plant growing up to three feet tall with large, green leaves forming a basal rosette from which grows a tall, packed spike of yellow-green flowers on a long, thin stalk (see also "Unicorn Root, True," p. 458) • wild but increasingly rare and difficult to cultivate • growing east of the Mississippi basin, in other southern states in the USA, and eastern Canada • magically use the roots and bulbous rhizome, which terminates suddenly into small, pale, wiry roots • the rhizome or roots, generally dried whole, can be bought already shredded or as powder online, ideal for instant spells and amulets

PLANET AND ELEMENT

Moon • Water

MAGICAL USES

male potency, fertility, pregnancy • stability in relationships • getting in touch with the cycles of the moon • an aphrodisiac charm hidden in the bedroom • prevents trickery and scams, especially romantic and financial • uncovering dishonesty

HOW TO USE

Use the dried rhizome and attached roots as a central focus in rituals with the full moon shining on it, to call fertility. Cast the whole root system into running water after the ritual. • Use chopped or shredded root in knotted white silk as an amulet for a safe pregnancy. • Burn the powder in an incense with juniper berries and dragon's blood resin or another fragrant resin, when you are questioning the honesty of a person or the genuine nature of an offer or deal. The answer will come, either immediately as an image in the smoke or your mind or in a dream.

CAUTION

Avoid ingesting during pregnancy or while breastfeeding and, if making an amulet, handle the rhizome or roots with great care. • Avoid ingesting if receiving conventional hormone treatment.

Unicorn Root, True

(*Aletris farinosa*)

MAGICAL FORMS

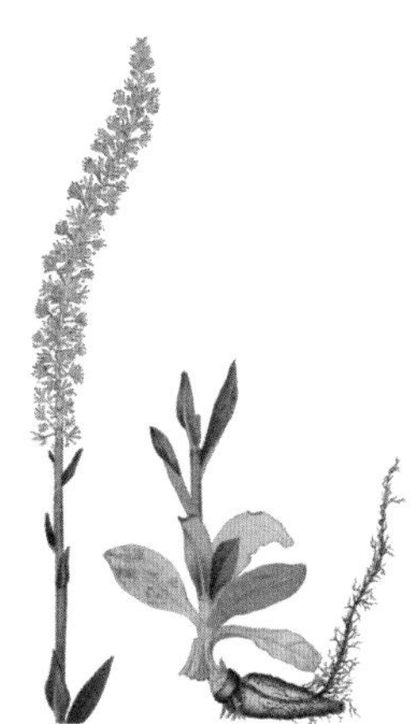

also called star grass • found in eastern North America, the southern part of Ontario, Southeast Asia, and China, wild and cultivated • an erect, round stem with rounded basal leaves near the base angled above like a unicorn horn, with a long spike of tubular, white flowers that appear to be covered in frost • magically use the dried root, stem, and dried leaves (with care as the leaves are spiky) • the leaves and root can be bought shredded or as a powder online • see also "Unicorn Root, False" (p. 457)

PLANET AND ELEMENT

Moon • Water

MAGICAL USES

astral projection • psychic dreaming • connection with magical animals • protection of young and teenage girls

HOW TO USE

If you are seeking your twin soul, hold the dried root or stripped stem in full moonlight like a wand and face the moon for flashes of insight into past worlds when you and your love have been together before and to call them across time. • The root is often used as a protective amulet, hung safely in a new infant's bedroom. • A decoction made from the root, sprinkled daily around a teenager's photo, offers a psychic shield if they are suffering bullying at school or undue sexual pressures.

CAUTION

Do not ingest or use topically if taking any medications that slow the nervous system, if you are pregnant or breastfeeding, or if you have stomach or intestinal disorders. • Use only in small quantities. • The fresh root is toxic if ingested.

Valerian

(*Valeriana officinalis*)

MAGICAL FORMS

perennial flowering plant • magically use the whole, growing plant; flowers; and oil

PLANET AND ELEMENT

Venus • Mercury

MAGICAL USES

love and love divination • dreams of a lover, known or unknown • reconciliation when relationships are parted by anger or circumstance • peaceful sleep • purification of home and any sacred space before ritual • protection against all harm to the home and family from earthly or paranormal sources

HOW TO USE

Worn in love sachets or carried as a sprig in a small, green drawstring bag, valerian can be used as a charm to attract lovers, the fresh plant replaced when it dries and loses fragrance. • Hang in the home above doorways or at windows to prevent lightning strikes, and to stop evil spirits and earthly intruders from entering. • Incense blends and oil diffusers attract animal spirits and power animals; mixed with catnip, they are effective for all cat spells. • Poppets filled with the dried herb and loosely tied face to face can mend quarrels with lovers or keep links with a lover far away. • Grow in the garden to create an aura of peace in the home and family.

CAUTION

Beware driving after working with the herb, as valerian can make you drowsy. • Do not use for prolonged periods, as valerian can cause depression.

Venus Flytrap

(*Dionaea muscipula*)

MAGICAL FORMS

a carnivorous fly- and small-insect-eating houseplant • *muscipula* is Latin for mousetrap • the trap is formed by modified two-lipped, flat, lobe-like leaves connected by a hinge • inside the plant is the nectar that lures the insects • once the insect triggers the trap's sensitive hairs, the plant then closes to trap them • there can be eight traps—sometimes more—on the same plant • Venus, the Roman love goddess, refers to the lovely white flowers but also gives a warning that love can be deceiving and cruel • native to North and South Carolina, Venus flytrap is grown as a houseplant all over the world • can be kept outside in summer • magically use the whole, growing plant

PLANET AND ELEMENTS

Venus • Earth/Water

MAGICAL USES

protection from overpossessive or destructive lovers, or on the internet, from those who deny or hide existing commitments • positively, to attract what you most need

HOW TO USE

Keep the plant near the computer or your tablet or smartphone when connecting to internet dating sites and to become aware of romance as well as financial scams. • If your plant is closed and there are not a lot of insects around, take it as a warning to be careful of sudden temptations in love or risky financial enterprises. • Surround the plant with a circle of gold-colored coins to draw money into your life. • Set a photo of a car, property, or even a person you desire (given the restrictions of free will for a would-be lover) to call these into your life.

Veronica

(*Veronica officinalis*)

MAGICAL FORMS

also known as common speedwell • magically, American speedwell (*Veronica americana*) has similar effects • like many of the five hundred forms of *Veronica*, is native to North America as well as Asia • veronica grows wild or in gardens • many are characterized by the celestial blue color that gives the veronica the alternative names angel's eyes or Christ's eyes • petals may drop off after a few days in more delicate varieties, hence the name speedwell or farewell • magically use the whole, growing plant; cut, fresh or dried flowers; and petals

PLANET AND ELEMENT

Saturn • Earth

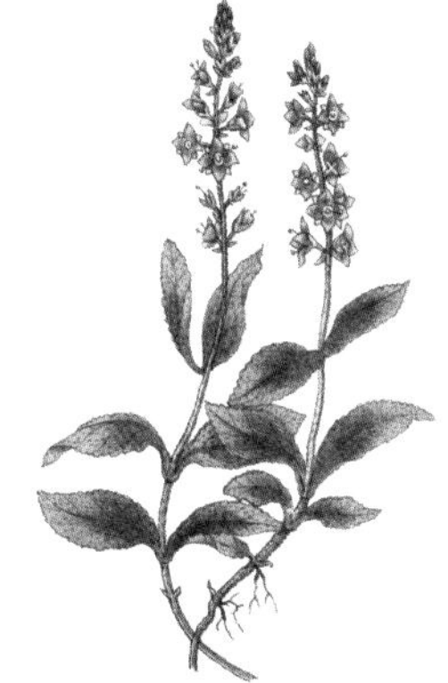

MAGICAL USES

healing • recovery from illness, because it was in times past considered an all-healer • house moves • the children's hymn "Daisies Are Our Silver" by Jan Struther in 1901 says, *While for shining sapphires we have the speedwell blue*, and so speedwell is regarded as one of nature's jewels • used in outdoor rituals or specially constructed nature altars for abundance when money is tight

HOW TO USE

The juice of veronica or speedwell is placed on eyelids to give psychic visions both of other worlds and of the realms of the fae. • Hold a large, celestial-blue flower or multiple flowers and gaze on them, or meditate on a growing bank of the smaller flowers. Superimposed in the aura around the flower or in your mind's vision, you may see the spiritual realms you most want to see. • Keep flowers on your altar or table where you practice divination to increase your clairvoyance and magical powers.

CAUTION

Do not consume while pregnant or breastfeeding.

Vervain

(*Verbena officinalis*)

MAGICAL FORMS

herbaceous perennial herb native to Europe • magically use the whole, growing plant; all aerial parts; and dried and fresh leaves and buds

PLANET AND ELEMENT

Venus • Earth

MAGICAL USES

often called the wizard's or druidic magical herb, vervain has been recognized for millennia for both attracting and defensive powers • for generating love that transforms enemies into friends and indifference into affection and warmth of feeling • financial security • preserves youthfulness • peaceful sleep • healing of fears and sorrows • protection • attracting the blessings of nature spirits and wights, who guard the land on which even urban homes are built

HOW TO USE

For protection from negativity against pets, weave into an amulet with pet hair and bury in the garden. • The herb is especially potent at midsummer when combined in a wreath with clover (see p. 127), St. John's wort (see p. 426), and dill (see p. 160) and hung on the front door; it is potent until it disintegrates. • When hung above a bed, dried vervain in a sachet keeps away nightmares, and in an infant's bedroom in a safe place promises both happiness and a lifelong love of learning. • Exchange with a friend or lover as a token of truth and faithfulness. • The dried plant tied in bunches is used to sweep a ritual area, and the infusion scattered as the Water element in rituals to recover what has been lost or stolen. • Vervain attracts money to the home or a business if planted near the entrance.

CAUTION

Vervain may cause vomiting in high doses and stimulate contractions of the womb, and so is not advisable in pregnancy.

Vetiver

(*Chrysopogon zizanioides*)

MAGICAL FORMS

also called vetivert • tall, clumping grass with very deep roots that are used medicinally • magically use the herb and essential oil

PLANET AND ELEMENT

Saturn • Earth

MAGICAL USES

brings good fortune, money, and necessary resources to the home and businesses • anti-theft • for finding new or self-employment • for all practical ventures, crafts, and hands-on skills • protective, growing in garden or pots in kitchen, against negativity and misfortune • love under difficulty

HOW TO USE

Keep a sachet of dried, fragrant roots with dollar bills to increase money. • Grow as part of a prosperity garden. • Burn as incense near lottery or other tickets for winning prizes. • Add to a charm bag to avoid misfortune. • Use the dried, chopped roots as an amulet in a bag hung outside the home on a tree or burned to overcome evil, or to deter thieves and break a hex or run of bad luck. • Place a sachet of dried leaves or roots in a cash register to improve business.

CAUTION

Do not use while pregnant, as it can bring on contractions. • Avoid if suffering from epilepsy or petit mal seizures. • Do not take the oil internally.

Vetiver, Bourbon

(*Vetiveria zizanioides* var. *Bourbon*)

MAGICAL FORMS

a grassy herb, Bourbon vetiver, though closely related to the more widely available vetiver, is found only on the island of Réunion, formerly known as Bourbon, a small tropical overseas territory of France in the Indian Ocean • sweeter, more subtle, and more refined than vetiver sourced in Haiti, India, and Indonesia, its roots provide essential oil and incense and are used in some perfumes • magically use as the incense, the oil, and in perfume

PLANET AND ELEMENT

Venus • Earth

MAGICAL USES

the oil as a sleep and relaxation aid in a diffuser with chamomile and sandalwood • as incense for astral travel and past-world experiences in meditation • the fragrance when you need to appear financially sound • Bourbon vetiver ointments are used to treat insect bites on the island of Réunion

HOW TO USE

In Réunion, its fragrance is called the *scent of money.* • Burn the oil or incense before speculating or applying for a favorable financial transaction. • Anoint your throat energy center at the base of the neck with any fragrance containing Bourbon vetiver when you have to use persuasion or negotiation for financial advantage or in a career interview or application for promotion.

CAUTION

When using the oil, dilute it well in coconut or jojoba carrier oil and carry out a patch test. • Do not use during pregnancy. • Avoid if suffering from epilepsy or petit mal seizures. • Do not take the oil internally.

Viola

(*Viola tricolor*)

MAGICAL FORMS

also known as Johnny jump up, heartsease, Jack-jump-up-and-kiss-me • close smaller relative of pansy • also called wild pansy, with five-petal blooms of purple, yellow, and white • the golden violet (*Viola pendulculata*) is found throughout California • magically use the whole, growing plant; cut flowers; or petals, fresh or dried

PLANET AND ELEMENTS

Venus • Water/Earth

MAGICAL USES

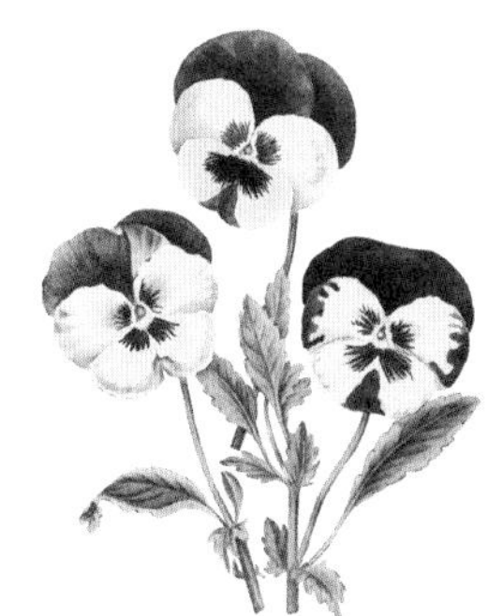

popular in Elizabethan gardens • in the language of flowers, it means *You fill my thoughts.* • Johnny (as in Johnny jump up) may well refer to Jack in the Green, who wooed the May Queen on May Day in the woodland wedding and fertility festival • use for love charms to fulfill unrequited love and prevent love temptations • for prosperity and good fortune

HOW TO USE

In magical cookery as *Viola tricolor*, it is an edible flower that can increase love, passion, and fertility if the food is shared by a couple, especially on May Day. • On any day, scatter the blossoms or dried flowers around the bed for romantic, gentle lovemaking if a lover is overly amorous. • To say goodbye to a love that cannot be or a destructive relationship, cast dried flowers into still waters and let them sink or remain motionless. • To replace them, buy or order any viola or violet flowers to plant or, if out of season, use the dried flowers in potpourri or incense mixed with rose petals and lavender heads to mark a new beginning.

Viola, Blue Elf

(*Viola tricolor* 'Blue Elf')

MAGICAL FORMS

a variation of Johnny jump up viola (see "Viola," p. 461, as they share many magical properties) • miniature pansy-like flowers in deep violet-blue with a tiny yellow eye in the center • up to twelve inches tall (Johnny jump up is three-colored purple, yellow, and white) • blue elf viola blooms in spring and fall, but may flower right through to midwinter • found wild in meadows and along roadsides in North America • also grown in other countries as well as the USA, as border plants or as cut flowers in bouquets for a young love or marriage • magically use the growing and cut flower and the flower essence, the most accessible and versatile form of blue elf viola

PLANET AND ELEMENTS

Venus • Water/Earth

MAGICAL USES

as its name suggests, a plant for connecting with elves and Earth spirits, especially around twilight if growing in the garden or planted as a miniature children's fairy garden indoors • the flower essence for relieving emotional repression that makes the user unable to express anger or resentment in a controlled effective way • ideal for teen and toddler tantrums

HOW TO USE

Take a drop or two of the essence four times a day for a few weeks to open your heart to release and vocalize love and gratitude you hold within. • Spritz a room with a few drops of the essence in water before a meeting or potential confrontation to talk through and resolve family conflicts and workplace tensions. • Add a little essence to the food or water of a perpetually bad-tempered pet or one who bites or scratches impulsively. • Plant the flowers in an indoor garden or just outside the door if certain family members always come home irritable and seeking a quarrel.

CAUTION

Nontoxic if used medicinally in moderation or as the flower essence.

Violet

(*Viola odorata*)

MAGICAL FORMS

flowering plant • magically use the whole, growing plant; leaf; flower; and oil

PLANET AND ELEMENT

Venus • Water

MAGICAL USES

the herald of spring • protection • luck • love spells • increased libido • wishes • peace • healing • wild violets increase happiness and enable us to be true to ourselves • potted violets prevent accidents and bring harmony • keeping secrets and secret love • white violets represent new love or restoration of trust • blue or purple are for loyalty, reliability, and support in good times and bad

HOW TO USE

Decorate cakes with sugar violets or add sugar to teas for romance with an undemonstrative partner. • The flowers in a wreath protect the home against malicious spirits and attract good luck and should be replaced when they lose their fragrance. • Violet oil mixed with lavender diluted with a carrier oil can be used for massage or added to a bath to attract or increase love and passion. • Picking the first violet seen in spring makes your dearest wish come true. • Carry a sachet of dried violet petals to ease the pain of unrequited love. • Keep violets in the home or plant in your garden to bring peace, healing, and protection against earthly spite or intolerance.

CAUTION

Avoid internal use of the oil, especially if suffering from the rare genetic disorder G6PD.

Violet, African

(*Saintpaulia ionantha*)

MAGICAL FORMS

an indoor prosperity garden area or garden plant • flowers have five rich, purple petals • magically use the whole, growing plant; flowers, fresh and dried; flower essence; and oil

PLANET AND ELEMENT

Venus • Water

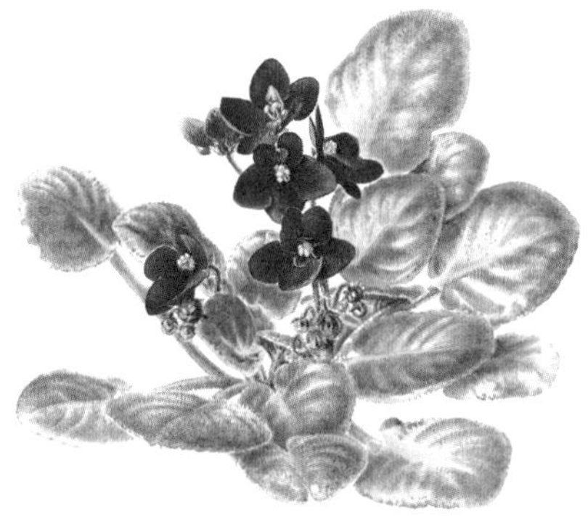

MAGICAL USES

wealth and growing prosperity, in feng shui, especially through increased status • cleansing negative atmospheres and bad habits • peace in the home and within a marriage • promotes abundance through attracting fey energies and benevolent house spirits, but drives away mischievous spirits

HOW TO USE

The five petals on each flower link with goddess energies and can be used in female-based rituals as offerings. • The dried flowers under pillows stop nightmares, and when carried in a sachet or hidden in the house, break and prevent hexes, ill-wishing, and curses.

CAUTION

The plant and oil should not be consumed, though the plant is not toxic to humans, cats, dogs, or horses.

Waffles/Pancakes

MAGICAL FORMS

when made with plants and plant extracts, pancakes and waffles form the ultimate natural magick spell, as each ingredient is named for its purpose while mixing and preparing • adding non-plant products such as eggs or milk generates new opportunities, leading to financial gain and unity with whoever is sharing the waffles or pancakes • above all, eating the finished result and absorbing the powers bring the possibility of manifesting what was or is desired or consciously wished while consuming • magically use as batter and as fully cooked pancakes or waffles

PLANET AND ELEMENTS

Sun • Fire/Earth/Air

MAGICAL USES

the act of mixing and cooking using Fire power brings together different, contrasting, and sometimes conflicting elements and people into a harmonious whole greater than the use of the separate ingredients • eaten on Fridays for love and on the crescent moon for new or better employment in the months ahead

HOW TO USE

Since sweet and savory fillings can be used, this opens the door magically to adding to the financial and property stability that comes from the flour (see p. 183) or the potato (see p. 361) if making potato waffles, or the strengths of different fruits, whether alone or in jellies. For example, the protective or memory-enhancing properties of blueberries (see p. 72) or the sweetening effect on tempers of maple syrup (see p. 281), which also attracts prosperity, can be used.

Wallflower

(*Erysimum* spp.)

MAGICAL FORMS

a genus containing more than 150 species of plants • members of the flowering cabbage family • growing flowers, especially clinging to walls • magically use the cut flowers and petals, dried and fresh

PLANET AND ELEMENT

Saturn • Earth

MAGICAL USES

happiness after misfortune • symbol of fidelity between a couple and given as bouquets since the Middle Ages • also to say thank you to someone who has helped your career or to parents who supported you through college • wallflower clings to walls to grow, and so it is magically associated with behind-the-scenes success, using the system and the influence and support of others to advance yourself (not "go it alone" magick) • progression from friendship to love • workplace advancement from a first job to a position of authority

HOW TO USE

Send a transitioning two-color plant or a selection of different, mixed-colored, vibrant wallflowers for a retirement, redundancy, or career change. • Inhale the scent of blossoming, fragrant wallflowers to awaken your psychic senses by placing the cut flowers on an altar or table where you are reading tarot cards. • To break a codependent or an overpossessive relationship, choose dying wallflowers clinging to a wall or trellis and shred the petals, naming not the person but the situation to be broken, then let the petals fall to the ground. • To beat a cigarette, recreational drug, gambling, or alcohol dependency, add a small symbol of the addiction—for example a gambling chip or crushed cigarette—to a bowl with dried wallflower petals you have already mixed, endowing the mix with your desire to quit the situation or habit. • Tip the contents into a dark, lidded glass jar or bottle. • Wrap well in cloth so burrowing animals will not cut themselves and bury it in a deep hole with stones on top.

CAUTION

Avoid if pregnant or breastfeeding.

Walnut Tree

(*Juglans* spp.)

MAGICAL FORMS

genus including English or common walnut (*Juglans regia*), black walnut (*Juglans nigra*), and white walnut (*Juglans cinerea*) • the English walnut is widespread throughout western Europe • cultivated since Roman times and brought to Britain by the Romans • taken to the USA by the settlers, where it grows in the east from Massachusetts to Ohio and in the west from the Pacific Northwest to New Mexico • the black walnut grows throughout eastern and central USA and the white walnut from Quebec to Tennessee • magically use the whole, growing tree; fresh and dried leaves; wood; and nuts

PLANETS AND ELEMENTS

Jupiter/Sun • Air/Fire

MAGICAL USES

fertility • abundance • money spells • as wands for weather magick, healing, and acquiring sudden wealth • Caraya, the ancient Greek prophetess, was transformed after her death into a walnut tree, and became associated with the wise goddess Artemis • by Roman times, she had evolved into Carmenta, goddess of childbirth and prophecy

HOW TO USE

Carefully break open the shell and eat a walnut to absorb its fertility, lasting love, and manifestation powers (naming your need or intention). • Set a small fire crystal, a blood agate, a garnet, a red jasper, or any bright-red crystal in the cracked-open nut. Tie the halves together with red twine and carry it in a red bag until your desire or wish is manifested. • Find nine walnuts beneath the tree, or if necessary purchase them. Shake them between your hands, asking a question of Caraya or Carmenta aloud about the future. Cast the nuts beneath the tree on a white cloth and you will hear the voice of Caraya, Carmenta, or Artemis in the rustling leaves or your inner voice.

CAUTION

While walnut trees are not considered toxic and the nuts are edible, the sap can be an irritant and opinion is divided over the toxicity of the leaves.

Walnut Tree, Black

(Juglans nigra)

MAGICAL FORMS

the black walnut grows throughout eastern and central USA as far west as California, and in Europe • native to central Asia • an ornamental tree that can grow up to a hundred feet high, with edible highly nutritious nuts • leaves that turn butter yellow in the fall and do not return until late May • magically use the growing tree and the nuts, either fallen from the tree or purchased still within the shell

PLANET AND ELEMENT

Jupiter • Air

MAGICAL USES

black walnut produces a natural herbicide from its roots that may extend fifty feet from the trunk, present in leaves and fruit husks that inhibit other plants growing nearby • magically a tree of self-sufficiency, if you work in a competitive environment or live in cramped accommodation

HOW TO USE

Hold a nut still within its inner shell and ask a question. Break open the nut and, if it is perfectly formed, it suggests a positive outcome. If not ripe, wait as it is too early to act. If the nut shatters or is broken within the shell, extreme care is needed in proceeding. If small or unformed, try another approach to the issue as the present one will come to nothing. • A very powerfully protective tree, burn the leaves crushed in incense or outdoors on a bonfire to cleanse the home spiritually and prevent all harm entering. • Burn dead or dying leaves to break the possessive hold of a lover or relative. • The leaves of this tree should not be burned, however, for destructive purposes such as in past times, breaking up someone's relationship, or hexing a rival as effects powerfully rebound.

CAUTION

Avoid if you have a tree nut allergy. • Do not take supplements containing black walnut if you are pregnant or breastfeeding as there is not enough evidence that these are safe.

Warri Tree

(Caesalpinia bonduc)

MAGICAL FORMS

shrubby vine native to Florida and the Caribbean islands • has casings with rough, hairy, spiny pods containing smooth, marble-like, egg-shaped, gray seeds known as fairy eggs, as well as nickernuts, Molucca beans or seeds, or sea pearls • the seeds from the warri tree wash up on shores in northern Europe as far away as Norway, especially to the Outer Hebrides, where they are used to make rum and are worn as amulets against evil • traditionally ground in tea or coffee and used medicinally to control blood sugar, colds, and stomach disorders, but in the modern world mainly used as protective jewelry and amulets • other varieties can be yellow, such as *Caesalpinia major* or *Caesalpinia ciliata* • magically use the seeds, which you can buy online, often as jewelry

PLANETS AND ELEMENTS

Mercury/Venus • Air/Water

MAGICAL USES

add all-purpose seed to amulets, talismans, charm bags, spell bags, wish jars, magical bottles, and poppets • since the smooth seed can be the size of a human palm (though light as a husk), choose size according to your needs • banishes all negative wishing, earthly and paranormal, and mind manipulation • connects with the fey

HOW TO USE

Wear a white or gray seed as a pendant to break and repel curses, hexes, and ill wishes. • Traditionally it is said that the seed will turn black to indicate the spell is broken, but in practice, if purchased commercially and treated, this won't happen. • Wear a bracelet on your left hand to guard against betrayal in love. • Hang a large seed in a net over the front door to keep away all malice. • Set a seed among flowers to make contact with the fey and hold a second one or touch your pendant as you gaze at the flowers through half-closed eyes to make a telepathic connection.

Wasabi

(*Wasabia japonica*)

MAGICAL FORMS

two feet tall with long, crisp stems • wasabi has been used medicinally and in cooking for many centuries in Japan, originally found wild along mountain streams and still mainly cultivated in Japan • grown also on a limited number of farms in New Zealand, the UK, the USA in Washington and New York, and British Columbia • leaves a burning sensation in the mouth • magically use the powdered spice, the grated rhizome, and as the green paste often accompanying sushi

PLANET AND ELEMENT

Mars • Fire

MAGICAL USES

added to recipes as sauce or powder to prevent procrastination and to open the channels to prophecy and psychological, as well as psychic, awareness

HOW TO USE

Traditionally, the powder is carried in a red "urgently needed success" or "fast money" bag if your way is being blocked, along with cinnamon and other Fire spices such as dried tarragon (see p. 443) and basil (see p. 53). As you tie three strong knots with red thread to secure it, state three times the bag's purpose and the time frame. • The wasabi-based spice bag can also be dedicated to an increase in passion, but should never be used to harm another, to take away a love that is not free or when angry.

CAUTION

Beware the very common fake wasabi, which is just colored horseradish. • Eat true wasabi only moderately while pregnant and with the advice of your doctor.

Water Lily

(*Nymphaea* spp.)

MAGICAL FORMS

genus encompassing multiple species of water lily, including the North American white water lily or pond lily (can also be pink), *Nyphaea odorata*, and the European white water lily (can also be red), *Nymphaea alba*, with large, fragrant flowers and yellow stamens • floats on the water or stands just above it with its lily pad (floating leaf) supporting it • each water lily lasts only three to five days but many new flowers are produced through the summer months • most water lilies open in the morning and close in the heat of the day or the evening • magically work with the floating plant; the closed, dried flower; the lily pad; and the flower essence

PLANET AND ELEMENT

Moon • Water

MAGICAL USES

the name *Nymphaea* links the water lily strongly with water nymphs, especially the freshwater, winged undines who sleep beneath water lilies and may be seen in the morning as the flower opens; they are said to bring love blessings because in some myths they are the spirits of women who died unloved • create a small pond or water feature where you can grow water lilies • leave an offering of a small flower or crystal on a large lily pad in the morning to ask the water lily for serenity and calm and not to react adversely to difficult people or situations in the day ahead

HOW TO USE

Carry the dried, closed flower in a sachet. • Alternatively, take the essence daily or mist the flower essence in a spray with rose (see p. 380) or lavender (see p. 252) water to reduce burning desires and impulsive behavior you might regret, especially in love or speaking out. • Meditate as the flower closes to let go of what or who can no longer be part of your life. • Return in the morning to see the new opening of possibility with the flower, remembering that although each individual flower is short-lived, many more will grow. • Put the flower essence daily on your inner wrist points to mend a broken heart and to reach out again like the unfolding lily.

CAUTION

Water lilies are toxic to humans and animals.

Water Violet

(*Hottonia palustris*)

MAGICAL FORMS

also known as featherfoil • a wild, aquatic flower native to northern and central Europe, Asia, and the USA, with small, violet or pale-pink flowers and feathery leaves that float on the surface of streams and ponds • flowering between May and June • oxygenate the water, preventing soil erosion and providing cover for fish eggs and small, aquatic creatures • can be planted in baskets in garden ponds, water gardens, and indoor aquariums • magically use the whole, growing plant in situ in water and as flower essence

PLANET AND ELEMENT

Venus • Water

MAGICAL USES

as the plant and flower essence, overcoming loneliness and a sense of alienation from others • for children who prefer their own company to learn to socialize • restoring trust after loss and betrayal • fulfilling modest ambitions • keeping secrets and secret love

HOW TO USE

Speak the name of a secret love as you kneel by the growing flowers outdoors or over the flowers in your aquarium, sinking crystals into the roots beneath the flowers or leaves, to keep love safe and growing, hidden from discovery. Ask that when the time is right, your love can be revealed or acknowledged. • Spritz a drop or two of the essence in water around children's school bags and coats each morning or add a single drop to older or teenage children's food or drink to build their confidence to reach out to and be welcomed by peers.

CAUTION

Though water violet is nontoxic, the plant is not considered safe for human consumption.

Watercress

(*Nasturtium officinale*)

MAGICAL FORMS

watercress is not related to the nasturtium flower but mustard and horseradish • aquatic or semiaquatic, near slow-moving water • fast-growing, clumped plants • introduced to the USA from Europe and found wild and cultivated in almost every state, especially the Pacific Northwest • spicy leaves two to five inches long • its cousin, garden cress, is even faster growing • magically, garden cress (also called "mustard and cress"; *Lepidium sativum*) can be used interchangeably with watercress, although they are different species • often the first plant grown by children, as it will grow on damp cotton, wool, or blotting paper and when cut, like watercress, will regrow • magically use the plant grown in well-watered containers indoors or outdoors and the cut plant, often in magical cookery

PLANET AND ELEMENT

Mars • Fire

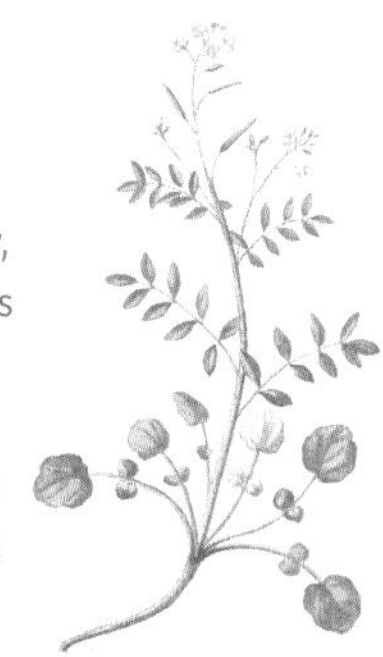

MAGICAL USES

traditionally associated with the military, watercress should be eaten on Tuesdays for strength and protection • sprigs were carried by Roman soldiers for safety and victory in battle • use garden cress or mustard for any urgent matters when results are required within the week

HOW TO USE

Eat watercress before any potential crisis or confrontation and to overcome bullying and intimidation. • Watercress can take as little as four weeks to grow, so it is useful for increasing what is needed, such as money, employment, health, or success within a relatively short period. • Let children plant, cut, and eat their own mustard and cress. Endow it with power as it is planted to overcome any teasing or intimidation. Let children take it to school or college in sandwiches to transfer the energies; constantly regrow and eat until the problem ends.

CAUTION

Watch out for water pollution if watercress is picked wild or from home ponds.

Watermelon

(*Citrullus lanatus*)

MAGICAL FORMS

a large, sweet fruit with a high water content, grown on a vine-like plant from the gourd family • developing from the ovary of the female • pale-yellow flower with green peel covering the white inner rind • red or pink flesh and numerous seeds, though some watermelons are being developed that are virtually seedless • native to South Africa and shown in ancient Egyptian art in hieroglyphs • grown all over the world in warm, frost-free climes • a watermelon can weigh from two and a half to forty-four pounds, and there are two to fifteen melons per vine • see also honeydew melon (p. 221) • magically use the whole melon, or melon sliced and deseeded

PLANET AND ELEMENT

Moon • Water

MAGICAL USES

as a water fruit, watermelon in juices or smoothies acts as a spiritual, as well as a physical, cleanser • the fruit can be shared by lovers to remove blockages in communication • the whole fruit is often cast into water, especially the ocean, as an offering to the water mothers such as the Yoruba or Santería goddess Yemaya and other Water spirits for love, fertility, good fortune, and prosperity

HOW TO USE

Eat a slice of watermelon still in the rind, afterward shredding a little of the outer green peel. • Mix with a gambling chip or a green dollar in a green bag for success in gambling. • In an adaptation of a traditional Hawaiian custom, when someone leaves your life in death or separation, roll a whole melon out of the front or back door, carrying grief and sorrow from the house. Do the same after a painful breakup for the release of anger. Find a place to bury the watermelon in your garden or an open space.

Wattle Tree, Black

(*Acacia mearnsii*)

MAGICAL FORMS

called black wattle because of the darkness of its bark • can bleed red resin • invasive in some lands • native to southeastern Australia and naturalized in China, Japan, India, southern Europe, and the southwestern USA • magically use the fresh or dried yellow flowers, fernlike leaves, bark, soft puff balls, and honey

PLANET AND ELEMENT

Saturn • Earth

MAGICAL USES

called the tree of trust, give or keep artifacts made of the wood or bark as tokens of freely expressing love and emotions • for creativity • to counteract prejudice and closed minds • improve memory • clear and accurate communication • focus • early shelters for European settlers in Australia were made out of black wattle branches and mud and flowering branches hung in huts to promote sleep (use dried flowers in sleep pillows) • enhances clairvoyance • the bark and leaves have been used medicinally for centuries by Australian Aboriginal people

HOW TO USE

Grow it as a tree of welcome to friends and strangers alike. • Break wattle twigs and cast them away to remove repressed anger and the effects of unfair criticism that linger in your mind. • Because black wattle regenerates fast after bush fires and deforestation, use the wand for recovering from loss. • Also use for defensive magick against those who are untrustworthy but mask their unreliability with false promises and reassurances. • Serve and eat the honey with friends or family or give some to a colleague to promote kinship and open, honest but kind communication.

CAUTION

Black wattle seeds are edible, but since some wattles can be toxic, take great care before ingesting parts of a wattle tree.

Wattle Tree, Golden

(*Acacia pycnantha*)

MAGICAL FORMS

the tree has existed for 35 million years • Australia's floral emblem—Wattle Day is celebrated on September 1 • grows in Australia and southern California, and can also be cultivated in Texas, Louisiana, Florida, and other areas in the southern USA, as well as in milder parts of the UK • naturalized in South Africa, Italy, Portugal, Indonesia, and New Zealand • introduced into the northern hemisphere in the mid-1800s • bright-yellow, fragrant, fluffy flower balls • flowers are sold in dried sprays online for bouquets and flower arrangements • magically use fresh or dried flowers, growing trees, seeds, and tree essence

PLANET AND ELEMENT

Sun • Fire

MAGICAL USES

perform rituals and meditation with the tree to feel empowered and in control • helps with expansion and perseverance in every area of life • reduces addictions and phobias • connects with universal energies

HOW TO USE

Make garlands from the flowers or use dried sprays to make certerpieces for solstice and equinox celebrations to welcome the sun and activate your inner sun power. • Spray home or workplace with golden wattle tree essence to lift a sour or critical mood and bring sunlight on even the gloomiest day.

CAUTION

Caution should be taken if pregnant, as golden wattle may reduce iron levels.

Wax Plant

(*Hoya carnosa*)

MAGICAL FORMS

a flowering plant from the dogbane family, found growing through tropical Asia and parts of Australia • worldwide, the wax plant is very popular as a houseplant because of its beautiful flowers • if you live in a tropical or semitropical zone in the USA, it may be possible to grow one outdoors • many species in *Hoya* are air plants, clinging to another plant or rocks, but some have shallow roots in soil • magically work with the whole plant; the stiff, waxlike leaves; and the star-shaped, white, clustered flowers that fade to pink with red or deep-pink centers

PLANET AND ELEMENT

Mercury • Air

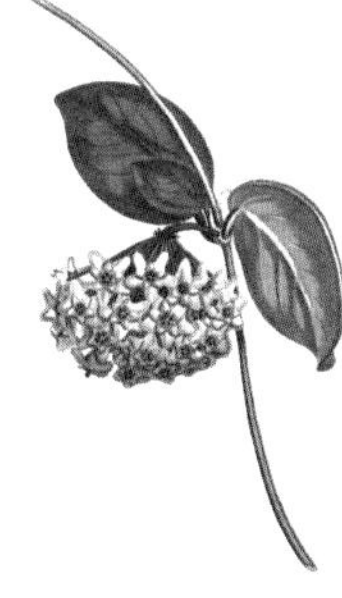

MAGICAL USES

the cut flowers are used in ritual magick because of their resemblance to a pentagram • the plant should be placed indoors near the entrance of the home so its entwining vine can tangle up harm, both paranormal and earthly • set fresh or dried star-shaped flowers in the center of the altar to give spells extra power and for planetary and zodiacal rites

HOW TO USE

For meditation, focus on each ascending star flower cluster on the growing plant in turn. If none is growing, make a stairway of particularly significant leaves on the plant. Inhale the night-time fragrance of the flowers; as you do so, open yourself to other dimensions and connect with Star beings, especially if you believe you are a Star Soul. • Using the point of a sharp stick, etch your desired lover's name on a single, heart-shaped leaf from a sweetheart wax plant (*Hoya kerrii*) on Valentine's Day morning. Press the etched leaf between two pieces of tissue paper (the leaf is already waxy, so you will not need wax paper). Copy a favorite love poem. Keep the leaf and poem together between the pages of a heavy book until love is fulfilled or you are ready to release the leaf and move on.

Weigela

(*Weigela* spp.)

MAGICAL FORMS

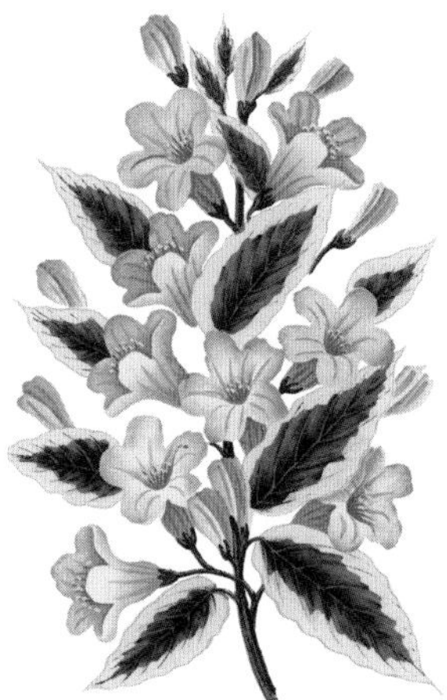

leafy shrubs, growing up to six to ten feet tall, though some of the cultivars are smaller • blooming in mid- to late spring and again in mid- to late summer with clusters of small, red and pink, trumpet- or funnel-shaped flowers • the *Weigela variegata* has cream and green leaves and rose pink flowers • cultivars are found also in red, blue, or purple • weigela plants flourish across the USA, the UK, and Europe as landscaping, for shrubberies, or, as compact varieties, in containers • magically use the growing or cut flowers and flower essence

PLANETS AND ELEMENTS

Sun/Venus • Fire/Earth

MAGICAL USES

signifying love and romance, the flowers and leaves are ideal for wedding bouquets and arrangements at informal weddings and commitment ceremonies • as the flower essence made from *Weigela florida*, because that variety is a hardy flower and adaptable to its environment, for dealing with shock and trauma, not only physically but emotionally

HOW TO USE

Use the flower essence to move on emotionally after unexpected events have shaken your world; it will help you reassess the future and what is now possible. • Meditate on the growing flowers or focus on the cut flowers to free yourself from inhibitions so you can explore and express what you really want from life, which may be very different from what you have been conditioned to think. • Grow the flowers in your garden or on patios to welcome joy, celebration, and people who make you feel good.

Wheat

(*Triticum aestivum*)

MAGICAL FORMS

variety of wheat, also known as common wheat, cultivated for culinary purposes • magically use the growing or dried plant with grains attached, separate grains, and as flour

PLANET AND ELEMENT

Venus • Earth

MAGICAL USES

ears of wheat or another grain, preferably found locally, can be added to a wedding bouquet for fertility, abundance, prosperity, and a secure home • used at Lammas, the first harvest that is traditionally in early August, in rituals for abundance in the months ahead • traditionally, when the first loaf is made from the first grain cut down, it represents the willing sacrifice of the grain god for the growth of the land

HOW TO USE

Sprinkle grain on the earth or scatter breadcrumbs on the altar as an offering for blessings, especially those concerning money or fertility. Repeat when the blessing has been received. This custom dates back to ancient Greek and Roman times, when wheat cakes were offered on altars to the deities. • Tie a small bundle of wheat together with red ribbon over the bed for conception. • Make a corn dolly or wheat knot at Lammas, again tied with red, to be preserved over the hearth until Twelfth Night and scattered on the garden or on nearby open land for continuing prosperity and health.

Wheatgerm

MAGICAL FORMS

the wheatgerm kernel is the embryo and internal part of the wheat grain, removed during processing unless a wheat product is marked 100 percent whole wheat grain • used widely in cookery, for example sprinkled on porridge, added to baked goods, or in veggie burgers • wheatgerm oil is extracted from the wheat germ as a carrier oil to mix with essential oils • the oil is a good mixer with other carrier oils, such as sweet almond or coconut, and essential oils like frankincense, helichrysum, lavender, or patchouli • the oil is too thick and sticky to use on its own • magically use the wheatgerm, often sold toasted, and the carrier oil (not very satisfactory in cooking)

PLANET AND ELEMENT

Saturn • Earth

MAGICAL USES

as oil, use for completeness • brings fulfillment and the successful completion of projects • can be empowered to enhance radiance, charisma, and youthfulness and magically magnify the effects of the physical properties of the vitamin E-rich carrier oil to aid dry, oily, or damaged hair or skin

HOW TO USE

Add wheatgerm to smoothies or cooking when you are in a David and Goliath situation, fighting a big organization or corrupt dealings from those who have unjust power. • Massage the soles of your feet and the tops of your thighs or the small of your back with wheatgerm oil and sweet almond or olive oil to activate your "go for it" energy center chakras before a major sporting event, to complete a project approaching a deadline, or for problems you urgently need to sort but for which you lack motivation and energy.

CAUTION

Wheatgerm is safe to eat in pregnancy but not to excess; seek medical advice before using the oil.

White Fringetree

(*Chionanthus virginicus*)

MAGICAL FORMS

also called old man's beard because of its feathery, beard-like flowers • small tree, native to the eastern USA, growing from New York and Pennsylvania south to Florida and Texas • George Washington planted white fringetrees on Mount Vernon • also found in eastern Asia • creamy, slightly fragrant flowers that hang like a fringe around the tree • dark-blue, egg-shaped, olive-like fruits (white fringetree is related to the olive, though it is not considered edible) • introduced into Europe and Great Britain in 1736, where the tree is now popular in parks and gardens • magically use the whole, growing tree; blossoms on the tree or still attached to the glossy leaves, fresh or dried; roots; root bark; and bark

PLANETS AND ELEMENT

Mercury/Jupiter • Air

MAGICAL USES

secrets • hidden love • the revelation of a mystery or truth • wisdom in later years or through intense early life experiences

HOW TO USE

Burn the shredded bark in an incense mix to uncover the truth about a matter or when you suspect deception. • Scatter the ash to the winds, asking that new information be revealed by the end of the day. • Collect the beard-like flowers dried on their leaves and sleep with them in a sealed sachet under or within a sleep pillow to dream of a beloved elderly relative who has passed and whose advice you need. • Subtly trail the dried blossoms along your path to a secret tryst. • When you are alone, sprinkle a circle of them around your phone, tablet, or computer if you suspect someone is reading your messages when you are not there or taking an undue interest in your private life or financial affairs (make sure you sweep up the blossoms and leave no trace).

White Gaura

(*Gaura lindheimeri*)

MAGICAL FORMS

originated in Texas and southern Louisiana, but now grown in temperate regions worldwide, both in the wild and gardens • especially as the 'Whirling Butterflies' cultivar, with numerous delicate, pure-white flowers that, when the wind blows on their tall stems, resemble visiting butterflies • nearly three feet tall, with arching, pink stems, the flowers open in succession a few at a time during the long flowering season, May to September and sometimes even longer • magically use the flowers swaying in the wind while exploring a botanical garden if you cannot find them locally

PLANET AND ELEMENT

Mercury • Air

MAGICAL USES

called the messenger flower, since butterflies are a form taken by beloved family souls returning • a symbol of transformation and a reminder to enjoy every day and not demand certainties about the future or lingering regrets from the past

HOW TO USE

Wait until you see real butterflies or other non-stinging pollinators near the flowers. Sway softly while watching their movements through half-closed eyes until you experience a light trance state and can experience out-of-body travel wherever you wish with your flying butterflies. Decide in advance where you wish to travel, which dimensions to visit, and whom to see. • If you need transformation in your life, every few days visit your plants and remove any flowers that have faded, naming what cannot or should no longer be in your life. Continue to link with the growth cycle of the plant until you have made the transformation, great or small, in your life.

CAUTION

White guara is nontoxic to humans but can be harmful to pets if ingested.

White Snakeroot

(*Ageratina altissima*)

MAGICAL FORMS

also called richweed or white sanicle • clump-forming plant up to three and a half feet tall, with flat-topped clusters of fluffy, bright-white flowers in summer and fall • long-stalked, nettle-like, gray-green leaves paired along the stem • both stem and leaves contain a highly poisonous alcohol, tremetol, which is dangerous to humans and animals • found as an ornamental in gardens • attracts bees, butterflies, and moths after other plants have ceased blooming • native to eastern and central North America, including Quebec and Ontario in Canada • so called because its roots were once considered as a poultice to cure snakebite • magically use the flowers and roots (but only with great caution, if at all, because of its toxicity)

PLANETS AND ELEMENTS

Saturn/Mercury • Earth/Air

MAGICAL USES

it was once believed that the smoke from the burning plant would revive an unconscious person, but its fumes are now considered unsafe • like many poisonous plants, the roots and flowers are occasionally kept dried in a locked box for banishing and protective magick in dire situations, one of the "last resort" herbs • should never be used in anger or revenge

HOW TO USE

Add the dried flowers and roots, not stems or leaves, to darkly colored, tighly sealed glass bottles with sour red wine and rusty nails. Store in an inaccessible place while there is any danger or threats to home or family. When the danger ceases, the bottle and its contents should be disposed of very carefully.

CAUTION

Handle the plant with care, only in gloves, and keep away from children and pets: it is highly toxic.

Wild Bergamot

(*Monarda fistulosa*)

MAGICAL FORMS

a native North American plant found growing profusely in gardens and hedgerows in Canada, the USA, and Europe • growing plant has a lemony smell • magically use the leaves, lavender-colored flowers, growing plant, and oil, often diluted as a carrier oil (available commercially as monarda bee balm)

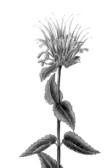

PLANET AND ELEMENT

Mercury • Air

MAGICAL USES

for successful property deals involving borrowing • encourages rapid returns on investment and attracts fast money • for business takeovers and swift expansion • offers opportunities in the area you most need them • attracts bees (associated with prosperity) and butterflies, and so enables abundance to flow freely in the garden and home

HOW TO USE

Wild bergamot can be made into a smudge stick for calling blessings of health, wealth, and happiness from all the directions. • The dried flowers and leaves, burned as an incense, heighten clear thinking and psychic intuition. • Growing areas of wild bergamot bring communication with nature spirits and returning family who loved the place in life.

CAUTION

Do not use while pregnant.

Wild Mustard Charlock

(*Rhamphospermum arvensis*)

MAGICAL FORMS

jagged leaves grow up to twelve inches long with a mustard-like scent when crushed • native to the Mediterranean, North Africa, Europe, and Asia • naturalized in temperate regions worldwide and extensively in fields in the USA since the eighteenth century • closely related to *Sinapis alba*, white mustard, from which culinary mustard is made • long pod fruits develop after the early flowering of the small yellow cruciform flowers, each containing ten to twelve long-lasting black seeds • magically use the seeds and the flower essence

PLANET AND ELEMENT

Mars • Fire

MAGICAL USES

the essence counteracts Peter Pan syndrome in those who are unwilling to assume adult roles and responsibility and rely on being liked and helpless • for young people who cling to the family nest rather than becoming independent and leaving home • in ancient Greek and Roman rituals, charlock signified fertility, love, and overcoming death • the crushed flowers were traditionally used in making magical yellow inks for petitions to deities of Fire, such as the Hindu household god Agni

HOW TO USE

Scatter the seeds over a map of the world, which can be bought online or taken naturally from the growing plant. • Spritz the essence in water each day around your computer, tablet, or smartphone if relatives, neighbors, or friends are constantly phoning for advice or sympathy.

CAUTION

The seeds may be poisonous to pets and livestock. • However, as with all alternative treatments, check with an expert and avoid while pregnant or breastfeeding without consultation.

Wild Teasel

(*Dipsacus fullonum*)

MAGICAL FORMS

also called common teasel • spiny, ridged stem, six to eight feet high • lance-shaped leaves • lilac-colored flowers, flowerheads containing numerous flowers tightly packed into coneheads • grows though Europe and western Asia and in many states of the USA • probably introduced in the 1700s for the cloth industry • usually found wild • stem leaves fuse around the flowering stems to form cups that catch rainwater, which was once used for healing and love • magically use the root and carefully removed spines, and in cut flower arrangements

PLANET AND ELEMENT

Mars • Fire

MAGICAL USES

defense against psychological attack and manipulation • contact with the fey through the fluffy structure of the seeds or spores when they fly

HOW TO USE

Add the whole spiky flowerheads or separate spikes to a magick defensive bottle with very sour wine or vinegar to protect yourself and loved ones if attack seems to come from many sources. • Keep the dried flowering plants in a display in the center of your home to keep away small, mischievous house spirits who cause chaos and hide and break objects when you most need them. • Because teasel is sacred to Hulda, the Norse goddess of spinning, weaving, and cloth making, for which the fiber was used, if life is chaotic, wrap a teasel head (wear gloves) in a tangle of red twine or thread, knotting the twine. In it, bind up all the chaos, unfinished tasks, and misunderstandings in your life. • Cut through the twine with sharp scissors and dispose of the teasel and cut twine in a biodegradable bag in a garbage bin away from your home right away.

CAUTION

Beware of the sharp spines, especially near children and pets. • It is not considered toxic but may interact if used medicinally with anti-inflammatory and antidepressant medication.

Willow Tree

(*Salix* spp.)

MAGICAL FORMS

including the white willow, with its silvery leaves (*Salix alba*); the traditional weeping willow (*Salix babylonica*); the coyote willow (*Salix exigua*), which grows from bush to shrub with leaves that turn silver green; and the black willow (*Salix nigra*) • magically use the whole, growing tree; branches that, where possible, have fallen naturally or were coppiced (cut back to ground level for growth stimulation); and leaves

PLANETS AND ELEMENT

Moon/Venus • Water

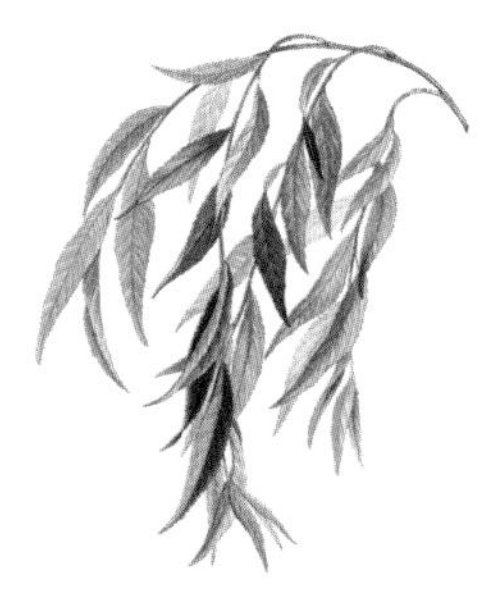

MAGICAL USES

a tree with a long history, growing on the banks of the River Babylon according to the Bible • in Celtic lore, Brigid the maiden goddess melted the winter snows with her willow wand at the early February festival • Native North American people hung willow branches in their tepees and boats to invoke protection of the Great Spirit • the wind whispering in willow trees is said to be elves and brings good luck • willow leaves are carried for shape-shifting

HOW TO USE

The weeping willow is associated with mourning rituals worldwide, possibly dating from when the Moon Mother was believed to carry deceased souls back to the moon. • In modern times, funeral caskets are increasingly woven out of willow. • Dried leaves and bark are burned on the waning moon to summon benign spirits. • On the crescent moon, weave three branches into a love wreath with silver ribbons, then set above the bed to preserve love or in the center of the home to attract a twin soul. • Willow is considered a symbol of eloquence: silver-tinged leaves can be dried and carried in a silver purse by those who work in communications or seek positions in the media.

CAUTION

Do not ingest if allergic to aspirin, are breastfeeding, or have gastric problems.

Wintergreen

(*Gaultheria procumbens*)

MAGICAL FORMS

small shrub that grows low to the ground • magically use the whole, growing plant; leaves; fruit; and oil

PLANET AND ELEMENT

Moon • Water

MAGICAL USES

planted in the garden, attracts good fortune and money on the waxing moon • reduces debts and bad luck on the wane • for healing • protection of mothers, babies, and children • deflects hostility from earthly and paranormal sources

HOW TO USE

Breaks and prevents hexes and curses if sprinkled on thresholds or near entrances. • Use an infusion of leaves with mint in floor washes and poured down water outlets to remove negative energies and entities from whatever source. • Keep in a small sealed sachet within the frame of photos of children to protect them from all harm and bring them good fortune. • Set sprigs of the fresh plant on your altar during healing spells and to attract benign spirits and wise guides to aid spells. • Burn like a smudge to purify atmospheres where there has been illness, anger, or sorrow. • Carry the dried leaves and fruit in a drawstring bag for successful gambling and speculation and to attract money. • A drop or two in a bath increases sensuality and well-being.

CAUTION

Avoid while pregnant or breastfeeding. • Do not use if allergic to aspirin or taking blood thinners, and do not use the oil internally; dilute the oil well to avoid skin irritation.

Winter Heliotrope

(*Petasites fragrans*)

MAGICAL FORMS

a wildflower with an intense vanilla fragrance, blooming with lilac-pink, pale-purple, or white very short petals, from November or December to early spring • native to North Africa but naturalized in temperate regions of the northern hemisphere, including North America, the UK, and Ireland • introduced into gardens in the nineteenth century because of its attractive powderpuff appearance, but rapidly escaped and spread to the wild and is now often considered invasive • a rich source of food for winter pollinators • found in perfumes and cosmetics • magically use the carpet of growing winter heliotrope in a wildlife garden or growing wild, or the dried or preserved flowers

PLANET AND ELEMENT

Venus • Air

MAGICAL USES

shares many of the same properties as the true summer blooming heliotrope, for example *Heliotropium arborescens* • winter heliotrope follows the movement of the sun during the day • for maximizing opportunities at the end of the year and the days before spring (it is said to stop blooming around March 1) • through the rest of the year, kept dried, it is a reminder that better times are coming

HOW TO USE

Walk among a fragrant carpet of flowers and absorb the scent as you name the particular sun you need to enter your life right now in the dark days of winter. • If you are experiencing hardship in the summer, scatter a few dried winter heliotrope flowers among growing summer heliotrope flowers or, if you cannot find any, among small, purple, pink, or white growing flowers to cast away misfortune, sickness, or doubt. • Sprinkle the last of the winter heliotrope blossoms at the beginning of March around your uncarpeted areas, boundaries, or on your doorstep and sweep outward to psychically spring clean your home, as you do so naming new beginnings.

CAUTION

No part of winter heliotrope should be ingested without expert medical advice.

Wintersweet

(*Chimonanthus praecox*)

MAGICAL FORMS

a flowering plant that in midwinter, January and February, produces an intense scent, a mix of jonquils and violets • small, yellow, pale, waxy stems appear bare before the leaves emerge • native to China but introduced to England in 1766 by Lord Cromer in his home at Croome Court in South Worcestershire in the Midlands of England • also found in parts of the USA, including California, Oregon, Washington, Virginia, and North Carolina • magically use the growing fresh or dried flowers and fragrances containing wintersweet

PLANET AND ELEMENT

Sun • Fire

MAGICAL USES

emerging as the sun even in the middle of winter, with promises of better times ahead and new beginnings • for achievements against all odds • in Japan, called "the flower of lonely love," the flower, fresh or dried, was kept by the bedside of a person whose love had gone away as a promise they would return

HOW TO USE

Keep the dried flowers in a yellow charm bag to call back an estranged lover or one when circumstances or others have caused the parting. Each week, cast a single flower from the bag into the wind until all are gone or your love returns. • Grow in the garden as a symbol of good fortune and health, especially when they are in bloom. • Apply the fragrance daily to your solar plexus energy center in the middle of and beneath your ribcage for happiness, whatever the weather, and for seduction.

CAUTION

Wintersweet is toxic and should not be ingested.

Wisteria

(*Wisteria* spp.)

MAGICAL FORMS

includes Chinese or Asian wisteria (*Wisteria sinensis*); Japanese wisteria (*Wisteria floribunda*); and the smaller American wisterias, such as *Wisteria frutescens*, which grows well in the eastern USA and southern Canada, and Kentucky wisteria (*Wisteria macrostachya*) • Asian wisteria is considered invasive in some American states, so keep well cut back • called the purple waterfall, though it can bloom in other colors; the flowers cascade down tightly knit vines • magically use the cut flowers; fresh and dried petals; oil, often sold in a blend (but beware synthetics); and flower essence

PLANET AND ELEMENT

Moon • Water

MAGICAL USES

for seeking educational advancement • longevity in love and life, for wisteria can thrive for more than a hundred years • on altars, attracts abundance and good fortune and ensures that results of rituals are long-lasting • in Korea, it is associated with romance and love, even that which transcends death • legend tells us of two sisters in love with the same man, who drowned themselves in a pool • one became the twisting vine, the other the flowers, since neither could let go • white wisteria signifies healing and health; mauve, intellect and devotion; pink, romance and platonic love; purple, prosperity; and blue, inspiration, intellect, and ambitions • to the Victorians, wisteria spoke of overwhelming desire and passion and they imported the flowers to add to bouquets and wedding decorations

HOW TO USE

Use in a bouquet or give as a potted plant on a wedding or anniversary to indicate love that will continue to grow through the years. • Anoint the Third Eye with a drop of diluted oil or the flower essence before sleep for astral travel and to recall dreams. • Since wisteria can sometimes form a free-standing tree, burn dried wisteria flowers as part of a mix or commercial incense sticks to break the possessive hold of a partner.

CAUTION

Do not ingest any part of wisteria as it is toxic to humans and pets.

Witchgrass

(*Panicum capillare*)

MAGICAL FORMS

also called witches' hair • a rough grass native to North America and the UK • a dense coat with fine soft hairs on leaves and stem with large flowering heads • probably grown around wisewomen's homes as a magical boundary, with defensive incantations to deter the curious • magically use the grass whole, but mainly dried and chopped, and the dried flowers

PLANETS AND ELEMENTS

Saturn/Jupiter • Earth/Air

MAGICAL USES

regarded as a weed, but as the name suggests, is a useful part of a witch's herb cabinet for defensive work and love spells • for calling love and removing curses, hexes, jinxes, and entities who disturb your sleep or home • a plant for working on the dark of the moon, when the moon is not visible in the sky, to leave behind what is no longer useful

HOW TO USE

Keep in a sachet under the mattress at night and take wherever you will encounter a person you desire. Sprinkle just a few grains from the sachet before entering the building where they are or will be. • On a night before the crescent moon appears in the sky, mix the dried, chopped grass with saffron and mugwort as incense on charcoal, then ask Hecate—goddess of the crossroads and the kindly grandmother goddess of past, present, and future—what you need to take from the past and present toward the future in the new lunar month. The answer may appear in the smoke or in your mind. If you prefer, ask a wise grandmother from your ancestral past instead. • Place two dried grasses in a diagonal cross where you know a person who has wished you ill or hexed you will walk (name them so the unhexing will affect no one else). As they walk across the witchgrass cross, the hex is broken. Kick the pieces into the undergrowth or off the sidewalk. • Anticipating the coming crescent, add the hairy parts to a bottle or jar for binding magick if you are being pestered or feel sexually harassed at work (as well as formally complaining of course!).

Witch Hazel

(*Hamamelis* spp.)

MAGICAL FORMS

grows slowly and can be cultivated as a shrub or in containers and kept cut back if space is limited • magically use the whole, growing plant; yellow or orange flowers blooming in winter; leaves; bark; and wood (twigs)

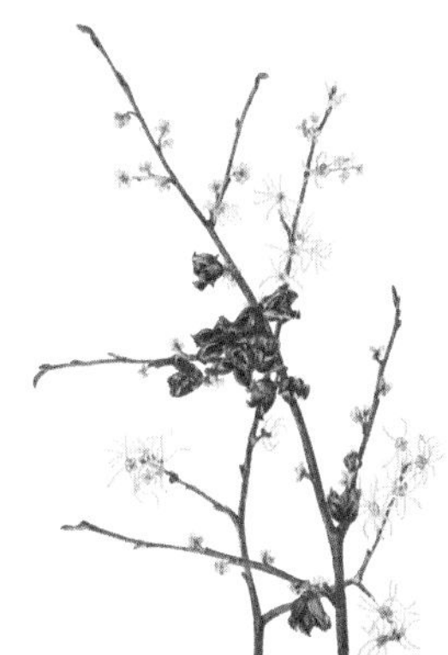

PLANETS AND ELEMENTS

Saturn/Sun • Earth/Fire

MAGICAL USES

a forked twig is a natural divining rod for finding water and lost objects or pets • overcomes grief and loss • draws love and clairvoyant powers • native to the Indigenous nations of eastern USA and Canada (also found in China and Japan) • its medicinal and dowsing powers were shared with the early Puritan settlers • use for Water and Earth magick and their elementals and nature spirits

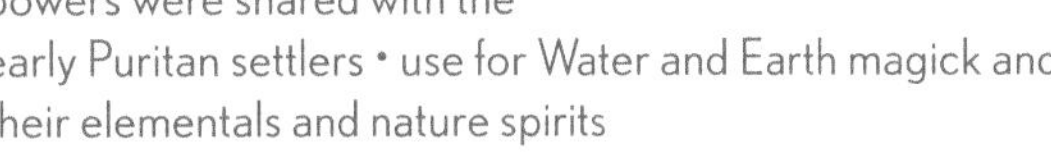

HOW TO USE

Add witch hazel twigs, leaves, seeds, petals, and bark in dishes at the main compass points surrounding the altar or as the Earth element to create boundaries to exclude hostile forces during divination and ritual, as well as to enhance psychic powers. • A witch hazel wand attracts and banishes equally; make the attracting end pointed with a moss agate crystal on the end. • A healing poppet can be filled with the dried leaves and flowers and the doll anointed with a drop of lavender essential oil. • If you lose something precious, a small, smoothed, forked branch will guide the direction and pull you to the location of what is missing or, if a pet, near where it is hiding. • Carry leaves in a brown sachet if brokenhearted, or shredded bark to end a relationship.

CAUTION

Use caution and consult a doctor before using if pregnant or breastfeeding.

Wolfberry

(*Lycium chinense*) and (*Lycium barbarum*)

MAGICAL FORMS

also called goji berry • shrub growing up to thirteen feet with bright-green leaves and scarlet berries • first recorded in Chinese medicine annals in the first century CE as promoting long life • a decoction is made from the berries or the fresh or dried root • berries are edible • the bush grows in several regions of the USA, including California, Oregon, Montana, Washington, New Mexico, Wyoming, and Utah, though in Montana and Wyoming in the wild it is considered a noxious weed • magically use the root and berries (berries are obtainable in supermarkets and health stores, the roots online or powdered as prepared tea)

PLANET AND ELEMENT

Saturn • Earth

MAGICAL USES

the tea is used in rituals against environmental pollution • in magical cookery, the berries are blessed and blended as smoothies or sprinkled on desserts, which can lift the mood of all present, so everything seems more possible • brew the tea at work to cheer a gloomy workplace

HOW TO USE

Drink the berry tea before chanting, meditation, and mindfulness and to connect with higher energies, especially wise guides from the Far East such as sages. Also drink if learning the *I Ching*. • Keep the dried berries or a root in a charm bag in the place where you store your *I Ching* divinatory coins or yarrow stalks. • On the root, etch the name of an older relative or friend about whom you worry. Keep this in an amulet bag with a green jade crystal, a sign of immortality. Each day, bless the bag for a long, healthy life.

CAUTION

Check with your midwife or obstetrician before consuming goji berries while pregnant.

Wood Betony

(*Stachys officinalis*)

MAGICAL FORMS

common name for several plants, also including *Betonica officinalis* and *Stachys betonica* • purple orchidlike flowers and unique toothed protective leaves • pick flowers before fully open • magically use the flowers and leaves, fresh and dried

PLANETS AND ELEMENTS

Mercury/Jupiter • Air/Earth

MAGICAL USES

called wood betony because it often grows wild in woodlands • also found in gardens to guard the home and those within, especially from the spite of human snakes and gossiping neighbors • against obsessions and addictions, particularly alcohol • purification • preserving love • improving memory • traditionally burned on midsummer fires • used medicinally from Roman times, Antonius Musa, physician to Emperor Augustus, claimed betony would heal forty-seven different illnesses

HOW TO USE

Mix the dried flowers and leaves with dried rosebuds and dried lavender heads, and place in a sleep pillow or a sachet beneath the pillow to protect against bad dreams and sexual demons, such as succubus and incubus. • Add it to purification and protection mixes and incenses. • The chopped fresh flowers and leaves can be scattered outside the home, especially around doors and windows, to create a protective wall against unwelcome or threatening visitors, such as unscrupulous debt collectors or gangs if you live in a dangerous area. • Burn dried betony on hearth fires, bonfires, and in incense with chamomile flowers, or add it to peace bottles and jars, to remove the effects of quarrels and family rivalries. • Carry the dried flowers and herbs in a blue sachet for success in examinations and tests, especially driving tests if you are very nervous and may panic.

CAUTION

Avoid if pregnant or breastfeeding or if you have low blood pressure.

Wormwood

(*Artemisia* spp.)

MAGICAL FORMS

plants from a large genus (see "Mugwort," p. 300, and "Davana," p. 154), including *Artemisia nivalis*, an herb native to the mountains of Europe and Asia, especially southwest Switzerland • a single stem and small, yellow flowers with a white center • grow up to three and a half feet high • wild or in gardens in cold climates • *Artemisia tilesii* has broad leaves and yellow flowers, reaching much higher than the nivalis kind • neutralizes acid rain • native from east Asia including Russia and Japan to northwest USA from Alaska east as far as Nunavut and south to Nevada • magically use the dried leaves and flowers, or as the mountain wormwood flower essence, which is made from *Artemisia tilesii*

PLANET AND ELEMENT

Mercury • Air

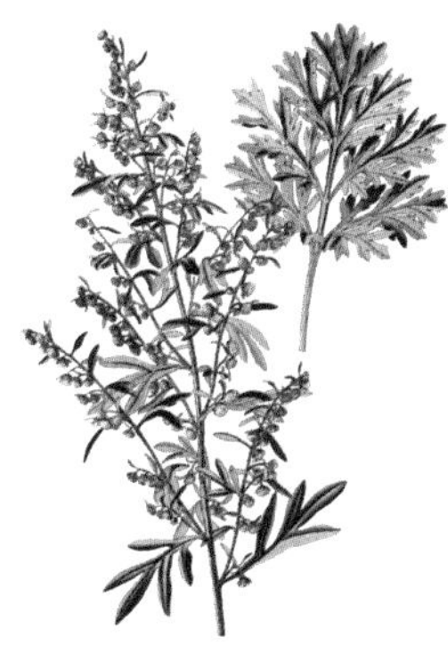

MAGICAL USES

both as the plant and the essence, diminishes unwarranted or undeserved guilt and blame for one's own and others' past behavior or attitudes • for healing emotional wounds even back to childhood and for overcoming current betrayal in relationships

HOW TO USE

Though *Artemisia tilesii* is popularly called stinkweed, it actually smells like a sweet sage. Perhaps *tilesii* is referred to as stinkweed because spirits are repelled by the smell. • *Nivalis* is a protective plant that can be dried and hung over doors or chopped and used in amulets to keep away harm and harmful spirits. • As the flower essence, it is the ultimate anti-guilt trip remedy when used in a humidifier or taken in water or under the tongue.

CAUTION

Some users may develop a skin allergy when touching, so handle with care.

Wormwood, Common

(*Artemisia absinthium*)

MAGICAL FORMS

also called "old woman" because of its association with the waning moon • once used to make the drink absinthe, which is no longer legal in many places, including the USA • magically use the whole, growing plant with its silvery-green leaves or the aerial parts dried and chopped

PLANET AND ELEMENT

Mars • Fire

MAGICAL USES

burned as incense to increase psychic awareness, especially mixed with sandalwood and for protection when working with the spirit world • in the past it was associated with summoning graveyard spirits, magical revenge, and more dubious practices • used wisely and with respect of the Otherworld, wormwood can make connection with ancestors and aid responsible mediumship

HOW TO USE

In modern magick, the dried plant is carried in a sealed amulet bag and placed in cars to prevent accidents and threats from aggressive drivers, and in the workplace to combat venomous colleagues. • Mix small quantities of the dried, chopped herb with lavender, rose petals, meadowsweet, and chamomile in a sleep pillow for astral travel during sleep and visions of future lovers or those from past worlds on the dream plane. • Wormwood is effective for waning moon divination: use it to capture the moon in a glass bowl of water in which a single wormwood plant is floating on a clear night, and use the water for scrying and seeing past lives and hidden realms.

CAUTION

Do not use while pregnant or breastfeeding. • Wormwood is toxic if ingested in anything except small amounts, so use only with extreme caution and on medical advice, always with the awareness that it can be hallucinogenic.

Yam, Cultivated

(*Dioscorea* spp.)

MAGICAL FORMS

cultivated forms of the yam, including the purple yam, *Dioscorea alata* • edible, thick tubers, formed from the base of the stem of a tropical vine growing more than seven feet tall • native to warmer regions of both hemispheres with more than 150 kinds of the cultivated tuber • eaten as a starchy vegetable instead of potatoes • often mistaken for the sweet potato, since though an individual yam can grow up to 150 pounds it can be as small as a potato • true yams have rough, dark skin and white to reddish flesh • magically use the tuber, often in magical cookery

PLANETS AND ELEMENT

Moon/Venus • Water

MAGICAL USES

like wild yam (*Dioscorea villosa*), of which only twelve varieties are edible and native to North America • cultivated yam is a fertility symbol • especially helpful to be shared by same-sex couples trying for a baby • promises good fortune, security to home life, a roof over your head, and stable relationships if there has been disruption

HOW TO USE

Round yams are associated with the anima and the oblong with the animus. Mix according to the balance you need within yourself or a love partnership; cook both kinds and mix and share them in a meal for a balanced, equal relationship. • Keep a basket of mixed-shape yams in your kitchen or on your altar until they grow roots. Make a hole in the tough skin on each. Press a small, silver or gold coin inside and plant them, asking the Earth Mother to bring sufficient material resources and a little more, as well as for the growth of love and health, to your life.

CAUTION

All yams are toxic if eaten raw.

Yam, Wild

(*Dioscorea villosa*)

MAGICAL FORMS

Twisting, tuberous vine, native to eastern North America, growing wild and cultivated from Texas and Florida as far north as Ontario and Massachusetts • magically use the root, bulb, and healing tea decoction made from chopped root, often with peppermint and stevia added

PLANET AND ELEMENT

Moon • Water

MAGICAL USES

for getting in touch with the anima side of the self, and for goddess rituals as an offering or as part of a celebratory meal, though wild yam can be bitter and need extra flavor (try roasting with butter) • add powdered to a protective amulet bag for women in hazardous jobs or who travel through uncertain places

HOW TO USE

The root of the wild yam is a fertility charm and can be helpful when same-sex couples, especially men, are seeking parenthood. • The tea can be shared in female rites of passage ceremonies, particularly during the transition to the wisewoman stage. • Use in moon rites on the waning moon, etching the root with words or an image representing whatever is to be removed, such as pain, sorrow, or ill wishes, and then burying it beneath stones or casting it into fast-flowing waters.

CAUTION

Avoid wild yam if additional estrogen will cause problems, such as in pregnancy and while breastfeeding.

Yarrow

(*Achillea millefolium*)

MAGICAL FORMS

flowering plant with small, white flowers • magically use the stalks, heads, dried flowers, growing plant, and oil

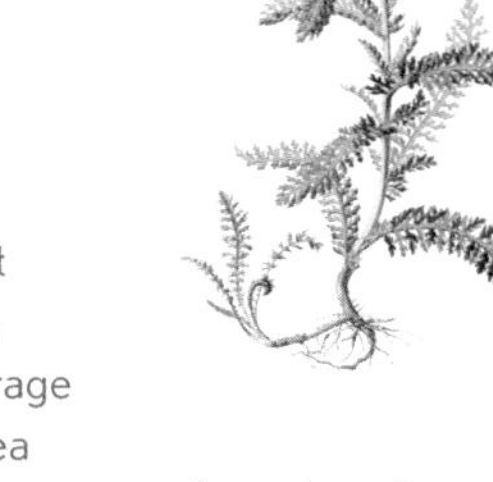

PLANET AND ELEMENT

Venus • Water

MAGICAL USES

for attracting friends and lovers from afar or the past • yarrow tea, when shared, brings enchantment • courage and protection when the tea is scattered around altars or rooms where there have been quarrels or malevolence

HOW TO USE

Hang a bunch of yarrow over the bed for lasting love, renewed every seven years as a love token. • Dried yarrow heads or stalks are cast as a divinatory method to determine in the *I Ching* which trigrams (three liners) combined with others answer questions. • Carry the dried heads or stalks in a red purse to call those you want to meet, adding a clove of garlic and a clear quartz point. Before sealing, pass the quartz over a letter or mail printout. • For protection, burn yarrow in incense, scatter around the home and entrances, or anoint door handles and window ledges with the oil or essence diluted in sunflower oil. • Use for protection and enhanced intuition if there is rivalry in the workplace.

CAUTION

Beware of skin allergies, avoid in pregnancy, and wash hands after use.

Yarrow, Pink

pink variety of (*Achillea millefolium*)

MAGICAL FORMS

much more sensitive spiritually than the white or yellow forms of yarrow • found in temperate regions of the northern hemisphere including Asia, Europe, and North America • wild, where pink flowers occur naturally, blooming from early to late summer • as cultivars, including the rose pink 'Pink Grapefruit' that fades with age, or the deep pink 'Cerise Queen' • magically use the cut or whole, growing plant for decoration; dried flowerheads or flowers; ferny aromatic leaves; and flower essence

PLANET AND ELEMENT

Venus • Earth

MAGICAL USES

as the flower and essence, for relieving anxiety, stress, and tension • creating emotional boundaries for those who give too much • for empaths, psychics, and healers who find it hard to not become exhausted by their work • for healing generational wounds and intergenerational conflicts

HOW TO USE

Add a drop or two of the essence to the cut yarrow in a vase, and set in a healing room or near a tarot table to shield the healer or diviner and allow the client to open emotionally in a safe space. • Hang the dried pink yarrow over the bed in traditional fashion for fidelity and unity, if the couple is young or there has been a parting followed by reconciliation, replacing whenever the flowers fade.

CAUTION

All yarrows can occasionally cause allergies and should not be ingested medicinally during pregnancy or breastfeeding.

Yeast

(*Saccharomyces cerevisiae*)

MAGICAL FORMS

a living single-cell fungus, used for baking bread (and brewing beer), dating back to 4000 BCE in ancient Egypt • magically use fresh yeast; active, dried granular yeast; instant yeast powder; nutritional yeast flakes; inactive yeast used for cooking or as toppings; and savory yeast extract spreads such as Marmite or Vegemite

PLANET AND ELEMENT

Jupiter • Air

MAGICAL USES

yeast added when making bread (see p. 79) increases business success and helps you rise financially • for gambling and speculation • yeast magick works best when you are increasing what you already have rather than starting from nothing • if using a yeast that requires dissolving in warm water, visualize the achievement of ambitions and the desired time frame until it bubbles • do the same when adding yeast to any mix to capture the energies of growth in your life or for loved ones (naming them aloud)

HOW TO USE

Mark the top of shaped, risen dough with a symbol of what you seek, then bake and eat to absorb its power. • If you are going to a casino, betting on horses, or participating in any other gaming or speculation, carry nutritional yeast flakes in a blue charm bag to make wise, fast, and calculated rather than impulsive choices to win and know when to go home with your winnings. • Eat or serve yeast extract spreads for conserving economy if you or a family member are a shopaholic to encourage wise purchases and savings.

Yellow Jessamine

(*Gelsemium sempervirens*)

MAGICAL FORMS

a twining, slender vine, climbing high even to the top of trees and the sides of buildings • indigenous to Southeast Asia, southeastern and south-central USA, Mexico, and Central America • also called Carolina jessamine because it is widespread through the Carolinas • resembles honeysuckle but is far more lethal • its fragrant, yellow flowers bloom in December and may continue until springtime • grown as ornamentals in spite of the toxicity • magically use the flowering vine, but only in dire defensive need, as there are many safer vines that serve a similar purpose

PLANET AND ELEMENT

Mercury • Air

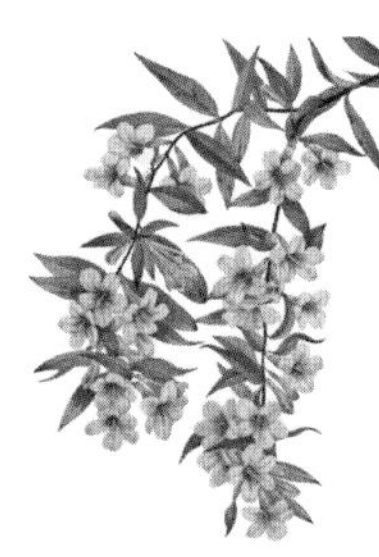

MAGICAL USES

because of its poisonous nature, used as a fierce psychic shield in defensive bottles and jars (handle with gloves and great care) • when grown in a safe place, creates an exclusion zone from danger and misfortune • traditionally proof against evil spirits

HOW TO USE

Meditate on the growing vine (not too near), especially when it is flowering, to psychically protect yourself from mind games, abuse, and manipulation by those who control you through what they call love. • Only with great care, cut away a piece of the vine, naming from whom or what you wish to be free. Chop it in pieces and place in a thick, brown cloth bag tightly sealed all around with yellow knotted threads once the contents are inside. Bury the bag deep where neither creature nor human can dig it up, placing a large stone on the spot, and say, *Rise no more.*

CAUTION

Although used in conventional and Indigenous medicine, since it is strychnine-related, all parts of this plant should be considered highly toxic, especially the flowers and root. • The smallest amount ingested can be fatal and even bees gathering nectar can be poisoned.

Yellow Rattle

(*Rhinanthus minor*)

MAGICAL FORMS

a wildflower with hooded, yellow, tubelike flowers, blooming May to September • so named because at the height of the summer when the wind blows, its tiny seeds rattle within the seed pods, which are dry capsules • semiparasitic • flowers until the fall • called "the meadow-maker" because it assists the growth of other plants by drawing water and nutrients from grasses so more traditional delicate wildflowers can compete • circumpolar, spanning Europe and the UK, Russia, and western Asia • up to almost twenty inches high • magically use the growing flowers in situ, seed-containing capsules, dried flowers, and seeds (when the capsules are opened)

PLANET AND ELEMENT

Saturn • Earth

MAGICAL USES

for the removal of what is restricting you and the growth or restoration of what you most need • to banish those who drain your energies • to gain mentors and those who will help your career or business to thrive

HOW TO USE

Fill a gourd or container with the seed pods and use for sound healing to pass as a rattle over a troubled person or rhythmically over a place where they experience pain. Shake your gourd as you walk through the flowers in situ or in a wildlife garden area in a park. If there is space, you can create your own yellow rattle garden, which will call those who will assist your path. • Break open some pods in a basket or bag and, turning around in all directions, let them fly, calling the freedom you need in your life. • Dry some of the flowers and keep in a yellow amulet bag to hold before or when talking electronically or face-to-face with someone who makes you feel guilty. Afterward, release the flowers and replenish the bag if there must be another encounter.

CAUTION

Yellow rattle may be mildly toxic to pets.

Yellowwood Tree

(*Cladrastis kentukea*)

MAGICAL FORMS

also called American yellowwood • native to North America through southeastern states, from Kentucky to North Carolina and bordering states, generally discovered in small areas • also grows in the UK and northern Europe • what has been described as a fragrant waterfall of white blossoms hanging down in clusters, in late spring and early summer • other species grow in east Asia • magically use the growing tree, which is worth seeking because of its bright-yellow leaves in the fall; yellow inner wood; and fresh and dried blossoms

PLANET AND ELEMENT

Mercury • Air

MAGICAL USES

for prosperity • for the fulfillment of a once-in-a-lifetime opportunity • for rediscovering the spontaneity of childhood and buried joy when you knew anything was possible

HOW TO USE

Carefully collect and dry the flower clusters if you are working toward a special dream or ambition. Add to them sturdy, broken twigs from which you have scraped the outer bark to reveal the yellow wood, or buy small pieces of the sawed wood from a specialty wood or craft store. Keep these in a sealed velvet bag hidden among your personal treasures. Hold the bag every Sunday morning, on your birthday, or when you have a special chance to further your dream and know it will come true. • Leap in a pile of yellow fall leaves as you did when you were a child, scrunching through them in spirals, tossing the leaves between your hands so that you are filled with their golden power and can claim or reclaim your place in the sun and the rebirth of the true inner self and possibilities.

CAUTION

Do not ingest any part of the yellowwood tree.

Yerba Mate

(*Ilex paraguariensis*)

MAGICAL FORMS

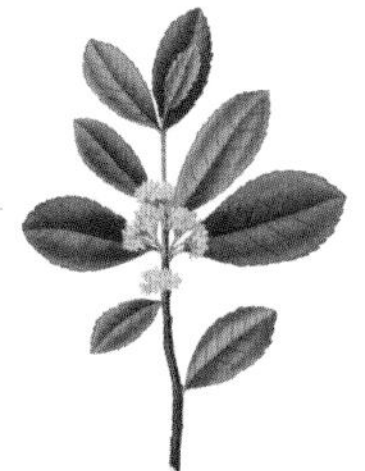

an evergreen tree from the holly family • the dried leaves can be made into a tea (which may be sold commercially roasted) • often consumed in a brew with ground-up twigs as part of social interaction in South America, made and drunk in a gourd through a special straw • native to subtropical South America, in the wild the tree can grow to twenty-six feet and beyond, needing substantial rainfall and warmth to grow • cultivated in the USA, the UK, and Australia, or as an indoor potted plant, ideal for magick • magically use the dried, organic, unroasted leaves for tea

PLANET AND ELEMENT

Venus • Water

MAGICAL USES

as tea, for astral travel, meditation, mindfulness, friendship, and group tea-drinking ceremonies • increases libido • encourages success in dieting and healthy eating programs • burn the dried leaves and ground twigs in incense at the spring equinox

HOW TO USE

Share the tea with a lover to increase passion and ensure lasting love. • To end a relationship, throw a trail of spilled tea after your lover when they have left your home. • Use the dried leaves (as organic tea leaves if necessary) in a health-bringing sachet if you suffer a lot of minor illnesses or are constantly exhausted. • When kept in a home or workspace, the potted plant increases creativity, brings ingenious solutions, and gives foresight of future results when brainstorming.

CAUTION

Avoid yerba mate in pregnancy and while breastfeeding. • Where possible, avoid smoked and roasted varieties by choosing organic varieties from health stores.

Yerba Santa

(*Eriodictyon californicum*)

MAGICAL FORMS

also called the Holy or Sacred Herb • evergreen, aromatic shrub, native to California, Oregon, and northern Mexico • thick, sticky leaves used medicinally for generations by Native Americans and Spanish missionaries, who regarded it as sacred because of its many healing properties • clusters of white or lavender flowers, blooming July to August • magically use the cut or whole, growing (fresh or dried) plant; leaves; fresh or dried flowers; as tea; and as incense

PLANET AND ELEMENT

Jupiter • Air

MAGICAL USES

for rising above the past, connection with higher energies, and healing the soul • detoxifies the self from being trapped in circular thinking about injustices that cannot be resolved and situations that must, for now, be accepted • as part of a healing incense or smudge mix, removes misfortune, bad atmospheres, and unfriendly entities and blesses people, artifacts, and altars

HOW TO USE

Drink the tea made by boiling the leaves, fresh or dried, before divination, meditation, magick, or mediumship to enhance psychic connection with spirits or when desiring to attain a state of mindfulness. • Drink also before sleep while holding a memento or photograph of a deceased relative who may appear in your dreams or give you a sign of their blessing the following day. • Hang the flowering, dried plant over the front door to keep away all harm, and to welcome the ancestors, place the chopped, dried plant as an altar offering, especially on the anniversary of a departed relative.

CAUTION

Yerba santa is generally regarded as safe, but it may have an unwanted diuretic effect. • Consult a doctor before using while pregnant or breastfeeding.

Yew Tree

(*Taxus* spp.)

MAGICAL FORMS

includes Canadian yew (*Taxus canandensis*) a sprawling shrub of central and eastern North America, especially north of Ohio, with relics from the ice age • Irish yew (*Taxus baccata* 'Fastigiata') • Ireland was originally home to two yews, which proliferated; now the trees grow in churchyards, gardens, and arboretums across western Europe • do not burn the wood or use in incense • magically add the wood, leaves, and berries in pouches as amulets for rituals and work with the living tree

PLANET AND ELEMENT

Saturn • Earth

MAGICAL USES

one of the Celtic sacred woods, for connecting with the wisdom of the ancestors and living older people • yews can live more than two thousand years, and as an evergreen the yew stands in graveyards as a symbol of immortality • Breton myths tell that the yew extends a root into the mouth of each body in a graveyard and breathes new life into them • for rituals for inevitable endings leading to new beginnings • facilitates aims that are slow to come to fruition and creates union between two people after difficulty

HOW TO USE

Yew is used to celebrate Samhain or Halloween—called the period of "no time" or "the time of the yew," from October 31 to November 2—when the gateway between the dimensions opens. During this period, the ancestors can be invoked through a yew tree wand or by meditating under the tree at midnight on Halloween. • It is also a winter solstice tree standing between two worlds; at the turn of the year, set symbolically next to the birch tree of new beginnings on the tree calendar. • Combine the two woods in a charm pouch, especially where the past needs to be released. • Conduct ceremonies near the living tree or cut branches on an altar for welcoming perimenopause or menopause, calling on the crone goddess grandmother of the yew.

CAUTION

All parts of the yew tree are poisonous, so use with caution. • Do not use while pregnant.

Yew Tree, Pacific

(*Taxus brevifolia*)

MAGICAL FORMS

native to the rainforests of western North America, from British Columbia to California • relatively small, growing in the shade of larger trees • red bark, needlelike leaves, winter buds covered in golden scales, and red, berrylike cones • long used in folk medicine by Indigenous people, the *taxol* within its bark was discovered in the 1960s to be helpful against some forms of cancer; this has led to many trees being felled • magically use the wood; living tree, often grown as a bonsai; and flower essence

PLANET AND ELEMENT

Saturn • Earth

MAGICAL USES

as the flower essence, for recovery from major illness or crisis, defensive of and resistant to attacks and intrusions of all kinds • the tree of music and musicians • as a bonsai tree, a reminder of tradition, the natural passage of time, and protection of home and all one holds dear because of its vital role in the forest and wildlife ecosystem • the bonsai restores natural energies if the owner is confined indoors because of chronic illness

HOW TO USE

If obtainable, Pacific yew wood makes a powerful protective wand, magically restoring the balance between the need for change and the preservation of what is of worth. • Pacific yew can be made into musical instruments by those who write or perform to allow the rhythms of the natural world and seasons to be expressed in their creations. • Use the flower essence in humidifiers and spritzers, and as a personal connection to restore the natural alignment between mind, body, and spirit.

CAUTION

While the Pacific yew has a lower toxicity than many other *Taxus* species, it should nevertheless not be ingested in any form. • Avoid in pregnancy unless medically advised to the contrary.

Ylang-Ylang Tree

(*Cananga odorata*)

MAGICAL FORMS

native to the Philippines, spreading to Malaysia, Indonesia, New Guinea, Queensland in Australia, the Solomon Islands, and the warmest parts of USA, such as southern Florida • can be up to sixty feet tall, but tends to be smaller in the USA • dwarf ylang-ylang trees (*Cananga odorata* var. *fruticosa*) will grow in containers in less tropical settings • magically use the whole, growing tree; fragrant, yellow flowers, fresh or dried; loose tea made from the flowers; essential oil; and as incense

PLANET AND ELEMENT

Venus • Water

MAGICAL USES

the oil, used in baths, in a diffuser, or diluted with sweet almond or jojoba oil for massage, enhances sensuality and can be used before sex magick • essential oil is called the oil of poets and is used for overcoming blocks in the flow of ideas • increases self-esteem and self-image and enhances personal radiance when sipped as a tea before a social event or when you need to shine in the workplace • ylang-ylang is burned in incense to cleanse a space after a quarrel or before a love ritual

HOW TO USE

In Indonesia, the fresh flowers are scattered on the marital bed after the wedding. • Mist sheets with a ylang-ylang water spray or burn a ylang-ylang incense stick in the bedroom while the room is empty for a similar effect. • Meditating while burning the oil, diffusing it, or sitting close to a tree brings calm and opens the pathways between earth and heavens. • For luck in business or personal success, anoint a white candle with a drop of the oil diluted with olive oil before lighting. • For seemingly insoluble problems, ask for the help of benevolent spirits and wise ancestors.

CAUTION

Do not ingest the oil; dissolve it in carrier oils for massage. • Ylang-ylang oils are safe to use during pregnancy; however, consult your doctor before drinking the tea if you are pregnant.

Yucca

(*Yucca* spp.)

MAGICAL FORMS

perennial shrub or tree • magically use the whole, growing plant; fibers; root; and flowers

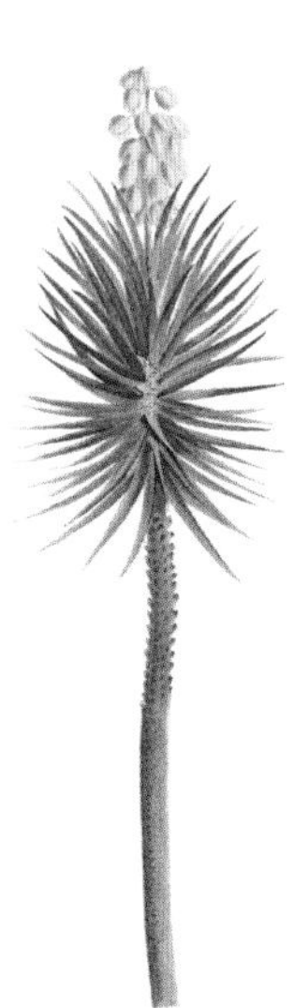

PLANET AND ELEMENT

Mars • Fire

MAGICAL USES

protects the home from evil • for shape-shifting into different forms including animals and so stimulating evolved magical and shamanic powers

HOW TO USE

Twist the fibers into a small wreath and add any flowers, then wear on your head to enable shape-shifting and astral projection and a safe return. • Hang a small fiber cross inside and over the entrance to your home or in a hearth space to prevent evil entities from entering. • Rub a slice of yucca root or stalk over your body to remove hexes, jinxes, and curses on the waning moon and afterward bury it at a crossroads or where nothing grows. Shower or bathe afterward. • Use a strong decoction of chopped yucca root or stalk to cleanse or asperge a ritual area before working with spirits or if there have been bad feelings among certain members of a group. • Keep yucca where you need the chi to flow freely, such as a a stagnant, inert workplace. • Burn, bury, or cast brown, dying leaves into water, naming what has not worked out.

CAUTION

Beware of eating raw yucca, which is highly toxic. • Avoid if pregnant or breastfeeding.

Yuzu

(*Citrus × junos*)

MAGICAL FORMS

upright, thorny, evergreen bush • naturally occurring hybrid of mandarin and lemon trees • grown mainly for the aromatic peel on its tangerine-size fruit that is made into the oil • small, white, highly aromatic flowers in spring, followed by bumpy, green fruit that passes through yellow to orange • highly prized in Japanese cuisine, though it originated in China • too strong to eat raw • magically use the fruit, occasionally to be found in Japanese or Chinese food stores; the juice; increasingly, as smaller yuzu plants in specialty garden centers worldwide or online; the essential oil, which has an exotic fragrance (a mixture of lime, grapefruit, and mandarin); and the thorns

PLANET AND ELEMENT

Moon • Water

MAGICAL USES

awareness of what is hidden • brings deep levels of relaxation and entry into spiritual awareness in breathwork, meditation, and yoga • for chronic fatigue and speeding convalescence • the thorns in protective jars against sarcasm, unfair criticism, and hidden malice

HOW TO USE

To clear trivial and redundant thoughts from your brain, diffuse the oil during spiritual work and in divination, especially with cards, where the heart of the matter can be revealed even if a client is blocking the process. • If you have unexpressed creativity or have hesitated to market your creations, add the juice or zest (if you can obtain a fruit) to drinks and desserts. • Burn the oil with other citrus oils to clear a spooky or gloomy atmosphere in a home or workplace or a new dwelling where the previous owners divorced or suffered misfortune.

CAUTION

If pregnant, consult your physician or midwife before using, as opinions vary; it is also unclear whether it is phototoxic.

Zinnia

(*Zinnia* spp.)

MAGICAL FORMS

flowering plant that blooms in a rainbow of colors • the Navajo call it the sacred elixir of life and Pueblo nation believe it makes children intelligent • magically use the whole, growing plant; cut flowers; and petals

PLANET AND ELEMENT

Sun • Fire

MAGICAL USES

connection with Indigenous wise men and wisewomen • acclaim for achievements • friendship • romance • farewells • celebrations such as weddings and reunions • a wish flower for a desire to reunite • flower psychometry

HOW TO USE

Give as a bouquet to a friend who is going away, whether for a short time or permanently, with the spoken or written wish that they will return. • Zinnias can be used at funerals to recall happy memories, sometimes left anonymously on a grave if the mourner is not able to share their grief, or regularly replaced if you have a memory table at home for your ancestors, especially if you are far from your roots. • Because zinnia is a long-blooming flower, the petals can be used for any matter that may take time to fix. • Carry the dried petals of the rarer green variety to fill a green purse if you have money troubles that will take months to resolve; each week, shed a few green petals in an open space until all are gone, taking with them your worries. As the purse empties, replace the green petals with orange and yellow zinnia petals for success and optimism. • If it is a slow-moving love matter, begin with pink petals in a pink bag and replace with red or fuchsia zinnia petals so your purse is never empty. • Grow a variety of colors in your garden or buy a mixed bunch of colors to ensure your home will always be abundant and filled with love. • Send the purple or rarer blue zinnia flowers as congratulations for an examination or career success.

CAUTION

Zinnia is nontoxic to adults, children, and pets, but some people have a skin reaction to the sap and hairy leaves with prolonged handling.

Zucchini

(*Cucurbita pepo*)

MAGICAL FORMS

also called courgette outside the USA • see also squash blossom and marrow (p. 284) • emerald to dark-green fruit, pale green to white flesh inside • cooked or eaten raw as a vegetable • an immature fruit that can be left on the vine to become a marrow • however, generally other cultivars are preferred for a stronger flavor • brought to North America from Italy in the 1920s • grows in temperate climes • magically use the raw and cooked vegetable and the flower essence

PLANETS AND ELEMENTS

Mercury/Moon • Air/Water

MAGICAL USES

as the essence, for women's concerns and anima concerns in both sexes, especially in pregnancy and after the birth for new parents • to bring bonding between mother and child after a difficult birth or if there are doubts and difficulties during pregnancy • calms anxiety when conception is slow • the plant, added to baked products or as a substitute for pasta or combined with pasta, brings prosperity and welcomes family members from or into a new relationship

HOW TO USE

Etch your love's name on the side of a zucchini and cook it to preserve fidelity in the relationship. If you are worried about unfaithfulness, freeze the uncooked zucchini containing the name. • While pregnant, to create a sense of harmony and connect with the unborn infant, add a drop or two of the essence to aloe vera cream for massage (the partner can massage the womb) or to bath water.

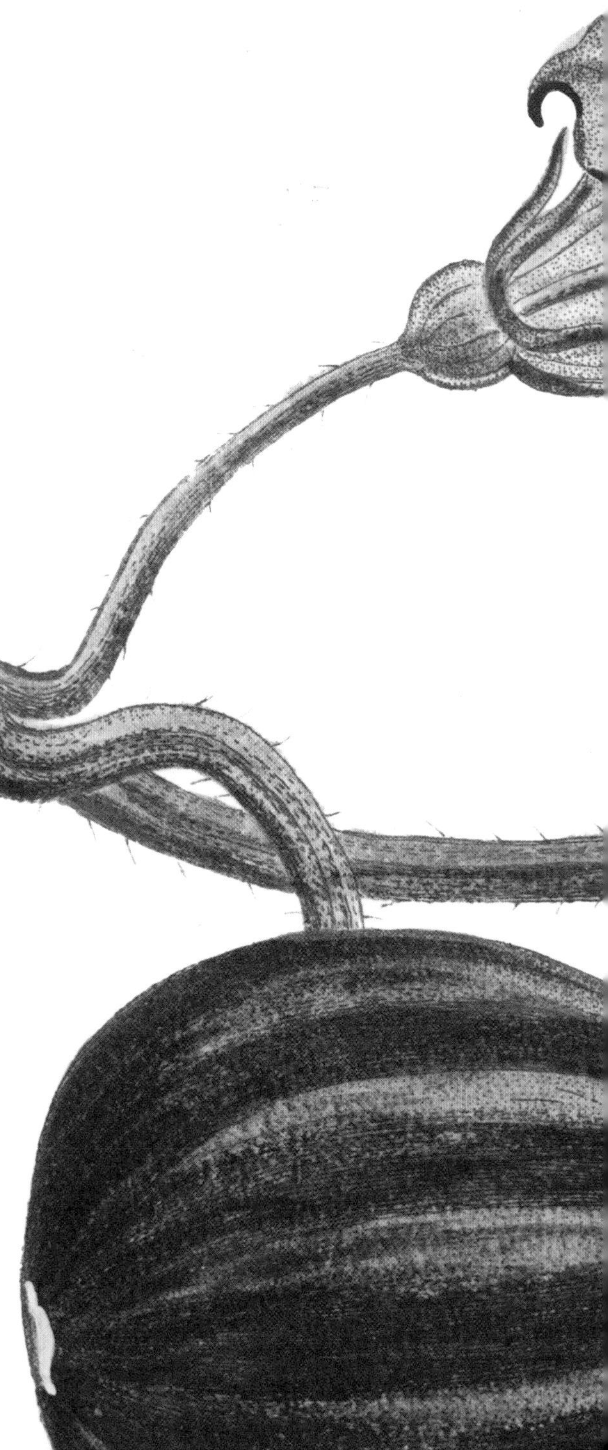

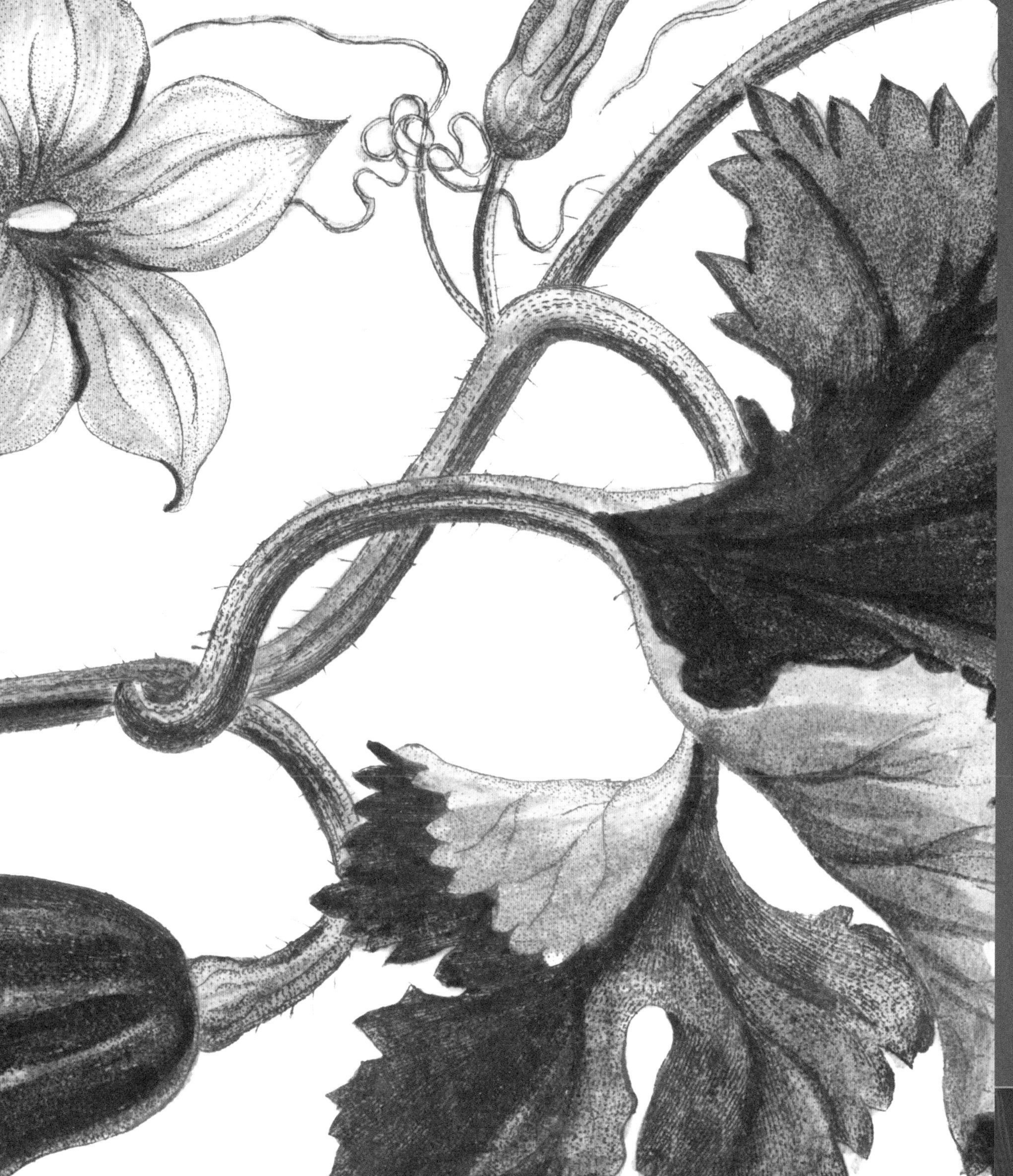

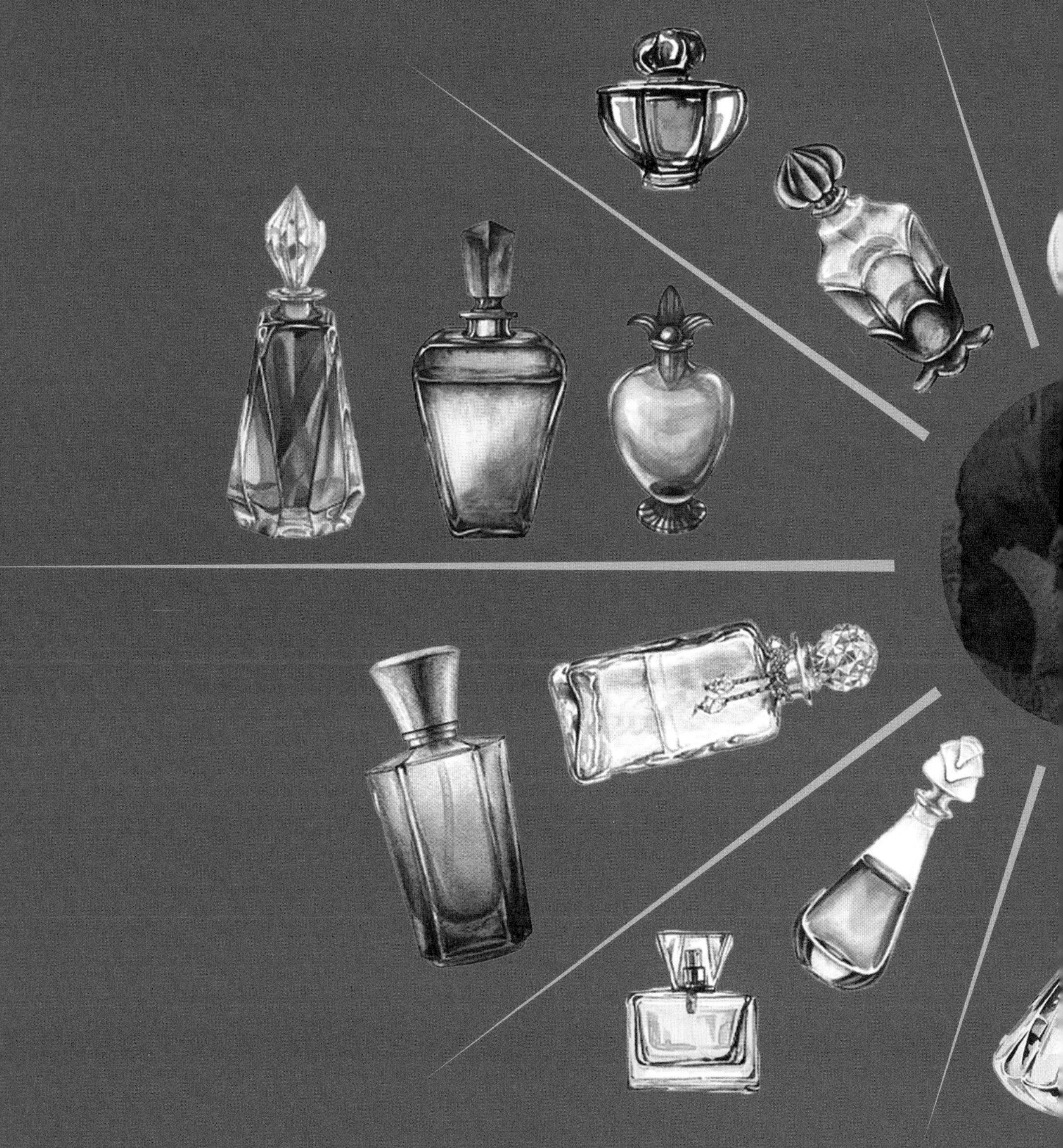

Magical Perfumes

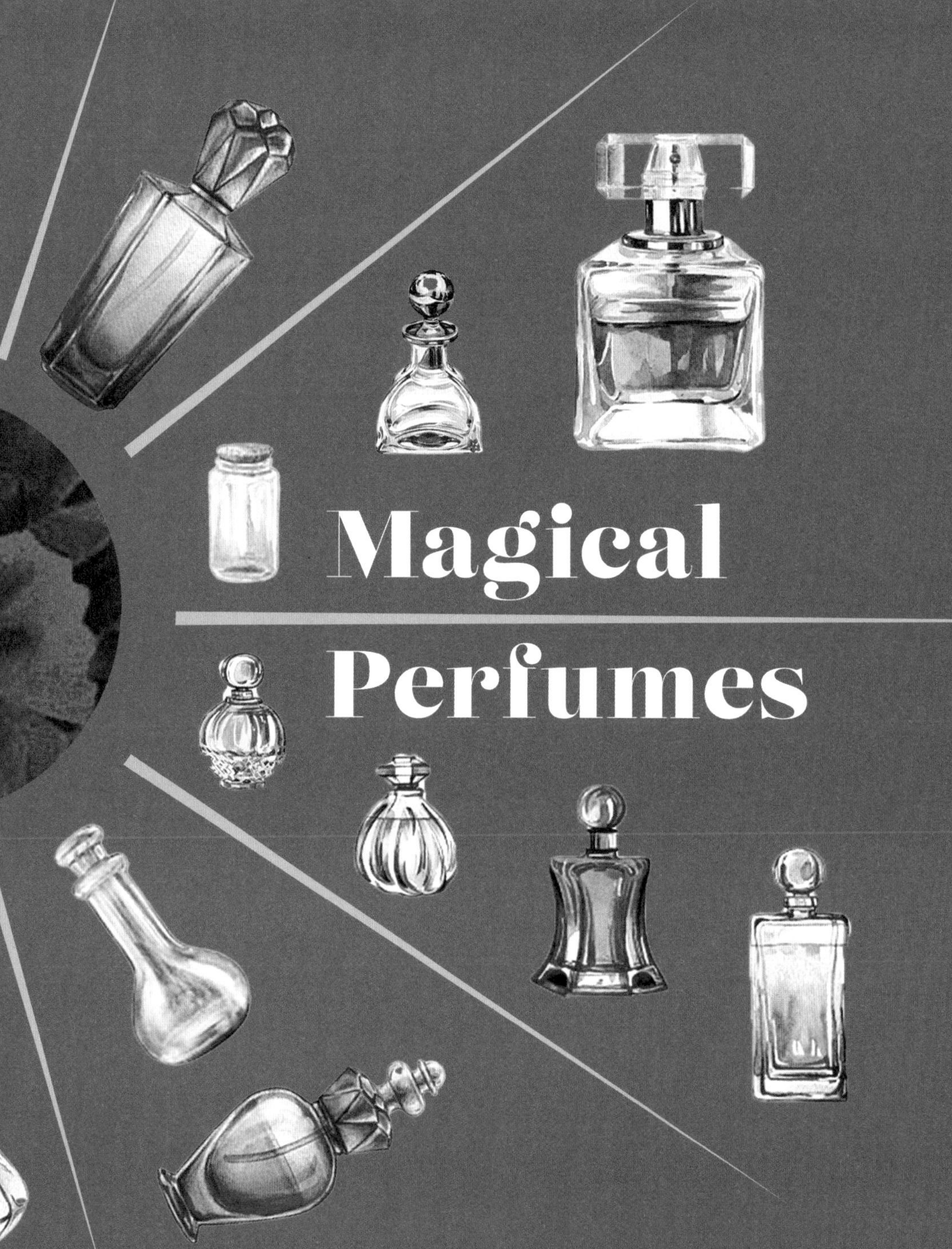

Alchimie

MAGICAL FORMS

Created in 1998 by Jacques Cavallier, this scent is characterized by a feel-good mesmeric factor so the wearer can awaken the senses of even the most hesitant or undemonstrative lover, especially if a rival or an ex will be present or for a work association to be cast in a new, dramatic, alluring light.

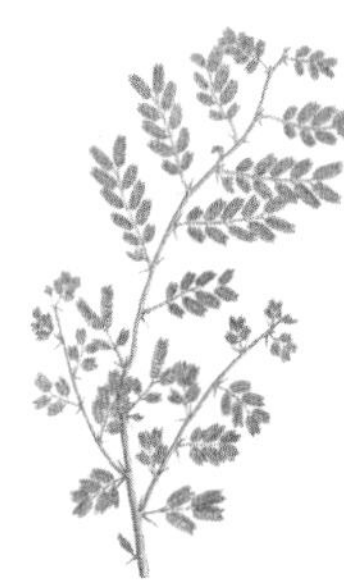

INGREDIENTS

TOP NOTES
Bergamot, cassia, cucumber, grapefruit, hyacinth, lilac, peach, plum, pear, lilac, mandarin

HEART NOTES
Acacia, coconut, heliotrope, jasmine, lily of the valley, passion flower, rose, wisteria

BASE NOTES
Amber, caramel, licorice, musk, sandalwood, tonka beans, vanilla

HOW TO USE

For enchanting a lover or the desired focus of your passion, recite their name as you twirl around in both directions, nine times, holding the sealed bottle, saying nine times, *Bewitched, bedazzled, enchanted, may you be by my Alchimie; alone me you shall see.* End by putting your lips to the bottle before applying the fragrance to pulse points. When you meet your lover or desired love, repeat the chant in your mind and touch your pulse points to connect with the magick.

Alien Eau de Parfum and Alien Goddess

MAGICAL FORMS

Alien was created in 2005 and Goddess in 2022. Alien is often chosen as a birthday, anniversary, or Christmas gift for a female partner, to say, *To me, you are beautiful, radiant, and of immense worth.* The newer Alien Goddess perfume continues the theme of linking with divine feminine energies that has made Alien prized by women exploring their goddess within. Alien and Alien Goddess create a strong sense of female mystery and of the woman as a spiritual being.

INGREDIENTS (ALIEN)

TOP NOTES
Jasmine sambac

HEART NOTE
Cashmere wood

BASE NOTE
White amber

INGREDIENTS (ALIEN GODDESS)

TOP NOTES
Coconut, bergamot

HEART NOTES
Jasmine flower, jasmine tea

BASE NOTES
Vanilla, benzoin, cashmere wood

HOW TO USE

Anoint the Third Eye, the center of the brow, and the crown energy center in the center of the hairline before any rituals that are centered on female energies, the goddess, and all-female magical groups.

Amarige

MAGICAL FORMS

A designer scent created by Dominique Ropion for Givenchy in 1991 that is long-lasting without being overpowering. It is an anagram of the French word *mariage*, and so is for a woman who wishes to tell the world she is in love and has found the right person or who is seeking a love who is worthy. It is also a great fragrance for a woman who loves herself as she is and for whom she is but welcomes whomever or whatever touches her with joy.

INGREDIENTS

TOP NOTES

Brazilian rosewood, mandarin, neroli, peach, plum, violet

HEART NOTES

Acacia farnesiana (sweet acacia), gardenia, jasmine, mimosa, red berries, tuberose, ylang-ylang

BASE NOTES

Amber or ambergris, cedar, musk, tonka bean, vanilla

HOW TO USE

Keep the fragrance surrounded by sparkling crystals or near a vase of fresh yellow flowers to fill it with life force and abundance. • Before a celebration or in situations when there is a chance to enrich yourself financially through a chance meeting, lightly spritz it in your aura energy field around the head and shoulders, picturing a shower of golden light beams entering your body. • Buy it at the airport for a happy vacation, which may include romance if you are unattached.

Anais Anais L'Original

MAGICAL FORMS

Called the fragrance of spring, this eau de toilette was created in 1978 by a group of perfumiers including Roger Pellegrino. It was Cacharel's first fragrance. Because of its incense-type scent, it works best for the woman who loves flowers, oils, and incenses. Women who are ready for new beginnings, no matter the time of the year or stage of life, are the right audience for Anais Anais, particularly a woman who is open to being romanced and retains youthful curiosity for what is around the next corner.

INGREDIENTS

TOP NOTES

Blackcurrant bud, citrus, galbanum, honeysuckle, hyacinth, lily of the valley, white Madonna lily

HEART NOTES

Grasse rose, iris, jasmine, orris root, orange blossom, tuberose, ylang-ylang

BASE NOTES

Amber, Bourbon vetiver (sometimes considered a heart ingredient), cedar, incense, patchouli, sandalwood

HOW TO USE

Anoint crystals or a crystal ball with a drop of the fragrance to gain visions of the future and, if you are not in love, of a future love. If you don't have crystals, anoint the center of your brow to open your psychic Third Eye for clairvoyant images in your mind or answers in tarot, angel, or oracle cards to reveal what lies over the horizon. • Put a drop behind your knees to let go of old sorrows or doubts and to walk forward to opportunity.

Baccarat Rouge 540

MAGICAL FORMS

A unisex fragrance created by Francis himself (of Maison Francis Kurkdjian) that provokes a *wow* reaction and ensures you won't be forgotten, whether socially, romantically, or in a business situation. Baccarat Rouge 540 is a long-lasting fragrance that makes the transition between day and evening and is especially suited for the fall and winter—when it is at its best—or in cool climates in summer. It is a fragrance for carving out your identity and for making positive impressions, especially in new situations or ones where you have previously felt undermined or invisible or are in a very competitive or overly macho environment.

INGREDIENTS

TOP NOTES
Jasmine, saffron

HEART NOTES
Amberwood, ambergris

BASE NOTES
Cedar, fir resin

HOW TO USE

Empower your fragrance with sound when you first purchase it, using bells, a small drum, or a singing bowl, moving all around it and chanting continuously at the same time as rhythmically using your instruments, saying, *Empower this hour, make me the center that I may enter every situation and radiate my power.* You will feel the bottle vibrating and know it is ready to use. • Re-empower your fragrance at any transition in your life, or when you want to stop the room on entering and make a strong impression.

BDK Oud Abramad Eau de Parfum

MAGICAL FORMS

A unisex perfume created in 2016 by David Benedek for BDK Parfums, this is a fragrance for the old soul, for natural healers and leaders to whom others will stop and listen. Its scent is ageless and timeless. Those wearing this perfume have a natural awareness of the cycles of the year and life and are most at home with others who are spiritual and questing for meaning.

INGREDIENTS

TOP NOTES
Saffron, ginger

HEART NOTES
Cumin, Turkish rose (damascene)

BASE NOTES
Agarwood (oud), labdanum, patchouli

HOW TO USE

To access other dimensions, wear the fragrance when visiting ancient and sacred places to tune into their energies. • Alternatively, anoint the center of your hairline with a drop or two to reach these spaces in meditation or astral travel to past worlds you may have once inhabited.

Black Opium Eau de Parfum

MAGICAL FORMS

Created for Yves Saint Laurent in 2019 by a group of perfumiers including Nathalie Lorson and Marie Salamagne, this is the espresso of the perfume world: an instant energizer and rocket boost for a grand entrance and attention-holding responses. It also naturally attracts all that is opulent and prosperous, personally and in front of others.

INGREDIENTS

TOP NOTES
Pear, pink pepper, mandarin essence

HEART NOTES
Almond, coffee, jasmine, licorice

BASE NOTES
Cashmere, cedar patchouli, vanilla

HOW TO USE

Keep this perfume in a gold-colored dish with a gold cloth lining or scarf, along with small pieces of gold and silver, such as earrings or lucky charms, and gold- and silver-colored coins. • Before using, place your hands around the bottle, saying, *Gold and silver to me come, silver of the moon and gold of the sun, that treasure however needed shall be won* (you can specify if, for example, you are networking at a career event).

Black Orchid Eau de Parfum

MAGICAL FORMS

Inspired by a black orchid, the darkest in the world, this perfume was created for Tom Ford, producer of the fragrance, by a Californian orchid grower. Black Orchid was first brought into being in 2006 by David Apel and Pierre Negrin of the fragrance company Givaudan. It contains a trace of the rare black orchid and so is best suited for strong, independent women who are at home in their bodies and with their sexuality and sensuality to enhance passion without guilt or inhibitions but always demanding respect.

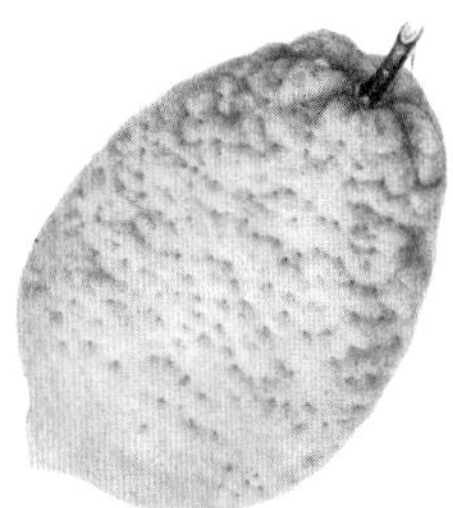

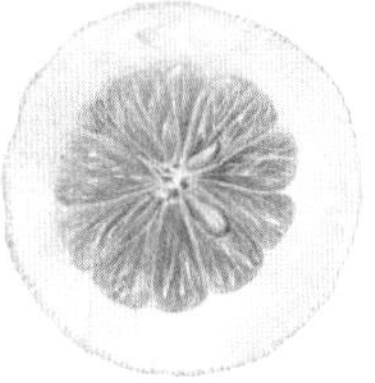

INGREDIENTS

TOP NOTES
Amalfi lemon, bergamot, black currant, jasmine, mandarin orange, osmanthus, tea, truffle, ylang-ylang

HEART NOTES
Gardenia, jasmine, lotus, spices, orchid, ylang-ylang

BASE NOTES
Mexican chocolate, incense, patchouli, vanilla vetiver, white musk

HOW TO USE

To feel good about your body before an occasion when you may choose to make love, massage your navel, the seat of your sacral energy center, to increase personal desire and to create the aura where you will be offered emotional as well as physical connection—or walk away.

Boss Bottled Elixir for Men

MAGICAL FORMS

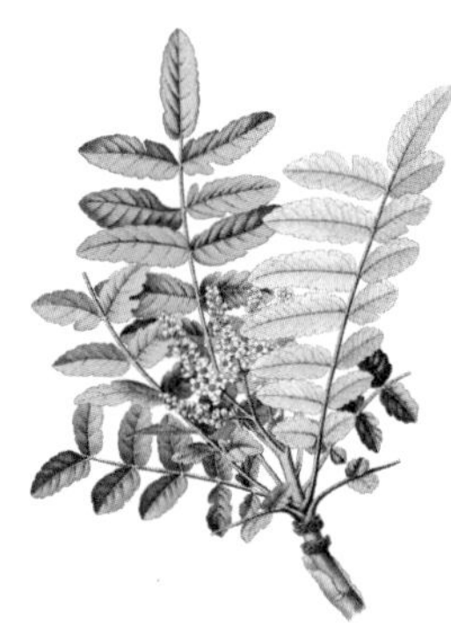

Created for Hugo Boss in 2023 by Amick Menardo and Suzy le Helley, Bottled Elixir was chosen to express inner confidence and to inspire trust in others. It is best suited for those who wish to be able to take charge of any situation at a moment's notice. The user will attract many would-be friends but is also very discerning—a partner or best friend, once chosen, will be for life.

INGREDIENTS

TOP NOTES
Frankincense, cardamom

HEART NOTES
Vetiver, patchouli

BASE NOTES
Labdanum, cedarwood

HOW TO USE

Bottled Elixir is very much a self-charging fragrance, as over time it will create a unique bond between itself and the wearer. For this reason, it is not one to lend or share with other guys in the locker room or even a best friend or partner. • Because it makes the user totally unself-conscious of creating an impression, it automatically deters any who would try to take advantage or intimidate others, especially when the fragrance is worn over time (it is not to be alternated with other fragrances!). • Before gifting the fragrance to a friend or partner, burn a red candle all the way through near the bottle to activate its energies.

Capricci

MAGICAL FORMS

Created for Nina Ricci in 1960 by Francis Fabron, this scent is for the businesswoman who wishes to be taken seriously and insists on equal opportunities without losing her femininity. It is ideal for the working mother who still has her eye on the top.

INGREDIENTS

TOP NOTES
Bergamot, green fragrances

HEART NOTES
Gardenia, hyacinth, jasmine, lily of the valley, narcissus, orris, rose, rosemary, ylang-ylang

BASE NOTES
Benzoin, musk, oakmoss, sandalwood, vetiver

HOW TO USE

Keep an emergency bottle in your office or workspace by taking a small vial filtered from a larger bottle. • Apply behind your ears when no one is listening or taking you seriously or to tune in to gossip when you know there is talk behind your back. Afterward, inhale the fragrance and feel strength and power flowing into your aura so you speak and act decisively and coolly, and gain or regain authority with charm and lightness of touch.

Chance Eau de Cologne

MAGICAL FORMS

Created for Coco Chanel by Jacques Polge in 2003, this scent is for manifesting unexpected chances and transforming daily life into an adventure by seeing and seizing possibilities you might have otherwise dismissed as impractical.

INGREDIENTS

TOP NOTES
Hyacinth, iris, patchouli, pineapple, pink pepper

HEART NOTES
Jasmine, lemon, rose

BASE NOTES
Musk, patchouli, vanilla, vetiver

HOW TO USE

Whether you are speculating, making a sudden decision based on new factors, or taking a risk financially, romantically, or in your career—or if you just sense positive change in the air—very gently cup your hands around the sealed bottle with your joined fingers at the top, saying nine times, *Take a risk, take a chance, Wheel of Fortune, for me dance.* End by putting the bottle against your heart, then applying a little perfume to your inner wrist points to fill your heart with anticipation of good times ahead. Afterward, go make your fortune!

Chanel N° 5 Eau de Parfum

MAGICAL FORMS

This perfume was created for Coco Chanel in 1921 by Ernest Beaux. Coco wanted something different, an abstract fragrance that had no dominant notes but gave an air of indefinable but unforgettable mystery. Chanel N° 5 is believed to contain over eighty ingredients. It is available as the original N° 5, as well as the Sensual N° 5 with citrus and vanilla, and in the N° 5 Woody fragrance, intertwined with sandalwood. Additionally, Airy is available with notes of ylang-ylang, and Fresh with vetiver and cedar.

INGREDIENTS

TOP NOTES
Grasse jasmine, aldehydes

HEART NOTES
May rose, ylang-ylang, iris

BASE NOTES
Amber, patchouli

HOW TO USE

Empower the fragrance by lighting a gold candle so the brightness reflects in the bottle, blowing softly into the flame, then saying, *The answer shall be yes*. Blow out the candle, filling yourself with the radiance. • Apply perfume to pulse points while picturing the desired outcome of a special occasion or situation.

CK Obsession for Men Eau de Toilette

MAGICAL FORMS

Created for Calvin Klein in 1986 by Robert Slattery. It's especially potent for a man who is not afraid to express his feelings. Wear with a twin soul perfume for a partner, CK Obsession for women if your partner is female or the male version if you have a male twin soul—this combination serves as a declaration of commitment to the world. This scent is an ideal Thanksgiving or Yuletide gift because of its cinnamon and pine notes. It is also perfect for those whose greatest wish is to fulfill their ambitions.

INGREDIENTS

TOP NOTES
Cinnamon, coriander, grapefruit, lavender, lime

HEART NOTES
Brazilian rosewood, carnation, myrrh, nutmeg, pine, sage

BASE NOTES
Amber, benzoin, patchouli, sandalwood, vetiver, vanilla

HOW TO USE

If there is a cause close to your heart, a burning desire, or talent as yet undeveloped, hold your CK bottle to generate its ability to aid in manifestation. Then pass a lighted incense stick in frankincense, cinnamon, or pine around the bottle in spirals clockwise in the air (make sure not to get too close to the bottle). As you do so, name your desire in a single word over and over again, faster and faster as you move the incense through the air. When you can go no faster, plunge the lighted incense stick into a dish of earth. Keep a symbol of your ambition with the bottle when not in use.

CK One Eau de Toilette

MAGICAL FORMS

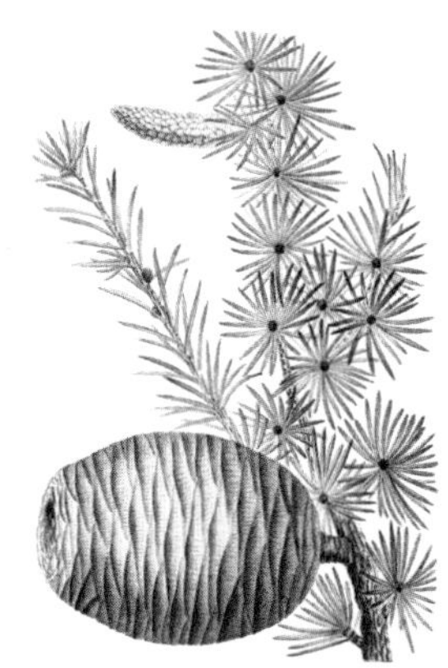

Created for Calvin Klein by Alberto Morillas and Harry Fremont in 1994, it is one of the first unisex fragrances to challenge the concept gender-specific fragrance. At an affordable price, it was meant to appeal to Generation X, those born between the 1960s and the early 1980s. It comes into its own as a hot weather perfume, so it is especially effective worn on summer vacations or when traveling to warmer destinations. It's best for carefree days, having fun, and for those to whom experiences and exploration of life are more important than possessions or settling down.

INGREDIENTS

TOP NOTES
Bergamot, cardamom, green fragrances, lemon, mandarin orange, papaya, pineapple

HEART NOTES
Freesia, nutmeg, jasmine, orris, rose

BASE NOTES
Amber, cedarwood, green tea, musk, sandalwood

HOW TO USE

To avoid being stereotyped or forced down a particular road through the expectations of family, the workplace, and society, carry the fragrance with you in a small vial or spray bottle, then head for the restroom and rub it on the soles of your feet and your thighs or the small of your back to awaken your resting Kundalini inner powerhouse for a positive immediate response to opportunities when a fast decision or action are needed.

Classique Eau de Parfum for Women

MAGICAL FORMS

Long-lasting and distinctive, this scent was created for Jean Paul Gaultier in 1992 by Jacques Cavallier. It's especially effective for those who wish to maintain an authoritative presence and the ability to make a lasting positive impression without being ostentatious. When worn, it aids in its wearer becoming memorable even in a crowd, whether at an audition, a performance, or among other candidates for a new job.

INGREDIENTS

TOP NOTES
Rose, rum

HEART NOTES
Daffodil, orchid, narcissus, vanilla

BASE NOTES
Amber, sandalwood, tonka bean, vanilla

HOW TO USE

The night before you speak during a significant video call with unknown or high-status people, take your place in a line of hopefuls to demonstrate your abilities, or face an individual on whom you wish to make an impression, surround your fragrance bottle with a circle of business cards or printed passport photos of yourself (make sure you're smiling in the pictures). In clockwise order, touch each with the index finger of your dominant hand (the one you write with) or the pointed end of a clear quartz crystal, saying for each, *See me, notice me, imprint me positively on your memory*. Leave them in place with the fragrance in the center of the ring overnight. The next morning, anoint the center of your brow with a drop of fragrance and carry one card or photo with you in a wallet or bag.

Cloud Eau de Parfum

MAGICAL FORMS

Created for performer Ariana Grande in 2018 by Clement Gavarry, this butterfly-aligned fragrance brings laughter, creating happiness and making every day fun. When this scent is worn, all the rain clouds in the sky will change to white fluffy ones. This fragrance attracts admirers and admiration effortlessly and then dances on. Its message is "enjoy today without regrets for the past or fears of the future—also, if you wish, aim for stardom in your own way."

INGREDIENTS

TOP NOTES
Bergamot, lavender blossom, pear

HEART NOTES
Crème de coconut, lavender blossom, praline, vanilla orchid

BASE NOTES
Ambroxan (which is a modern synthetic with a dry amber, musky fragrance, a mix of plant-based and synthetic musk), cashmeran (a synthetic, smelling like soft new wool)

HOW TO USE

Spritz above your head to brighten aura energies and on pulse points to increase personal allure. • Wear for fun, flirtation, and romance. • Wrap your perfume in colored ribbons, surrounding it with bright flowers, and dance and sing around it, which lets wishes come true quite spontaneously.

Coach for Men Eau de Toilette

MAGICAL FORMS

This scent was created in 2017 for Coach by Anne Flipo and Bruno Jovanovic. Like the luxury brand of accessories of the same name, Coach has the smell of understated opulence. It can be worn in any situation and at any time of the year, works well in day or evening, and is just as effective for work as it is for pleasure. It produces a fresh perspective and stress-free approach to life and works best for those who wish to assume the best about everything and everyone. It makes the user totally unself-conscious in any situation.

INGREDIENTS

TOP NOTES
Asian (Nashi) pear, bergamot, kumquat

HEART NOTES
Cardamom, coriander, geranium

BASE NOTES
Ambergris, cedar, amber wood, vetiver

HOW TO USE

Allow the bottle to breathe freely on display, not shut in a cupboard, so when it is applied, it offers an instant and ongoing "wake up world!" message. • The more frequently the fragrance is used, the more it projects the wearer as someone to be trusted and whose opinions should be taken seriously—someone who never lacks a suggestion or solution, seemingly without effort.

Coco Mademoiselle Eau de Parfum

MAGICAL FORMS

Created in 2001 for Chanel by Jacques Polge, this is a chameleon perfume for the ever-changing moods and aspects of personality of an independent yet caring woman. It is for the woman who protects those she loves but also challenges them—without malice. It's for those who can tease and provoke without causing hurt, for the young or young-at-heart sophisticate who constantly reinvents herself and her life so that she can explore new situations.

INGREDIENTS

TOP NOTES
Bergamot, grapefruit, mandarin orange, orange blossom

HEART NOTES
Lychee, iris, jasmine mimosa, Turkish rose (damascena)

BASE NOTES
Opoponax, patchouli, vanilla, tonka bean, vetiver, white musk

HOW TO USE

Place a little of the fragrance beneath your pillow for magical dreams of walking and running through fields of flowers, where you may glimpse someone you know or have yet to meet who may become significant to you. If you are lucky, you will be able to talk with that person heart-to-heart on the astral plane. • For those who are older, the scent brings dreams of being young and free again, dancing and moving close to others and then tantalizingly away, so that you'll seem to float over the earth and maybe fly, awakening refreshed and full of hope for the day ahead.

Daisy Eau de Toilette

MAGICAL FORMS

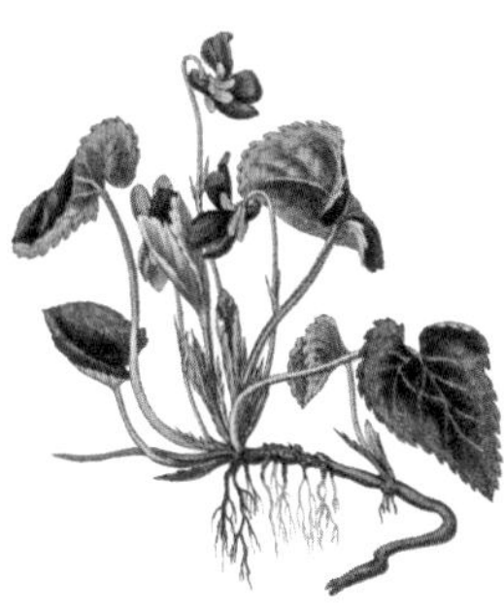

Created for Marc Jacobs in 2007 by Alberto Morillas, this is a fresh yet sophisticated fragrance for fun, spontaneous days in the sun and for all female friendships, parties, vacations, and girls' nights. It is a wonderful gift that speaks to appreciation between women of all ages for their "besties" and particularly for younger women who delight in their femininity and enjoy sharing confidences and secrets with trusted female friends.

INGREDIENTS

TOP NOTES
Grapefruit, jasmine, strawberries, violet leaf, wild berries

HEART NOTES
Gardenia, jasmine, white violet

BASE NOTES
Musk, vanilla, white woods

HOW TO USE

When you first obtain it, surround your bottle with a circle of daisies, whether garden daisies, Michaelmas daisies, or the more exotic African or Gerbera kind, according to which fits your persona, or a mixture if you have many aspects to reveal or conceal. When the flowers fade, scatter the shredded petals outdoors in a high or open space to express your love of freedom and pleasure in making the world around you fit your unfettered desired lifestyle.

Dior Sauvage Elixir for Men

MAGICAL FORMS

Created for Christian Dior in 2021 by Francois Demachy, this scent is full of fire—an "action man" fragrance inspired by ideas and original approaches to existing problems. Wearing it will energize, remove inertia, maximize opportunities, and make unlikely solutions work.

INGREDIENTS

TOP NOTES
Nutmeg, cinnamon, cardamom, grapefruit

HEART NOTE
Lavender

BASE NOTES
Licorice, sandalwood, amber patchouli, Haitian vetiver

HOW TO USE

Burn a ring of small, red candles around the unopened bottle, especially if you are buying the fragrance to give to your man to make him more dynamic. • Personally adopt the fragrance to assert your presence and rights when it is most needed, and for making a fast decision rather than sitting on the fence. • Wear this if you are naturally reticent and stay in the background, to help you express deeply held beliefs and opinions that may run contrary to the status quo.

DKNY Be Delicious Eau de Parfum

MAGICAL FORMS

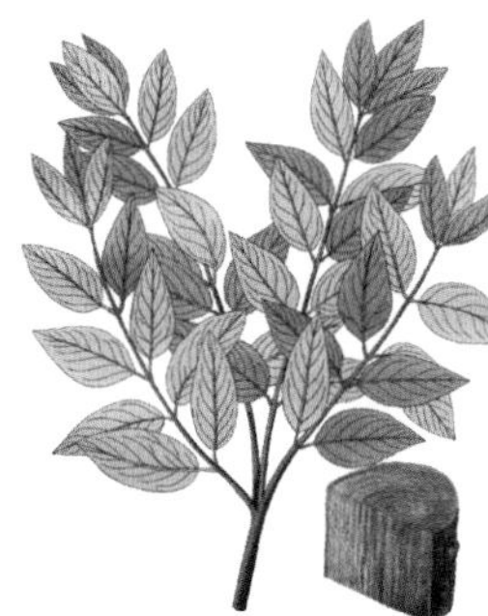

Created for Donna Karan in 2004 by Maurice Roucel, this perfume is perfect for wearing in the workplace and in your social life to manifest—behind the smile and encouraging words—a powerful agenda that can be achieved to mutual satisfaction and with minimum dissension.

INGREDIENTS

TOP NOTES
Cucumber, grapefruit, magnolia

HEART NOTES
Apple, lily of the valley, rose, tuberose, violet

BASE NOTES
Amber, musk, woods (especially sandalwood)

HOW TO USE

Bury your bottle in a basket or bowl of fresh, fragrant fruit, placing your hands on either side of the basket and then bringing them closer, then farther away, for a minute or two. As you do so, recite softly, *Be fragrant, be sweet, that all our desires may meet, in mutual satisfaction without disagreement or distraction*. Then remove the bottle and apply the fragrance first to the inner pulse points of your wrists and then to your throat for a mix of head and heart energy. Whenever you have a specific purpose, repeat the action, adapting the words accordingly.

Eau de Campagne

MAGICAL FORMS

A unisex fragrance created for Sisley in 1976 by Jean-Claude Ellena, this perfume is for men and women who love the outdoors and seek to recreate the same freshness indoors or who need but lack that pure life flow.

INGREDIENTS

TOP NOTES
Bergamot, basil, lemon, wild herbs, galbanum

HEART NOTES
Tomato leaves, lily of the valley, jasmine, geranium plum

BASE NOTES
Oakmoss, patchouli, vetiver, musk

HOW TO USE

Keep fresh greenery near your fragrance when you are not using it. • To empower the fragrance, on a full moon, set the bottle where it will absorb lunar energies. • Purchase the fragrance at the airport when going on vacation and give to a workaholic partner to encourage their enthusiasm for the exploration of new lands, flowers, forests, seashores, and mountains rather than staying by the pool or in the bar plugged into office technology.

Eau Dynamisante

MAGICAL FORMS

Created in 1987 by Jacques Courtin-Clarins, this scent is a harmonizing, healing unisex fragrance to wear when a couple goes out socially to be recognized and accepted in a new relationship whenever there may be resistance, perhaps because of loyalty to an ex.

INGREDIENTS

TOP NOTES
Caraway, coriander, lemon, orange, petitgrain

HEART NOTES
Cardamom, carnation, rosemary, thyme

BASE NOTE
Patchouli

HOW TO USE

Whenever you need energy or your immune system is not protecting you from numerous minor ailments, add the fragrance to a diffuser or aroma lamp. • If you are not using this specific perfume, a little rosemary, thyme, and patchouli oil (all ingredients in the scent) will do the same job. • To empower the perfume, allow the smoke or steam to waft around the bottle, activating its healing properties. Wear your empowered fragrance if you have a physically or emotionally challenging day or evening ahead.

English Pear & Freesia Cologne

MAGICAL FORMS

Created for Jo Malone in 2010 by Christine Nagel, this is an "all through the year" fragrance for celebrations, especially those connected with the seasons, festivals, and family milestones. It is an ideal gift for a woman who has just had a baby or who is trying for one, especially if she is older or has been using contraception for many years and feels anxious to harmonize her cycles with those of the natural world.

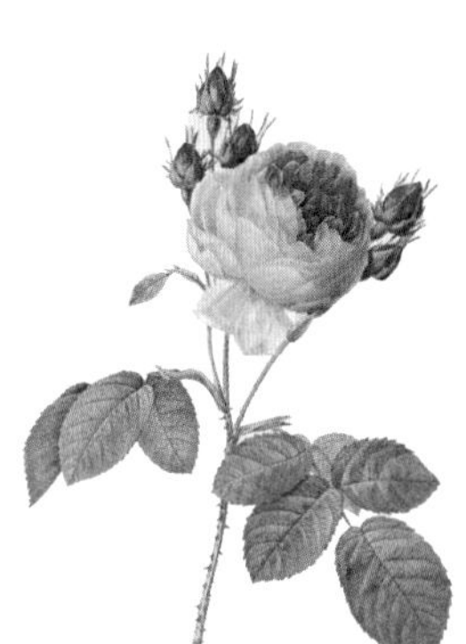

INGREDIENTS

TOP NOTES
King William pear, melon

HEART NOTES
Rose, white freesia

BASE NOTES
Amber, patchouli, rhubarb, white musk

HOW TO USE

Surround your fragrance when new with fragrant blossoms from any tree, flowering white freesias, or any white flowers. Inhale the fragrance and the life force of the flowers, breathing out all worries or what disturbs you. When you feel at peace, open the bottle and anoint your inner wrists to fill your heart with love of life, and set your flowers free outdoors.

Flowerbomb Eau de Parfum

MAGICAL FORMS

Created for Viktor & Rolf in 2005 by designers including Olivier Polge and Carlos Benaïm, this scent could be described as an ever-changing bouquet, sophisticated when the occasion demands for dressed-to-the-nines champagne evenings, but with a hidden element that, whatever a woman's age, allows her to feel and act girly and feminine when she encounters flirtation or a promise of romance.

INGREDIENTS

TOP NOTES
Bergamot, osmanthus, green tea

HEART NOTES
Freesia, jasmine, orange blossom, orchid, rose

BASE NOTES
Musk, patchouli, vanilla

HOW TO USE

Release this flower bomb before a special occasion when someone significant will be present or before going out for the day, by spritzing lightly around yourself, saying as you do so, *I walk among the flowers, my fascination more irresistible hour by hour, magnetic, unmissable, my radiance do I empower.* Wear your empowered perfume with your favorite flower or carry a velvet sachet of the fresh petals when seduction is the name of the game.

Giorgio Beverly Hills

MAGICAL FORMS

Created for Giorgio in 1981 by Bob Aliano, this fragrance is intense, long-lasting, and unforgettable, especially for the woman who has known for years this is *her* perfume and has no intention of changing it or her "get up and go" lifestyle.

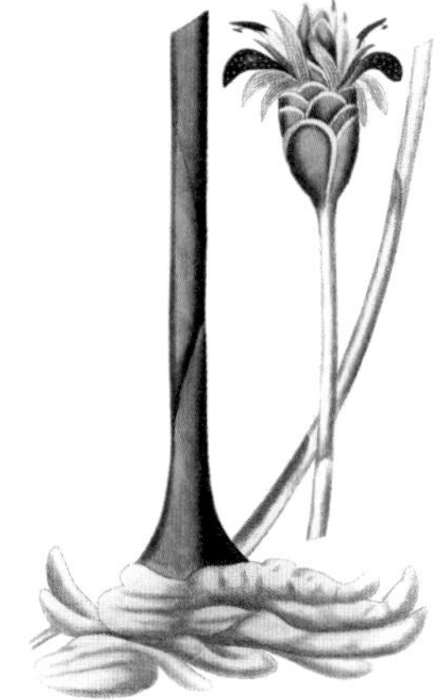

INGREDIENTS

TOP NOTES
Bitter grape, grapefruit, melon, pineapple

HEART NOTES
Gardenia, ginger, orchid, peach, peony

BASE NOTES
Sandalwood, vetiver

HOW TO USE

Put a very small amount of the fragrance in a tiny bowl when you have an especially active day ahead, setting a yellow mercurial candle on either side of the bowl. First, light the left-hand candle, and from it the right-hand one. Blow out the left-hand candle fast, then relight it from the right-hand one. Continue the lighting and blowing out sequence until your aura is buzzing. Blow out the remaining candle, sending the light into the bowl and your own energy field. Dab the fragrance on the soles of your feet, the inside of your ankles, and your wrists, and anoint the handle of the front door with any remaining fragrance before you take on the world.

Good Girl Eau de Parfum

MAGICAL FORMS

Created for Carolina Herrera in 2016 by Louise Turner and Quentin Bisch, this is a provocative, sexy, classy scent worn for pleasure rather than work. It is a party fragrance, offering anyone who wears it the confidence to become the center of any gathering. It comes into its own in the fall and winter, especially on dark nights indoors.

INGREDIENTS

TOP NOTES
Almond, bergamot, coffee, lemon

HEART NOTES
Jasmine sambac, orange blossom, orris, rose, tuberose

BASE NOTES
Cacao, cedar, cinnamon, patchouli, praline, sandalwood

HOW TO USE

Apply slowly and sensuously to pulse points and close to erotic zones after a bath or shower for the feel-good factor, whether heading out for a celebration or a date or staying home with chocolates, wine, and a racy novel.

Impact Spark Eau de Toilette for Men

MAGICAL FORMS

Created for Tommy Hilfiger and launched in 2022, this scent is more citrusy than the original Impact. It's great for seizing the moment, giving way to a sudden desire to go and sometimes just to keep going. The fragrance lights the spark of adventure and curiosity to see what is over the next horizon. If you are still footloose, Impact Spark will attract a similarly minded partner for travel and exploration, who, regardless of their gender, may borrow your fragrance and claim it as their own.

INGREDIENTS

TOP NOTES
Bergamot, bitter orange, fig, lemon, violet leaf

HEART NOTES
Cardamom, French cypress, green tea

BASE NOTES
Akigalawood (a spicy, woody extract of patchouli), cedar, sandalwood

HOW TO USE

Men may be attracted initially to the fragrance because it is like a breath of fresh air—really more like a wind tunnel!—stirring life after a mental hibernation. • Wear it on a windy day, on the soles of the feet and on ankles and knees to remove doubts and on the small of the back to wake the slumbering Kundalini serpent power and see where your feet take you.

J'adore Eau de Parfum

MAGICAL FORMS

Created for Christian Dior in 1999, it has, since then, appeared in various concentrates, including a Parfum d'eau consisting of flowers and water without alcohol. Made from flowers from around the world, J'adore Eau de Parfum contains the rare Grasse jasmine. It's great for first dates, especially if you are older and revisiting the dating scene, as it combines elegance and sophistication radiating from the aura to attract compliments and, if wanted, the right kind of romance.

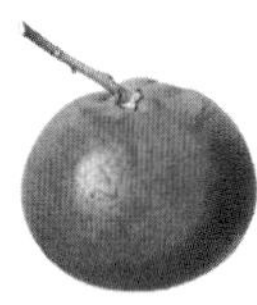

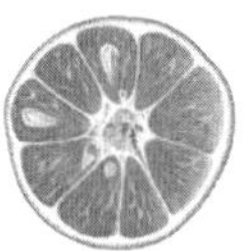

INGREDIENTS

TOP NOTES
Bergamot, magnolia, mandarin, melon, orange, peach, pear

HEART NOTES
Freesia, jasmine, lily of the valley, magnolia, mandarin, orchid, plum, tuberose, violet

BASE NOTES
Blackberry, cedar, musk, vanilla

HOW TO USE

Buy a bouquet of mixed flowers, fragrances, and colors as a sign to yourself and the world that you are ready for the right love, placing it in a vase. Then set your perfume in front of the vase until the first petals start to fall on and around it, indicating that your fragrance has been activated.

Jimmy Choo Eau de Parfum for Women

MAGICAL FORMS

Created as the first perfume for Jimmy Choo in 2011 by Olivier Polge, this fragrance becomes part of the woman and acts for the wearer as a magnet for would-be lovers, friends, and business associates, and is especially good at breaking down competitive barriers between women. This versatile scent can be used in all seasons, all settings, and all times of the day.

INGREDIENTS

TOP NOTES
Green fragrances, mandarin orange, pear

HEART NOTE
Tiger orchid

BASE NOTES
Indonesian patchouli, sweet toffee

HOW TO USE

This fragrance needs no special empowerment, as over time Jimmy Choo perfume absorbs and mingles with the essence of the woman using it. • It will never create exactly the same fragrance for two wearers and so is an ideal signature fragrance. • Add to the inside of your ankles to enable you to walk with confidence into unfamiliar settings or where others flaunt status.

Jo Malone Red Roses

MAGICAL FORMS

A timeless fragrance that appeals to old souls or those with a love of tradition, historical fantasy, or visiting gardens in old houses, churches, or formal areas in botanical gardens, this perfume was created in 2001 for Jo Malone by Lucien Piquet and Patricia Bilodeau and has an authentic pure rose fragrance. The addition of beeswax, violets, and mint invokes the sense of being in a country garden in warm summer sunshine.

INGREDIENTS

TOP NOTES
Lemon, mint

HEART NOTES
Bulgarian rose, violet leaf

BASE NOTE
Beeswax

HOW TO USE

Linked with past worlds, the red rose fragrance dates back thousands of years and is present in many different cultures and lands. To travel back to other lives and worlds where red roses were once featured, inhale the perfume or spritz it around your aura while focusing on a vase of fragrant red roses during meditation.

La Vie Est Belle Eau de Parfum

MAGICAL FORMS

Redefined and recreated for Lancôme in 2014 by Dominique Ropion and Anne Flipo, its title translates to "life is beautiful" or "life is good." The fragrance encourages a woman to live by her own unique definition of happiness and fulfillment, which may mean going against what is conventionally seen as having beauty or of monetary value. It encourages a life close to nature as a source for joy rather than a chance to seek material advantage or possessions.

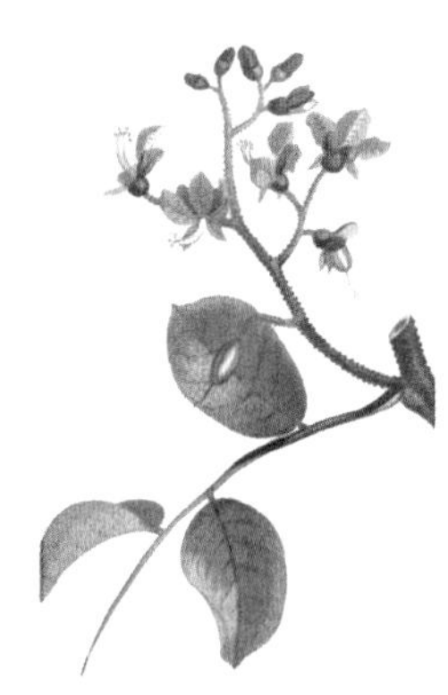

INGREDIENTS

TOP NOTES
Magnolia, almond

HEART NOTES
Iris, patchouli, white flowers

BASE NOTES
Spun sugar, praline, patchouli, tonka bean

HOW TO USE

Obtain flowering magnolia or, if not available, diffuse or burn magnolia oil near your bottle with a single white, large, fragrant flower next to it to empower the fragrance with fresh energies that make every day a new beginning. Keep your flower until it fades with the perfume.

Lady Million Eau de Parfum

MAGICAL FORMS

Created for Paco Rabanne in 2010 by designers including Anne Flipo and Beatrice Piquet, as a result of the successful male Million Dollars fragrance, this is a dressy perfume for attending or aiming to one day attend high-power work meetings, corporate dinners, interstate and international courses, or conferences. It is great to wear while networking with those who might be able to help further your ambitions. This is a fragrance that radiates the message "this woman is heading for the top," even if at this stage you are struggling up a corporate ladder. It manifests the impression of looking and feeling like a million dollars.

INGREDIENTS

TOP NOTES
Bitter orange, lemon, neroli, raspberry

HEART NOTES
Gardenia, jasmine, orange blossom

BASE NOTES
Amber, patchouli, white honey

HOW TO USE

When not in use, keep the bottle in a gold-colored basket lined with gold silk, along with glittering crystals such as rainbow quartz, goldstones, and entrepreneurial sparkling citrine, plus some real gold, such as earrings. If starting off your career, fill your basket with anything that glitters. • Before wearing your empowered fragrance, say, *I seek gold, riches untold, a million dollars to have and hold, let wealth this day/night for me unfold*. Then anoint your solar plexus, the power center at the base of your ribcage, with the fragrance, repeating the words.

Light Blue Eau Intense Pour Homme

MAGICAL FORMS

This perfume was created as a more intense version of the original for Dolce & Gabbana in 2017 by Alberto Morillas and contains salt water. Intense is particularly effective for men who love the ocean with a passion, including sailing, water sports, or overseas ventures. It's for all seasons, day to night, with energies evoking the ebbing, flowing, and resting tides that shift with the changing moods of the user.

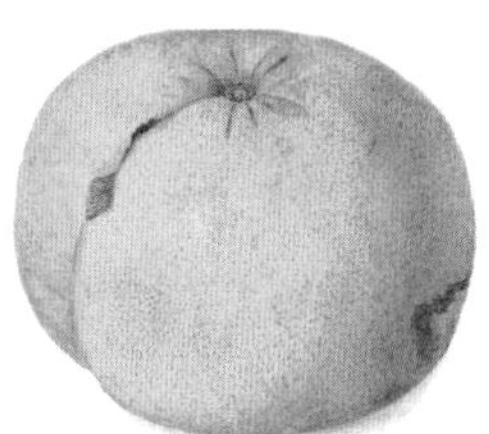

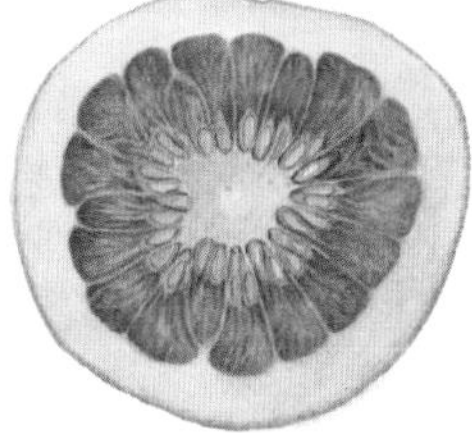

INGREDIENTS

TOP NOTES
Grapefruit, mandarin orange

HEART NOTES
Sea water, juniper

BASE NOTES
Musk, amberwood

HOW TO USE

After you first purchase the fragrance, take powdered kelp or any other seaweed plant powder and sprinkle in three circles, moving outward around the bottle. Leave it for a full twenty-four-hour cycle—if near the ocean, match with tide times—and then, afterward, scoop up the powder and dissolve it in any source of running water or the ocean. This purifies the fragrance, removing the energies of those who have made, packed, or sold it. Connect, like a sea breeze, anew every day.

Michael for Men Cologne

MAGICAL FORMS

Created for Michael Kors in 2001 by Harry Fremont, this scent is for a man not influenced by others to keep up with trends. He has an air of financial stability, whether acquired through career or family, and may be interested in or currently renovating property. This is a fragrance for cold winter days by the fireside or the local inn after a long walk. There are newer Michael Kors fragrances for men, including a spicier amber version, just called Michael Kors for Men, which came out in 2014. However, many remain loyal to the traditional blend, described here, that contains notes of tobacco.

INGREDIENTS

TOP NOTES
Bergamot, cardamom, coriander, elemi, star anise, thyme

HEART NOTES
Incense, tobacco, suede

BASE NOTES
Dark plum, dried fruits, patchouli, sandalwood

HOW TO USE

On a cold evening, light a *real* fire using untreated wood, adding a few spices to the unlit wood before igniting. Wearing the fragrance on your wrists and soles of the feet, pass briefly through the smoke created by this fire, mingling your fragrance with the smoke to activate your own energetic capacity to function effortlessly in the boardroom or office.

Miss Dior Eau de Parfum

MAGICAL FORMS

This perfume contains the rare fragrant Grasse rose (see p. 385) that—mixed with iris, peony, and lily of the valley—creates within the fragrance a heady bouquet, taking a woman from first awakening, to love, to her wedding or commitment day, and honeymoon. This new version was recreated for Dior in 2021 by Francois Demachy for romantics, including those who have never given up on love. Wear it to evoke those energies, or give to the woman you are romancing. Pick up this perfume when you need flowers, flowers, and more flowers.

INGREDIENTS

TOP NOTES
Iris, peony, lily of the valley

HEART NOTES
Apricot, centifolia (Grasse) rose, peach

BASE NOTES
Vanilla, musk, tonka bean, sandalwood, benzoin

HOW TO USE

To activate this fragrance, sit among fragrant flowers on a sunny day, holding your bottle to your heart, and call the love you seek or seek to increase. • When using the fragrance for a special occasion or seeking the return of a lost love, place the bottle in rose petals for a few minutes, adding a drop or two of the perfume. When you feel ready, hold it once more to your heart.

Missing Person Eau de Parfum for Men and Women

MAGICAL FORMS

Created for Phlur in 2022 by Constance Georges-Picot as a unisex fragrance, this perfume is considered a fragrance for intimacy between a couple on a spiritual as well as physical level as twin souls coming together to complete their missing halves. When apart by necessity, lovers should both wear this perfume to remain close on the astral or dream plane. It's a lovely fragrance for LGBTQ couples to share if circumstances or prejudice sometimes seems to conspire to keep them apart.

INGREDIENTS

TOP NOTES
Bergamot, jasmine, musk

HEART NOTES
Cyclamen, neroli, orange blossom

BASE NOTES
Australian sandalwood, white musk and white woods, vetiver, patchouli

HOW TO USE

Add a drop or two of the fragrance to sacred or holy water from an ancient well or spring for spiritual uplift, as well as to reconnect with what shamans called "soul loss" or a part of yourself you have, perhaps out of necessity, sacrificed or not developed because of others' needs. • When you use the fragrance, you will be offered opportunities to regain your lost powers and develop those missing gifts.

Mystique Shimmer for Women, Limited Edition

MAGICAL FORMS

A new addition to the Shimmer range that includes Midnight Shimmer (2016) and Starlight Shimmer (2019, released in 2020), the Kors Shimmer range promises glamour from dusk to dawn. Mystique is the most intriguing, hinting of mystery, hidden fire, and promise, but above all it's an elusive scent, so others will seek to know more about the wearer.

INGREDIENTS

TOP NOTES
Black pepper, bergamot

HEART NOTES
Saffron, floral notes

BASE NOTES
Woody notes, amber, musk

HOW TO USE

To empower your fragrance when first acquired, wear it—where else?—under the stars, ideally in a location where there is no light pollution. Hold the bottle toward your favorite star or constellation and then close to your heart, repeating this motion slowly and languorously until you feel the hidden power within you mingle with the fragrance (this also works well if you are empowering the Starlight Shimmer fragrance). • When not in use, keep the bottle wrapped in silver or iridescent cloth to maintain its power.

Nuit et Confidences Eau de Parfum for Women

MAGICAL FORMS

A new version of this fragrance, inspired by Parisian nights or as Goutal says by "champagne bubbles and sequin dresses," Nuit et Confidences was created in 2017 by Camille Goutal (daughter of legendary perfumer Annick Goutal) and Mathieu Nardin. It retains the warmth and reassurance of the most exotic Goutal fragrances, but adds something new and exciting—it reveals that the user has desires she trusts with just a few; someone with a secret part of her life known only to her closest confidantes. It's best for the woman of any age who dreams of being wooed, adored, and feted and exudes this aura even on the most unglamorous occasion. It inspires the wearer to fulfill her dreams.

INGREDIENTS

TOP NOTES
Black pepper, bergamot

HEART NOTES
Tonka beans, incense, white flowers

BASE NOTES
Vanilla, white musk

HOW TO USE

Buy the fragrance at the airport on the way to a romantic weekend or to a city known for its connection to love, such as Paris, even if you have to take the family along or are alone. • To empower the scent, whisper your dreams and desires into the bottle, and then apply the fragrance to your skin, letting the warmth of future, if not immediate, fulfillment flow through you. As you wear it at your destination, feel yourself filling the bottle with memories or what may as yet still be fantasies.

Obsession Eau de Parfum for Women

MAGICAL FORMS

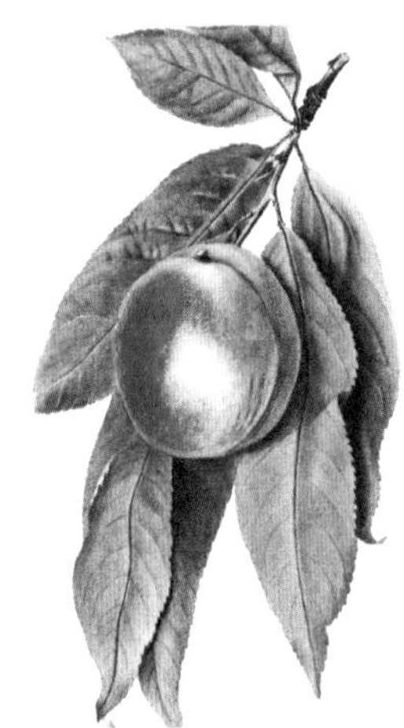

This is a fragrance for the fulfillment of burning dreams and desires that exclude everything else, whether creative, career based, or a twin soul love (even one that cannot yet be fulfilled or acknowledged). Created in 1985 for Calvin Klein by Jean Guichard, Obsession is perfect in the fall, especially on cooler evenings. It is for women meeting or seeking a partner the second or third time around or a little later in life.

INGREDIENTS

TOP NOTES
Basil, bergamot, lemon, mandarin orange, peach

HEART NOTES
Cedar, coriander, jasmine, orange blossom, rose, spices

BASE NOTES
Amber, civet (synthetic), incense, musk, oakmoss, vetiver

HOW TO USE

If you wish to increase commitment in a relationship, mix a drop or two of this fragrance with the men's equivalent (Obsession for Men) into oil for a mutual massage. If you are in a same-sex relationship, use the Obsession fragrance of your choice. • Wear each other's Obsession or mix them if you are meeting disapproving friends or relations, as this will enhance your joined aura energy field that even the most insensitive person must recognize and feel positive toward.

The Only One Eau de Parfum

MAGICAL FORMS

A 2018/2019 update of The One, which was first released in 2006, described by Dolce & Gabbana as "capturing the essence of a sophisticated hypnotizing femininity." This scent is a contrasting blend of fruity, floral, and gourmand ingredients that vary with the mood and the current situation in which the fragrance is being worn. It's best for those with quicksilver temperaments who wish to seize the moment, embracing life and worrying about consequences later.

INGREDIENTS

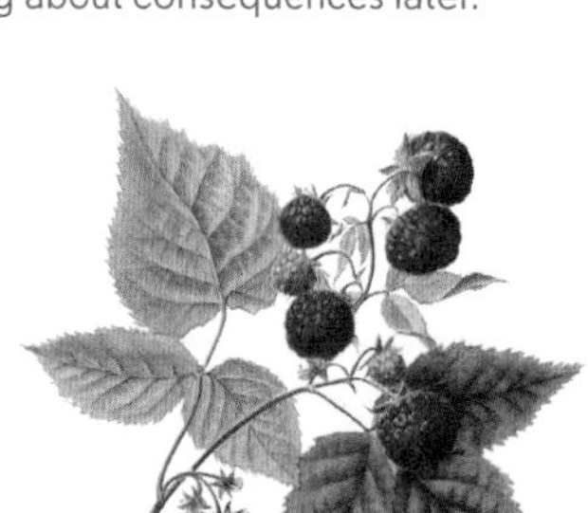

TOP NOTES
Bergamot, violet, pear, berries

HEART NOTES
Coffee, iris

BASE NOTES
Patchouli, vanilla

HOW TO USE

To empower the fragrance, place the unopened bottle in a bowl of unpeeled fruit, fragrant petals, vanilla pods, and coffee beans, and inhale the blending fragrances. Add the petals, the coffee beans, and vanilla pods to a bowl of potpourri with just a little of the perfume. Eat or share the peeled fruit and plan an adventure or carry out some major networking to sell your unique talents, using your enhanced charisma.

Perfect Eau de Toilette

MAGICAL FORMS

Created by Domitille Michalon Bertier for Marc Jacobs in late 2022/early 2023 to supplement the original fragrances Perfect Eau de Parfum and Perfect Intense, this variety is lighter and fresher. With lucky charms on the lid, this new Perfect celebrates the joy of loving yourself and following *your* definition of perfection. It builds up self-esteem in those who have acquired or have been given a poor self-image through others' insensitivity, to restore confidence.

INGREDIENTS

TOP NOTES
Polygonum (knotweed), pink pepper

HEART NOTES
Narcissus, white daffodil

BASE NOTES
Cedarwood

HOW TO USE

Hold your bottle, whether new or already being used, enclosing the charms on the lid as the bottle sits upright on a table, saying, *I make my own good fortune, by sun and moon, by every star, no one shall bar me from fulfilling my destiny, I am myself, perfect in my own light and henceforward shall be.* Repeat the words and actions every time you use your fragrance to build or reinforce your own sense of perfection no matter what others say to make you doubt it.

Princess Eau de Toilette

MAGICAL FORMS

Created for Vera Wang in 2006 by Ilias Ermenidis and Harry Fremont, this is a fragrance for a woman in her teens, twenties, or early thirties who sees herself as a princess or would like to be treated as one. It's perfect for flirty people who love dressing up and emphasizing their femininity. When you wear this perfume, you'll be popular, a natural focus at any party, but kind enough to include anyone left out–it's for anyone who loves her pets and takes care of them well. She's fun but nevertheless knows exactly what she is doing, where she is heading, and the effect she has on others.

INGREDIENTS

TOP NOTES
Apricot, apple, water lily, mandarin orange

HEART NOTES
Guava, dark chocolate, tuberose

BASE NOTES
Amber, vanilla

HOW TO USE

Wear this fragrance at a fairground, a theme park, festival, or rock concert for the first time or when you get a new bottle, to merge its bubbly "get up and go" energies with your "ready for anything" aura. When you get home, surround the bottle with trinkets and souvenirs from the event.

Santal 33 Eau de Parfum, Unisex

MAGICAL FORMS

Created in 2011 by Frank Voelkl, Santal 33 is a very relaxed fragrance, inspired by the old American West–the pioneers, explorers for gold–evoking the sense of sitting by an open fire under the stars, letting the day flow away. This scent will be beloved by the man with a pioneering spirit released temporarily by days away from the city or vacations in the wilderness. Some women like to wear the fragrance to express their own desire for the wide-open plains and an untamable spirit, or they may buy it for their cowboy who spends too much time watching sports on TV.

INGREDIENTS

TOP NOTES
Cardamom, violet seeds

HEART NOTES
Cedar, iris, sandalwood

BASE NOTES
Ambroxan (synthetic ambergris), papyrus, white musk

HOW TO USE

Wear on a wilderness vacation, camping (especially "glamping"), or horse riding or ranch weekends, and if with a partner, share the fragrance to recreate life on the prairies. If you can't manage this, watch old movies together or alone, having spritzed the room with a little of the fragrance in water or use one or more of the associated products.

Sì Eau de Parfum

MAGICAL FORMS

This is a lighter version of the fragrance recreated in 2015 by Julie Massé from the classic 2013 Sì for Armani. This perfume always prompts the wearer to say *yes* to what life offers right now, even sometimes what has been regarded as forbidden fruit, casting off restrictions and inhibitions, not carelessly but as a daring, independent life choice.

INGREDIENTS

TOP NOTES
Black currant or cassis liqueur, Sicilian bergamot, mandarin orange, vanilla

HEART NOTES
Freesia, Egyptian jasmine, rose de Mai or rose centifolia

BASE NOTES
Oakmoss, patchouli, vanilla absolute

HOW TO USE

List five dreams you have that have been dismissed by others as risky or unwise. Steer your own path ahead, and each time you wear your perfume, take a step—however small—toward fulfilling one of your desires until all are completed.

Viva la Juicy le Bubbly Eau de Parfum

MAGICAL FORMS

In 2020, Viva la Juicy le Bubbly joined the party: All a woman needs, it is said, is her little black dress and this fragrance to be a showstopper, whether at a party or networking with the executives at a workplace event. Wearing the perfume guides the woman by instinct, impulse, intuition, and magical inspiration to give the solution while others are puzzling over the question. The original was created in 2008, complete with matching body lotions, cream, and bath products.

INGREDIENTS

TOP NOTES
Mandarin orange, wild pink berries

HEART NOTES
Gardenia, jasmine, vanilla orchid, honeysuckle

BASE NOTES
Caramel, praline, amber, sandalwood, vanilla

HOW TO USE

Obtain an invitation to an upmarket event if you aren't already part of the "upwardly mobile" crowd. Dress with understated elegance and put the fragrance on your pulse points. By the time you are through your first glass of champagne and being offered the second, you will feel your radiance growing. Keep circulating and collecting the contact numbers of those who will open the right doors.

Yardley's English Lavender Eau de Toilette

MAGICAL FORMS

Probably the best known of all the Yardley fragrances, this perfume is beloved by great-grandmothers, grandmothers, mothers, and daughters through many years. It is still thriving, though younger woman may consider it old-fashioned. It first launched in 1801 and updates innovate on the beloved fragrance while keeping its traditional core scent. It's known to calm the mind at bedtime but can gently energize through the day as well, whether worn on pulse points or spritzed around the home or workplace using a few drops in a spray bottle of water. It's especially effective at bringing peace to any confrontational situation. If you are homesick and far from home or family or feeling alone, the fragrance is like a gentle aura hug.

INGREDIENTS

TOP NOTES
English lavender, eucalyptus, rosemary, bergamot

HEART NOTES
Clary sage, cedar, geranium

BASE NOTES
Musk, tonka bean, oakmoss

HOW TO USE

Along with Yardley's rose fragrance, this fragrance is the ultimate past-life channel, since lavender (see p. 252) is common to many cultures and time periods. Obtain some old-fashioned lavender or beeswax furniture polish. Add the fragrance to your pulse points, especially your inner wrist points that link with your heart. Polish a piece of furniture slowly and rhythmically using a soft cloth in clockwise and counterclockwise movements. As you do so, allow visions of old worlds to flow into your mind where once you walked among lavender. Maybe you will see a beloved ancestor recognized from a faded photo. The scenes you see may give you the answer to present-day questions. • Anoint door and window catches with the fragrance to bring harmony and abundance to your home.

Yardley's English Rose Eau de Toilette

MAGICAL FORMS

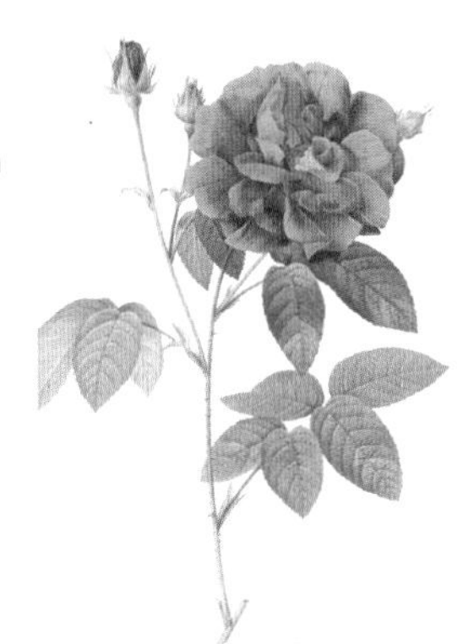

A very traditional classic fragrance by Yardley, worn by many generations, it is also available as soap, talcum powder, and lotion, as well as other bath products, in addition to the fragrance. A contemporary edition was launched in 2015, though it is still considered by some to be old-fashioned and not for younger women. But whether in new or classical form, it is still one of the most authentic and subtle rose scents. It creates a gentle aura of love, kindness, and goodwill around the user that extends to enclose everyone the wearer encounters, whether friend, family, or stranger.

INGREDIENTS

TOP NOTES
Rose, tea, citruses

HEART NOTES
Rose, magnolia, cassis, violet

BASE NOTES
Musk, patchouli

HOW TO USE

To empower your fragrance, wear it when visiting a rose garden. Sit quietly among the flowers, allowing your aura to absorb both the scent of the living flowers and your rose perfume. • Refresh it at any time by setting the bottle in a bowl of dried rose petals or rose-based potpourri.

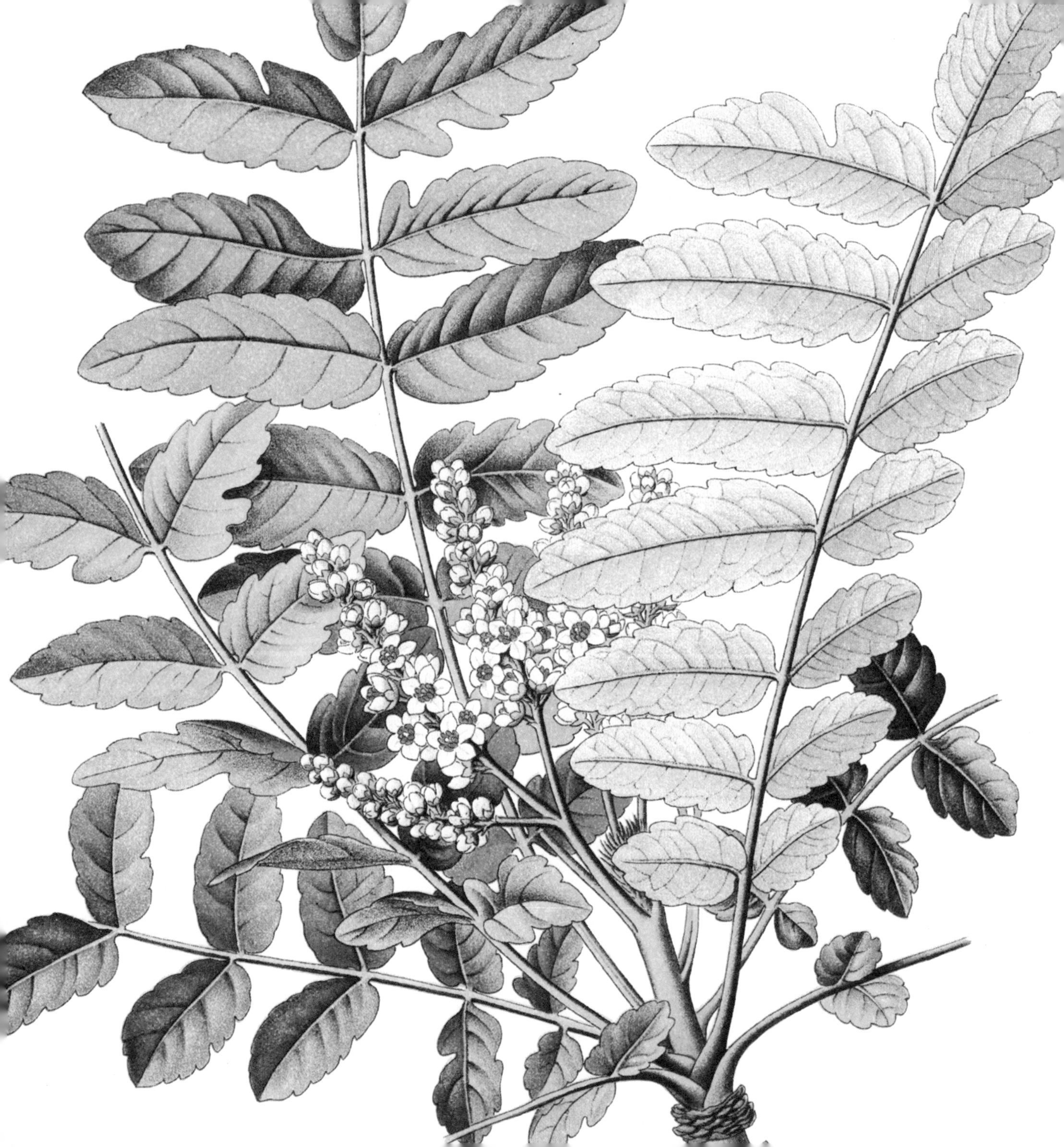

Alphabetical Index

S

T

U

V

W

Y

Z

General Index

D

E

F

G

H

I

J

K

L

M

Y

Acknowledgments

To my beloved children, Tom, Jade, Jack, Miranda, and Bill, and my beautiful grandchildren, Freya, Holly, Oliver, and Sophie. To John Gold, my subeditor, protector, and mentor, and Kornelia Gold, my inspiration and wonderful friend. Finally, my sincere gratitude to Kate Zimmermann, executive editor at Union Square & Co., who has kept faith with me throughout the many years I have written for Sterling/Union Square.

Picture Credits

Courtesy of Artvee: cover, 3, 5, 7, 142, 13, 14, 25, 29, 35, 43, 52, 58, 62, 70, 72, 117, 119, 124, 132, 139, 140, 141, 142, 145, 157, 158, 173, 181, 185, 198, 205, 214, 221, 223, 228, 230, 247, 257, 262, 265, 273, 275, 279, 280, 282, 301, 328, 332, 346, 372, 376, 389, 394, 400, 402, 418, 426, 429, 431, 441, 453, 456, 464, 467, 477, 482, 484, 488, 492, 495, 497, 503, 506, 508, 511, 512, back cover

Getty Images: *Digital Vision Vectors:* ivan-96: 19, 27; mashuk: 213; Nastasic: cover, 3, 12, 21 (allspice); ZU-09: 6, 11; *iStock/Getty Images Plus:* Tatiana Arefyeva: 490, 491; El_Suhova: 490, 491; NSA Digital Archive: 31, 32, 105, 192, 196; Alexandra Romanova: 490, 491; wacomka: 490, 491

Courtesy of Hathi Trust: 325

Courtesy of Internet Archive: cover, 3, 13, 22, 75, 81, 153, 258

Courtesy of Rawpixel: 12, 13, 34, 38, 42, 44, 47, 55, 61, 66, 67, 88, 91, 92, 97, 100, 101, 102, 108, 113, 114, 122, 126, 129, 131, 135, 147, 149, 155, 160, 169, 187, 188, 191, 203, 207, 212, 215, 217, 218, 224, 226, 232, 237, 241, 253, 260, 263, 267, 269, 272, 277, 285, 294, 303, 304, 305, 312, 317, 321, 323, 338, 342, 350, 353, 354, 358, 363, 364, 366, 369, 373, 374, 380, 386, 391, 406, 409, 415, 432, 434, 439, 449, 450, 454, 455, 461, 470, 474, 486, 501, 504, 544

Shutterstock.com: Foxyliam: 425

Courtesy of Wikimedia Commons: 36, 49, 65, 69, 76, 78, 83, 85, 87, 98, 115, 120, 128, 136, 138, 147, 150, 162, 166, 171, 175, 177, 201, 210, 229, 239, 243, 245, 246, 248, 255, 271, 286, 289, 290, 236, 296, 307, 310, 327, 330, 334, 336, 348, 351, 367, 370, 378, 385, 397, 398, 404, 410, 412, 421, 422, 440, 443, 445, 446, 459, 479, 481, 496, 498, 515, 516, spine; Biodiversity Heritage Library: 30, 41, 50, 94, 106, 110, 164, 179, 182, 190, 194, 209, 234, 250, 299, 314, 318, 340, 345, 356, 361, 392, 416, 437, 458, 469, 473, 502, 507; Roger Culos: 57; Felloni claire: 463; Metropolitan Museum of Art: 382; National Gallery of Canada: 12

About the Author

CASSANDRA EASON is one of the most prolific and popular authors of our time, writing on all aspects of spirituality and magic, in addition to lecturing, broadcasting, and facilitating workshops throughout the world. During the past forty years, Cassandra has written over 130 titles, many of which have been translated into numerous languages, including Japanese, Russian, Hebrew, Portuguese, German, Dutch, and Spanish.

Cassandra was a teacher and university lecturer for ten years; however, her life path was to change following a vision by her three-year-old son, who accurately described a motorcycle accident in which his father was to be involved and which subsequently occurred within minutes of the vision.

Following a great deal of research into this phenomenon, Cassandra went on to write the bestselling *The Psychic Power of Children*, followed by many others, including *A Spell a Day, A Little Bit of Palmistry, The Complete Book of Women's Wisdom, A Complete Guide to Magick and Ritual*, and *The Modern Day Druidess* to name just a few. In the 1001 series, in addition to this book, Cassandra has written *1001 Spells, 1001 Dreams, 1001 Tarot Spreads*, and *1001 Crystals*.

Her books have been serialized around the world, including in the *Daily Mail*, the *Daily Mirror*, the *Daily Express, People, The Sun*, the *News of the World, Spirit & Destiny, Fate & Fortune, Prediction, Best, Bella, Better Homes and Gardens, Good Housekeeping, Woman's Day*, and *New Idea*. She had her own psychic column in the national women's magazine *Best* and in *Writers' News* for two years, and for eighteen months produced a monthly psychic master class for *Beyond* magazine.

In the UK, Cassandra had her own weekly miniseries, *Sixth Sense*, on United Artists Cable Network for a number of years, before moving on to the Granada Breeze lifestyle channel, where she was resident white witch for over two years on *Psychic Live Time.* She acted as psychic consultant/resident expert on the successful ITV *Magic and Mystery* series and has also analyzed dreams on the UK's *Big Brother* seasons 3 and 4 and *Celebrity Big Brother.*

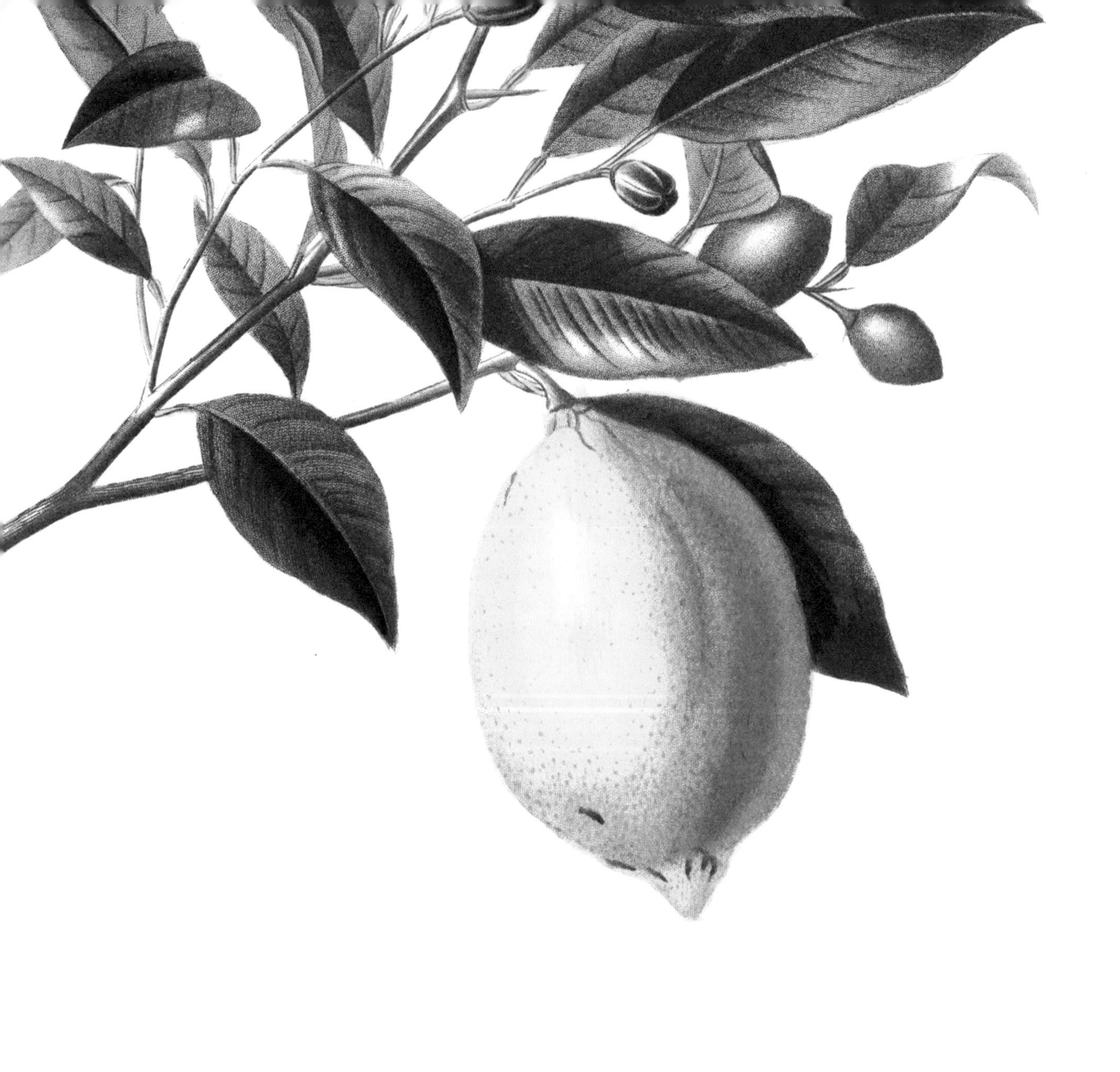